Latest Research on Breast Cancer - Molecular Insights, Diagnostic Advances and Therapeutic Innovations

Edited by Ana Carolina Monteiro and Lulu Wang

Published in London, United Kingdom

Latest Research on Breast Cancer - Molecular Insights, Diagnostic Advances and Therapeutic Innovations
http://dx.doi.org/10.5772/intechopen.1003587
Edited by Ana Carolina Monteiro and Lulu Wang

Contributors
Abhiram Kumar, Ahmed Subhy Alsheikhly, Aise Chatzi Ismail Mouchterem, Ana Carolina Monteiro, Ana Lilia Remirez-Castellanos, Anam Mehmood, Anastasia Bothou, Andreou Sotiris, Armando Gamboa-Dominguez, Arya Rajesh, Athar Shams Rana, Ceylan Hepokur, Chao Lu, Chhavi Dhiman, Chikezie O. Madu, Christos Damaskos, Cindy Chavira-Macias, Delour Haj, Eftymios Oikonomou, Emran Habibi, Evan Easley, Falak Sharma, Fernando Candanedo-Gonzalez, Fábio B. Canto, Georgios Iatrakis, Hadi Hassannia, Hesamoddin Arabnozari, Hira Riffat, ia Asghar, Javairia Rafique, Konstantinos Nikolettos, Kotanidou Sonia, Kritsotaki Nektaria, KuanHui Ethan Chen, Kyriaki Chalkia, Kyriakou Dimitrios, Lulu Wang, Madhaw Kumar, Mani Sharma, Maria Eduarda Globa Masset, Mazin Ahmed Subhy Alsheikhly, Mei Li, Micah Gustafson, Mikiyas Amare Getu, Mohini Rawat, Nalmpanti Athanasia-Theopi, Navita Somaiah, Nemala Siva Kumar, Nicholas Deleon, Nicholas Pascuzzi, Nikolaos Garmpis, Nikolaos Nikolettos, Noura Al-Zeheimi, Omer A. Idris, Osman Akidan, Panagiotis Tsikouras, Rama Satya Sri Kotipalli, Reagan Farrell, Reza Taghipour, Ryan Panchal, Sema Misir, Serap Ozer Yaman, Seyed Ehsan Enderami, Shakil Khan, Sirin A. Adham, Spanakis Vlasios, Stefanos Zervoudis, Sy Bogutski, Tiantian Zhang, Ursula Salazar-Gomez, Uzma S, Wilfredo Valenzuela-Gonzalez, Xianbin Zhang, Yashna Nadkarni, Yi Lu, Ying Qian, Yue Zhang, Yuksel Aliyazicioglu, Yumeng Liu, Zoya Iqbal

First published in London, United Kingdom, 2025 by IntechOpen
IntechOpen is the global imprint of INTECHOPEN LIMITED, registered in England and Wales, registration number: 11086078, 167-169 Great Portland Street, London, W1W 5PF, United Kingdom

For EU product safety concerns: IN TECH d.o.o., Prolaz Marije Krucifikse Kozulić 3, 51000 Rijeka, Croatia, info@intechopen.com or visit our website at intechopen.com.

British Library Cataloguing-in-Publication Data
A catalogue record for this book is available from the British Library

Latest Research on Breast Cancer - Molecular Insights, Diagnostic Advances and Therapeutic Innovations
Edited by Ana Carolina Monteiro and Lulu Wang
p. cm.

This title is part of the Oncology Book Series, Volume 4
Series Editor: Thomas J. FitzGerald

Print ISBN 978-0-85466-464-1
Online ISBN 978-0-85466-463-4
eBook (PDF) ISBN 978-0-85466-465-8
ISSN 3049-8864

IntechOpen Book Series
Oncology
Volume 4

Aims and Scope of the Series

The field of oncology has undergone extraordinary change and progress over the past several decades. Today, information is evolving at a rapid rate, with standards of management far different than standards of care applied during the training of most practicing oncologists. Oncology practitioners in all disciplines must remain current to optimize patient care. Basic and translational science remain critical in developing process improvements for patient care. The closer we understand the mechanism, the more we can improve targeted therapies and apply them to patient care. The pace of information is moving faster than at any previous time in history, and all oncology disciplines must remain current to provide excellent service to patients. The modern oncologist must be fluent in using big data and the volume of information generated in clinical trials. As we move closer to personalized patient care based on genomics and molecular biomarkers, the modern oncologist has to be nimble in assessing all available information and how this would be applied to each patient, balanced by the clinical status and medical co-morbidities of each patient. Targeted therapies can bring new and different sequelae, and oncology teams need to remain fluent in managing the consequences of therapy and primary management. In this book series, we will present how modern care has progressed in multiple disease areas and how modern oncology teams need to adapt in order to manage the cancer patients of today successfully. Surgery, radiation therapy, and medical oncology are practiced today with the support of exceptional modern technology, and in this series, we will review how these improvements are applied to each disease site to maintain excellence in patient care.

Meet the Series Editor

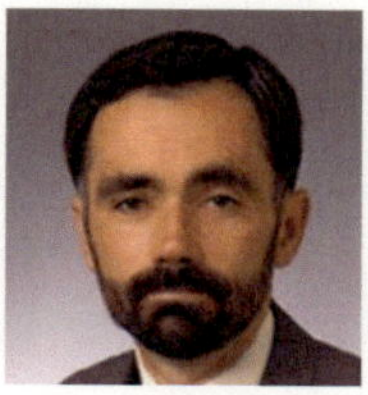

Dr. FitzGerald is the professor and chair of the Department of Radiation Oncology at UMass Chan Medical School in the USA. He serves as one of the principal investigators of the Imaging and Radiation Oncology Core (IROC) service for the National Cancer Institute clinical trials program and is directly involved in the quality assurance of clinical trials in the National Clinical Trials Network (NCTN). Dr. Fitzgerald manages NCTN clinical trials with a real-time pre-therapy review of imaging and radiation therapy treatment objects to ensure the care plan complies with study objectives and the patient stage has been assigned to the correct study. His basic science interest is in hematopoietic stem cell biology and cellular adhesion molecules as they pertain to therapeutic resistance and mitigation of injury from therapy.

Meet the Volume Editors

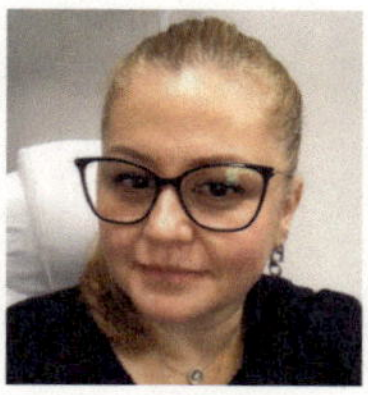

Ana Carolina Monteiro is an Associate Professor of Immunobiology at the Fluminense Federal University (UFF), Brazil, where she coordinates the Laboratory of Osteoimmunology and Tumor Immunology (LOIT). She holds a Ph.D. in Biological Sciences (Biophysics) from the Federal University of Rio de Janeiro (UFRJ), with postdoctoral training in tumor immunology and bone metastasis. Her research focuses on adaptive immune responses in cancer, bone metastasis, and osteoimmune interactions. She is a member of the Research Ethics Committee at the UFF School of Medicine and teaches undergraduate and graduate courses in Immunobiology, Tumor Immunology, and Osteoimmunology.

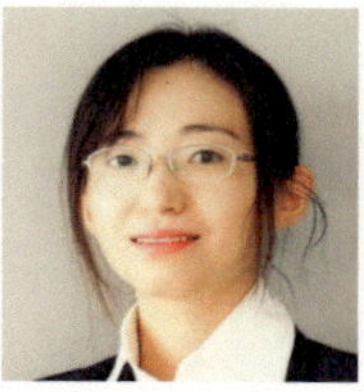

Dr. Lulu Wang holds a Full Professorship in the Department of Engineering at Reykjavík University in Iceland. In addition, she serves as a Visiting Professor in the Department of Physiology and Biomedical Engineering at the Mayo Clinic in Rochester, USA, and as a Professor Extraordinarius in the College of Science, Engineering, and Technology at the University of South Africa. Dr. Wang's interdisciplinary research spans the areas of electromagnetic sensing and imaging, artificial intelligence (AI) for healthcare, and the development of innovative medical devices. Her work is driven by the pursuit of translational impact, with numerous findings having progressed beyond the laboratory to successful commercialization. She has published over 100 peer-reviewed scientific articles and is the author of three academic books. In recognition of her contributions to the field, she also served as the editor for five additional volumes. Her inventive capacity is reflected in her portfolio of 35 granted patents. Dr. Wang's achievements have been recognized by several esteemed scientific and engineering societies. She is a Fellow of the American Society of Mechanical Engineers (ASME Fellow), a Full Member of the scientific research honor society Sigma Xi, and a Professional Member of the Royal Society of New Zealand. Furthermore, she has been selected as a Nominator for the prestigious VinFuture Prize, underscoring her international reputation and commitment to advancing science for the global good. Since 2021, Dr. Wang has been consistently listed among Stanford University and Elsevier's compilation of the world's top 2% of scientists.

Contents

Preface

Breast cancer remains one of the most studied and yet most challenging malignancies in modern oncology. The biological heterogeneity of breast tumors, the diversity of their clinical manifestations, and the evolving landscape of therapeutic resistance continue to drive innovation in both research and care. This volume, *Latest Research on Breast Cancer – Molecular Insights, Diagnostic Advances and Therapeutic Innovations*, aims to provide readers with an updated and integrated view of the scientific and clinical advances that are shaping the future of breast cancer diagnosis and treatment.

The book opens with Chapter 1, *A Comprehensive Review of Breast Cancer and the Latest Advancement in Diagnosis and Treatment*, which offers a foundational overview of breast cancer, covering historical milestones, current practices, and future research directions.

Chapter 2, *Breast Cancer Heterogeneity and Its Implication in Precision Therapy*, dives into the genomic, epigenomic, and transcriptomic variability of tumors and how this complexity informs personalized medicine.

Chapter 3, *The Role of Estrogen Receptors and Signaling Pathways in Breast Cancer*, examines key molecular mechanisms and their implications for endocrine therapy, while Chapter 4, *Precision Medicine Approaches in Breast Cancer: Current Strategies and Future Directions*, details how biomarker-based classification is transforming treatment decisions.

Chapter 5, *Recent Breakthroughs in Breast Cancer Endocrinology and Tumor Microenvironmental Interactions*, explores the metabolic and cellular dynamics of hormone receptor-positive tumors.

The second section of the book focuses on diagnostic innovation. Chapter 6, *Screening and Diagnosis Imagery in Breast Cancer: Classical and Emergent Techniques*, covers a wide range of imaging approaches from digital tomosynthesis to magnetic resonance spectroscopy. Chapters 7 through 9—*AI-Assisted Breast Imaging*, *Advances in Breast Ultrasound Imaging: Enhancing Diagnostic Precision and Clinical Utility*, and *Application of Magnetic Resonance Imaging in Breast Cancer Patients*—highlight the use of artificial intelligence and advanced imaging modalities to improve early detection and diagnostic accuracy.

Chapter 10, *BCNet: A Novel Deep Learning Model for Enhanced Breast Cancer Classification Using Histopathological Images*, exemplifies how deep learning can revolutionize pathology.

In the third section, the focus shifts toward therapeutic innovation. Chapter 11, *Neuropilin-1: A Promising Therapeutic Target for Triple-Negative Breast Cancer*, and

Chapter 12, *miRNA-Based Therapeutic Strategy and Its Application in Breast Cancer*, both emphasize molecular targets and regulatory RNAs.

Chapter 13, *Natural Polysaccharides in Breast Cancer: Fucoidan's Role in Enhancing Cisplatin Cytotoxicity and Reducing Chemotherapy Resistance*, presents a novel approach combining natural compounds with conventional chemotherapy.

Chapters 14 and 15 provide a broader view of systemic treatment. *Key Landmark Clinical Trials Transforming the Therapeutic Landscape of Metastatic Breast Cancer: From Precision Medicine to Immunotherapy* reviews clinical progress and *Innovations in Drug Delivery Strategies for Breast Cancer* and addresses advanced delivery systems and nanotechnology.

Finally, Chapter 16, *Understanding the Relationship Between Bone-Remodeling T Cells and Microbiota in Breast Cancer Bone Metastases*, introduces a unique perspective on the immunological and microbiological dimensions of bone metastasis, emphasizing the translational importance of immune cell phenotypes and host-microbiota interactions in metastatic progression.

This book reflects the collaborative efforts of a global community of researchers, clinicians, and contributors committed to advancing breast cancer science and care. I want to express my sincere gratitude to all authors and reviewers for their dedication and to the IntechOpen team for their professional support throughout the editorial process.

Ana Carolina Monteiro
Department of Immunobiology,
Fluminense Federal University (UFF),
Niterói, Brazil

Lulu Wang
Department of Engineering,
Reykjavík University,
Reykjavik, Iceland

Department of Physiology and Biomedical Engineering,
Mayo Clinic, Rochester, USA

Section 1

Foundations and Molecular Complexity

Chapter 1

A Comprehensive Review of Breast Cancer and the Latest Advancement in Diagnosis and Treatment

Ahmed Subhy Alsheikhly and Mazin Ahmed Subhy Alsheikhly

Abstract

Breast cancer, a significant global health challenge, remains a leading cause of cancer-related morbidity and mortality worldwide, necessitating comprehensive strategies for diagnosis, treatment, and survivorship care. Early detection through modalities such as mammography, ultrasound, MRI, and tissue sampling is crucial. Genetic testing, on the other hand, identifies hereditary risks. Tissue sampling and biopsy provide a definitive histopathologic diagnosis. Breast cancer care aims to diagnose timely and achieve optimal outcomes while preserving quality of life. Surgical approaches remain integral to treatment, with options ranging from breast-conserving surgery (lumpectomy) to mastectomy based on tumor stage, size, and patient preference. Oncoplastic breast surgery combines oncologic resection with plastic surgical techniques to optimize esthetic outcomes without compromising cancer control. Breast reconstruction, using autologous tissue or implants, further enhances physical and psychological recovery. Surgical approaches often precede adjuvant therapies such as chemotherapy, radiation, and hormone therapy, which aim to reduce the risk of recurrence and improve survival rates. Prognosis varies based on factors such as tumor stage, grade, hormone-receptor status, and involvement of lymph nodes. Disparities in care exist based on factors such as socioeconomic status, race, and geographic location, affecting access to quality treatment and impacting prognosis. Ongoing research focuses on improving diagnostic accuracy, innovations in surgical techniques and systemic therapies, developing personalized therapies, and addressing healthcare inequities to improve outcomes for all women with breast cancer. This review highlights the importance of a holistic approach in optimizing outcomes and survivorship for patients with breast cancer.

Keywords: breast cancer, reconstruction, oncoplastic, breast conserving, prognosis, mammogram

1. Introduction

Breast cancer, a frequently diagnosed malignancy and a leading cause of death in women, describes a malignant change to the breast tissue in which neoplasia of cells occurs within the milk ducts or the milk-producing lobules of the breast. It often presents as a lump or mass that is hard and immobile with some distortion in breast shape, such as dimpling of the skin or significant asymmetry, a newly inverted nipple, bloody nipple discharge, or skin irritation with redness or scaly patches of skin noted by the patient, which raises concern regarding breast cancer and encourages the patient to seek medical attention. However, with the advancement in the awareness and screening programs of breast cancer, many are detected early and perhaps even before the formation of lobulated cancerous mass in the breast.

Breast cancer remains multifactorial. There are many risk factors, which include modifiable and non-modifiable risk factors. Modifiable factors includes nulliparity and/or late pregnancy, smoking, alcohol consumption, radiation exposure as well as obesity with BMI ≥30 kg/m^2; evidence suggests that women with higher BMI have an increased risk of developing postmenopausal breast cancer [1]. Nulliparity and/or late pregnancy. Consumption of alcohol as well as smoking and history of radiation exposure. Non-modifiable factors include female sex, advanced age, and a strong family history of breast cancer.

According to Global Cancer Statistics 2020, which is the latest major cancer statistic up to date, breast cancer represents the second most common cancer in females after lung cancer and the fourth most common cause of mortality in cancer-related deaths, with almost 670,000 deaths globally [2]. It is estimated that, even in countries where screening programs are widely available, about 15% of patients who develop breast cancer are diagnosed with a breast mass that was not detected on screening imaging modalities such as mammograms [3]. In countries where such programs are not well established, or women do not have easy access to such programs, they often present with locally advanced diseases [3].

1.1 Workup and diagnosis

The approach to workup and diagnosis of breast cancer has developed well and progressed from simply depending on suspicious physical examination findings or abnormal imaging to well-established Triple Assessment Clinics (TAC). TAC is considered the current gold standard in evaluating patients for suspicious breast cancer. It aims to provide a rapid outpatient approach to the diagnosis of breast cancer and allow for its early intervention and management. The cornerstone of TAC depends on detailed history and physical examination, suitable imaging according to the patient's age, and tissue biopsy. Thus, it is necessary to ensure that all aspects of the triple assessment process are specific and sensitive to ensure accurate results are delivered [4]. Perhaps one of the main points in working with a patient with suspicious findings is deciding the best imaging modality for the patient.

2. Imaging modalities

Multiple imaging modalities are available to assist clinicians in screening and detecting breast cancer. Patient age and breast tissue quality play a significant role in deciding the imaging modality. Breast imaging modalities keep evolving, and their strengths and drawbacks are continually being assessed to develop recommendations and guidelines for clinical practice.

2.1 Breast ultrasound

Breast ultrasound, which utilizes the reflection of acoustic waves in the tissue, is a valuable adjunct and diagnostic tool in screening for breast cancer. Breast ultrasonography is the first (and usually sufficient) tool for evaluating young, pregnant, and breastfeeding individuals who exhibit clinical symptoms. In this cohort, ultrasonography accurately distinguishes benign findings from those that require biopsy. However, ultrasound should be supplemented with mammography in patients with very dense or heterogeneously dense breasts. Also, axillary ultrasound must be done to stage breast cancer [5].

According to the National Comprehensive Cancer Network (NCCN) and the American College of Radiology (ACR), ultrasound is the imaging modality of choice for patients aged 30 and younger, while mammogram is the primary one for patients aged 40 and older. However, there has also been a popular combination of Ultrasound and mammograms in young patients ranging in the age bracket of 30 to 39, as dense breasts in this age group make mammograms more difficult to interpret.

2.2 Mammogram/mammography

A mammogram is an X-ray of the breast soft tissue using low doses of ionizing radiation (**Figure 1**). It has the superiority in detecting early changes and aids in diagnosing breast cancer early when it is still a limited disease and has not yet exhibited invasiveness. Mammography is mostly used in staging to assess microcalcifications, which may not be visible in other modalities and may indicate a ductal carcinoma *in situ* (DCIS) component [5].

Classically, there are two main types of mammography. The first is film screen mammography, in which X-rays pass through breast tissue, are converted to light, and are displayed on film in the form of grayscale images. This has been replaced with digital mammography, wherein the image is displayed on the radiologist's workstation [7]. Digital mammography (DM) has been the standard of care for imaging as it is proven to have higher sensitivity in detecting breast cancer and carries fewer false-positive results [8].

Lately, the addition of digital breast tomosynthesis (DBT), or 3D mammography, has been gaining popularity in screening programs by converting 2D studies electronically to reconstruct a three-dimensional image using computer algorithms, thus enhancing the parenchymal distortion features and multiple slices of the breast. This has been studied in screening settings only, and some studies highly support the addition of DBT to conventional digital mammography with an increased rate of detecting ductal carcinoma *in situ*, yet not for invasive cancers [8, 9]. The Oslo screening trial, published in 2019, showed superiority in screening programs that combine DBT + DM with significant improvement in sensitivity and specificity [10].

However, mammography is not always suitable for all breast tissue. Mammography requires an abundance of fatty tissue in the breast to provide the best imaging quality and guide the workup accordingly.

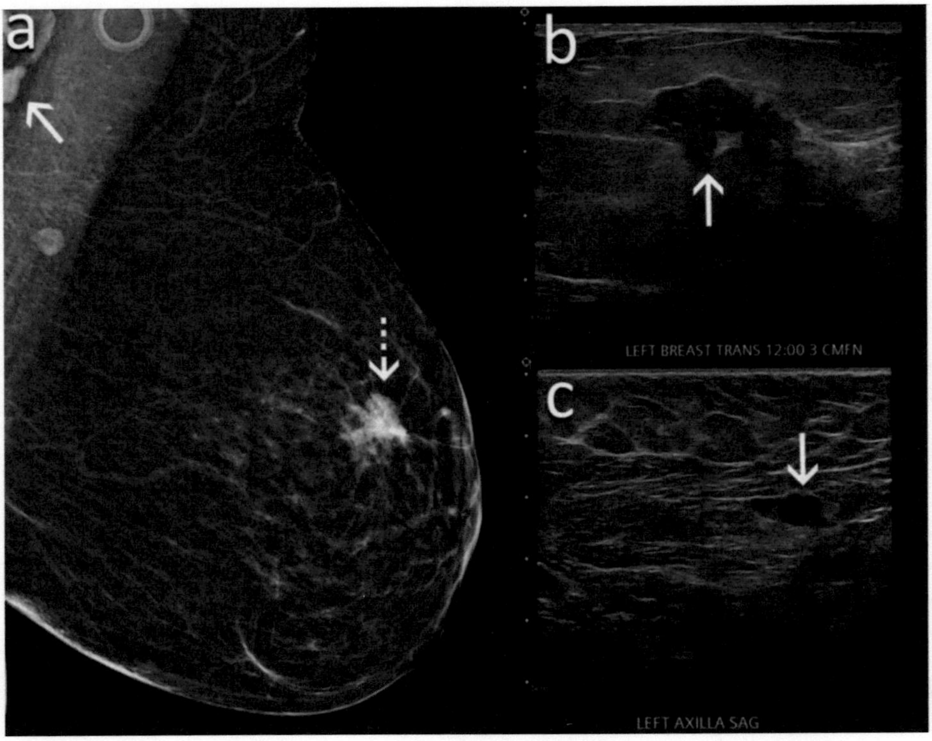

Figure 1.
Mammogram showing breast cancer and axillary lymphadenopathy [6].

2.3 Magnetic resonance imaging (MRI)

Breast MRI is an established method for detecting lesions not visible to other imaging modalities. It creates breast images by measuring and processing the signal changes in the movement of protons in water and fat by applying changing magnetic fields. Its use in breast cancer detection is based on the concept of tumor neovascularity or angiogenesis. MRI remains one of the most useful diagnostic tools used to screen women who are at higher-than-average risk of breast cancer, patients post-excision who are found to have a positive margin, and further surgical planning is required, as well as women post breast conservative therapy undergoing surveillance. MRI is very beneficial in these patients as it provides a clearer image of the breast tissue without exposing it to radiation. Due to its high sensitivity, it is considered superior to mammography and ultrasound in detecting a multifocality or DCIS component [5].

3. Tissue sampling

Biopsy should be done on any lesion found during imaging wherein malignancy cannot be ruled out. A breast tissue biopsy is obtained to provide histopathological evidence of the disease and describe its characteristics. Different receptors found on cells will shape chemotherapy and hormonal therapy differently for each patient.

3.1 Core needle biopsy (CNB)

CNB is the preferred choice as it provides adequate tissue for analysis. Some biopsies will be image-guided, either US-guided or stereotactic, according to the lesion targeted. To facilitate the subsequent management in patients who will undergo neoadjuvant therapy, or if more than one lesion were biopsied, a clip can be inserted at the time of CNB. This will help to guide neoadjuvant treatment and follow the lesion subsequently before planning surgical excision. Local surgical excision can also benefit from these clips; a preoperative localizing clip can be inserted guided by the previous clip in the lesion cavity; these clips are magnetized and can be detected by a probe designed to pick up signals from the clip to provide better breast conservative surgery. Many different types of clips are available; perhaps the most famous lately are the magnetized clips. Some prefer wire localization of the lesion, yet many struggle with wires dislodging from the lesion mid-surgical excision; hence, with its revolution in guiding conservative breast surgery, preoperative clip localization has been gaining wide acceptance in breast-conserving surgery. Its main pitfall, perhaps, is clip migration, which has been reported to an extent, yet it still does not overcome the huge advantage that it provides [11].

3.2 Fine needle aspiration

Fine needle aspiration still carries a significant role in diagnosis as well. Histology can be obtained using a fine needle such as a Trucut or Corecut biopsy device under local anesthesia. A needle of 21 or 23 gauge with a syringe is usually used with multiple passes targeting the area of suspicion while keeping the syringe withdrawn to maintain a negative suction effect and effectively collect a cytological sample for analysis. The sample is then placed on a slide, smeared, and analyzed by an expert pathologist. This helps establish cell diagnosis using a minimally invasive approach. However, many problems can arise from aspiration alone. False-negative results are expected, which can be due to errors in targeting or aspirating the area of suspicion. Also, aspiration samples often fail to distinguish an invasive cancer from an *in situ* disease; this remains the most significant limitation depending on this modality; hence, CNB biopsy is the modality of choice [11].

4. Genetic testing

Specific genetic mutations that may be familial have been very well studied, and it established the increased risk of breast cancer; hence, many women will undergo genetic testing in cases where such gene mutations are suspected to reduce the risk of the remaining family member by early screening and detection. The most common genetic mutations that are inherited in high penetrance and increase breast cancer risk are BRCA1, BRCA2, and PALB-2. Women with such genetic mutations are encouraged to consider risk-reduction surgical interventions as well as chemoprevention strategies [12]. Specific tools, such as the Gail Model, have been developed to aid in stratification and estimate the risk of certain individuals with a family history of the disease. Overall, patients with a family history of breast cancer are at increased risk for the disease. Yet, there are inherited genetic mutations that some are born with that place them in a bracket of very high risk on statistically inevitable risk of developing the disease.

An established part of medical practice is genetic testing to assess for cancer susceptibility. Until recently, testing was limited to patients with a significant family history of cancer and focused on a small number of genes linked to a high risk of cancer or specific cancer syndromes. A large-scale study consisting of 113,000 women conducted by the Breast Cancer Association Consortium in 2020 evaluated the coding variation in putative breast cancer susceptibility genes and found a strong association with breast cancer risk and the five protein-truncating gene variants (ATM, BRCA1, BRCA2, CHEK2, and PALB2) [13]. Genetic findings may help guide screening and prevention with risk-reducing surgery or medication per national standards. However, all genetic testing shares many ethical considerations, such as the basic questions of distributive justice in resource distribution and fairness in test availability.

4.1 Aims of breast cancer care

1. Cure the disease by accepting that recurrence in some patients is possible. It is essential to keep the treatment's aims and goals realistic.

2. Accurately diagnose and control any local disease in the breast or axilla.

3. Focus on conserving local shape, form, and function as much as possible.

4. Prevention and reduction of local recurrence.

5. Breast cancer treatment

The approach to breast cancer treatment remains multidisciplinary, with the patient at the center of the treatment. Treatment should start with excellent doctor-patient communication, and a physician should develop their skills in bad news-breaking conversations. This plays a vital role in reducing patient anxiety, building trust, and preparing the patient for what is to come next. Participation of the patient in treatment decisions is crucial in breast cancer management. Pre- and postoperative involvement of an expert counselor alongside a physiotherapist to provide psychological and emotional support coupled with planned physiotherapy sessions offers a significant improvement in patient well-being and quality of life following the diagnosis and treatment of breast cancer. A multidisciplinary approach to the treatment and care of breast cancer patients has proven to be the gold standard with the collective efforts of the surgeon providing the surgical resection, oncologist providing needed chemotherapy and/or hormonal therapy, radiotherapist with radiotherapy, and other professionals such as clinical nurse specialists and coordinators to streamline a smooth experience for the patient.

6. Surgical approach

Surgical treatment remains at the center of breast cancer management. There has been a gradual shift toward more conservative techniques. This helps alleviate the considerable psychological morbidity and provides minimal disfiguration of the breast shape. It has offered equal, if not superior, reduction risk of local recurrence with an estimate of 2% at 10 years [14].

The risk of recurrence risk is increased in positive surgical margins, node positivity, absence of postoperative radiation therapy, and aggressive features of cancer cells. Positive margin is considered a modifiable or controllable risk factor as re-excision is mandated in positive margin excisions. In cases of ductal carcinoma *in situ*, the acceptable negative margin is defined as 2 mm+ [15, 16], and there is no tumor on ink for invasive cancer or stage I–II cancer [17]. The risk reduction in local recurrence and margin guidelines are dependent on the fact that breast conservative surgery is strictly followed by adjuvant radiotherapy except in selected patients such as, but not restricted to, elderly with stage I node-negative disease with hormone receptive positive who will undergo endocrine therapy postoperatively, it may be a reasonable option to exclude radiotherapy [18]. It is worth noting that almost all breast-conserving surgery includes axillary sampling, which aims to confirm the negativity of spread into axillary lymph nodes.

As mentioned, surgery in breast cancer holds a central role in treatment, between establishing diagnosis and workup, neoadjuvant therapy, and adjuvant therapy. Surgery aims to excise the diseased tissue and, most recently, is accompanied by reconstructive efforts, namely breast once-reconstructive surgery, where the surgery re-establishes and orients the breast tissue cosmetically in the same setting of surgery or a two-step surgery. The choice for breast surgery depends on lesion characteristics and patient preferences. Some factors include tumor size, location, and spread.

6.1 Mastectomy

Mastectomy describes the surgical excision of breast tissue, which may include local or regional lymph nodes. It is sometimes performed as a risk-reduction intervention for women with high risk and who have genetic inheritance.

Mastectomies may be nipple-sparing or skin-sparing mastectomy. Nipple-sparing mastectomy describes the excision of cancerous breast tissue with the preservation of breast skin and nipple-areola complex. Meanwhile, the skin-sparing mastectomy technique excises the breast tissue with the nipple-areola complex, leaving the remaining breast skin in place with either closure of the skin or immediate reconstruction.

Mastectomy is now only strictly indicated for large tumors, central tumors beneath or involving the nipple, multifocal disease, local recurrence, patient preference, or if conservative breast surgery is contraindicated. Halstead mastectomy (created in 1882) is no longer indicated, providing evidence of excessive morbidity with no survival benefits (**Figure 2**). Modified radical (Patey) mastectomy is more commonly performed when indicated (**Figure 3**).

Some indications that prefer mastectomy over breast-conserving surgery include inflammatory breast cancer, multicentric disease, diffuse microcalcifications, previous breast radiation, pregnancy as it is contraindicated to radiate breast tissue in pregnancy, and inability to achieve negative margins after reasonable attempts of re-excision. However, some patients will elect and insist on mastectomy, in which case, their choice is respected after proper education on the benefits of breast-conserving surgery.

Following mastectomy, immediate vs. delayed reconstruction can be planned according to its indication. Immediate reconstruction can be safe in selected patients who undergo oncological resection [21]. In prophylactic resection, immediate reconstruction will provide the patient with minimal image distortion and support their psychological recovery.

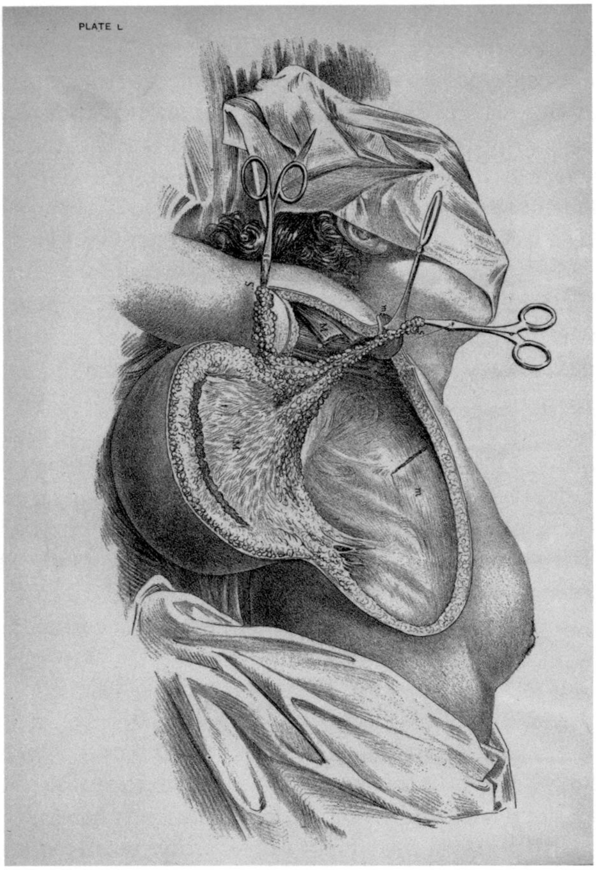

Figure 2.
William Stewart Halsted radical mastectomy [19].

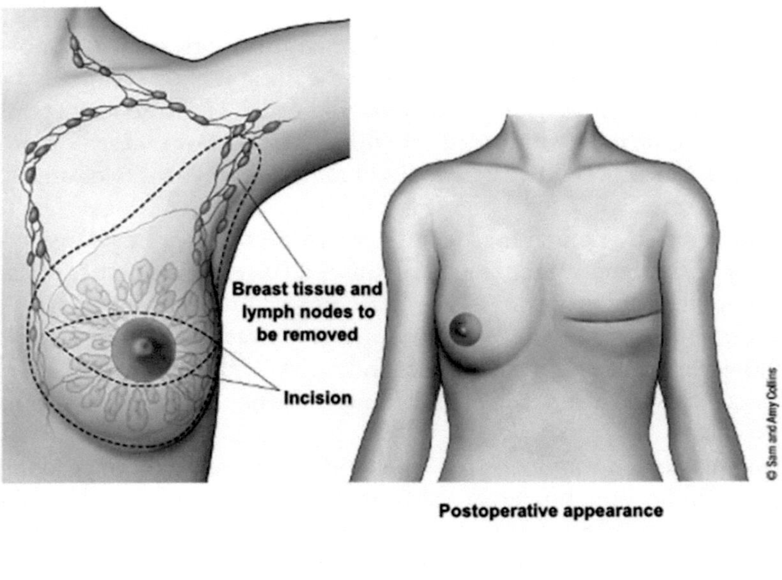

Figure 3.
Modified radical (Patey) mastectomy [20].

6.2 Lobectomy

Lobectomy is the base of breast conservative surgery. It is the surgical removal of the tumor, with minimal surrounding breast tissue, to establish negative margins, and often is accompanied by reconstructive measures with local flap advancement. Lymph node sampling is a significant part of such surgery as positivity will change the surgical management. This option is often used for small, early-stage cancers where no contraindications to breast conservative surgery are present.

7. Breast reconstruction and oncoplastic breast surgery

Breast reconstruction and oncoplastic surgery provide the patient with a positive quality of life. The aim is to preserve the shape of the breast while achieving oncological resection of the diseased tissue. Oncoplastic surgery has taken the lead over classic breast-conserving surgery with a lower rate of positive margins and a lower rate of re-excision [14]. Breast reconstruction can be in many different forms, such as autologous expanders or immediate implants. There has been a shift toward autologous flap-based reconstruction as it reutilizes the body's tissue to reshape the breast, which provides a very natural feel to the new breast tissue. Many different flaps have been developed for this purpose, such as DIEP flap—deep inferior epigastric perforator—and TRAM flap—transverse rectus abdominis myocutaneous. The main downfall to such flaps is the preservation of blood supply, which can be challenging in some patients, especially smokers. The most recent approach has been utilizing rotational flaps with the established blood supply and no need for microvascular reconstruction. The main challenge remains in careful patient selection, possible morbidities of flap necrosis, and the need for re-operation.

Patients who have enough breast skin remaining after a mastectomy may be suited for direct or delayed implant breast reconstruction. Direct implants allow patients to recover from their surgery and wake up to a well-defined breast shape [14]. This, however, can be challenging if the patient requires postoperative radiotherapy. Expanders are implants that are more suitable for patients who need radiotherapy and/or patients who are more fit for delayed reconstruction. Tissue and skin can adjust slowly to the effect of radiotherapy while preserving space for future implants.

Other forms of reconstruction can be based on prostheses with specifically made bras and attached prosthetics. However, these do not provide satisfaction for the patient as they remain flat-chested and can alter the patient's image of themselves.

Reconstruction can go beyond breast shape only. Newly developed fields of microvascular reconstruction in breast surgery aim to reduce the burden of lymphedema that accompanies axillary dissection with careful reconstruction of lymphatic vessels and improve sensory function in the nipple-areolar complex by reconstructing the fourth or fifth intercostal sensory nerve using an extended allograph.

7.1 Oncoplastic breast-conserving surgery (OCBS)

OCBS was developed by combining the facets of reconstructive plastic surgery with more traditional resection techniques. It provides an alternative surgical option for patients who are not candidates for full mastectomy or vast local excisions. OCBS allows adequate resection of tumor margins, providing better cosmesis than a modified radical mastectomy. In 2020, a meta-analysis of 22 studies comparing the oncological safety of OCBS with traditional techniques showed no significant difference in the re-operation rate and recurrence of cancer [22].

Multicentric disease is a contraindication for breast conservative surgery, yet some recent studies are challenging that. The Alliance Z11102 trial conducted by the American College of Surgeons evaluated closely the possibility of breast conservative surgery in multicentric disease that qualifies for local excision of the cancerous focus, which includes 2 or 3 foci separated by 2 cm+. The trial aimed to evaluate whether breast-conserving surgery with adjuvant radiation that includes lumpectomy will yield an acceptably low 5-year local recurrence rate for multiple ipsilateral breast cancer. The trial presented promising results with acceptable and comparable local recurrence rates at 5-year intervals [23]; this practice is yet to be accepted as more evidence is required.

7.2 Lymphedema and rehabilitation

Lymphedema management can be complex and challenging, with incidence close to 30% occurrence post-axillary dissection, and some studies also suggest a high incidence of lymphedema post-axillary sampling. The main aim of the treatment in such cases with the abscess of experience in lymphovascular reconstruction is the conservative management of specific and focused physical therapy and rehabilitation that focuses on improving lymphatics flow early postoperatively and preventing fluid accumulation within the tissues. Postoperative rehabilitation and physical therapy go beyond reducing the risk of developing lymphedema to include the patient's overall well-being and providing psychological support when needed.

8. Adjuvant therapy

Adjuvant therapy for breast cancer includes chemotherapy, radiotherapy, and endocrine therapy. Immunotherapy is under development as adjuvant therapy for stubborn invasive cancers where classic adjuvant therapy is not a fit.

8.1 Radiotherapy

Radiotherapy delivers high-energy or ray particles to eliminate cancer cells. It is commonly combined with a specific chemotherapy regimen to complement each other as they play a significant role in reducing the local recurrence rate. Many factors will determine the type of adjuvant therapy and whether neoadjuvant treatment was taken. Radiotherapy is indicated in, but not excluded, breast-conserving surgery to reduce recurrence in the breast or nearby lymph nodes after mastectomy, especially with large cancers or in cases of lymph node metastasis and cases of distance metastasis.

Some patients may also be eligible for intraoperative radiation therapy, which is a new take on radiotherapy delivery in cancer; it delivers high-dose radiation treatment during surgery targeted toward the cancer bed. The hope for this kind of treatment is for the patients to skip the standard 6 weeks of radiation therapy that follow a lumpectomy. Many Phase II and Phase III trials are undergoing to try and establish the efficacy of such intervention; however, it is still to prove itself as a replacement for neoadjuvant radiotherapy [24].

8.2 Chemotherapy

Chemotherapy has been well established as an adjunct treatment of cancer; many different chemotherapies have been developed to target cancer cells. Chemotherapy targets all rapidly dividing cells, specifically cancer cells, as they have a high rate of turnover. Several treatment regimens aim to reduce the risk of recurrence and eliminate remnant cancer cells that might not have been excised surgically. They also aim to halt the progression or even reduce the disease burden to provide a better surgical approach.

Indication for chemotherapy, whether neoadjuvant or adjuvant, depends on the receptor status of cancer cells, estrogen receptor (ER), progesterone receptor (PR), human epidermal growth factor receptor 2 (HER2), tumor stage and grade, and histological features of high risk such as lymphovascular invasion. Triple-negative breast cancer, that is, all three receptors are negative in expression, is one of the main indications of chemotherapy in breast cancer.

Targeted therapy, which is the preferred type of chemotherapeutic in breast cancer, selectively attacks cancer based on specific characteristics of the breast cancer cells. In cases of HER2-positive cells, targeted therapy is employed as it specifically targets these cells according to the receptor expression. Such therapeutics include herceptin alongside other agents. Each patient will have a regimen based on histological features. This has greatly decreased the use of unnecessary chemotherapeutics that do not reduce the recurrence rate and reduce the burden on the patient.

8.3 Immunotherapy

Immunotherapy aims to stimulate the patient's immune system to target cancer cells from within. Immunotherapy hopes to provide better management of cancer and provide longer progression-free survival, especially in triple-negative breast cancer. Many trials are testing such agents, yet more is needed to establish substantial evidence of treatment. Most immunotherapeutics are being tested alongside or in addition to already established chemotherapy regimens. Pembrolizumab is being tested extensively as an adjunct to chemotherapy. It has been proven to result in significantly longer overall survival compared to chemotherapy alone [25]. Most Immunotherapy does require specific tumor expressions to be present on the cancer cell; for example, pembrolizumab requires cancer cells to express Programmed Death Ligand 1 (PD-L1); it remains the only approved agent in combination with chemotherapy for early stage triple-negative high-risk breast cancer.

8.4 Hormonal therapy

Breast cancer tissue often relies on hormones to fuel its growth. Hormones such as estrogen and progesterone are the main hormones that play a role in such mechanisms. Treatment that decreases hormonal production may help slow or halt the disease. Endocrine therapy is a crucial part of treatment after surgery in patients with positive hormonal receptors to reduce cancer recurrence. The current recommendation for endocrine therapy is a minimum of 5 years for women with stage I to III breast cancer with hormonal receptor positivity. Some more recent trials advocate for up to 8 years of endocrine therapy for such patients.

9. Disparities in breast cancer care

Advances in standardized screening and improved diagnosis and treatment of breast cancer have not translated into optimum survival in women. Disparities in access to quality screening and result interpretation faced by distinct populations pose significant challenges to the creation of equitable breast cancer care and outcomes. Many have investigated and reported barriers and disparities in access to care that have resulted in suboptimal application of standards of care across populations and groups. Lack of insurance and general socioeconomic disadvantage go hand in hand with delayed treatment, which leads to poor and limited adherence, ultimately impacting breast cancer survival. It is well-studied that rural women have difficulty receiving adjuvant therapy and surgical interventions. Racial disparities remain a worrying factor in breast cancer care, given that minorities are disproportionately affected by socioeconomic disadvantages that increase barriers to receiving optimal care [26]. Overall, the etiology of the various disparities in breast cancer outcomes is complex and multifactorial. It is paramount to recognize that the intersectionality of multiple factors may cumulatively impact the experience and survival of breast cancer patients, especially those from marginalized communities.

10. Prognosis

The prognosis of breast cancer depends on the stage of the disease at the time of diagnosis; however, with the advancement of treatment modalities, most of the locally advanced cancers can be treated successfully. Challenges remain with cases of distant metastasis and late presentation of the disease. Prognostic factors can involve the histological grade, hormone receptors, tumor proliferation, growth factor analysis, involvement of local and regional lymph nodes, and metastasis. On the bright side, breast cancer mortality has reduced tremendously due to the advancement of diagnostic modalities and, most importantly, awareness and early detection. In an analysis comparing breast cancer mortality in the US, there has been a reduction of almost 58% mortality in 2019 compared to 1975 of stage I to stage III breast cancer with close to 30% reduction in metastatic breast cancer mortality rate [27]. However, breast cancer mortality rates have risen in sub-Saharan Africa and are now among the world's highest. While 5-year survival rates for breast cancer approach 90% in most high-income nations, this statistic was 66% for the 12 sub-Saharan African countries combined. According to the GLOBACAN database, the global burden of breast cancer remains concentrated in women aged 50 and older, accounting for more than 70% of all new cases and 81% of all deaths. However, the age distribution of cases and fatalities varied significantly around the world, with Middle Africa accounting for 43% of cases and 49% of deaths, while Northern America, Western, and Northern Europe accounted for more than 80% of cases and 90% of deaths.

11. Conclusion

To conclude, we have come a long way in the treatment of one of the deadliest cancers known to humanity. The fight still goes on. Many new therapies are on the rise, and there has been a massive advancement in treating breast cancer. Innovation is on the rise in the surgical and medical management of this disease. The hope is high. We encourage our patients to trust their physicians and surgeons and to trust that they are not alone. We encourage physicians and surgeons to keep innovating and thinking outside the box to further develop and invent treatments, follow the latest evidence-based management, and always keep the patient in mind.

Author details

Ahmed Subhy Alsheikhly[1*] and Mazin Ahmed Subhy Alsheikhly[2]

1 Hamad Medical Corporation, Weill Cornell Medicine, Qatar

2 General Surgery Department, Hamad Medical Corporation, Qatar

*Address all correspondence to: ahmadmomz@yahoo.com

References

[1] Lauby-Secretan B, Scoccianti C, Loomis D, Grosse Y, Bianchini F, Straif K, et al. Body fatness and cancer–viewpoint of the IARC working group. The New England Journal of Medicine. 2016;**375**(8):794-798. DOI: 10.1056/NEJMsr1606602

[2] Sung H, Ferlay J, Siegel RL, Laversanne M, Soerjomataram I, Jemal A, et al. Global cancer statistics 2020: GLOBOCAN estimates of incidence and mortality worldwide for 36 cancers in 185 countries. CA: A Cancer Journal for Clinicians. 2021;**71**(3):209-249. DOI: 10.3322/caac.21660. Epub 2021 Feb 4

[3] Esserman LJ, Shieh Y, Rutgers EJ, Knauer M, Retèl VP, Mook S, et al. Impact of mammographic screening on the detection of good and poor prognosis breast cancers. Breast Cancer Research and Treatment. 2011;**130**(3):725-734. DOI: 10.1007/s10549-011-1748-z. Epub 2011 Sep 4

[4] Maha R, Alison J, Michael S, Manvydas V. Triple assessment breast clinics: The value of clinical core biopsies. Irish Journal of Medical Science (1971-). 2024;**193**(2):565-570

[5] Steyerova P, Burgetova A. Current imaging techniques and impact on diagnosis and survival—A narrative review. Annals of Breast Surgery. 2022;**6**:4-6

[6] Wolfson S, Kim E, Plaunova A, Bukhman R, Sarmiento RD, Samreen N, et al. Axillary adenopathy after COVID-19 vaccine: No reason to delay screening mammogram. Radiology. 2022;**303**(2):297-299

[7] Yaffe MJ, AAPM tutorial. Physics of mammography: Image recording process. Radiographics. 1990;**10**(2):341-363. DOI: 10.1148/radiographics.10.2.2183301

[8] Pisano ED. Digital compared with screen-film mammography: Measures of diagnostic accuracy among women screened in the Ontario breast screening program–Evidence that direct radiography is superior to computed radiography for cancer detection. Radiology. 2016;**278**(2):311-312. DOI: 10.1148/radiol.2015152344

[9] Skaane P, Bandos AI, Gullien R, Eben EB, Ekseth U, Haakenaasen U, et al. Comparison of digital mammography alone and digital mammography plus tomosynthesis in a population-based screening program. Radiology. 2013;**267**(1):47-56. DOI: 10.1148/radiol.12121373. Epub 2013 Jan 7

[10] Skaane P, Bandos AI, Niklason LT, Sebuødegård S, Østerås BH, Gullien R, et al. Digital mammography versus digital mammography plus tomosynthesis in breast cancer screening: The Oslo tomosynthesis screening trial. Radiology. 2019;**291**(1):23-30. DOI: 10.1148/radiol.2019182394. Epub 2019 Feb 19

[11] Guenin MA. Clip placement during a sonographically guided large-core breast biopsy for mammographic-sonographic correlation. AJR. American Journal of Roentgenology. 2000;**175**(4):1053-1055. DOI: 10.2214/ajr.175.4.1751053

[12] World Health Organization: WHO, World Health Organization: WHO. Breast Cancer [Internet]. 2024. Available from: https://www.who.int/news-room/fact-sheets/detail/breast-cancer

[13] Breast Cancer Association Consortium. Breast cancer risk

genes—Association analysis in more than 113,000 women. New England Journal of Medicine. 2021;**384**(5):428-439

[14] Keelan S, Flanagan M, Hill ADK. Evolving trends in surgical management of breast cancer: An analysis of 30 years of practice changing papers. Frontiers in Oncology. 2021;**4**:622621. DOI: 10.3389/fonc.2021.622621

[15] Tadros AB, Smith BD, Shen Y, Lin H, Krishnamurthy S, Lucci A, et al. Ductal carcinoma in situ and margins <2 mm: Contemporary outcomes with breast conservation. Annals of Surgery. 2019;**269**(1):150-157. DOI: 10.1097/SLA.0000000000002439

[16] Van Zee KJ, Subhedar P, Olcese C, Patil S, Morrow M. Relationship between margin width and recurrence of ductal carcinoma in situ: Analysis of 2996 women treated with breast-conserving surgery for 30 years. Annals of Surgery. 2015;**262**(4):623-631. DOI: 10.1097/SLA.0000000000001454

[17] Moran MS, Schnitt SJ, Giuliano AE, Harris JR, Khan SA, Horton J, et al. Society of Surgical Oncology-American Society for Radiation Oncology consensus guideline on margins for breast-conserving surgery with whole-breast irradiation in stages I and II invasive breast cancer. Journal of Clinical Oncology. 2014;**32**(14):1507-1515. DOI: 10.1200/JCO.2013.53.3935. Epub 2014 Feb 10

[18] Kunkler IH, Williams LJ, Jack WJ, Cameron DA, Dixon JM, PRIME II Investigators. Breast-conserving surgery with or without irradiation in women aged 65 years or older with early breast cancer (PRIME II): A randomised controlled trial. The Lancet Oncology. 2015;**16**(3):266-273. DOI: 10.1016/S1470-2045(14)71221-5. Epub 2015 Jan 28. Erratum in: Lancet Oncol. Mar 2015;**16**(3):e105. DOI: 10.1016/S1470-2045(15)70094-X

[19] Akl MM, Ahmed A. [Commentary] Impact of total mastectomy on the lymphatic pathway and the limitation of PET imaging in breast cancer surveillance. 2024

[20] Surgery: Cancer of the Breast. Wellcome Collection; n.d. Available from: https://wellcomecollection.org/works/sncrzk6s?wellcomeImagesUrl=%2Findexplus%2Fimage%2FL0076910.html

[21] Munhoz AM, Montag E, Filassi JR, Gemperli R. Immediate nipple-areola-sparing mastectomy reconstruction: An update on oncological and reconstruction techniques. World Journal of Clinical Oncology. 2014;**5**(3):478-494. DOI: 10.5306/wjco.v5.i3.478

[22] Kosasih S, Tayeh S, Mokbel K, Kasem A. Is oncoplastic breast conserving surgery oncologically safe? A meta-analysis of 18,103 patients. The American Journal of Surgery. 2020;**220**(2):385-392

[23] Boughey JC, Rosenkranz KM, Ballman KV, McCall L, Haffty BG, Cuttino LW, et al. Local recurrence after breast-conserving therapy in patients with multiple ipsilateral breast cancer: Results from ACOSOG Z11102 (alliance). Journal of Clinical Oncology. 2023;**41**(17):3184-3193

[24] Pilar A, Gupta M, Ghosh Laskar S, Laskar S. Intraoperative radiotherapy: Review of techniques and results. Ecancermedicalscience. 2017;**11**:750. DOI: 10.3332/ecancer.2017.750

[25] Cortes J, Rugo HS, Cescon DW, Im SA, Yusof MM, Gallardo C, et al. Pembrolizumab plus chemotherapy in advanced triple-negative breast cancer. The New England Journal of Medicine.

2022;**387**(3):217-226. DOI: 10.1056/NEJMoa2202809

[26] Wilkerson AD, Gentle CK, Ortega C, Al-Hilli Z. Disparities in breast cancer care—How factors related to prevention, diagnosis, and treatment drive inequity. Healthcare. 2024;**12**(4):462. DOI: 10.3390/healthcare12040462

[27] Caswell-Jin JL, Sun LP, Munoz D, Lu Y, Li Y, Huang H, et al. Analysis of breast cancer mortality in the US-1975 to 2019. Journal of the American Medical Association. 2024;**331**(3):233-241. DOI: 10.1001/jama.2023.25881

Chapter 2

Breast Cancer Heterogeneity and Its Implication in Precision Therapy

Fernando Candanedo-Gonzalez, Ana Lilia Remirez-Castellanos, Ursula Salazar-Gomez, Wilfredo Valenzuela-Gonzalez, Cindy Chavira-Macias and Armando Gamboa-Dominguez

Abstract

Breast cancer (BC) is the most common cancer among women worldwide, with a progressive increase in its incidence. It is the second leading cause of cancer-related death in women, with most cases due to metastatic disease and its heterogeneity. Tumor heterogeneity is associated with differences in molecular characteristics, which regulate hormonal receptor expression, HER2 amplification, proliferation, metastatic potential, drug resistance, etc. Molecular heterogeneity in BC presents multiple clinical challenges to accurately characterize and treat the disease. BC heterogeneity represents a challenge in selecting the most appropriate therapy for each patient and predicting prognosis. In this review, we discuss the different types of heterogeneity in BC, including imaging features, histopathological and immunohistochemical characteristics, the mechanisms involved, some molecular tests that allow exploring heterogeneity, and new treatment options.

Keywords: breast cancer, heterogeneity, precision therapy, genomic, epigenomic, transcriptomic

1. Introduction

1.1 Normal anatomy, histology, and biology

Mammary glands in humans are a paired, highly specialized organ. The mammary tissue consists of milk-producing glands, called lobules, which transport milk through ducts to the nipple (**Figure 1A**). The terminal duct-lobular unit is composed of a duct and acini (**Figure 1B**). This unit constitutes the milk-secreting part and the region with the highest proliferation rate [1]. The ducts and lobules are made of two layers of cells. The inner layer contains luminal epithelial cells, while the outer layer is composed of myoepithelial cells, in contact with the basement membrane (**Figure 1C**). The stroma surrounding the terminal duct-lobular units is made of fibroadipose tissue, blood vessels, lymphatic vessels, and fibroblasts.

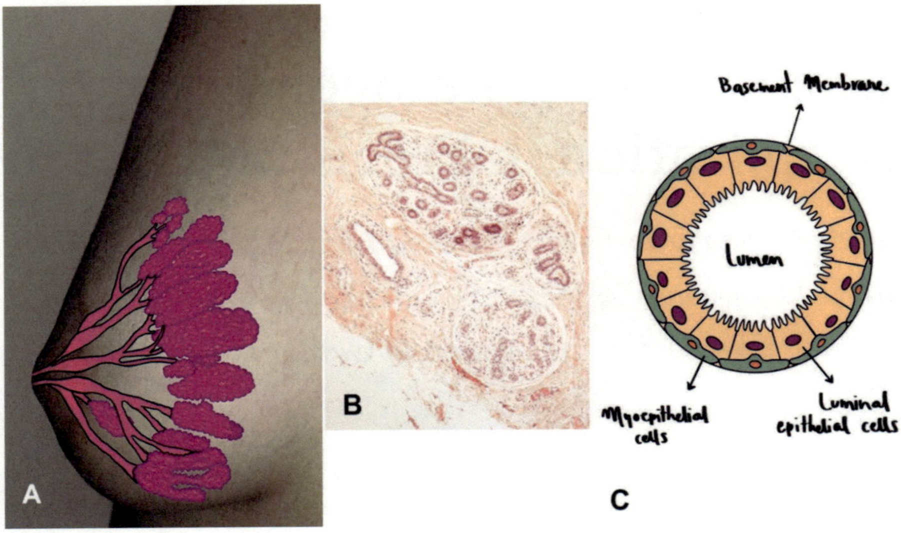

Figure 1.
Mammary gland: (A) It is composed of ducts that branch; (B) In the deeper portion, it is made of terminal duct-lobular units; (C) An acinus is the functional milk-producing unit.

During the normal development of the mammary gland, estrogens, progesterone, and epidermal growth factor (EGF) are required. The alpha estrogen receptor (ER-α) promotes the growth and elongation of ducts embedded in mammary adipose tissue, while progesterone receptors (PR) induce the development of terminal units or acini (alveologenesis), located at the end of the ducts. In addition, EGF promotes the proliferation of terminal buds, synergizing estrogen-induced duct growth and progesterone-induced branching [2–4].

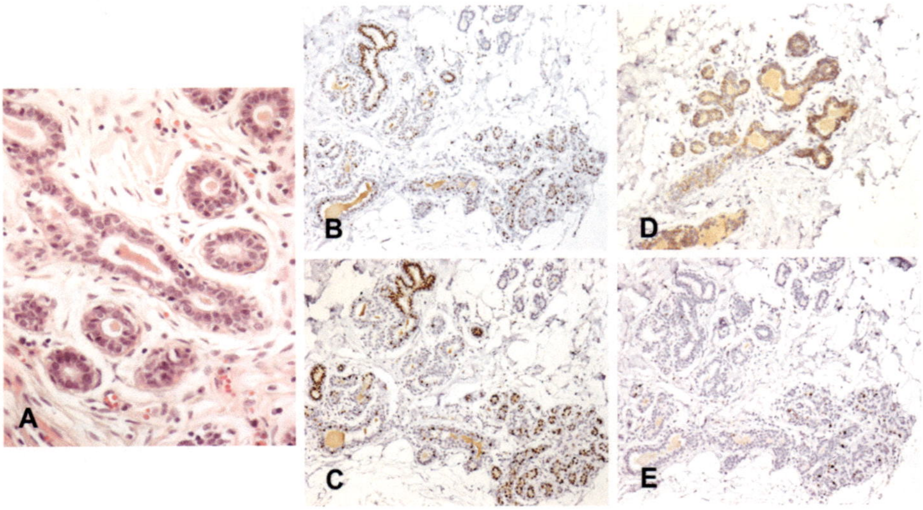

Figure 2.
(A) Terminal duct-lobular unit in a histological section stained with hematoxylin and eosin; (B) ER expression less than 10%; (C) PR expression less than 10%; (D) Focal EGFR expression; (E) Ki-67 proliferation index of 1%.

In adult mammary tissue, cells expressing estrogen receptors (ER) and PR represent 7–10% of the epithelial cell population (**Figure 2**). There is evidence that the extracellular matrix (ECM) has tumor-suppressing functions by maintaining the basement membrane intact, providing a physical barrier between epithelial cells and the surrounding stroma, and preserving cell polarity. The ECM also produces substances with paracrine effects, such as growth inhibitors, and factors that affect invasion and angiogenesis [5].

Breast cancer (BC) can originate from any cellular type from the mammary tissue. However, the most frequent tumors arise from the epithelium lining the terminal duct-lobular units [6]. In relation to the above, 80% of all malignant tumors are classified as invasive ductal carcinoma. It is proposed that the process begins with an accelerated and dysregulated proliferation of cells in the terminal duct-lobular region, leading to the formation of cellular clusters, which over time develop into a tumor [7].

2. Epidemiology

BC is the most common cancer among women worldwide, with a progressive increase in its incidence [8, 9]. Despite significant advances in our understanding and treatment of BC, it remains a public health issue and continues to raise major challenges globally. Over the past decades, the classification and treatment of BC have primarily been based on clinical-pathological characteristics, tumor size, histological subtype, histological grade, multifocality, and lymph node status. Even so, BC constitutes a heterogeneous group of tumors with marked variation in clinical presentation, biological behavior, morphology, immunophenotype, molecular characteristics, and treatment response [10]. Due to its heterogeneity, it is also the second leading cause of cancer-related death among women. This progression of BC involves underlying mechanisms, new research methods to measure BC heterogeneity, and treatment strategies considering this heterogeneity.

3. Definition of heterogeneity

Tumor heterogeneity shows in different forms. Firstly, tumor heterogeneity can arise from cells of an individual tumor, known as intratumoral heterogeneity [11, 12]. Intratumoral heterogeneity, in turn, can be either spatial or temporal. While spatial heterogeneity occurs in different areas of the same primary tumor, temporal heterogeneity can present differences in the tumor over time during follow-up [13, 14]. Secondly, intermetastatic heterogeneity is the variety between different metastatic lesions in the same patient. Thirdly, there is a type of intrametastatic heterogeneity that can affect different cells within a single metastasis. This type of heterogeneity can promote resistance to therapy and disease recurrence [15]. Finally, there is also heterogeneity between tumors from different patients, known as intertumoral heterogeneity, which requires personalized treatments adapted to each patient. Intertumoral heterogeneity is due to differences in genetic, epigenetic, transcriptomic, and proteomic features in each patient. These features provide each tumor with varying capacities to proliferate, migrate, invade, metastasize, and respond to therapy. Heterogeneity in BC presents multiple clinical challenges in order to accurately characterize and treat the disease [16–19]. It increases the difficulty of an early diagnosis, choice of treatment, and prognosis prediction.

4. Heterogeneity by imaging

There are several imaging techniques for the detection and diagnosis of BC [20]. Mammography has been widely utilized in BC detection and allows to obtain information about the presence of tumor and/or microcalcifications, morphological characteristics, mass shape, whether it is round, oval, lobulated, or irregular (**Figure 3A**). Nevertheless, its usefulness in detecting intertumoral or intratumoral heterogeneity is not well understood. Elastography allows the analysis by imaging the stiffness of tissues. In BC, this stiffness translates into interactions between neoplastic cells and cells of the stroma and ECM. These properties are associated with heterogeneity. Some elastographic characteristics are associated with histological grade [21, 22]. However, it is not useful for the correlation between mechanical elasticity and BC subtype. On the other hand, due to its excellent soft tissue contrast and high sensibility, MRI is used as a complementary technique to mammography and ultrasound (**Figure 3B–D**) [23]. MRI images can provide parameters such as tumor size, morphology, and shape (**Figure 3E**). Dynamic contrast-enhanced MRI (DCE-MRI) allows investigation of microvascular structure and kinetic characterization, as well as statistical measurement from texture enhancement. These parameters reflect intratumoral characteristics, including growth patterns, angiogenesis, and permeability. Different BC subtypes exhibit various patterns of growth and angiogenesis. Therefore, it is possible to correlate MRI parameters with molecular subtypes of BC. MRI is also a powerful tool for predicting the heterogeneity of the response to neoadjuvant therapy. Hence, MRI is a viable instrument for assessing BC heterogeneity.

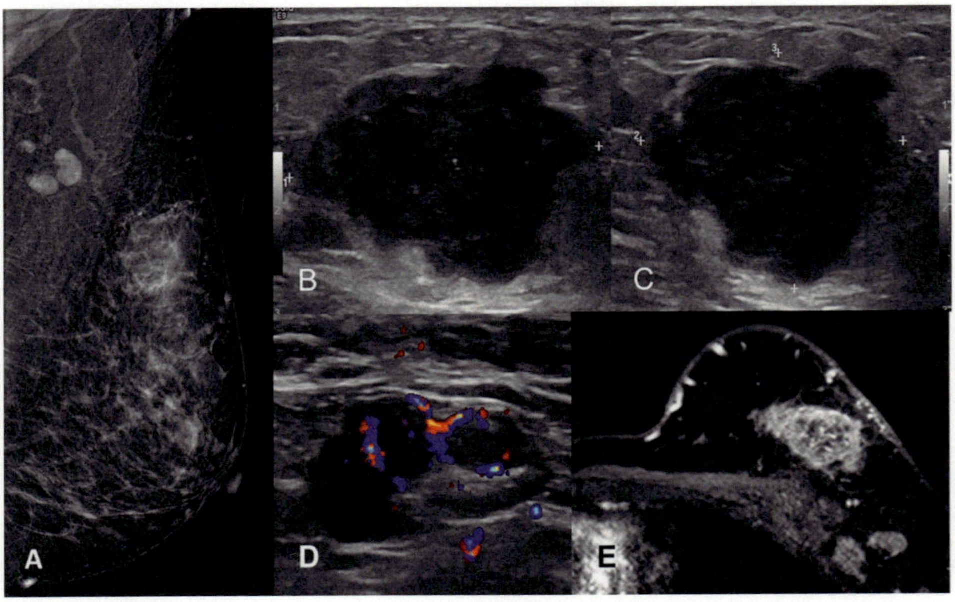

Figure 3.
(A) Triple-negative right breast cancer in the upper outer quadrant with a lobulated nodule with architectural distortion and dense lymph nodes with cortical thickening and loss of the fatty hilum; (B and C) Irregular ultrasound, angled margins, hypoechoic and posterior acoustic enhancement; (D) Right axillary lymph node with cortical thickening and increased vascularity on color Doppler; (E) T1-weighted MRI with contrast showing a lobulated nodule with heterogeneous enhancement and axillary nodes at level I with cortical thickening and loss of the fatty hilum.

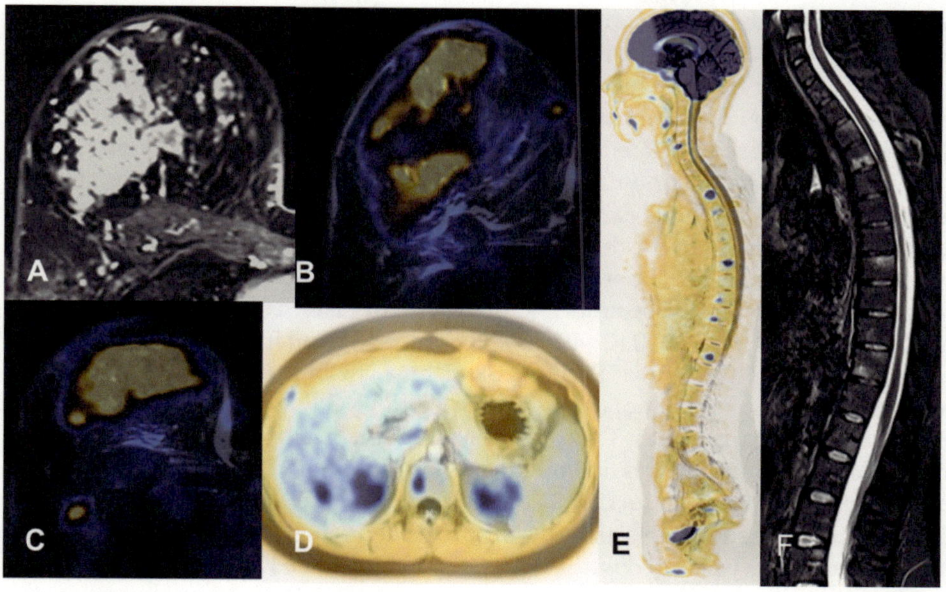

Figure 4.
PET-MR of multicentric HER2+ invasive ductal carcinoma of the right breast with tumor activity in ipsilateral lymph nodes, liver, and bone. (A) and (B) Right axial T1 with contrast shows nodules in the upper quadrants with irregular morphology and margins with heterogeneous enhancement with hypermetabolism SUmax of 7.7; (C) Right axillary lymph node at level I with increased metabolic activity; D) Hypermetabolic hepatic lesions in segments 4 and 7 SU max of 2.6. (E) and (F) Multiple bone lesions in the axial and appendicular skeleton.

Positron emission tomography (PET) is the most widely used molecular imaging technique with significant use for detecting intratumoral and intertumoral expression patterns of key molecules in breast cancer. Molecular imaging relies heavily on labeled biomarkers. By analyzing these labeled biomarkers, we can evaluate the heterogeneity of biochemical changes, cellular physiology, cellular function, and metabolism. PET is an imaging method that allows evaluating various tumor properties such as tumor metabolism, tumor proliferation, and the ER status through the use of specific radiotracers for each tumor characteristic. In this regard, 18F-fluorodeoxyglucose (18F-FDG) is used to analyze tumor metabolism [24], 18F-fluorothymidine (18F-FLT) is employed to assess tumor proliferation characteristics, and PET with 18F-estradiol (18F-FES) is useful for evaluating the ER status. Therefore, it is an imaging method that enables the study of dynamic changes related to intratumoral heterogeneity in BC. On one hand, 18F-FDG PET uptake has been associated with a high Ki-67 index in triple-negative BC. Conversely, 18F-FES PET uptake helps determine the necessary dose for ER antagonists to completely eliminate ER. Lastly, 18F-FLT PET uptake allows for imaging of intratumoral proliferation heterogeneity to assess the response to neoadjuvant chemotherapy (**Figure 4**) [25, 26].

5. Histopathobiology of heterogeneity

The morphological analysis of the tumor provides useful information about its biological behavior and the type of treatment required. BC can be classified into different subgroups according to histological type and histological grade using the Nottingham Grading System. Histological grade not only determines the level of differentiation, tubular formation, nuclear pleomorphism, and mitotic index of a tumor; but is also a prognostic factor independent of tumor size and the number of positive lymphatic nodes, which evaluates the neoplasm's biological behavior and response to therapy [27]. Histological type refers to the morphological growth pattern of tumors, which are associated with different clinical presentations and prognoses.

BC is divided into carcinoma in situ and invasive carcinoma. Carcinoma *in situ* represents 15–30% of all BC cases. Carcinoma *in situ* consists of a population of neoplastic cells limited to the ductal and lobular lumens, without invasion of the basement membrane. On the other hand, invasive carcinoma infiltrates beyond the basement membrane and accounts for 70–85% of all cases. These are divided into invasive ductal carcinoma (IDC; 40–75%) (**Figure 5A**) and invasive lobular carcinoma (ILC; 15–20%) (**Figure 5B**). Approximately 75% of tumors are classified as invasive ductal carcinoma, not otherwise specified (NOS). Special subtypes represent 25% of all ductal carcinomas. This group includes infiltrating tubular carcinoma, cribriform, mucinous, infiltrating micropapillary carcinoma, with apocrine differentiation, with neuroendocrine differentiation, and metaplastic carcinoma. Some histological types, such as tubular or cribriform carcinoma, are associated with a good prognosis and may be treated with endocrine therapy alone [10, 28].

BC can be categorized by immunohistochemistry (IHC) based on the status of ER and PR, HER2, and the proliferation index with Ki-67 into luminal A, luminal B, HER2+, and triple-negative BC (TNBC) subtypes (**Table 1**) [29]. These IHC subgroups are similar to the subtypes defined by gene expression studies, with specific responses to therapy and different prognoses [15, 30–32]. Therapeutic decisions in BC are based on the type of expression of ER, PR, HER2, and the proliferation index with Ki-67. Between 70 and 80% of all tumors are positive for hormone receptors and are classified as luminal A or luminal B. The main biological difference between ER+ Luminal A and ER- Luminal B BC is their proliferation index (**Figure 6**), with higher

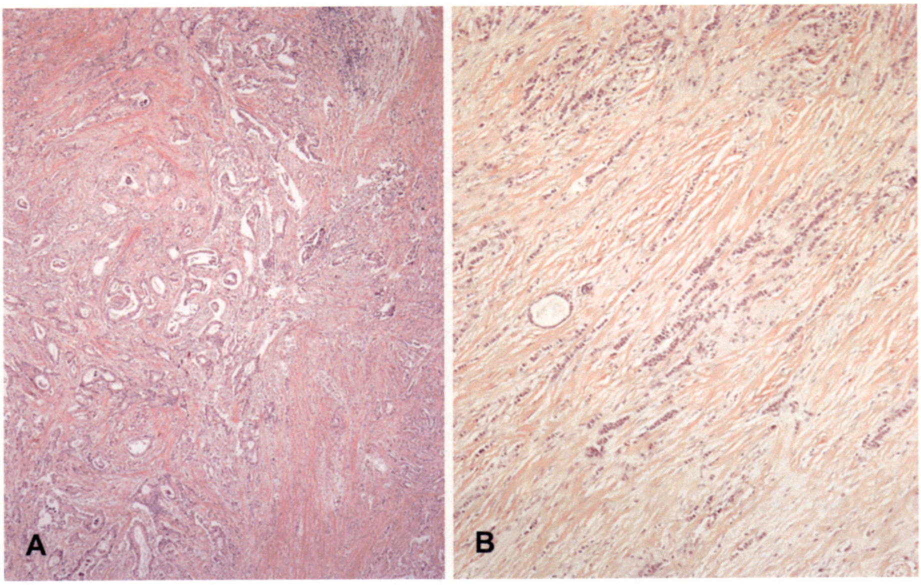

Figure 5.
Breast cancer: (A) Invasive ductal carcinoma with a tubular growth pattern embedded in desmoplasia; (B) Invasive lobular carcinoma with a row growth pattern.

	Luminal-A	Luminal-B	HER2+	Triple negative
Hormone Receptors HER2 Ki-67	ER+ and/or PR + HER2- < 20%	ER+ and/or PR + HER2+/– >20%	ER-,PR-HER2+++	ER-,PR-, HER2-
Prevalence among populations				
• All		8–18%		
• Non african	47–61%			
• African	26–27%		15–23%	27–37%
• Asiatic			19–36%	
• Caucasic			14–19%	
• Other				8–20%
Most common mutated genes				
• PIK3CA	48%	30%	33%	
• CDH1	22%			
• GATA3	15%	20%		
• MAP3K1	14%			
• TP53		36%	71%	90%
• TTN		20%	29%	24%
• MUC1			19%	
• BRCA1				8%
• NF1				5%
Most common copy number alterations				
• CCND1	17%	26%		
• FGF3	17%	24%		
• FGF4	17%	24%		
• FGF19	17%			
• FGFR1		19%		
• ERBB2			71%	
• MYC				36%
Biological pathway	ER signaling ECM	ER signaling ECM	HER-2 signaling Proliferation Immune response Tumoral invasion	Immune response ECM Proliferation

Table 1.
Epidemiological, phenotypic, and genetic differences of BC subtypes.

expression of genes such as CCNB1, MK167, and MYBL2 in luminal B tumors and a worse prognosis [29]. Additionally, HER2+ and HER2- tumors exhibit different clinical and molecular characteristics (**Figure** 7) [32]. In this context, the expression by IHC of ER, PR, HER2, and Ki-67 can vary between different areas of the same tumor.

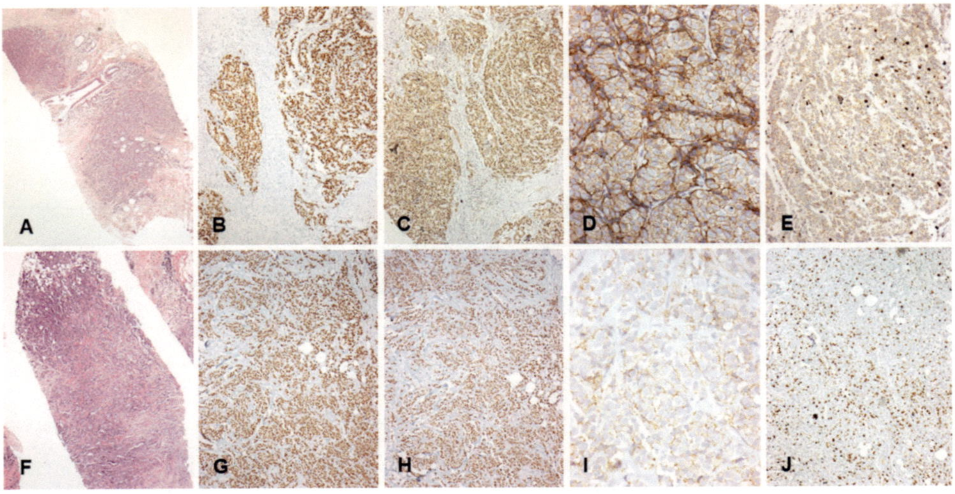

Figure 6.
Guided core-needle biopsies in breast cancer: (A) Case 1: Invasive ductal carcinoma with a non-specific pattern (luminal A); (B) ER+ by IHC; (C) PR+; (D) HER21+; (E) Ki-67 proliferation index <10%; (F) Case 2: invasive ductal carcinoma with a non-specific pattern (luminal B); (G) ER+ by IHC; (H) PR+; (I) HER2 1+; (J) Ki-67 proliferation index >20%.

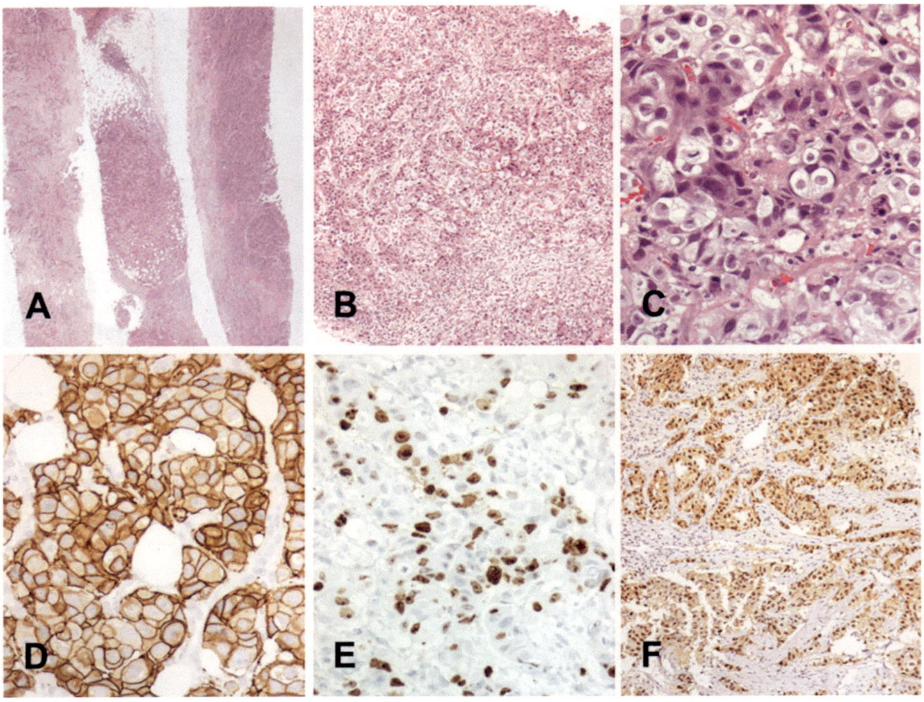

Figure 7.
Core-needle biopsy of BC: (A) Invasive ductal carcinoma with apocrine component; (B) High-grade solid growth pattern; (C) Neoplastic cells with nuclear pleomorphism and high mitotic index; (D) Her2 expression 3+; (E) Proliferation index with Ki-67 > 30%; (F) Positive for androgen receptor.

We may also observe discordance between the expression in the primary tumor and its metastases, as part of tumor heterogeneity [33]. Consequently, at the beginning of the evaluation of a patient with suspected BC, it is necessary to obtain serial biopsies guided by imaging to assess the BC phenotype, both in the primary tumor and in metastatic sites. They also enable the analysis of tumor heterogeneity in unifocal, multifocal, and/or bilateral cases through IHC, which aids in planning neoadjuvant therapy [34, 35].

The evaluation of other prognostic markers such as stage, multifocality, bilaterality, lymphovascular invasion, margin status, and identification of precursor lesions guides subsequent management and complements BC classification. The staging system used is the one from the American Joint Committee on Cancer (AJCC). This construct includes tumor size (T), regional lymph node status (N), and the presence of distant metastases (M) [36, 37].

6. Tumor heterogeneity and clonal evolution

Whole-genome and exome sequencing of human tumor samples has revealed the existence of an extensive intratumoral genetic heterogeneity [38–40]. This promotes the appearance of biologically more resistant subclones. In clonal evolution, subclones with greater growth capacity in a hostile microenvironment will survive and eventually expand, while less adapted subclones will die [41]. Studies in BC have shown that due to the early emergence of driver mutations and genetic alterations, genetic variations arise with the expansion of multiple subclones [42]. As a result, significant changes occur during breast cancer progression in the number and size of clones and in the emergence of new subclones within and between primary and secondary tumors [43]. Dominant clones of primary tumors do not necessarily contribute to the development of metastases, and it is important to distinguish those dependent on primary tumors but not yet forming metastases from true metastatic seed cells, indicating that therapeutic strategies should target selected subpopulations [44].

7. Cellular plasticity as a source of tumor heterogeneity

Genetic, epigenetic, transcriptomic, and proteomic features of a cell are not fixed determinants. The microenvironment also stimulates gene expression in cancer cells, which can transition from one phenotypic state to another through cellular plasticity. Cellular plasticity is the ability of cells to change their phenotype without genetic mutations in response to environmental signals. In pathological conditions such as BC, high reactivity to external and internal signals has been associated with increased cellular plasticity, which may contribute to cancer initiation, progression, and therapy resistance [45]. The epithelial-mesenchymal transition (EMT) and its reverse process, the mesenchymal-epithelial transition (MET), are fundamental processes of high cellular plasticity during embryonic development, tissue repair, and cancer progression [46]. Neoplastic cells during EMT acquire a mesenchymal, dedifferentiated phenotype with reduced cell adhesion, which enhances their ability to migrate, invade, and metastasize. This process has been associated with greater

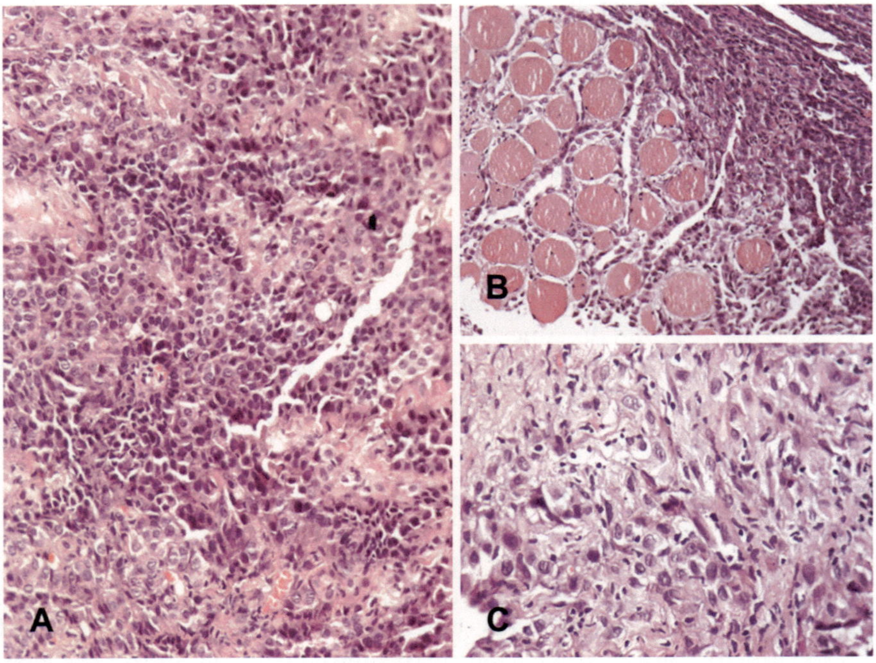

Figure 8.
Triple-negative breast cancer: (A) Tumor with solid high-grade growth pattern; (B) Skeletal muscle infiltration; (C) Neoplastic cells with epithelioid and fusiform appearance.

resistance to chemotherapy and immunotherapy [46, 47]. In fact, EMT is a process that can potentially be induced in different cell types and at various stages of differentiation. TNBC is the prototype of BC that exhibits changes similar to EMT, with a highly dedifferentiated mesenchymal phenotype, which contributes to increased chemotherapy resistance (**Figure 8**) [48].

Another source of heterogeneity lies in cancer stem cells (CSCs) with a high degree of cellular plasticity. CSCs are subpopulations of cancer cells that share characteristics with normal stem cells, such as self-renewal and multi-lineage differentiation capacities, which promote tumor growth, progression, and heterogeneity. Evidence suggests that EMT is related to the generation of CSCs in BC [49].

8. Genomic analysis

Genomic analysis is an important tool for analyzing tumor heterogeneity. In situ hybridization (ISH) is a technique used to detect alterations in gene copy numbers by identifying a specific DNA sequence using labeled probes [50]. The importance of HER2 status in breast cancer treatment has led to the development of molecular tests that allow for a high degree of certainty in evaluating HER2 amplification status. Fluorescence in situ hybridization (FISH) assay is the gold standard for assessing HER2 gene status in BC patients [51]. It also allows the identification of heterogeneity in gene copy numbers and gene distribution. Moreover, the development of the multicolor FISH (mFISH) assay enables the simultaneous detection of intertumoral and intratumoral heterogeneity in multiple genes [52]. Another test is Silver-enhanced in situ hybridization (SISH), which is a rapid and automated assay that

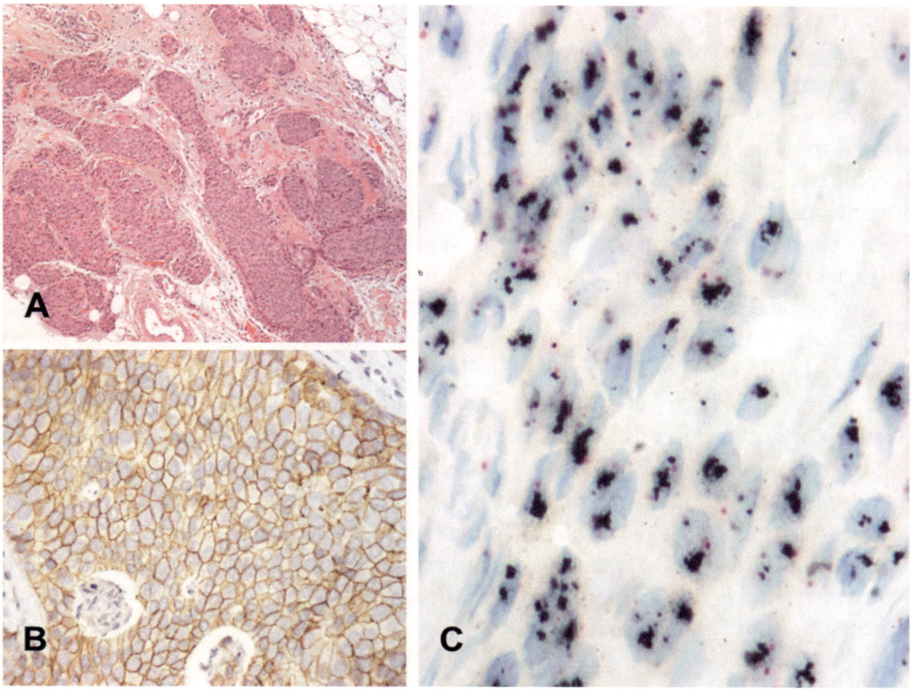

Figure 9.
Breast biopsies: (A) High-grade invasive ductal carcinoma; (B) By IHC HER2 2+ (indeterminate); (C) Silver-enhanced in situ hybridization (SISH): At high magnification, the centromeres of chromosome 17 (red-chromogen) and the HER2 gene (black-silver) are recognized in the nuclei of neoplastic cells with cluster formation (amplified case) (1000X).

provides permanently stained tissue mounted on slides, allowing for evaluation under a conventional light microscope by a pathologist (**Figure 9**) [53].

DNA microarrays, also known as DNA chips or biochips, and the 21-gene expression assay are two molecular tests useful for identifying heterogeneity in patients with BC. A DNA microarray contains thousands of microscopic DNA spots that allow the measurement of gene expression and DNA genotype. It is based on the DNA's ability to find and bind reversibly and specifically to its complementary sequence [54]. The technique can simultaneously measure the expression levels of thousands of genes and identify genes expressed differentially among different cancer patients [55]. In this regard, Perou et al. [30] used DNA microarrays on BC patient samples to stratify patients into five groups: luminal A, luminal B, HER2-enriched, claudin-low, and basal. These tests can also be used to predict response to chemotherapy and the risk of recurrence by analyzing genes associated with resistance and recurrence [56].

9. Clonal selection and resistance

The use of targeted therapies can generate new mutations in metastatic cells that are associated with disease progression and recurrence. In BC, there are several examples of clonal selection and resistance. Through DNA sequencing of individual cells from TNBC, before and after neoadjuvant chemotherapy, it has been observed that resistance to neoadjuvant chemotherapy arises from pre-existing clonal selection [57]. On the other hand, in BC, expressing hormonal receptors, endocrine therapy remains the core of treatment in both early and advanced stages. Approximately 30% of BC patients treated with tamoxifen become refractory to treatment within 2 to 5 years or develop drug resistance during treatment [58]. Point mutations in the *ESR1* gene, which encodes for ER-α, particularly acquired mutations in the ligand-binding domain of *ESR1*, represent one of the main mechanisms of resistance to endocrine therapy [59]. The identification of *ESR1* mutations can be performed using a conventional biopsy of the primary tumor. However, this is an invasive method, and also, mutations are less likely to be present in the initial tumor. Currently, the identification of *ESR1* mutations during follow-up can be done using liquid biopsy, based on the analysis of circulating free DNA in plasma [60]. Additionally, epigenetic regulation through hypermethylation of cytosine-guanine (CpG) dinucleotides in the *ESR1* gene is associated with decreased or loss of ER-α expression and consequently with acquired resistance [59]. Another way to acquire resistance to specific drugs is through the activation of alternative signaling pathways [61]. One mechanism of action of trastuzumab and T-DM1 is the inhibition of the PI3K signaling pathway. In that sense, mutations in PIK3CA and PTEN can contribute to the acquisition of resistance to these agents [61]. In addition, overexpression and heterodimerization of EGFR, HER3, HER4, IGF-1R, and MET can confer resistance to anti-HER2 therapies by restoring the original downstream signaling pathways activated by HER2 overexpression and amplification [62].

10. Epigenetic modifications

In addition to genetic heterogeneity, tumors can present epigenetic changes. Epigenetic modulation plays a role in the regulation of gene expression during tumorigenesis [63]. It does so through promoter gene methylation, global hypomethylation, and histone methylation and deacetylation. This results in a selective effect on certain clones, leading to specific outcomes such as the inactivation of tumor suppressor genes. Moreover, epigenetic heterogeneity allows for the development of cellular subpopulations that are tolerant to cytotoxic and targeted therapies. In the case of basal-like BC, it has been observed that after treatment with the MEK inhibitor (Trametinib) and the PI3K/mTOR inhibitor (BEZ235), neoplastic cells persist [64]. Additionally, it has been found that genes involved in the SWI/SNF chromatin remodeling complex (ARID1A, ARID1B, and ARID2) are mutated in metastatic recurrences of BC resistant to treatment [65]. These observations suggest that epigenetic changes can create drug-tolerant states that allow the survival of small subpopulations that would otherwise be sensitive to treatment. For this reason, drugs targeting epigenetic enzymes can reduce intratumoral cellular heterogeneity and reverse treatment resistance when combined with chemotherapy or targeted therapies.

11. Tumor microenvironment

The tumor microenvironment (TME) refers to the space in which tumor cells coexist with the stroma, blood vessels, immune cells, fibroblasts, and the extracellular matrix. The TME is crucial for regulating tumor growth, progression, and metastasis development and plays a role in resistance to targeted therapy. The TME participates in intratumoral heterogeneity by favoring the growth of specific subclones that are better adapted. This selection process involves hypoxia, inflammation, and a fibrotic state [18]. Hypoxia activates a set of adaptive transcriptional responses that enable neoplastic cells to survive in a hostile microenvironment and activate drug resistance genes. In addition, stromal and inflammatory cells release pro-inflammatory cytokines that induce epigenetic modifications [18].

Tumorigenesis is a complex process involving dynamic interactions between neoplastic cells and the stroma. Fibroblasts are the main component of the stroma (**Figure 10A**). Normal fibroblasts can have suppressive functions against neoplastic cells through direct cell contact, paracrine signaling of soluble factors, and the integrity of the ECM. Nonetheless, during tumor progression, neoplastic cells induce a change in normal fibroblasts to cancer-associated fibroblasts (CAFs), causing them to lose their suppressive functions [66]. CAFs have high plasticity and ability to remodel the tumor microenvironment. CAFs are a heterogeneous population; they play an important role in tumor growth, invasion, metastasis, and resistance to therapy. Besides, they can communicate with immune cells, helping neoplastic cells evade immune detection. Four subtypes of CAFs have been identified in BC. The CAF-S1 subtype is present in TNBC with an immunosuppressive function [67].

The presence of tumor-infiltrating lymphocytes (TILs) is associated with a favorable prognosis in BC (**Figure 10B**) [68, 69]. Nonetheless, there is heterogeneity in the composition of the subset, the functional state, and the spatial location of immune cells within the tumor [70]. Tumors with low inflammatory infiltration are considered "cold" tumors. In mixed tumors, a combination of inflammatory cells and neoplastic cells can be observed. Nevertheless, in compartmentalized tumors, inflammatory cells and neoplastic cells are found separately [71]. Approximately 70% of BC cases have TILs [72, 73]. These TILs, along with macrophages and fibroblasts, express PD-L1 at a high percentage, whereas PD-L1 expression is much lower in neoplastic cells [74]. This expression pattern involves PD-1/PD-L1 signaling between tumor cells and immune cells, which is important for the action of antibodies targeting PD-1/PD-L1 (**Figure 10C**) [75]. Recently, several transcriptomic signatures associated with immune infiltrates in BC have been described and seem to be useful in predicting a favorable outcome in TNBC after neoadjuvant therapy [76, 77].

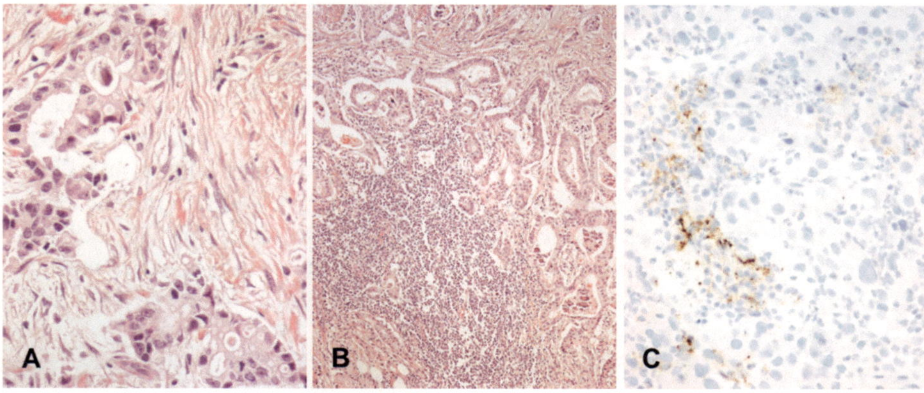

Figure 10.
Tumor microenvironment and immune system: (A) Fibroblasts are part of the stroma, in close contact with neoplastic cells; (B) Presence of tumor-infiltrating lymphocytes (TILs) among the neoplastic cells. (C) Expression of PD-L1 in intratumoral lymphocytes by IHC (Clone SP 142 Assay). PD-L1 is an emerging biomarker for breast cancer immunotherapy.

There are differences between the TME of the primary tumor and its metastases [78]. One difference is that metastatic neoplastic cells can negatively regulate the immune response, evading immune surveillance [79]. Additionally, the presence of TILs and PD-L1 expression is substantially lower in metastases, affecting the response to immune checkpoint inhibition with anti-PD1/PD-L1 antibodies [79]. Tumors lacking inflammatory response and an immunosuppressive microenvironment are significant obstacles to therapy with checkpoint inhibitors. Tumors with low mutational burden and low immunogenicity may be resistant to immunotherapy [18].

12. Heterogeneity and precision medicine

Driver molecular alterations promote tumor generation and progression. The response to a therapeutic agent depends on genetic heterogeneity within the primary tumor and between the primary tumor and its metastases. The presence of a different clone lacking the driver gene mutation will promote resistance. There are approximately 40 to 60 recurrent driver alterations in BC [80]. In advanced BC, the presence of alterations in *ERBB2, PIK3CA, AKT1, ESR1*, and *NTRK* genes helps to stratify patients for targeted therapies [81]. These genetic abnormalities have been classified into six levels based on the level of clinical benefit observed from treating specific alterations [82]. Level 1 is considered when targeted therapy provides clinical benefit based on better outcomes observed in clinical trials [80]. Therefore, these patients should have access to targeted therapy as a standard of care. Level 1 includes *ERBB2* amplification, *BRCA1/2* germline mutations, *PIK3CA* mutations, *NTRK* translocations, and microsatellite instability (MSI) [80].

13. Conclusions and perspectives

Pathological analysis plays an important role in diagnosis. However, BC is characterized by a notable degree of morphological heterogeneity. Therefore, it is important to correlate with IHC markers and molecular tests. This analysis provides a deeper understanding of BC heterogeneity and allows the identification of subgroups of patients with different treatment responses. There is a wide range of sources of biological heterogeneity in BC, including the formation of subclones with different biological capacities, tumor plasticity, clonal selection, epigenetic modifications, and the microenvironment, all of which contribute to progression and resistance to therapy. Therefore, a multidisciplinary approach is important to improve therapy and outcomes in breast cancer. It is probable that in the future, BC patients will be treated with combination therapy involving several drugs aimed at targeting different oncogenic drivers present in various populations of tumor cells. In addition, these therapies could be combined with others, such as those that enhance immune responses against tumors. There is still much work to be done to achieve personalized treatment for each patient.

Acknowledgements

The authors would like to thank Dr. Maria del Carmen Lara Tamburrino and Dr. Nadia Millan Sanchez from the Breast Unit of the CT Scanner Group, San Angel®,

We also thank Jean Michelle Martínez Nava from molecular biology area of Pathology Department, Oncology Hospital CMN Siglo XXI, Mexico City, Mexico, for sharing PD-L1 immunohistochemistry samples for illustration.

Author details

Fernando Candanedo-Gonzalez[1,2]*, Ana Lilia Remirez-Castellanos[3], Ursula Salazar-Gomez[1,4], Wilfredo Valenzuela-Gonzalez[5], Cindy Chavira-Macias[1] and Armando Gamboa-Dominguez[6]

1 Department of Pathology, Instituto Nacional de Ciencias Medicas y Nutricion Salvador Zubiran (INCMNSZ), Mexico City, Mexico

2 Department of Pathology, UMAE Hospital de Oncologia CMN Siglo XXI, IMSS, Mexico City, Mexico

3 Department of Radiology, UMAE Hospital de Oncologia, Centro Medico Nacional Siglo XXI, IMSS, Mexico City, Mexico

4 Social Service in Research, Department of Pathology, INCMNSZ, Mexico City, Mexico

5 Faculty of Medicine, Universidad Autonoma de Sinaloa, Sinaloa, Mexico

6 Chief of the Department of Pathology, INCMNSZ, Mexico City, Mexico

*Address all correspondence to: fa_candanedo@yahoo.com.mx

References

[1] Biswas SK, Banerjee S, Baker GW, Kuo CY, Chowdhury I. The mammary gland: Basic structure and molecular signaling during development. International Journal of Molecular Sciences. 2022;**23**(7):2883

[2] Candanedo GF, Pérez SE. The role of progesterone in breast cancer. GAMO. 2012;**11**(3):182-188

[3] Candanedo GF, Galindo HO, Serna MN, Espinosa NR, Soto GA, Cortes RP, et al. Progesterone induces NF B DNA binding activity through a PI3K/Akt-dependent pathway in MCF-7 breast cancer cells. Journal of Cancer Research. 2014;**2**(4):63-69

[4] Haslam SZ, Countermand LJ, Nummy KA. Effects of epidermal growth factor, estrogen, and progestin of DNA synthesis in mammary cells in vivo are determined by the developmental state of gland. Journal of Cellular Physiology. 1993;**155**(1):72-78

[5] Polyak K, Hu M. Do myoepithelial cells hold the key for breast tumor progression? Journal of Mammary Gland Biology and Neoplasia. 2005;**10**(3):231-247

[6] Schnitt SJ. The transition from ductal carcinoma in situ to invasive breast cancer: The other side of the coin. Breast Cancer Research. 2009;**11**(1):1-2

[7] Russo J, Russo IH. Breast development, hormones and cancer. Advances in Experimental Medicine and Biology. 2008;**630**:52-56

[8] Siegel RL, Miller KD, Fuchs HE, Jemal A. Cancer statistics, 2021. CA: a Cancer Journal for Clinicians. 2022;**72**(1):7-33

[9] Yi M, Li T, Niu M, Luo S, Chu Q, Wu K. Epidemiological trends of women's cancer from 1990 to 2019 at the global, regional, and national levels: A population-based study. Biomarker Research. 2021;**9**(1):55

[10] Romero UA, Osuna RJF, Candanedo GF, Ramirez ZMG, Peñuelas JE. Cáncer de mama: Entidad patológica de biología heterogénea. Archivos de Salud de Sinaloa. 2014;**8**(3):109-116

[11] Reiter JG, Baretti M, Gerold JM, Mahon MAP, Lacobuzio DA, Donahue CA, et al. An analysis of genetic heterogeneity in untreated cancers. Nature Reviews. Cancer. 2019;**19**(11):639-650

[12] Vogels B, Papadopoulos N, Velculescu VE, Zhou S, Diaz LA, Kinzler KW. Cancer genome landscapes. Science. 2013;**339**(6127):1546-1558

[13] Dagogo JI, Shaw AT. Tumor heterogeneity and resistance to cancer therapies. Nature Reviews. Clinical Oncology. 2018;**15**(2):81-94

[14] Ellsworth RE, Blackburn HL, Shriver CD, Soon SP, Ellsworth DL. Molecular heterogeneity in breast cancer: State of the science and implications for patient care. Seminars in Cell and Developmental Biology. 2016;**64**:65-72

[15] Fumagalli C, Barberis M. Breast cancer heterogeneity. Diagnostics (Basel). 2021;**11**(9):1555

[16] Guo L, Kong D, Liu J, Zhan L, Luo L, Zheng W, et al. Breast cancer heterogeneity and its implications in personalized precision therapy.

Experimental Hematology & Oncology. 2023;**12**:3

[17] Luond F, Tiede SCG. Breast cancer as an example of tumour heterogeneity and tumour cell plasticity during malignant prEllsworthogression. British Journal of Cancer. 2021;**125**(2):164-175

[18] Baliu PM, Pandiella A, Ocana A. Breast cancer heterogeneity and response to novel therapeutics. Cancers (Basel). 2020;**12**(11):3271

[19] Annaratone L, Cascardi E, Vissio E, Sarotto I, Chmielik E, Sapino A, et al. The multifaceted nature of tumor microenvironment in breast carcinomas. Pathobiology. 2020;**87**(2):125-142

[20] Son JL, Chen C, Yuan JP, Sun SR. Progress in the clinical detection of heterogeneity in breast cancer. Cancer Medicine. 2016;**5**(12):3475-3488

[21] Lee SH, Moon WK, Cho N, Chang JM, Moon HG, Han W, et al. Shear-wave elastographic features of breast cancers: Comparison with mechanical elasticity and histopathologic characteristics. Investigative Radiology. 2014;**49**(3):147-155

[22] Evans A, Sim YT, Thompson SK, Jordan L, Purdie C, Vinnicombe SJ. Shear wave elastography of breast cancer: Sensitivity according to histological type in a large cohort. Breast. 2016;**26**:115-118

[23] Moy L, Elias K, Patel V, Lee J, Babb JS, Toth HK. Is breast MRI helpful in the evaluation of inconclusive mammographic findings? AJR. American Journal of Roentgenology. 2009;**193**(4):986-993

[24] Vriens D, Disselhorst JA, Oyen WJG, Geus-Oei LF, Visser EP. Quantitative assessment of heterogeneity in tumor metabolism using FDG-PET. International Journal of Radiation Oncology, Biology, Physics. 2012;**82**(5):e725-e731

[25] Willaime JM, Turkheimer FE, Kenny LM, Aboagye EO. Quantification of intra- tumour cell proliferation heterogeneity using imaging descriptors of 18F fluorothymidine-positron emission tomography. Physics in Medicine and Biology. 2013;**58**(2):187-203

[26] Kenny L. The use of novel PET tracers to image breast cancer biologic processes such as proliferation, DNA damage and repair, and angiogenesis. Journal of Nuclear Medicine. Feb 2016;**57**(Suppl. 1):89S-95S

[27] Rakha EA, Reis-Filho JS, Boehner F, Dabbs DJ, Decker T, Eusebi V, et al. Breast cancer prognostic classification in the molecular era: The role of histological grade. Breast Cancer Research. 2010;**12**(4):207

[28] Aleskandarany MA, Vandenbergue ME, Marchio C, Ellis IO, Sapino A, Rakha EA. Tumours heterogeneity of breast cancer: From morphology to perzonalized medicine. Pathobiology. 2018;**85**(1-2):23-34

[29] Leong ASY, Zhuang Z. The changing role of pathology in breast cancer diagnosis and treatment. Pathobiology. 2011;**78**(2):99-114

[30] Perou CM, Sorlie T, Elsen MB, Rijn MV, Jeffrey SS, Rees CA, et al. Molecular portraits of human breast tumors. Nature. 2000;**406**(6796):747-752

[31] Candanedo GF, Cordova JC, Smeke SJ, Valenzuela GW, Gamboa DA. Agreement between incisional and excisional biopsies for hormone receptors and her2 in breast cancer. Cirugia y Cirujanos. 2023;**91**(4):451-456

[32] Hou YH, Nitta H, Li Z. HER2 intratumoral heterogeneity in breast cancer, an evolving concept. Cancers (Basel). 2023;**15**(10):2664

[33] Liang Y, Zhang H, Song X, Yang Q. Metastatic heterogeneity of breast cancer: Molecular mechanisms and potential therapeutic targets. Seminars in Cancer Biology. 2020;**60**:14-27

[34] Li A, Keck JM, Parmar S, Patterson J, Labrie M, Creason AL, et al. Characterizing advanced breast cancer heterogeneity and treatment resistance through serial biopsies and comprehensive analytics. npj Precision Oncology. 2021;**5**(1):28

[35] Remírez CAL, Herrera KJ, Quintana CM, Candanedo GF. Image features in correlation with biopsy in diabetic mastopathy associated with diabetes type 2. Revista Médica del Instituto Mexicano del Seguro Social. 2018;**56**(3):323-328

[36] Giuliano AE, Edge SB, Hortobagyi GN. Eight editions of the AJCC cancer staging manual: Breast cancer. Annals of Surgical Oncology. 2018;**25**(7):1783-1785

[37] Corso G, Magnoni F, Provenzano E, Girardi A, Iorfida M, De Scalzi AM, et al. Future Oncology. 2020;**16**(8):395-412

[38] Ellis MJ, Perou CM. The genomic landscape of breast cancer as a therapeutic roadmap. Cancer Discovery. 2013;**3**(1):27-34

[39] Shah SP, Roth A, Goya R, Oloumi A, Ha G, Zhao Y. The clonal and mutational evolution spectrum of primary triple-negative breast cancers. Nature. 2012;**486**(7403):395-399

[40] Banerji S, Cibulski K, Rangel-Escareno C, Brown KK, Carter SL, Frederick AM, et al. Sequence analysis of mutations and translocations across breast cancer subtypes. Nature. 2012;**486**(7403):405-409

[41] Nowell PC. The clonal evolution of tumor cell populations. Science. 1976;**194**(4260):23-28

[42] Nik-Zainal S, Alexandrov LB, Wedge DC, Loo PV, Greenman CD, Raine K, et al. Mutational process molding the genomes of 21 breast cancers. Breast cancer Workin Group of the International Cancer Genome Consortium. Cell. 2012;**149**(5):979-993

[43] Nguyen LV, Cox CL, Eirew P, Knapp DJ, Pellacani D, Kannan N, et al. DNA serially passaged xenografts. Nature Communications. 2014;**5**(5871):5871

[44] Merino D, Weber TS, Serrano A, Vaillant F, Liu K, Pal B, et al. Barcoding reveals complex clonal behavior in patient-derived xenografts of metastatic triple negative breast cancer. Nature Communications. 2019;**10**(1):766

[45] Gupta PB, Pastushenko I, Skibinski A, Blanpain C, Kuperwasser C. Phenotypic plasticity: Driver of cancer initiation, progression, and therapy resistance. Cell Stem Cell. 2019;**24**(1):65-78

[46] Nieto MA, Huang RY, Jackson RA, Thiery JP. EMT:2016. Cell. 2016;**166**(1):21-45

[47] Yan J, Antin P, Berx G, Blanpain C, Brabletz T, Bronner M, et al. Guidelines and definitions for research on epithelial-mesenchymal transition. Nature Reviews. Molecular Cell Biology. 2020;**21**(6):341-352

[48] Lawson DA, Bhakta NR, Kessenbrock K, Prummel KD, Yu Y, Taki K, et al. Single-cell analysis

reveals a stem-cell program in human metastatic breast cancer cells. Nature. 2015;**526**(7571):131-135

[49] Ye X, Tam WL, Shibue T, Kaygusuz Y, Reinhardt F, Eaton EN, et al. Distinct EMT programs control normal mammary stem cells and tumour- initiating cells. Nature. 2015;**525**(7568):256-260

[50] Lambros MBK, Natrajan R, Reis-Filho JS. Chromogenic and fluorescent in situ hybridization in breast cancer. Human Pathology. 2007;**38**(8):1105-1122

[51] Horii R, Matsuura M, Iwase T, Ito Y, Akiyama F. Comparison of dual-color in- situ hybridization and fluorescence in-situ hybridization in HER2 gene amplification in breast cancer. Breast Cancer. 2014;**21**(5):598-604

[52] Li C, Bai J, Hao X, Zhang S, Hu Y, Zhang X, et al. Multi-gene fluorescence in situ hybridization to detect cell cycle gene copy number aberrations in young breast cancer patients. Cell Cycle. 2014;**13**(8):1299-1305

[53] Papouchado BG, Myles J, Lloyd RV, Stoler M, Oliveira AM, Downs-Kelly E, et al. Silver in situ hybridization (SISH) for determination of HER2 gene status in breast carcinoma. Comparison with FISH and assessment of interobserver reproducibility. The American Journal of Surgical Pathology. 2010;**34**(6):767-776

[54] Schena M, Shalon D, Davis RW, Brown PO. Quantitative monitoring of gene expression patterns with a complementary DNA microarray. Science. 1995;**270**(5235):467-470

[55] Wu X, Zahari MS, Renuse S, Jacob HK, Sakamuri S, Signal M, et al. A breast cancer cell microarray (CMA) as a rapid method to characterize candidate biomarkers. Cancer Biology & Therapy. 2014;**15**(12):1593-1599

[56] Korde LA, Lusa L, McShane L, Lebowitz PF, Lukes L, Camphausen K, et al. Gene expression pathways analysis to predict response to neoadjuvant docetaxel and capecitabine for breast cancer. Breast Cancer Research and Treatment. 2010;**119**(3):685-699

[57] Kim C, Gao R, Sei E, Brandt R, Hartman J, Hatschek T, et al. Chemoresistance evolution in triple-negative breast cancer delineated by single-cell sequencing. Cell. 2018;**173**(4):879-893.e13

[58] Roggins RB, Schrecengost RS, Guerrero MS, Bouton AH. Pathways to tamoxifen resistance. Cancer Letters. 2007;**256**(1):1-24

[59] Fan W, Chang J, Fu P. Endocrine therapy resistance in breast cancer: Current status, possible mechanisms and overcoming strategies. Future Medicinal Chemistry. 2015;**7**(12):1511-1519

[60] Betz M, Massard V, Gilson P, Witz A, Dardare J, Harlé A. *ESR*1 gene mutations and liquid biopsy in ER-positive breast cancers: as, all step forward, a giant leap for personalization of endocrine therapy? Cancers (Basel). 2023;**15**(21):5169

[61] Pagliarini R, Shao W, Sellers WR. Oncogene addiction: Pathways of therapeutic response, resistance, and road maps toward a cure. EMBO Reports. 2015;**16**(3):280-296

[62] Chandarlapaty S, Sakr RA, Giri D, Patil S, Heguy A, Morrow M, et al. Frequent mutational activation of the PI3K-AKT pathway in trastuzumab-resistant breast cancer. Clinical Cancer Research. 2012;**18**(24):6784-6791

[63] Feinberg AP. The key role of epigenetics in human disease prevention and mitigation. The New England Journal of Medicine. 2018;**378**(14):1323-1334

[64] Risom T, Langer EM, Chapman MP, Rantala J, Fields AJ, Boniface C, et al. Differentiation-state plasticity is a targetable resistance mechanism in basal-like breast cancer. Nature Communications. 2018;**9**(1):3815

[65] Yates LR, Knappskog S, Wedge D, Farmery JHR, Gonzalez S, Martincorena I, et al. Genomic evolution of breast cancer metastasis and relapse. Cancer Cell. 2017;**32**(2):169-184e7

[66] Alkasalias T, Moyano GL, Arsenian HM, Lehti K. Fibroblast in the tumor microenvironment: Shield or spear? International Journal of Molecular Sciences. 2018;**19**(5):1532

[67] Costa A, Kieffer Y, Scholer DA, Pelon F, Bourachot B, Cardon M, et al. Fibroblast heterogeneity and immunosuppressive environment in human breast cancer. Cancer Cell. 2018;**33**(3):463-479.e10

[68] Adams S, Gray RJ, DeMaria S, Goldstein L, Perez EA, Shulman LN, et al. Prognostic value of tumor-infiltrating lymphocytes in triple-negative breast cancers from two phase III randomized adjuvant breast cancer trials: ECOG 2197 and ECOG. Journal of Clinical Oncology. 2014;**32**(27):2959-2966

[69] Denkert C, Loibl S, Noske A, Roller M, Müller BM, Komor M, et al. Tumor-associated lymphocytes as an independent predictor of response to neoadjuvant chemotherapy in breast cancer. Journal of Clinical Oncology. 2010;**28**(1):105-113

[70] Gruosso T, Gigoux M, Manem VSK, Bertos N, Zuo D, Perlitch I, et al. Spatially distinct tumor immune microenvironments stratify triple-negative breast cancers. Journal of Clinical Investigation. 2019;**129**(4):1785-1800

[71] Keren L, Bose M, Marquez D, Angoshtari R, Jain S, Varma S, et al. A structured tumor-immune microenvironment in triple negative breast cancer revealed by multiplexed ion beam imaging. Cell. 2018;**174**(6):1373-1387.e19

[72] Pelekanou V, Barlow WE, Nahleh ZA, Wasserman B, Lo YC, Von WMK, et al. Tumor-infiltrating lymphocytes and PD-L1 expression in pre- and prosttreatment breast cancers in the SWOG S0800 phase II neoadjuvant chemotherapy trial. Molecular Cancer Therapeutics. 2018;**17**(6):1324-1331

[73] Li X, Warren S, Pelekanou V, Wali V, Cesano A, Liu M, et al. Immune profiling of pre- and post-treatment breast cancer tissues from the SWOG S0800 neoadjuvant trial. Journal for Immunotherapy of Cancer. 2019;**7**(1):88

[74] Cimino-Mathews A, Thompson E, Taube JM, Ye X, Lu Y, Meeker A, et al. PD-L1 (B7- H1) expression and the immune tumor microenvironment in primary and metastatic breast carcinomas. Human Pathology. 2016;**47**(1):52-63

[75] Tang F, Zheng P. Tumor cells versus host immune cells: Whose PD-L1 contributes to PD-1/PD-L1 blockade mediated cancer immunotherapy? Cell & Bioscience. 2018;**8**:34

[76] Noblejas-LMDM NJC, García SM, Pérez PJ, Nuncia CM, Andrés PF, Galán MEM, et al. Expression of MHC class I, HLA-A and HLA-B identifies immune-activated breast tumors with favorable outcome. OncoImmunology. 2019;**8**(10):e1629780

[77] Pérez PJ, Fekete JT, Páez R, Baliu PM, García SJA, García BV, et al. A transcriptomic immunologic signature predicts favorable outcome in

neoadjuvant chemotherapy treat triple negative breast tumors. Frontiers in Immunology. 2019;**10**:2802

[78] Comen EA. Tracking the seed and tending the soil: Evolving concepts in metastatic breast cancer. Discovery Medicine. 2012;**14**(75):97-104

[79] Szekely B, Bossuyt V, Li X, Wali VB, Patwardhan GA, Frederick C, et al. Immunological differences between primary and metastatic breast cancer. Annals of Oncology. 2018;**29**(11):2232-2239

[80] Condorelli R, Mosele F, Verret B, Bachelot T, Bedard PL, Cortes J, et al. Genomic alterations in breast cancer: Level of evidence for actionability according to ESMO scale for clinical actionability of molecular targets (ESCAT). Annals of Oncology. 2019;**30**(3):365-373

[81] Kratz J, Burkard M, O'Meara T, Pusztai L, Veitch Z, Bedard PL. Incorporating genomics into the care of patients with advanced breast cancer. American Society of Clinical Oncology Educational Book. 2018;**38**:56-64

[82] Mateo J, Chakravarty D, Dienstmann R, Jezdic S, Gonzalez PA, Lopez BN, et al. A framework to rank genomic alterations as targets for cancer precision medicine: The ESMO scale for clinical actionability of molecular targets (ESCAT). Annals of Oncology. 2018;**29**(9):1895-1902

Chapter 3

The Role of Estrogen Receptors and Signaling Pathways in Breast Cancer

Arya Rajesh, Evan Easley, Chikezie O. Madu and Yi Lu

Abstract

Breast cancer is the leading cancer found in females today. Although breast cancer can be broken down into various subtypes, the most prominent type is hormone receptor (HR) breast cancer. Hormones especially effective in females, such as progesterone and estrogen, may stimulate cancer cell proliferation. The four main breast cancer subtypes are HR+/HER2-, HR-/HER2+/−, HR-/HER2+, and HR-/HER2-, each characterized by the presence or absence of certain hormone receptors. HR breast cancers, due to high levels of progesterone and estrogen that promote cell proliferation and human epidermal growth factor receptors, grow by controlling gene transcription, cell division, and migration. Estrogen, a sex hormone primarily found in the female ovaries, binds to its associated receptors throughout the menstrual cycle and pregnancy. Various genes encode estrogen receptors, which regulate the expression of their respective genes. Estrogen causes ER-positive breast cancer growth via the continual binding of the hormone to cancer cell receptors. Conversely, ER-negative breast cancers are tumors that form due to the depletion of estrogen receptors from cancer cells. These cancers are regulated by two receptor types: ERα and ERβ. Recent treatment includes endocrine therapy, surgery, and epigenetic therapy.

Keywords: estrogen, reception, breast cancer, signaling, cancer, endocrine therapy, progesterone signaling

1. Introduction

Breast cancer is characterized by the formation of malignant cells in mammary epithelial tissue, and it is the most common cancer found in females [1]. Over the last three decades, breast cancer has become increasingly common [2]. Through the stimulation of carcinogenic factors, benign tumors and metastatic carcinomas may develop [3]. Carcinogenesis may occur as a result of epigenetic functions, genetic predispositions, and environmental factors such as certain lifestyles, including later pregnancies, a lack of physical activity, and inadequate diets [2, 3].

These factors can be categorized into non-modifiable and modifiable risk factors. Non-modifiable factors include sex, age, race, genetic mutations, and family history, while modifiable factors include alcoholism, smoking, exposure to dangerous chemicals, and insufficient vitamin supplements [2]. Breast cancer is often found in older women who have late menopause, lack breastfeeding, have a positive family history, or have dense breast tissue [1]. Additionally, genetic mutations that occur on BRCA1 on chromosome 17 and BRCA2 on chromosome 13 are linked to cancer progression [2].

Current treatment for breast cancer includes systemic endocrine treatment, immunotherapies, chemotherapy, and radiation [1]. A lumpectomy, the excision of the tumor from the breast, can be performed through breast-conserving therapy only if the patient can undergo radiotherapy, a treatment that uses radiation to reduce tumor growth and kill cancer cells [4]. Systemic chemotherapy is often recommended for high-risk patients to lower cancer growth [4].

2. Breast cancer diagnosis

Early diagnosis is the best prevention method for breast cancer, but tumors often metastasize and spread to other parts of the body, preventing such prompt diagnosis [3]. Current screenings and imaging allow a pathway to recognize early breast cancer [5]. Mammography, breast ultrasounds, and breast magnetic resonance imaging (MRI) are all procedures for detection [5]. Mammography is the most common screening method, and it allows for efficient, minimal technical setup diagnosis of breast cancer [5]. The simplicity of this method allows mammography to be used in several countries for early diagnosis [5]. Breast ultrasounds provide an enhanced screening of breast tissues, but the quality of screenings depends on the patient's breast size, tissue density, and exposure to previous radiation [5]. Breast MRIs offer the most accurate examination for breast cancer but are the most expensive option [5].

Following these examinations, areas with a lump, microcalcification, or swelling can be identified [5]. The presence of microcalcifications in mammograms is associated with premalignancy and malignancy, but pleomorphic and fine linear microcalcifications are especially associated with these outcomes [6]. Furthermore, they are associated with worse outcomes in eight-year survival rate, lymph node involvement, and tumor width [6].

Due to the multitude of causes and effects of breast cancer, various subtypes exist to categorize the broad area of breast cancer. Such subtypes include metrics such as tumor size, lymph node size, pathologic type, molecular subtype classification, and more recently, receptor status classification [7]. In many cases, microRNA (mRNA) gene expression levels determine molecular subtypes [2]. Receptor status classification considers the role of estrogen receptors, progesterone receptors, and human growth factor receptors (HER2) in breast cancer patients [7].

The recent usage of biosensors and biomarkers as an early detection tool has been extensively studied and is promising on account of their relatively low cost and efficiency [8]. Exosomes and various immune biomarkers have produced promising data for their potential usage in diagnosis and treatment, though full therapies have not yet been tested or developed [9, 10]. MicroRNA expression levels are affected in many cancers, leading to effects on disease progression, severity, and recovery; for these reasons, tracking microRNA levels as a biomarker may prove useful for early detection [11]. Novel apparati, such as that shown by Parchekani et al. [11], can detect microRNAs as biomarkers at a zeptomolar concentration. Furthermore, microwave imaging (MI) techniques have also proven highly promising, as some clinical trials using MI have been successful [8].

3. Hormone receptor breast cancers

Hormone receptor (HR-positive) breast cancer occurs when hormones—especially estrogen and progesterone—attach to their respective receptors and stimulate rapid cancer growth [12]. HR-positive breast cancer requires specific hormones for progression and occurs when cancer cells have embedded proteins that act as signaling molecules that bind to specific hormones [13]. This category of tumors constitutes over 70% of breast cancers [13, 14].

HR-negative breast cancer occurs when cancer cells grow without the presence of these hormones [15]. These cancer cells do not have specific receptors for estrogen, progesterone, or human epidermal growth factor receptor-2 for growth [15]. This cancer involves the absence or overexpression of progesterone, estrogen, and/or human epidermal growth factor receptor-2 in individuals diagnosed with this cancer [7]. Gran et al. have shown that patients with HR-negative tumors have a higher risk of mortality than those with HR-positive tumors [16, 17].

3.1 Mechanism of progesterone in HR breast cancer

Progesterone is an ovarian steroid hormone that plays a crucial role in the female menstrual cycle and pregnancy and is essential for normal breast development [18, 19]. Progesterone receptors (PR) are prevalent among HR-positive breast

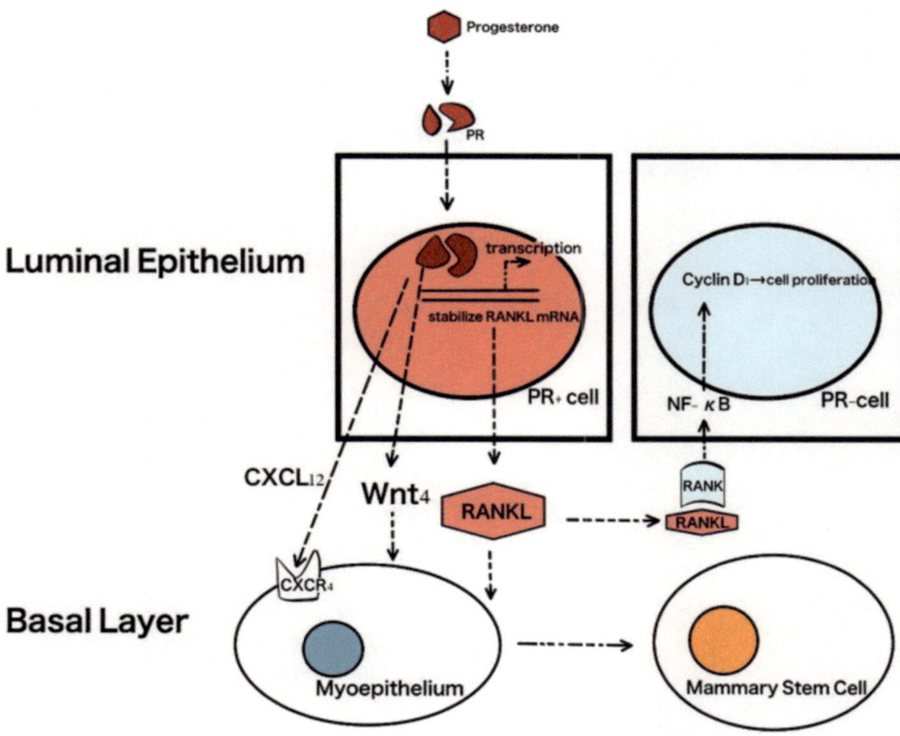

Figure 1.
Progesterone signaling pathway. The reception of progesterone leads to increased nuclear factor κB (NF-κB) ligand (RANKL) through the transcription or stabilization of RANKL mRNA; this increased RANKL leads to the increased proliferation of progesterone receptor-negative luminal cells (adapted from Ref. [19]).

cancers. As progestins, synthetic ligands, and progesterone bind to the PR, a signaling pathway is initiated (**Figure 1**) [18]. This binding initiates PR signaling and regulates gene transcription [20]. As ligands bind to PR in cancer cells, cancer cell proliferation increases. Increased exposure to progesterone increases the risk of breast cancer through the development of HR-negative tumors [19]. Endogenous progesterone, progesterone metabolites, and interactions with estradiol result in a 16% increase in the risk of breast cancer for postmenopausal females [21].

3.2 Role of estrogen in the body

Estrogen is a sex steroid hormone that plays a crucial role in the sexual and reproductive development of females and plays a minor role in male reproductive development [22]. It is essential in various other biological systems, including the vascular, skeletal, and immune systems [22]. Estrogen production in females occurs in the ovaries and may occur in other tissues via androgen synthesis (**Figure 2**) [24]. Estrogen in females can be found in various forms, such as estrone, estradiol,

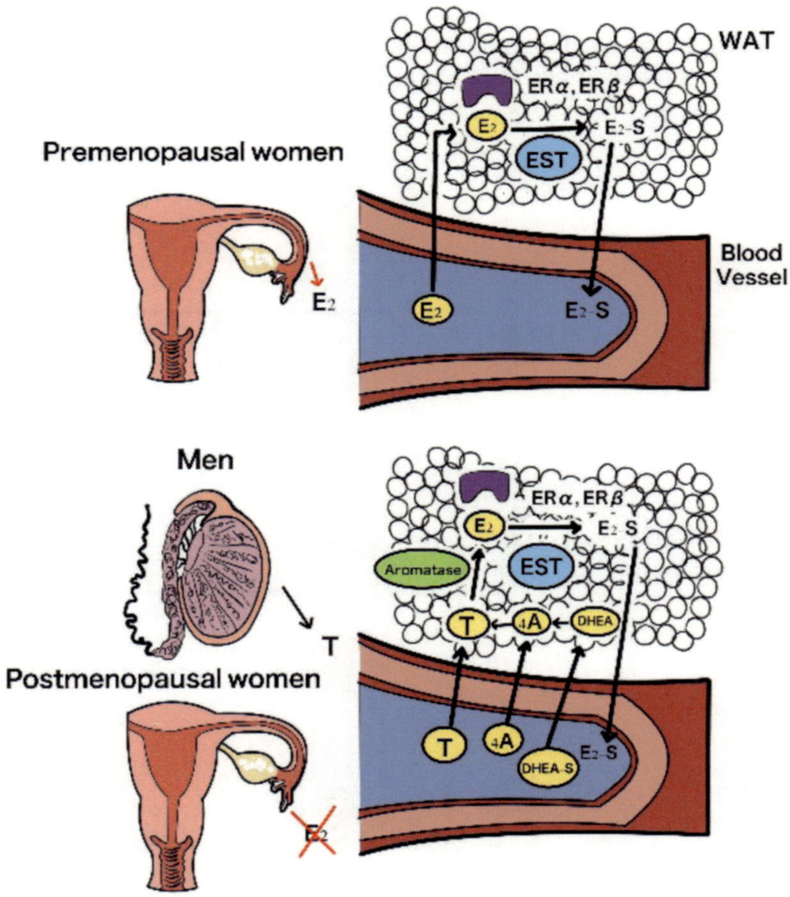

Figure 2.
Origin of circulating and tissue estrogens. In premenopausal women, estrogen is secreted directly from the ovaries. In postmenopausal women and in men, it is instead produced from androgenic precursors such as testosterone (adapted from Ref. [23]).

and estriol, with each molecule varying in structure and activity level throughout the female reproductive cycle [25]. These estrogens act as signaling molecules that bind to receptor molecules during different periods of the menstrual cycle and pregnancy [25].

In postmenopausal females, estradiol is not produced as abundantly due to the ovaries failing [23]. Instead, estradiol is produced in extragonadal sites, including the breasts, brain, muscles, bones, and adipose tissues [23]. In men, circulating estrogens are not produced; instead, biosynthesis occurs via circulating androgens [23]. This leads to the regulation of estrogen through tissue metabolism or inactivation of circulating estrogen, specifically through tissue estrogen sulfotransferase (EST). This enzyme prevents the binding of estrogen to their respective receptors [23].

4. Mechanism of HER2 in HR breast cancer

HR-positive breast cancer may also arise due to the upregulation of the human epidermal growth factor receptor (HER2), a membrane tyrosine kinase receptor [26, 27]. HER2 overexpression promotes cancer cell growth by promoting cell division, differentiation, and migration [28]. Phosphorylated tyrosine kinases activate HER2, leading to eventual cell cycle progression and proliferation [28]. The HER2 is part of a signaling pathway composed of three layers: membrane receptors and their ligands, protein kinases, and transcription factors (**Figure 3**) [29]. The first layer of receptors takes in the

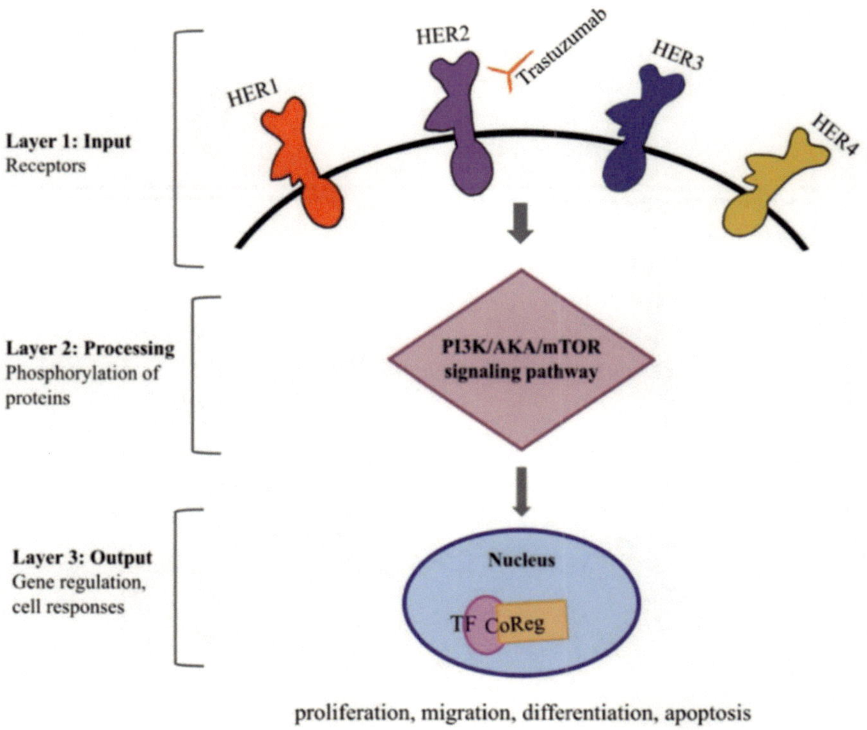

Figure 3.
HER2 signaling pathway. The pathway consists of three layers in order to regulate proliferation, migration, differentiation, apoptosis, and angiogenesis (adapted from Ref. [29]).

signal, the second layer involves the phosphorylation of protein kinases that transmit signals to the nucleus, and the final layer regulates genes for proper cellular function [29]. Although the input layer consists of four tyrosine kinases HER1–4, breast cancer research primarily focuses on the HER2 tyrosine kinase receptor [29].

HER2 overexpression occurs through HER2 amplification, which increases cell proliferation rates, lowers estrogen and progesterone levels, promotes aneuploidy, and causes resistance to endocrine therapy [28, 29]. Due to this resistance, HER2-targeted therapy controls the expression of growth factors [30]. Trastuzumab is a cancer drug developed to target HER2 protein kinases in the early stages of breast cancer by attaching to HER2 proteins to prevent cancer cell growth and proliferation (**Figure 3**) [29, 30].

Although HER2 and PRs in cancer cells can cause hormone receptor breast cancers, estrogen receptor signaling in cancer cells is the most prevalent cause of breast cancer. Impaired estrogen receptors and signaling are responsible for a high percentage of breast cancer cases [7].

5. Estrogen receptors and signaling

Estrogen receptors (ERs) are nuclear proteins found in cells that regulate the expression of specific genes [31]. Various genes encode these receptors, but they can be expressed in the same tissues [31]. Dimer formation is important for the function of estrogen receptors to regulate gene expression, as it is for many steroid hormones [32]. Circulating estrogen is regulated by two estrogen receptors: ERα and ERβ (**Figure 4**) [31]. These receptors can bind to agonist, agonist–antagonist, or full antagonist molecules [31].

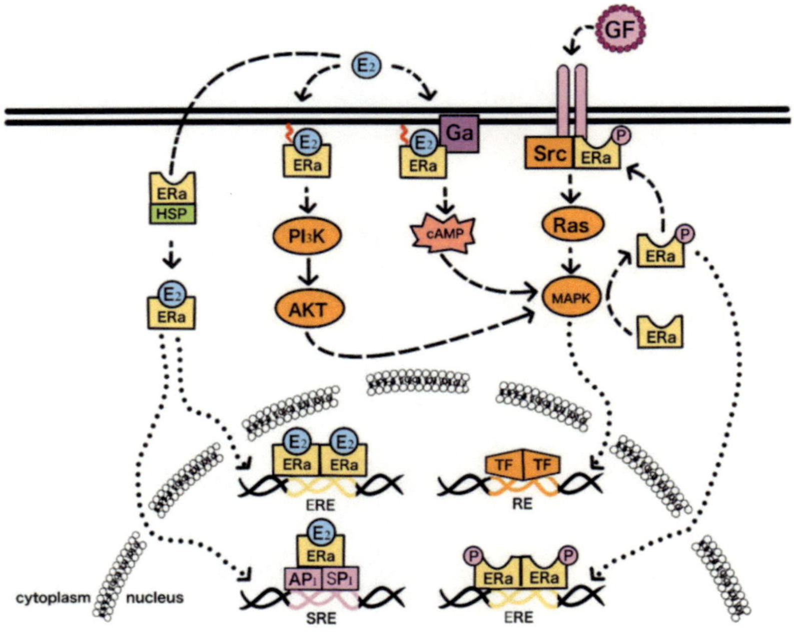

Figure 4.
ERα signaling pathway. The regulation of transcription of target genes is completed in the genomic activity of ERα, while the activation of transcription factors relating to cell proliferation and survival is done in the non-genomic activity of ERα (adapted from Ref. [33]).

Estrogen regularly binds to its receptors in breast cells; however, when cancer cells are present with the same receptors, estrogen binds to these proteins and causes rapid cancer growth in the affected individual [23]. ERs function as ligand-activated transcription factors; when the ligand attaches to the receptor, a conformational change occurs in the protein [34]. The resulting transcription factor is translocated to the nucleus, where it attaches to estrogen response elements—which are specific DNA sequences—to regulate the transcription of target genes [34]. Further, mutations may occur in the receptors that cause them to lose the ability for ligands to bind and thereby the ability for transcription to occur.

Estrogen receptors contain different distinct amino acid compositions that allow for specific 17β-estradiol [E2] signaling [35]. Estrogen receptor-ligand-binding domains (LBDs) are made up of a three-layer α-helical fold [35]. Estrogen receptors contain unstructured carboxyl-terminal extensions—an extra domain—to maintain their structure [35]. ERα LBDs have a helical arrangement of 12 helices that create a site for ligands to bind [35, 36]. The LBD domains in ERα allow for the regulation of transcription, coactivators, dimerization, and stability [35]. ERα also contains a globular LBD that holds hormone-binding and coregulator interaction sites [36]. E2, as a natural ligand, binds easily in a hydrophobic environment [36]. Such hydrophobic interactions between molecules and estrogen receptor helices allow for the formation of specific LBD structures, subsequently allowing estrogen to bind (**Figure 5**) [36, 37]. Synthetic ligands are currently being developed to overcome various diseases [37]. ERβ has a similar structure to an arbitrary coil, but little is known of the function [35].

Estrogen receptor-DNA binding domains (DBDs) are usually found central to estrogen receptors and provide the ability to bind to estrogen response elements (EREs) [35]. EREs are palindromic DNA sequences that allow estrogen receptors to bind as a transcriptional regulator [2]. Zinc finger domains regulate ERE interactions and dimerization in DBDs [36]. Three amino acids found in the zinc finger domains

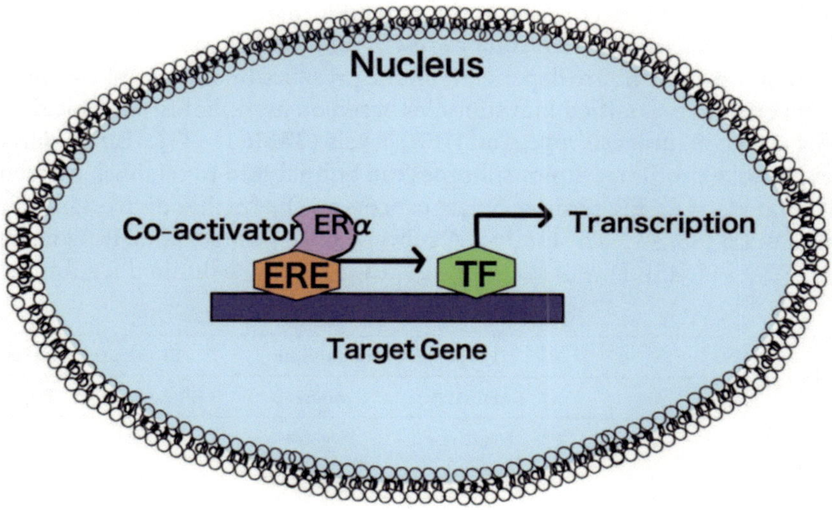

Figure 5.
17β-estradiol [E2] signaling. In this pathway, an ER bound to E2 interacts with a G-protein (GP) that results in kinase activation, further leading to co-regulatory proteins (CR) and transcription factors (TF) alongside the ER complex altering gene expression (adapted from Ref. [36]).

determine the interaction with EREs and the glucocorticoid response element (GRE) [36]. Depending on the amino acids, the transcriptional activity can be mediated by EREs or GREs [36].

Following reception and dimerization, the estrogen receptor complex translocates to the nucleus; though the specific mechanism through which this translocation occurs is currently unclear, the general transport of nuclear hormone receptors to the nucleus is facilitated by the interactions between nuclear localization signals with importins and microtubule-associated motor proteins [36].

Transcriptional activity of estrogen receptors occurs through the interactions between two activation function domains: AF1 and AFR2 [36]. AF1, located in the N-terminal domain, can function without the presence of a hormone, and AF2, located in the LBD, only functions in the presence of a hormone [36, 38]. In a study conducted using mice by Couse et al., ERαAF2 activity was observed, and the results suggested the essential role of AF2 in E2 transcriptional activity [38, 39].

G protein-coupled estrogen receptors (GPERs) are crucial to breast cancer progression, in which they bind to estrogens and other molecules; this binding results in the modulation of genes involved in cell proliferation, metastasis, apoptosis, and migration [40]. Specifically, G protein-coupled estrogen receptor 1 (GPER-1) in patients with triple-negative breast cancer is associated with shorter overall survival and relapse-free survival in premenopausal patients [40]. GPER-1 and ERβ facilitate estrogen responsivity in triple-negative breast cancer despite the lack of ERα expression [41]. Furthermore, measuring GPER expression or its cellular distribution may provide new avenues in diagnosis for ER or estrogen-related diseases [42].

6. Estrogen receptors in breast cancer

6.1 ER-positive and ER-negative breast cancers

ER-positive breast cancer is the most common form of breast cancer (**Table 1**) [33]. Estrogen acts as a signal for tumor growth [33]. ER breast cancers, also known as luminal breast cancers, are dependent on the presence or absence of estrogen [43]. Breast cancer can be classified into subtypes based on immunohistochemical staining regarding estrogen, progesterone, and HER2 levels (**Table 1**) [43]. Using microarray-based expression profiling, tumor subtypes can be analyzed to establish molecular classification [43, 44]. ER-positive breast cancers can be further divided into subtypes luminal A and B [43, 44]. The luminal A subtype is PR positive and HER2 negative (HR+/HER2-) [44, 45]. Due to lower proliferation rates, the luminal A subtype has a

	ER-positive breast cancer		ER-negative breast cancer	
	Luminal A	**Luminal B**	**ER-negative**	**Triple negative**
HER2	Negative	Negative	Positive	Negative
Hormone receptor	Positive	Positive/Negative	Negative	Negative
Proportion of breast cancer cases (%)	60	10	20	10

Table 1.
Breast cancer subtypes. Proportion of breast cancer cases organized into subtypes: Luminal A, Luminal B, HER2 positive, and triple negative (adapted from Ref [33]).

lower relapse rate after treatment; this lower relapse rate is indicated by low levels of Ki67, the proliferating cell nuclear antigen [44]. The luminal A subtype has high levels of ER and high expression of luminal epithelial cytokeratins 8 and 18, ER1 markers, and the LIV1, FOXA1, XBP1, GATA3, and BCL2 genes [44]. Furthermore, luminal-A breast cancer has a relatively low expression of genes associated with cell proliferation compared to its luminal-B counterpart, leading to such cancers being slow-growing and low-grade and to such cancers having the best prognosis [2]. Luminal B cancers are PR-negative and HER2-positive or negative (HR-/HER2+/−) [43–45]. The luminal B subtype has higher proliferation rates, indicating high levels of Ki67 [43]. This subtype has increased expression of the proliferation-related genes GGH, v-MYB, LAPTMB4, NSEP1, and CCNE1 [44].

There is evidence that androgen receptors (AR) play a role in the formation and proliferation of cancer cells [33]. In ER-positive breast cancer, AR can both stimulate and hinder the growth of cancer cells. AR has also been found to use Src protein kinase and PI3K—a pathway discussed later in this review—to promote the proliferation of ER-negative cancer cells [33].

ER-negative breast cancers are tumors that form due to the depletion of estrogen receptors from cancer cells [33]. Breast cancer grows rapidly in the absence of estrogen and thus there are fewer cancer prevention treatments for this disease, leading to patients diagnosed with ER-negative breast cancer generally having a lower chance of survival due to both this rapid growth and poor tumor differentiation [46]. Due to this, ER-negative breast cancer tumors are commonly identified at a young age [47]. Studies from Sharma et al. have shown that epigenetics—how environment and behavior affect and change a heritable phenotype but not DNA itself—may affect the onset of ER-negative breast cancer [46, 47]. Epigenetic factors include poor diet quality, which can stimulate stress through the low intake of fruits and vegetables as well as low intake of vitamins, decreasing DNA methylation [47].

ER-negative cases are commonly paired with PR expression [48]. For this reason, estrogen resistance can be classified into two categories: de novo and acquired [48]. De novo resistance occurs in the absence of both estrogen receptors and progesterone receptors in cells [48]. In these cases, the lack of estrogen in the body may be caused by long-term activation of growth factor signaling pathways that are no longer able to produce any signal at all or one that is sufficient to produce successive molecules [48]. On the other hand, acquired resistance occurs when there is initial estrogen responsiveness but later unresponsiveness [48]. Several drugs that attempt to battle the relapse of ER-positive breast cancer can unexpectedly cause ER-positive tumors to develop resistance to that drug and become ER-negative tumors [48].

HER2-positive cases occur when tumors are ER negative and PR negative but HER2 positive (HR-/HER2+) (**Table 1**) [33]. The HER2 receptors are overactive in these cases, causing cell proliferation through several signaling pathways such as PI3K/AKT, as described later in this review [33]. HER2 ER-negative breast cancers are more aggressive due to increased development of metastasis [33].

Triple-negative breast cancer (TNBC) is ER, PR, and HER2 negative (HR-/HER2-) [43–45, 49, 50]. Triple-negative breast cancer is usually basal subtype tumors that have an unfavorable prognosis [43]. These tumors are treated with chemotherapeutic agents due to difficulties with using a targeted drug for endocrine treatment [43]. Basal-like subtypes have higher rates of metastasis to the brain and lungs due to the growth of infiltrating ductal tumors [44]. Although most are established as basal-like through molecular classification, not all TNBCs are basal-like [43, 44].

Data shows that TNBC patients have larger tumor sizes, greater proliferation rates, and more aggressive metastasis than other breast cancers [50].

6.2 Estrogen receptor type: ERα

ERα is an estrogen receptor type found in the mammary epithelium [51]. ERα consists of an N-terminal domain, a DNA-binding domain, and a C-terminal ligand-binding region where the estrogen binds [51]. The C-terminal ligand-binding region consists of an antiparallel α-helical fold that maintains a ligand-binding cavity for the receptor [31]. The gene for this receptor is on q24-a27 of chromosome 6 [31]. ERα travels to the nucleus once estrogen is bound and regulates gene transcription of its associated genes [34]. Transcription may be disrupted by mutations in dimerization [31]. Specifically, ERα specializes in regulating the genes that control cell proliferation, differentiation, and migration [52]. ERα is modulated by extranuclear signaling, coregulators, post-translational modifications, and microRNA and can be affected by deregulated expressions of these factors [52]. This fragility makes the mammary epithelium easily susceptible to cancer cell development [52].

One example of a coactivator of ERα is CDKN1A-interacting zinc finger protein 1 (CIZ1), which responds to circulating estrogen [53]. CIZ1 is considered a coactivator rather than an oncoprotein because no mutations of CIZ1 have been found to cause cancer [54]. CIZ1 increases the expression of estrogen in target genes by binding to estrogen receptors in cancer cells [54]. The coactivator increases the activity of cyclin-dependent kinase 2 (CDK2) by binding to estrogen-induced protein DLC1 [54]. CDK2, in turn, causes the rapid growth of breast cancer cells [54]. Several coactivators and ERα activate transcription factors in the presence of estrogen on a target gene (Figure 6) [53].

Extracellular signals are transmitted through G-proteins that are linked to membrane ERα [55]. The deregulation of specific signaling pathways begets disorder in cell interactions and development, contributing to breast cancer in individuals [52]. In a study conducted by Manavathi et al. [53] to determine the role of ERα, deletion of this receptor causes the ductal system to fail to expand in mice due to the lack of regulation of circulating estrogen in their systems. After the maturation of the mice, however, there was little to no mammary gland development in female mice [53]. ERα interaction with target genes may occur through estrogen response elements or DNA transcription factors [53]. A receptor may either positively or negatively mediate target gene transcription [53].

Extranuclear signaling occurs through ERα activation by circulating estrogen, which causes rapid cytoskeletal reorganization and the development of filopodia and ruffles in motile cells [56]. ERα extranuclear signaling affects breast cancer motility as it promotes the stimulation of Src kinase, mitogen-activated protein kinase, phosphatidylinositol 3-kinase (PI3K), and protein kinase C [56]. Breast cancer cell migrations occur through kinases activated by ERα extranuclear signaling while other signaling pathways play roles in the invasion and metastasis of these cells [56]. ERα works with growth factor receptors such as HER2 to reorganize the cytoskeleton in breast cells; the dysregulation of the growth factor in cells can promote cytoplasmic sequestration of ERα [56]. ERα may be methylated through post-translational modifications by methyltransferase G9a [56]. Depletion of G9a in breast cancer cell lines decreases estrogen signaling and slows down cell proliferation and transformation in cells [56]. Increases in extranuclear signaling may be responsible for breast cancer cell migration and metastasis [56].

In ER-positive breast cancer, estrogen initiates the PI3K/AKT/mTOR signaling pathway [55]. When it is targeted, the PI3K/AKT- protein kinase Cα signaling pathway activates, which results in the increased expression of the signaling pathway as well as tumor invasion and metastasis, causing cancer to spread [55, 57]. Additionally, breast cell apoptosis occurs while cancer cells proliferate [55]. Cyclic adenosine monophosphate (cAMP) levels increase as a result of the activation of these signaling pathways, causing a rapid increase in the presence of estrogen [55]. Consequently, the C-terminal of ERα is activated and interacts with signaling molecules to amplify its signaling pathway [55]. This activation increases HER2 levels and epidermal growth factor receptor levels, causing further cancer growth [55]. Similar disease progression by the overexpression of ERα has been linked to other cancers such as prostate cancer [55].

Rajhans et al. have shown the retention of ERα in metastatic tumors, indicating the correlation between ERα-positive tumors and metastasis [56, 58]. Metastatic ER-positive cancers commonly spread to the bone, bone marrow, lymph nodes, lungs, liver, and skin [33]. Specifically, studies by Koenders et al. have shown a correlation between ERα-positive tumors and bone metastasis in breast cancer patients [56, 59]. Metastasis occurs when tumor cells migrate from the stroma into the bloodstream and progress through epithelial-mesenchymal transitions (EMT) to increase the mobility of cancer cells [60]. Once in the bloodstream, tumor cells attach to organs, spreading cancer to another part of the body [60].

Studies by Borough et al. show the correlation between rapidly spreading tumors and oncogenic signaling pathways that contribute to anabolism and metabolism [17, 60]. Lowered levels of glutaminolysis, glycine, lactate, and glutamate in ER-positive tumors indicate the role of estrogen receptors in tumor metabolism [60]. The PI3K/AKT/mTOR signaling pathway works in conjunction with estrogen receptors to allow for tumor stabilization [60]. The process of glycolysis may be altered in periods of high glucose conditions by estradiol, and glucose availability may also alter the programming of metabolism by ERα [60].

6.3 Estrogen receptor type: ERβ

ERβ, like ERα, is an estrogen receptor type found in the nuclear transcription factor family [49]. It is encoded by the ESR2 gene, which has eight encoding exons and is found predominantly in breast epithelial cells [49]. As with ERα, ERβ has an N-terminal activation function-A that stabilizes ligand-independent transcription as well as multiple domains for ligand binding [49]. ERβ, unlike ERα, does not target the uterus or mammary gland but instead regulates signaling in the ovary, immune system, and prostate [61]. The N-terminal domain contains a repressor function in ERβ that decreases ERβ-mediated activity; this domain plays a role in regulating interactions between ERβ and cellular pathways in the body [61]. In the presence of estradiol, ERβ inhibits transcription, while ERα activates transcription on AP-1-driven promoters [61].

As the levels of ERβ increase, levels of cell proliferation decrease, serving as a tumor suppressor [62]. Breast cancers display decreased levels of ERβ [62]. The downregulation of these estrogen receptors exhibits EMT in cancer cells and prevents cancer cell migration [62]. This downregulation is done by inhibiting receptor tyrosine kinases and activators of transcription signaling pathways of cancer cells [63]. ERβ carries tumor-suppressor characteristics by inhibiting transforming growth factor (TGF) signaling and decreasing the expression of genes in the extracellular matrix, cell invasion, and vitamin metabolism [63]. ERβ has also been shown to play an inhibitory effect on cell cycle progression [63]. By decreasing levels of ERβ, cancer cells elevate cyclin levels needed for cell cycle progression and cause rapid proliferation and growth [63].

Studies by Paruthiyil et al. have identified a network of genes in the G2 stage of breast cancer cells [63]. Targeting this specific stage in the cell cycle, ERβ represses cyclin D1, cyclin A, and c-myc gene transcription while increasing the expression of Cip1 and Kip1 to inhibit cell proliferation before progressing toward mitosis [63, 64]. Cyclin-dependent kinases, regulatory enzymes necessary for the progression through the cell cycle, are also inhibited by ERβ [63].

ERβ isoforms in mRNA can form through alternative splicing of exons 8 and 9, deletion of a coding exon, or the use of untranslated exons [65]. ERβ isoforms are differentially expressed and associated with breast cancer tumor growth [66]. In an experiment conducted to observe the role of ERβ in therapy for triple-negative breast cancer, ERβ isoforms ERβ2/ERβ5 and ERβ1 were shown to serve different functions in cancer cells [67]. The different outcomes of the subgroups are due to the various mRNA and protein expressions from different ERβ isoforms [66].

The role of ERβ is versatile in providing an antiproliferative role when in the presence of ERα. At the same time, some data correlate the growth of breast cancer with ERβ as in experimental studies by Förster et al. [68, 69]. Through treatment of mice in a 48-hour study, they presented the mediation of tissue-specific cell proliferation with colocalization of ERβ in mammary epithelial cells (Couse et al.) [38, 39]. However, this data presented that ERβ1, the functional isoform, did not inhibit the proliferation of cells in some circumstances [38]. The presence of ERβ in some breast cancer tumors indicates the lack of a role of ERβ in halting cancer growth [65]. Rody et al. have associated the methylation of ERβ promoters in cancer cells with the depletion of ERβ in breast cancer cells [65, 70]. In *in vitro* studies, the lack of ERβ in breast cancer tumors supports that ERβ is a tumor suppressor gene [65]. The role of ERβ is continually being studied due to the duality it presents in various studies [68]. Due to this uncertainty, ERα is measured to determine the treatment and identification of the type of breast cancer for a patient [65].

6.4 Difference in receptor types

During the progression of tumors, ERβ levels decrease, serving as a tumor suppressor [61]. This suggests a role opposite of ERα which promotes cancer cell proliferation [61]. Malignant tumors show a higher expression of ERα and a lower expression of ERβ; however, as discussed in a previous study, the presence of ERβ levels in breast cancer patients is still being studied [38, 65, 71]. Due to this, ERβ expresses an anticancer effect and is used in therapies for breast cancer treatment [63]. ERα and ERβ levels are responsible for the signaling pathways that mediate cell proliferation and therapy response [72, 73].

The interaction between these receptor types can affect the transcription and downregulation of breast cancer cells [73]. Transcription is upregulated in the presence of the AP-1 binding element with ERα but downregulated in the presence of estradiol with ERβ [74]. Although similar in their structure and their role in controlling estrogen signaling by binding to an ERE, the function of each receptor differs [71]. The ligand-binding domain of both receptors also differs, allowing for subtype selectivity [71]. Other factors such as transcriptional activation and cofactor interactions cause different effects of ERα and ERβ in tissues [71].

7. Recent progress: Treatment

7.1 Endocrine therapy

Endocrine therapy (ET) is a common form of treatment used for estrogen receptor-positive cancers in conjunction with surgery [31]. This therapy can be categorized into three groups: ovarian function suppression, estrogen receptor modulators and down-regulators, and aromatase inhibitors [31].

Ovarian function suppression (OFS) is a form of therapy used to decrease and stop the production of estrogen by the ovaries [31]. This therapy lowers the level of estrogen in the body and prevents the overexpression of estrogen that causes cancer cells to grow [75]. Through luteinizing hormone-releasing (LHRH) hormone agonists or radiation therapy, OFS can be used to treat tumors [75]. LHRH targets G-protein coupled receptors in pituitary glands to reduce ovarian hormone production in the long term for premenopausal females [75]. OFS is used with adjuvant endocrine therapy to treat ER-positive breast cancer patients [76].

Selective ER modulators (SERMS) and down-regulators (SERDS) are also used to stop estrogen receptor function and signaling [31]. A common selective ER modulator, Tamoxifen (TAM), is used to treat both pre- and postmenopausal patients [31]. TAM acts as a competitive receptor inhibitor—blocking estrogen from binding in the site—in breast tissues by blocking the signaling of estrogen receptors and is commonly used for premenopausal women [49, 76]. SERMS are dependent on the activity of an estrogen receptor agonist or antagonist to determine the complexity of the compound [77]. SERMs use target-site specificity to interact with either of the two subunits that an estrogen receptor is composed of [77]. SERDs act as ER antagonists, blocking the function and signaling of receptors by degradation [31]. Those who are resistant to first hormone therapy—commonly those with luminal metastatic breast cancer—have been treated using the SERD fulvestrant [78]. Although oral administration is currently being developed, fulvestrant is usually administered through an intramuscular injection in postmenopausal women [78]. Approved by the FDA in January 2023, elacestrant is an oral SERD for ER-positive breast cancers [33, 79]. The EMERALD trial conducted by Aditya Bardia et al. found an improvement in phase III patients in using elacestrant for hormone therapy with an overall 30% reduction in the progression of the cancer in the study population [79].

Aromatase inhibitors block aromatase enzyme activity by decreasing the circulation of estrogen in the bloodstream, thereby reducing the frequency of estrogen receptor binding [31]. However, aromatase inhibitors have been shown to only be effective in postmenopausal females [31]. These inhibitors do not function in females whose ovaries are active, as they increase estrogen production [31]. The STAGE study conducted by Masuda et al. has shown that 70.4% of postmenopausal patients who undergo aromatase inhibitor and OFS therapy have a response to treatment [31, 80].

Endocrine therapy has proven to be beneficial for ER-positive patients; however, mutations present in ERα can lead to endocrine resistance [55]. ERα is affected by post-translational modifications, often getting degraded through ubiquitination [55]. Endocrine resistance can cause ER-positive patient relapse due to changes in protein expression from ERα alterations [55]. One mutation that exists is the Y537S mutation that causes endocrine resistance against Tamoxifen in MCF7 cells, according to studies performed by Fiorillo et al. [81]. Results show that the Y537S mutation creates Tamoxifen resistance through refined mitochondrial metabolism and increased levels of glycolysis due to increased mitochondrial oxygen intake [81].

7.1.1 Endocrine therapy induced osteoporosis

Aromatase inhibitors are chosen as the primary treatment for postmenopausal women by blocking the production of estrogen from androgens [80, 82]. Endocrine therapy is used to inhibit the growth of tumor cells by reducing the levels of estrogen. This therapy will prevent estrogen from binding to estrogen receptors on tumor cells [82]. However, the reduced estrogen levels stimulate osteoporosis—the loss of bone density with decreased estrogen levels—in older women and hinder bone formation and growth [82]. This development is commonly induced by the anti-estrogenic drugs and aromatase inhibitors mentioned previously [82].

There has been recent progress in the use of cyclin-dependent kinase inhibitors for these women. Specifically, CDK4 and CDK6 inhibitors prevent tumor cell growth and proliferation [82]. Cyclin-dependent kinases are key in controlling the progression of the cell cycle. Normally, the cyclin D-CDK4/6 complex phosphorylates Rb, the retinoblastoma protein, allowing for the release of E2F, which binds to promote growth. Without the presence of CDK4/6, these cells cannot progress from the G1 to S phase, preventing the growth of these cells [83]. CDK4/6 inhibitors include Abemaciclib, Palbociclib, Ribociclib, and Trilaciclib [82]. These inhibitors are mostly used for HR+/HER2- patients, and specifically palbociclib is used in conjunction with aromatase inhibitors to treat postmenopausal patients [83]. However, as with many other breast cancer treatments, acquired resistance to CDK inhibitors can still occur, necessitating future research into CDK inhibitors and how such resistance arises [83]. One novel CDK inhibitor, Dalpiciclib, has shown promise for lengthening progression-free survival of HR+/HER2- patients that have been heavily pretreated; furthermore, it also displays some synergistic effects when used in combination with other therapies [84]. Nevertheless, further research into CDK inhibitors as a therapeutic option may prove beneficial [83].

7.2 Surgery

Surgery is used to treat ER-negative cancers to directly target tumor growth [85]. Surgery for cancer prevention allows for enhanced tissue retrieval and local and regional control of solid cancers [85].

HR-negative breast cancers are commonly treated through lumpectomy [86]. Lumpectomy treats centrally located tumors on the breast through surgical removal of the tumor and surrounding tissue [86, 87]. This surgery is performed to conserve the breast and remove the cancerous tumor and tissues. Radiation therapy is used after lumpectomy to reduce the recurrence rate of breast cancer [88]. Although these surgeries are low risk, in the case that a lumpectomy fails, a re-excision or a mastectomy may be required [87]. A mastectomy removes all breast tissue due to the large size of tumors and the spread of the cancer. In low-income countries, mastectomy is the preferred surgical treatment due to the late stage of breast cancer diagnosis and the prevalence of the disease [85].

7.3 Epigenetic therapy

Epigenetics is known to play a substantial role in many normal developmental functions, but its role in cancer initiation and development has only recently been researched [89]. In breast cancer, epigenetic modifications such as rapid DNA methylation, cytosine-phosphate-guanine (CpG) promoter methylation, and histone modification may lead to its initiation, promotion, or metastasis; furthermore, other epigenetic functions may result in the silencing of tumor suppressor genes, contributing to epigenetics' role in cancer development [89, 90].

Epigenetic drugs (epi-drugs) are chemical agents that inhibit these epigenetic changes [89, 90]. The most common method is for epi-drugs to reactivate tumor suppressors and DNA repair elements by inhibiting DNMTs-DNA methyltransferase which inhibits CpG island methylation [90, 91]. The drug, DNMTi creates an apoptotic response for cancer cells [90, 91]. Similarly, histone deactetylases (HDACs) are inhibited by the HDACi epi-drug, which normalizes histone acetylation through decreasing activation of zinc-dependent enzymes [91].

Consequently, many epi-drugs have been developed to tackle breast cancer from the epigenetic angle; however, many so far have been confined only to hematological malignancies and have had little success with solid tumors [92]. Preclinical and clinical evidence supports that epi-drugs may have a synergistic effect when used in conjunction with radiotherapy, immunotherapy, and endocrine therapy [92]. The most common types of epigenetic therapy for breast cancers are histone deacetylase inhibitors, DNA methyltransferase inhibitors, and RNA inhibitors, which ultimately aim to restore normal expression of tumor suppressor genes [93]. Some studies have shown that such therapy may be especially effective for hormone-resistant breast cancer [93].

DNMTi and HDACi epi-drugs have low specificity, causing scientists and providers to look for a more selective option [94, 95]. A lysine-specific demthylase 1 (LSD1) inhibitor called Iadademstat has made progress in proving to be an epigenetic treatment for breast cancer by targeting SOX-2 [94, 95]. SOX-2 is prominent in differentiating adult cells and therefore, in high levels, proliferates cancer cells [95].

8. Conclusion

Estrogen is a hormone that can control breast cancer growth through the presence or depletion of it in the body. Regularly, estrogen circulates in the bloodstream as produced by the ovaries and aids in the progression through the menstrual cycle and pregnancy. The role of estrogen receptors and signaling in breast cancer is crucial to understanding hormone receptor breast cancer, as ER breast cancer comprises two-thirds of all breast cancer cases. ER-positive breast cancers are attributed to the necessary presence of estrogen in the body for cancer cell growth to progress. Estrogen receptors and their signaling can cause cancer cell proliferation and tumor growth.

ER-negative breast cancers occur when in the absence of the hormone, cancer growth occurs, as these cells cannot proliferate in the presence of estrogen. Metastasis of breast cancer may also occur as a result of both cancers spreading to several places in the body. ERα and ERβ are estrogen receptor types that bind with estrogen to function in the cell. Although these receptor types are similar in structure, the function differs in that ERα mediates estrogens in the mammary gland, promoting growth, while ERβ inhibits cell proliferation.

One future treatment includes tumor cell apoptosis, which would slow tumor progression, potentially making it an effective tool to treat ER-breast cancer [96]. Lok et al. have developed a potential method of BCL2 inhibition, which is an apoptotic mechanism, to slow the progression of ER-positive breast cancer [96, 97].

By inhibiting the activity of BCL2, the apoptotic processes in tumor cells can be restored [96]. Similar drugs are being developed to target ER-positive tumor cells [96].

The reception and signaling of estrogen receptors play a key role in the development of breast cancer. Treatments using endocrine therapy and other therapies are being developed to medicate those affected by ER breast cancer.

Acknowledgements

Funding for publication of this paper was made possible by a grant from the Assisi Foundation of Memphis. Brown, Chester, PhD (PI). We also thank Yirui Tang and Annie Wu for drawing the figures used in this paper.

Conflict of interest

The authors have declared that no conflict of interest exists.

Author details

Arya Rajesh[1], Evan Easley[2], Chikezie O. Madu[3] and Yi Lu[4*]

1 University of Virginia, Charlottesville, VA, USA

2 Departments of Biology, White Station High, Memphis, USA

3 Departments of Biological Sciences, University of Memphis, Memphis, USA

4 Department of Pathology and Laboratory Medicine, University of Tennessee Health Science Center, Memphis, USA

*Address all correspondence to: ylu@utshc.edu

References

[1] Trayes KP, Cokenakes SEH. Breast cancer treatment. American Family Physician. 2021;**104**(2):171-178 Available from: www.aafp.org/pubs/afp/issues/2021/0800/p171.html

[2] Łukasiewicz S, Czeczelewski M, Forma A, Baj J, Sitarz R, Stanisławek A. Breast Cancer-Epidemiology, Risk Factors, Classification, Prognostic Markers, and Current Treatment Strategies-An Updated Review. 2021. Available from: https://www.ncbi.nlm.nih.gov/pmc/articles/PMC8428369/

[3] Sun Y, Zhao Z, Yang Z, Xu F, Lu H, Zhu Z, et al. Risk Factors and Preventions of Breast Cancer. 2017. Available from: https://www.ncbi.nlm.nih.gov/pmc/articles/PMC5715522/

[4] Moo T, Sanford R, Dang C, Morrow M. Overview of Breast Cancer Therapy. 2018. Available from: https://www.ncbi.nlm.nih.gov/pmc/articles/PMC6092031/

[5] Becker S. A Historic and Scientific Review of Breast Cancer: The Next Global Healthcare Challenge. 2015. Available from: https://www.sciencedirect.com/science/article/pii/S002072921500154X

[6] Logullo AF, Prigenzi KCK, Nimir CCBA, Franco AFV, Campos MSDA. Breast microcalcifications: Past, present and future (review). Molecular and Clinical Oncology. 2022;**16**(4):81. DOI: 10.3892/mco.2022.2514

[7] Xue M, Zhang K, Mu K, Xu J, Yang H, Liu Y, et al. Regulation of Estrogen Signaling and Breast Cancer Proliferation by an Ubiquitin Ligase TRIM56. 2019. Available from: https://www.nature.com/articles/s41389-019-0139-x

[8] Wang L. Early diagnosis of breast cancer. Sensors. 2017;**17**(7):1572. DOI: 10.3390/s17071572

[9] Sukumar J, Gast K, Quiroga D, Lustberg M, Williams N. Triple-negative breast cancer: Promising prognostic biomarkers currently in development. Expert Review of Anticancer Therapy. Feb 2021;**21**(2):135-148. DOI: 10.1080/14737140.2021.1840984

[10] Jia Y et al. Exosome: Emerging biomarker in breast cancer. Oncotarget. 2017;**8**(25):41717-41733. Available from: www.ncbi.nlm.nih.gov/pmc/articles/PMC5522217/

[11] Parchekani J, Hashemzadeh H, Allahverdi A, Siampour H, Abbasian S, Moshaii A, et al. Zepto molar miRNA-21 detection in gold Nano-islands platform toward early cancer screening. Sensing and Bio-Sensing Research. 2021;**34**:100449. DOI: 10.1016/j.sbsr.2021.100449

[12] Mohanty S, Sahoo C, Padhy R. Role of Hormone Receptors and HER2 as Prospective Molecular Markers for Breast Cancer: An Update. 2020. Available from: https://www.sciencedirect.com/science/article/pii/S2352304220301628

[13] Goldberg J, Pastorello R, Vallius T, Davis J, Cui Y, Agudo J, et al. The Immunology of Hormone Receptor Positive Breast Cancer. Available from: https://www.frontiersin.org/articles/10.3389/fimmu.2021.674192/full

[14] Reinert T, Barrios C. Optimal Management of Hormone Receptor Positive Metastatic Breast Cancer in 2016.

2015. Available from: https://www.ncbi.nlm.nih.gov/pmc/articles/PMC4622303/

[15] Jiao Q, Wu A, Shao G, Peng H, Wang M, Ji S, et al. The Latest Progress in Research on Triple Negative Breast Cancer [TNBC]: Risk Factors, Possible Therapeutic Targets and Prognostic Markers. 2014. Available from: https://www.ncbi.nlm.nih.gov/pmc/articles/PMC4178098/

[16] Dunnwald L, Rossing M, Li C. Hormone Receptor Status, Tumor Characteristics, and Prognosis: A Prospective Cohort of Breast Cancer Patients. 2007. Available from: https://www.ncbi.nlm.nih.gov/pmc/articles/PMC1851385/

[17] Ogundiran T, Ayandipo O, Ademola A, Adebamowo C. Mastectomy for Management of Breast Cancer in Ibadan, Nigeria - BMC Surgery. 2013. Available from: https://bmcsurg.biomedcentral.com/articles/10.1186/1471-2482-13-59

[18] Lange C, Yee D Progesterone and Breast Cancer. 2008. Available from: https://www.ncbi.nlm.nih.gov/pmc/articles/PMC4038907/#:~:text=Progesterone%20action%20in%20human%20breast%20cancer%20cells&text=Progesterone%20acts%20to%20sensitize%20breast,D%20and%20E%2C%20p21

[19] Li Z, Wei H, Li S, Wu P, Mao X. The role of progesterone receptors in breast cancer. Drug Design, Development and Therapy. 2022;**16**:305-314. DOI: 10.2147/DDDT.S336643

[20] Horwitz K, Sartorius C. 90 Years of Progesterone: Progesterone and Progesterone Receptors in Breast Cancer: Past, Present, Future. 2020. Available from: https://jme.bioscientifica.com/view/journals/jme/65/1/JME-20-0104.xml?body=fullhtml-10207

[21] Trabert B, Bauer D, Buist D, Cauley J, Falk R, Geczik A, et al. Association of Circulating Progesterone with Breast Cancer Risk Among Postmenopausal Women. 2020. Available from: https://www.ncbi.nlm.nih.gov/pmc/articles/PMC7182797/#:~:text=Conclusions%20and%20Relevance,the%20risk%20of%20breast%20cancer

[22] Hamilton K, Hewitt S, Arao Y, Korach K. Estrogen Hormone Biology. 2017. Available from: https://www.ncbi.nlm.nih.gov/pmc/articles/PMC6206851/

[23] Mauvais-Jarvis F, Clegg D, Hevener A. The Role of Estrogens in Control of Energy Balance and Glucose Homeostasis. 2013. Available from: https://www.ncbi.nlm.nih.gov/pmc/articles/PMC3660717/

[24] Estrogen Production and Action - Journal of the American Academy of ... n.d.. Available from: https://www.jaad.org/article/S0190-9622[01]45314-X/abstract

[25] The Embryo Project Encyclopedia. n.d.. Available from: https://embryo.asu.edu/pages/estrogen-and-menstrual-cycle-humans

[26] Department of Pathology and Laboratory Medicine. HER2 in Breast Cancer: A Review and Update: Advances in Anatomic Pathology. n.d.. Available from: https://journals.lww.com/anatomicpathology/Abstract/2014/03000/HER2_in_Breast_Cancer__A_Review_and_Update.4.aspx

[27] Mitri Z, Constantine T, O'Regan R. The HER2 Receptor in Breast Cancer: Pathophysiology, Clinical Use, and New Advances in Therapy. 2012. Available from: https://www.ncbi.nlm.nih.gov/pmc/articles/PMC3539433/

[28] Schlam I, Swain S. Her2-Positive Breast Cancer and Tyrosine Kinase

Inhibitors: The Time is Now. 2021. Available from: https://www.nature.com/articles/s41523-021-00265-1

[29] Gutierrez C, Schiff R. HER2: Biology, Detection, and Clinical Implications. 2011. Available from: https://www.ncbi.nlm.nih.gov/pmc/articles/PMC3242418/

[30] Wang J, Xu B. Targeted Therapeutic Options and Future Perspectives for HER2-Positive Breast Cancer. 2019. Available from: https://www.nature.com/articles/s41392-019-0069-2

[31] Lumachi F, Santeufemia D, Basso S. Current Medical Treatment of Estrogen Receptor-Positive Breast Cancer. 2015. Available from: https://www.ncbi.nlm.nih.gov/pmc/articles/PMC4549764/

[32] Gourdy P, Guillaume M, Fontaine C, et al. Estrogen receptor subcellular localization and cardiometabolism. Molecular Metabolism. 2018;**15**:56-69. DOI: 10.1016/j.molmet.2018.05.009

[33] Clusan L, Ferrière F, Flouriot G, Pakdel F. A basic review on estrogen receptor signaling pathways in breast cancer. International Journal of Molecular Sciences. 2023;**24**(7):6834. DOI: 10.3390/ijms24076834

[34] Alluri P, Speers C, Chinnaiyan A. Estrogen Receptor Mutations and their Role in Breast Cancer Progression - Breast Cancer Research. 2014. Available from: https://breast-cancer-research.biomedcentral.com/articles/10.1186/s13058-014-0494-7

[35] Farzaneh S, Zarghi A. Estrogen Receptor Ligands: A Review [2013-2015]. 2016. Available from: https://www.ncbi.nlm.nih.gov/pmc/articles/PMC5064234/

[36] Yaşar P, Ayaz G, User S, Güpür G, Muyan M. Molecular Mechanism of Estrogen-Estrogen Receptor Signaling. 2016. Available from: https://www.ncbi.nlm.nih.gov/pmc/articles/PMC5715874/#:~:text=Estrogen%20receptors%2C%20as%20other%20members,different%20tissues%20at%20varying%20levels

[37] Kumar R, Zakharov M, Khan S, Miki R, Jang H, Toraldo G, et al. The Dynamic Structure of the Estrogen Receptor. 2011. Available from: https://www.ncbi.nlm.nih.gov/pmc/articles/PMC3268042/

[38] Saji S, Jensen EV, Nilsson S, Rylander T, Warner M, Gustafsson J. Estrogen Receptors α and β in the Rodent Mammary Gland. n.d. Available from: https://www.pnas.org/doi/full/10.1073/pnas.97.1.337

[39] Masuda N, Sagara Y, Kinoshita T, Iwata H, Nakamura S, Yanagita Y, et al. Neoadjuvant Anastrozole Versus Tamoxifen in Patients Receiving Goserelin for Premenopausal Breast Cancer (Stage): A Double-Blind, Randomised Phase 3 Trial. n.d. Available from: https://pubmed.ncbi.nlm.nih.gov/22265697/

[40] Vivacqua A. GPER1 and microRNA: Two players in breast cancer progression. International Journal of Molecular Sciences. 2020;**22**(1):98. DOI: 10.3390/ijms22010098

[41] Treeck O, Schüler-Toprak S, Ortmann O. Estrogen actions in triple-negative breast cancer. Cells. 2020;**9**(11):2358. DOI: 10.3390/cells9112358

[42] Prossnitz ER, Barton M. Estrogen biology: New insights into GPER function and clinical opportunities. Molecular and Cellular Endocrinology. 2014;**389**(1-2):71-83. DOI: 10.1016/j.mce.2014.02.002

[43] Johnston S. New Strategies in Estrogen Receptor–Positive Breast Cancer. 2010. Available from: https://aacrjournals.org/clincancerres/article/16/7/1979/76026/New-Strategies-in-Estrogen-Receptor-Positive

[44] Gao J, Swain S. Luminal a Breast Cancer and Molecular Assays: A Review. 2018. Available from: https://www.ncbi.nlm.nih.gov/pmc/articles/PMC5947456/

[45] Zwart W, Theodorou V, Carroll JS. Estrogen receptor-positive breast cancer: A multidisciplinary challenge. Wiley Interdisciplinary Reviews. Systems Biology and Medicine. 2011;**3**(2):216-230. DOI: 10.1002/wsbm.109

[46] Putti T, El-Rehim D, Rakha E, Paish C, Lee A, Pinder S, Ellis I. Estrogen Receptor-Negative Breast Carcinomas: A Review of Morphology and Immunophenotypical Analysis. 2004. Available from: https://www.nature.com/articles/3800255

[47] Hidaka BH, Boddy AM. Is Estrogen Receptor-Negative Breast Cancer Risk Associated with a Fast Life History Strategy? 2016. Available from: https://www.ncbi.nlm.nih.gov/pmc/articles/PMC4716563/

[48] Gajulapalli V, Malisetty V, Chitta S, Manavathi B. Oestrogen Receptor Negativity in Breast Cancer: A Cause or Consequence? 2016. Available from: https://www.ncbi.nlm.nih.gov/pmc/articles/PMC5180249/

[49] Mal R, Magner A, David J, Datta J, Vallabhaneni M, Kassem M et al. Estrogen Receptor Beta [ERB]: A Ligand Activated Tumor Suppressor. Available from: https://www.frontiersin.org/articles/10.3389/fonc.2020.587386/full

[50] Yersal O, Barutca S. Biological Subtypes of Breast Cancer: Prognostic and Therapeutic Implications. 2014. Available from: https://www.ncbi.nlm.nih.gov/pmc/articles/PMC4127612/

[51] Arnal J, Lenfant F, Metivier R, Flouriot G, Henrion D, et al. Membrane and Nuclear Estrogen Receptor Alpha Actions: From Tissue Specificity to Medical Implications. 2017. Available from: https://journals.physiology.org/doi/full/10.1152/physrev.00024.2016

[52] Paterni I, Granchi C, Katzenellenbogen J, Minutolo F. Estrogen Receptors Alpha [ERA] and Beta [ERB]: Subtype-Selective Ligands and Clinical Potential. 2014. Available from: https://www.ncbi.nlm.nih.gov/pmc/articles/PMC4192010/

[53] Manavathi B, Dey O, Gajulapalli V, Bhatia R, Bugide S, Kumar R. Derailed Estrogen Signaling and Breast Cancer: An Authentic Couple. 2013. Available from: https://www.ncbi.nlm.nih.gov/pmc/articles/PMC3565105/

[54] Liu Q, Niu N, Wada Y, Liu J. The role of CDKN1A-Interacting Zinc Finger Protein 1 [CIZ1] in DNA Replication and Pathophysiology. 2016. Available from: https://www.ncbi.nlm.nih.gov/pmc/articles/PMC4783944/

[55] Liu Y, Ma H, Yao J. ERA, A Key Target for Cancer Therapy: A Review. 2020. Available from: https://www.ncbi.nlm.nih.gov/pmc/articles/PMC7073439/

[56] Saha Roy S, Vadlamudi R. Role of Estrogen Receptor Signaling in Breast Cancer Metastasis. 2011. Available from: https://www.hindawi.com/journals/ijbc/2012/654698/

[57] Porta C, Paglino C, Mosca A. Targeting PI3K/AKT/mtor Signaling in Cancer. Available from: https://www.frontiersin.org/articles/10.3389/fonc.2014.00064/full

[58] Boroughs L, DeBerardinis R. Metabolic Pathways Promoting Cancer Cell Survival and Growth. 2015. Available from: https://www.ncbi.nlm.nih.gov/pmc/articles/PMC4939711/

[59] Rajhans R, Nair S, Holden A, Kumar R, Tekmal R, Vadlamudi R. Oncogenic Potential of the Nuclear Receptor Coregulator Proline-, Glutamic Acid–, Leucine-Rich Protein 1/Modulator of the Nongenomic Actions of the Estrogen Receptor. 2007. Available from: https://aacrjournals.org/cancerres/article/67/11/5505/533197/Oncogenic-Potential-of-the-Nuclear-Receptor

[60] Wang L, Zhang S, Wang X The Metabolic Mechanisms of Breast Cancer Metastasis. Available from: https://www.frontiersin.org/articles/10.3389/fonc.2020.602416/full

[61] Deroo B, Buensuceso A. Minireview: Estrogen Receptor-Beta: Mechanistic Insights from Recent Studies. 2010. Available from: https://www.ncbi.nlm.nih.gov/pmc/articles/PMC5417404/

[62] Pesapane F, Downey K, Rotili A, Cassano E, Koh D. Imaging Diagnosis of Metastatic Breast Cancer - Insights into Imaging. 2020. Available from: https://insightsimaging.springeropen.com/articles/10.1186/s13244-020-00885-4

[63] Zhou Y, Liu X. The Role of Estrogen Receptor Beta in Breast Cancer. 2020. Available from: https://www.ncbi.nlm.nih.gov/pmc/articles/PMC7487630/

[64] Koenders P, Beex L, Langens R, Kloppenborg P, Smals A, Benraad T. Steroid Hormone Receptor Activity of Primary Human Breast Cancer and Pattern of First Metastasis - Breast Cancer Research and Treatment. n.d.. Available from: https://link.springer.com/article/10.1007/BF01975440

[65] Estrogen Receptor β: An Overview and Update - Sage Journals. n.d.. Available from: https://journals.sagepub.com/doi/10.1621/nrs.06003

[66] Choi Y, Kim H, Pollack S, ERB Isoforms have Differential Clinical Significance in Breast Cancer Subtypes and Subgroups. 2022. Available from: https://www.mdpi.com/1467-3045/44/4/107

[67] Yan S, Dey P, Ziegler Y, Jiao X, Kim SH, Katzenellenbogen JA, Katzenellenbogen BS. Contrasting Activities of Estrogen Receptor Beta Isoforms in Triple Negative Breast Cancer. n.d.. Available from: https://pubmed.ncbi.nlm.nih.gov/33001337/

[68] Leygue E, Murphy L. A Bi-Faceted Role of Estrogen Receptor β in Breast Cancer. 2013. Available from: https://erc.bioscientifica.com/configurable/content/journals$002ferc$002f20$002f3$002fR127.xml?t%3Aac=journals%24002ferc%24002f20%24002f3%24002fR127.xml

[69] Paruthiyil S, Parmar H, Kerekatte V, Cunha G, Firestone G, Leitman D. Estrogen Receptor β Inhibits Human Breast Cancer Cell Proliferation and Tumor Formation by Causing a G2 Cell Cycle Arrest. 2004. Available from: https://aacrjournals.org/cancerres/article/64/1/423/511266/Estrogen-Receptor-Inhibits-Human-Breast-Cancer

[70] Förster, C., Mäkela, S., Wärri, A., Kietz, S., Becker, D., Hultenby, K., et al. Involvement of Estrogen Receptor β in Terminal Differentiation of Mammary Gland Epithelium. 2022. Available from: https://www.pnas.org/doi/full/10.1073/pnas.192561299

[71] Zhou Y, Liu X. The role of estrogen receptor beta in breast cancer. Biomarker Research. 2020;**8**:39. DOI: 10.1186/s40364-020-00223-2

[72] Madeira M, Mattar A, Logullo, Soares F, Gebrim L Estrogen Receptor Alpha/Beta Ratio and Estrogen Receptor Beta as Predictors of Endocrine Therapy Responsiveness–a Randomized Neoadjuvant Trial Comparison Between Anastrozole and Tamoxifen for the Treatment of Postmenopausal Breast Cancer - BMC Cancer. 2013. Available from: https://bmccancer.biomedcentral.com/articles/10.1186/1471-2407-13-425

[73] Sellitto A, D'Agostino Y, Alexandrova E, Lamberti J, Pecoraro G, Memoli D, et al. Insights into the role of Estrogen receptor β in triple-negative breast cancer. Cancers (Basel). 2020;**12**(6):1477. DOI: 10.3390/cancers12061477

[74] Zhao Z, Wang L, James T, Jung Y, Kim I, Tan R, et al.. Reciprocal Regulation of ERA and ERB Stability and Activity by Diptoindonesin G. 2015. Available from: https://www.sciencedirect.com/science/article/pii/S1074552115004159

[75] Lu Y, Wong A, Kim H. Ovarian Function Suppression with Luteinizing Hormone-Releasing Hormone Agonists for the Treatment of Hormone Receptor-Positive Early Breast Cancer in Premenopausal Women. 2021. Available from: https://www.ncbi.nlm.nih.gov/pmc/articles/PMC8477635/

[76] Xie X, Yao Y, Zhang D. Ovarian Function Suppression Plus Aromatase Inhibitors or Tamoxifen in Premenopausal HR-Positive Breast Cancer. 2020. Available from: https://www.scientificarchives.com/article/ovarian-function-suppression-plus-aromatase-inhibitors-or-tamoxifen-in-premenopausal-hr-positive-breast-cancer

[77] An K. Selective Estrogen Receptor Modulators. 2016. Available from: https://www.ncbi.nlm.nih.gov/pmc/articles/PMC4995266/

[78] Lok SW, Whittle JR, Vaillant F, Teh CE, Lo LL, Policheni AN, et al. A Phase IB Dose-Escalation and Expansion Study of the BCL2 Inhibitor Venetoclax Combined with Tamoxifen in ER and BCL2-Positive Metastatic Breast Cancer. n.d.. Available from: https://pubmed.ncbi.nlm.nih.gov/30518523/

[79] Center for Drug Evaluation and Research. "FDA Approves Elacestrant for ER-Positive." U.S. Food and Drug Administration. Available from: www.fda.gov/drugs/resources-information-approved-drugs/fda-approves-elacestrant-er-positive-her2-negative-esr1-mutated-advanced-or-metastatic-breast-cancer

[80] Rody A, Holtrich U, Solbach C, Kourtis K, Minckwitz G, Engels K, et al. Methylation of Estrogen Receptor β Promoter Correlates with Loss of ER-β Expression in Mammary Carcinoma and is an Early Indication Marker in Premalignant Lesions. 2005. Available from: https://erc.bioscientifica.com/view/journals/erc/12/4/0120903.xml

[81] Fiorillo M, Sanchez-Alvarez R, Sotgia F, Lisanti MP. The ER-alpha mutation Y537S confers tamoxifen-resistance via enhanced mitochondrial metabolism, glycolysis and rho-GDI/PTEN signaling: Implicating TIGAR in somatic resistance to endocrine therapy. Aging (Albany NY). 2018;**10**(12):4000-4023. DOI: 10.18632/aging.101690

[82] Xu J, Cao B, Li C, Li G. The recent progress of endocrine therapy-induced osteoporosis in estrogen-positive breast cancer therapy. Frontiers in Oncology. 2023;**13**:1218206. DOI: 10.3389/fonc.2023.1218206

[83] Sheikh MS, Satti SA. The emerging CDK4/6 inhibitor for breast cancer treatment. Molecular and Cellular Pharmacology. 2021;**13**(3):9-12

[84] Dalpiciclib extends progression-free survival in HR+/HER2- advanced breast cancer. The Oncologist. 2021;**26 Suppl 3**(Suppl. 3):S9-S10. DOI: 10.1002/onco.13865

[85] Breast Cancer Surgery - Statpearls - NCBI Bookshelf. n.d.. Available from: https://www.ncbi.nlm.nih.gov/books/NBK553076/

[86] Aysola K, Desai A, Welch C, Xu J, Qin Y, Reddy V, et al. Triple Negative Breast Cancer - An Overview. 2013. Available from: https://www.ncbi.nlm.nih.gov/pmc/articles/PMC4181680/

[87] Holli K, Saaristo R, Isola J, Joensuu H, Hakama M. Lumpectomy with or Without Postoperative Radiotherapy for Breast Cancer with Favourable Prognostic Features: Results of a Randomized Study. 2001. Available from: https://www.nature.com/articles/6691571

[88] Authors A, Blichert-Toft M. Long-Term Results of Breast Conserving Surgery vs. Mastectomy for Early Stage Invasive Breast Cancer: 20-Year Follow-Up of the Danish Randomized DBCG-82TM Protocol, n.d.. Available from: https://www.tandfonline.com/doi/full/10.1080/02841860801971439

[89] Wu Y, Sarkissyan M, Vadgama JV. Epigenetics in breast and prostate cancer. Methods in Molecular Biology. 2015;**1238**:425-466. DOI: 10.1007/978-1-4939-1804-1_23

[90] Kim A, Mo K, Kwon H, Choe S, Park M, Kwak W, et al. Epigenetic regulation in breast cancer: Insights on Epidrugs. Epigenomes. 2023;7(1):6. DOI: 10.3390/epigenomes7010006

[91] Erdmann A, Halby L, Fahy J, Arimondo PB. Targeting DNA methylation with small molecules: What's next? Miniperspective. Journal of Medicinal Chemistry. 2015;**58**(6):2569-2583. DOI: 10.1021/jm500843d

[92] Garcia-Martinez L, Zhang Y, Nakata Y, Chan HL, Morey L. Epigenetic mechanisms in breast cancer therapy and resistance. Nature Communications. 2021;**12**(1):1786. DOI: 10.1038/s41467-021-22024-3

[93] Szczepanek J, Skorupa M, Jarkiewicz-Tretyn J, Cybulski C, Tretyn A. Harnessing epigenetics for breast cancer therapy: The role of DNA methylation, histone modifications, and MicroRNA. International Journal of Molecular Sciences. 2023;**24**(8):7235. DOI: 10.3390/ijms24087235

[94] Noce B, Di Bello E, Fioravanti R, Mai A. LSD1 inhibitors for cancer treatment: Focus on multi-target agents and compounds in clinical trials. Frontiers in Pharmacology. 2023;**14**:1120911. DOI: 10.3389/fphar.2023.1120911

[95] Dey A, Kundu M, Das S, Jena BC, Mandal M. Understanding the function and regulation of Sox2 for its therapeutic potential in breast cancer. Biochimica et Biophysica Acta (BBA) - Reviews on Cancer. 2022;**1877**(2):188692. DOI: 10.1016/j.bbcan.2022.188692

[96] Estrogen Receptor Null Mice: What have we Learned and Where Will They ... n.d. Available from: https://www.researchgate.net/profile/Kenneth-Korach/publication/12929821_Estrogen_Receptor_Null_Mice_What_Have_We_Learned_and_Where_Will_They_Lead_Us/links/5a1c3d2845851514b530503f/Estrogen-Receptor-Null-Mice-What-Have-We-Learned-and-Where-Will-They-Lead-Us.pdf

[97] Rozeboom B, Dey N De P. Er+ Metastatic Breast Cancer: Past, Present, and a Prescription for an Apoptosis-Targeted Future. 2019. Available from: https://www.ncbi.nlm.nih.gov/pmc/articles/PMC6943351/

Chapter 4

Precision Medicine Approaches in Breast Cancer: Current Strategies and Future Directions

Omer A. Idris, Nicholas Deleon, Micah Gustafson, Delour Haj and Tiantian Zhang

Abstract

Precision medicine has revolutionized the approach to breast cancer treatment by leveraging molecular subtyping, biomarker identification, genomic profiling, and targeted therapies. This comprehensive review explores the significance of breast cancer subtypes—Luminal A, Luminal B, HER2+, and triple-negative—and their respective molecular characteristics and prognoses. It discusses the pivotal role of biomarkers such as HER2, estrogen receptors (ER), and progesterone receptors (PR) in predicting prognosis and therapy response. The review delves into advanced genomic profiling techniques, including next-generation sequencing (NGS) and fluorescence *in situ* hybridization (FISH), and their implications for personalized treatment plans. Furthermore, it highlights the potential of liquid biopsies and circulating tumor DNA (ctDNA) in non-invasive cancer diagnostics and monitoring. The integration of machine learning and artificial intelligence in predictive modeling and treatment algorithms is examined, along with the challenges posed by tumor heterogeneity and access to genomic testing. Future prospects, such as the expansion of CRISPR-based technologies and machine learning, are also discussed. Finally, strategies for integrating precision medicine into clinical practice and future innovations in the field are highlighted, emphasizing the importance of collaboration, patient education, and shared decision-making.

Keywords: precision medicine, breast cancer, cancer therapy, targeted therapies, biomarkers

1. Introduction

Breast cancer is a heterogeneous and diverse disease that presents significant challenges in its diagnosis, treatment, and prognosis due to its variability across patients and tumor types. Precision medicine has emerged as a promising approach in the field of oncology, particularly in the management of breast cancer. By customizing medical care based on individual characteristics such as genetic makeup, molecular subtype of the tumor, and specific biomarkers, precision medicine aims to enhance treatment outcomes while minimizing adverse effects [1]. Breast cancer is a global health concern, being the most diagnosed cancer type and a leading cause of cancer-related mortality among women worldwide [2, 3]. The diagnosis of breast cancer in its early stages is crucial for successful treatment [4]. Metastatic breast cancer, where the primary tumor spreads to other parts of the body, represents the most severe form of the disease [5]. It is now well-established that breast cancer comprises a diverse spectrum of diseases, each characterized by unique biological behaviors and clinical outcomes, necessitating personalized therapeutic approaches. Various biomarkers play essential roles in breast cancer diagnosis and treatment. For instance, microRNAs (miRNAs) have shown potential for diagnosing and monitoring breast cancer [6, 7]. Additionally, circulating tumor DNA methylation patterns and changes in the methylation level of microRNA genes have been explored as sensitive biomarkers for breast cancer [8, 9]. Moreover, tRNA-derived fragments have been proposed as novel diagnostic biomarkers for breast cancer, offering potential for early detection [10]. The identification of biomarkers such as miR-25-3p and miR-411 has provided insights into tumor biology and potential targets for breast cancer treatment [11, 12]. Furthermore, the discovery of a two-microRNA signature in plasma has shown promise as a novel biomarker for the early diagnosis of breast cancer, emphasizing the importance of early detection in improving patient outcomes [13]. This review provides an in-depth exploration of the key components of precision medicine in breast cancer treatment. It begins by categorizing breast cancer into four primary molecular subtypes—Luminal A, Luminal B, HER2+, and triple-negative—each with distinct molecular and clinical features. The identification and role of biomarkers, such as human epidermal growth factor receptor 2 (HER2), estrogen receptors (ER), and progesterone receptors (PR), are examined in the context of predicting prognosis and guiding treatment decisions. The advancements in genomic profiling techniques, including next-generation sequencing (NGS) and fluorescence in situ hybridization (FISH), are discussed, highlighting their impact on personalized treatment strategies. Moreover, the review addresses the emerging role of liquid biopsies and ctDNA in non-invasive cancer diagnostics and monitoring, which holds promise for early detection and real-time assessment of treatment efficacy. The integration of machine learning and artificial intelligence in predictive modeling and treatment algorithms is also explored, showcasing their potential to revolutionize breast cancer management. Despite the significant progress, challenges such as tumor heterogeneity and limited access to genomic testing persist, necessitating further research and innovative solutions.

2. Molecular subtyping and biomarker identification

2.1 Molecular subtypes

Breast cancer consists of three distinct tumor subtypes, each differentiated by variations in estrogen or progesterone receptors and HER2 gene expression [14].

2.1.1 Luminal A

Luminal A breast cancer accounts for over 50% of all breast cancer cases, making it the most common subtype [15]. Luminal A has a better prognosis compared to Luminal B, due to higher levels of PR and the upregulation of ER target genes [16].

2.1.2 Luminal B

Luminal B breast cancer expresses fewer hormone receptors, has a higher histologic grade than Luminal A, and exhibits more proliferation markers [17]. The prognosis for Luminal B is poorer, primarily due to lower PR levels [16]. Early differentiation between Luminal A and Luminal B subtypes is crucial for treatment, as each has unique molecular characteristics [18]. Research has shown that distinct treatment strategies are required for Luminal A and Luminal B cancers to address their respective molecular signatures [17].

2.1.3 HER2+

HER2+ BC is characterized by the overexpression of the HER2 gene, leading to abnormal proliferation and division of breast tissue cells [19]. This subtype is aggressive and spreads rapidly, but therapies like Herceptin® (trastuzumab) have been highly effective [19]. Identifying HER2-amplified tumors and developing new strategies to manage resistance have become a significant topic in ongoing research [20].

2.1.4 Triple-negative breast cancer (TNBC)

TNBC lacks ER, PR, and HER2 expression [21]. TNBC is prone to relapse, has a poor prognosis, and exhibits high metastatic potential [21]. TNBC is known for its aggressive

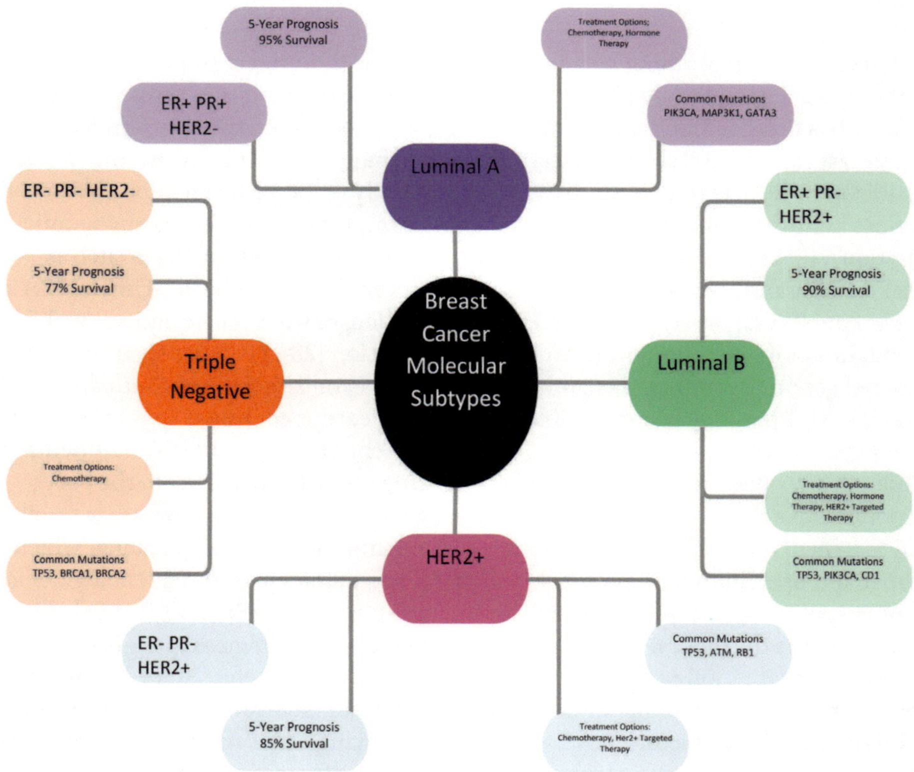

Figure 1.
Characteristics and treatment options for breast cancer molecular subtypes.

clinical behavior and is more commonly found in women of Hispanic or African descent [22]. Due to limited treatment options, ongoing research is focused on developing novel therapies, including immunotherapies, for TNBC patients (**Figure 1**) [16].

2.2 Biomarkers

Tumor biomarkers for clinical use should be able to predict prognosis and therapy response [23]. HER2 is a prognostic biomarker not only for breast cancer but also for stomach and colon cancers [24]. It has been associated with increased survival benefits when combined with chemotherapy and anti-HER2 therapy in advanced or recurrent disease cases [24].

The use of estrogen receptors (ERs) as biomarkers remains controversial, primarily due to much of the research being conducted with inadequately validated antibodies [25]. Nevertheless, ERs, along with PR and HER2, are currently the most common biomarkers used by oncologists to guide treatment plans [26]. Selective progesterone receptor modulators (SPRMs) are designed to target PR with agonist/antagonistic properties [26]. In ER-positive cases, PR remains a prognostic marker, and the American Society of Clinical Oncology continues to endorse ER testing in invasive breast cancer cases [27].

3. Tumor genomic profiling and targeted therapies

3.1 Genomic profiling techniques

Gene expression profiling techniques have become essential in breast cancer treatment [28]. Assessing family history for hereditary cancer syndromes through genomic profiling has become standard practice in many cases of malignancies or advanced-stage breast cancers [28]. Next-generation sequencing (NGS) and fluorescence *in situ* hybridization (FISH) remain the two most commonly employed techniques. While NGS provides high-throughput sequencing, enabling comprehensive analysis of genomic alterations, FISH is more suited to detecting specific genetic abnormalities such as translocations and amplifications. A balanced approach utilizing both technologies can offer enhanced diagnostic precision. However, challenges such as cost and accessibility remain significant hurdles for wider implementation [28]. NGS has significantly impacted genomic profiling, becoming more effective, reliable, and cost-effective [29]. Although NGS has only been available for about 15 years, it continues to gain support and is expected to grow rapidly [30]. NGS can sequence millions of DNA fragments without prior sequence knowledge, revolutionizing the field compared to the previous polymerase chain reaction (PCR) method, which could only analyze a few small DNA fragments [29]. NGS models are categorized into short-read sequencing, which is cheaper and uses Illumina® protocols and machines, and long-read sequencing, which is more expensive and utilizes PacBio® or Roche® platforms [29]. Until 2017, short-read sequencing was the most widely used NGS method due to its low cost per gigabase and precision. However, long-read sequencing has become more preferred for its advantages in bioinformatics pipeline alignment, making it more suitable for DNA selection and various chromosomal factors [29]. Long-read sequencing offers precise comprehension of full-length (FL) isoforms, eliminating the need for reference-based transcription [30]. Despite the advances in NGS efficiency and accuracy, further research is required before it can be standardized [31]. FISH also plays a crucial role in genomic profiling.

FISH has demonstrated proficiency in personalized medicine by detecting abnormalities related to translocations, insertions, inversions, deletions, and amplifications [32]. Advances in FISH methods have enabled the deciphering of RNA transcription and degradation rates [33]. FISH involves combining fixed-point cells with fluorescent oligonucleotide probes, which permeates the cell and binds to the RNA of interest. These probes create fluorescent spots within tumor cells, which can be numerically assessed for RNA location and type [34]. Practical applications of FISH have been successful in HER2 enumeration and assessing heterogeneity among HER2 signaling, although challenges remain with poor image quality and high background instances [35]. Precision medicine is fundamentally based on the idea that aligning targeted therapies with the molecular subtypes of patients enhances efficacy, reduces toxicity, and ultimately improves clinical outcomes. To address the heterogeneity inherent in existing breast cancer classification systems [36], there was a need for more robust subgroups. This led Perou et al. [37] to develop an integrated genome-driven classification within the METABRIC cohort. This innovative classification combines genomic and transcriptomic profiles of breast cancer to define 10 integrative clusters, each characterized by unique clinical outcomes and subtype-specific candidate drivers. Recent advancements in high-throughput genomics, particularly through the application of massively parallel sequencing (MPS), have substantially improved our understanding of the genomic complexity of breast cancer. These technologies have allowed for comprehensive exploration of somatic changes in breast cancer, such as gene mutations, structural variants, copy number alterations, transcriptional dysregulation, and epigenetic modifications [38–41]. By combining genomic and transcriptional data, new breast cancer subgroups with distinct clinical outcomes were identified. This integration led to the development of a robust molecular taxonomy that refines and enhances existing classification systems [37]. As shown in **Figure 2**, next-generation sequencing (NGS) and fluorescence *in situ* hybridization (FISH) methodologies each have distinct applications, advantages, and limitations that contribute to advancements in genomic research and diagnostics.

3.2 Targeted therapies

Targeted therapies in breast cancer management have become invaluable due to their ability to attack cancer cell proteins with chemotherapeutic agents [42]. Endocrine therapies, such as HER2-targeted treatment, have advanced precision medicine in breast cancer treatment [43]. The success of anti-HER2 therapies, particularly trastuzumab, underscores the potential of targeted treatments. However, resistance remains a critical challenge, often arising from mutations in downstream signaling pathways like PI3K/AKT. Addressing these resistance mechanisms through novel therapeutic combinations is essential for improving outcomes [43]. Since early-stage breast cancer is considered potentially curable, advances in anti-HER2 targeting and chemotherapy hold promise for long-term control of the disease [44]. As of 2023, HER2 has become a significant target in breast cancer therapy. The effectiveness of the HER2 approach was established through repeated testing of anti-HER2 antibody-drug conjugates [45]. Molecular biology research and immunotherapy have enabled the design of patient-specific treatments based on HER2 status [46]. Despite initial skepticism and extensive debate among a 32-panel multidisciplinary team from nine countries, HER2-targeted therapy successfully launched, leading to the development of trastuzumab deruxtecan (T-DXd, Ds-8210), a recombinant antibody targeting HER2 [45, 46]. T-DXd has shown promising results in breast cancer patients. In the phase 2 DESTINY-Breast01 trial, T-DXd achieved a 60.9% response rate and a median progression-free survival

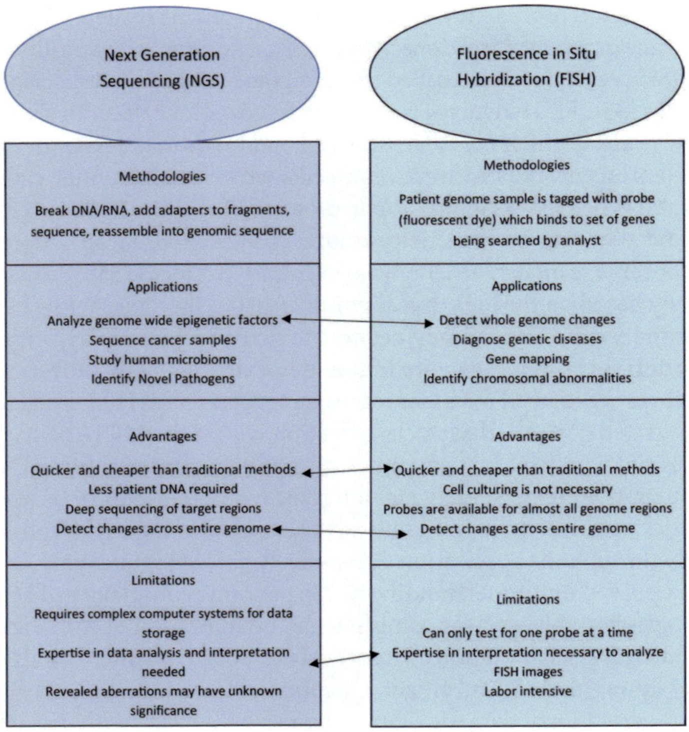

Figure 2.
Comparative overview of NGS and FISH methodologies in genomic research.

of 16.4 months, offering hope for HER2 metastatic breast cancer patients who had received at least two prior anti-HER2-based regimens [47]. However, approximately 50% of HER2+ breast cancer patients do not respond to HER2-targeted therapy, and about 20% experience relapse [48]. For HER2-overexpressing breast tumors, poly (ADP-ribose) polymerase (PARP) inhibitors play a role in destabilizing replication forks by trapping PARP on DNA, leading to cell death through stress-induced mitotic catastrophe [49]. PARP consists of 17 members, with PARP-1 being the primary enzyme involved in DNA repair, and PARP-2 and PARP-3 serving as essential overlapping repair units [50]. Resistance to PARP inhibitors, like other targeted therapies, presents challenges. Although the interaction between PARP inhibitors and BRCA synthetic lethality has been shown to selectively kill cancer cells, the mechanisms behind the development of resistance to PARP inhibitors have also been investigated. These include mutations in BRCA genes, the emergence of resistant BRCA-defective tumor cells, and the involvement of DNA repair proteins. While these discoveries have shed light on resistance pathways, additional research is desired to enhance their effectiveness in combination therapies [51]. Another important inhibitor is 2-deoxy-4β-propylcarbamate-pulchellin (P-13), which has proven effective in managing STAT3 signaling and overall cancer cell growth [46]. In cases of HER2 overexpression, estrogen receptors and co-activator proteins can lead to tamoxifen resistance. P-13 can engage signaling pathways to develop endocrine resistance, making it a potential target for overcoming therapy resistance [52]. As summarized in **Table 1**, PARP inhibitors, CDK inhibitors, HER2 inhibitors, and angiogenesis inhibitors each have distinct mechanisms of action and targets that contribute to their anti-cancer effects.

	PARP inhibitors	CDK inhibitors	HER2 inhibitors	Angiogenesis inhibitors
Mechanism of action	Small molecule that diffuses into cell and stops cell's DNA repair	Small molecule that diffuses into cell to stop cell signaling	Monoclonal antibody that attaches to cell surface to cause desired effect	Monoclonal antibody which prevents tumor from forming new blood vessels
Target	Poly (ADP-ribose) polymerase (PARP)	Cyclin-dependent kinase (CDK)	HER2 transmembrane protein	Vascular endothelial growth factor (VEGF)
Effect on cancer cells	Cell death	Cell death	Reduced ability to divide and grow	Cancer cells unable to access nutrients

Table 1.
Examples of targeted therapy modalities for breast cancer.

4. Tumor detection: Liquid biopsies and circulating biomarkers

4.1 Liquid biopsies

Liquid biopsy technologies are transforming breast cancer diagnostics by providing non-invasive monitoring tools. These methods not only offer early detection of relapse but also allow for real-time tracking of treatment efficacy. However, integration into clinical practice requires overcoming challenges related to standardization and ensuring broad access, especially in low-resource settings [53, 54]. Breast cancer is a highly heterogeneous disease, making its treatment more complex and presenting many challenges [55]. Approximately 90% of cancer therapy-related deaths are due to drug resistance, whether through traditional chemotherapy or new targeted drugs [56]. Drug resistance mechanisms include increased metabolism of xenobiotics, enhanced drug efflux, growth factors such as VEGF and EGF that promote cell survival and proliferation, increased DNA repair capacity, and certain genetic factors. These growth factors activate downstream signaling pathways such as PI3K/AKT and MAPK, which enhance cell resistance to therapy. However, liquid biopsies have shown the potential to identify better treatments non-invasively, offering hope in this area of precision medicine [56]. Previously, liquid biopsies were inadequate for analyzing breast cancer comprehensively, but new techniques have significantly improved their effectiveness. This innovation now allows clinicians to discern early diagnoses, predict prognoses, enable serial sampling, facilitate screening, and offers several other useful features [57]. When working with free circulating tumor DNA, liquid biopsies have become a sought-after, non-invasive alternative to other high-cost, high-risk diagnostic options [58]. As treatments are adopted and combined with liquid biopsy technology, monitoring the progression of treatment remains crucial. To monitor disease progress and therapy response, circulating biomarkers have been extremely beneficial in detecting changes in mutation and tumor quality [59]. Biomarkers are now regarded as proper prognostic and predictive factors in breast cancer [60]. One of these biomarkers is circulating tumor DNA.

4.2 Circulating biomarkers

Circulating tumor DNA (ctDNA), composed of "naked" DNA molecules released from cancer cells, has been paired with liquid biopsies to help identify breast cancer mutations [61]. These DNA particles can serve as a replacement for tumor tissues, allowing for effective treatment response predictions and counter-resistance solutions, making them favorable over traditional biopsies [61]. ctDNA analysis functions non-invasively as a biomarker and shows promise in early-stage breast cancer detection, complementing tissue biopsy as a biomarker [62]. Minimal residual disease (MRD) has been detected using ctDNA, aiding in determining relapse periods in advanced cancers [63]. MRD, associated with relapse and particularly found in individuals showing no signs of metastasis, could otherwise lead to undetected recurrence [64]. In this context, ctDNA has further potential to facilitate adequate clinical trialing with minimal risk factors [65]. Fragment size analysis, a noteworthy subcategory of ctDNA, has proven successful in exploiting different fragment lengths of circulating DNA for higher sensitivity yield from ctDNA. This analysis has identified significant mutations and copy number alterations that could otherwise go unnoticed, highlighting the vast potential for further research into ctDNA [66].

5. Cancer treatment algorithms and predictive modeling

5.1 The use of machine learning and artificial intelligence in predicting treatment outcomes

Artificial intelligence (AI) and machine learning (ML) hold great promise in revolutionizing cancer care by predicting treatment outcomes based on genomic and clinical data. Early models, such as deep learning algorithms, have already demonstrated superior performance compared to traditional predictive models. Future advancements in AI will likely focus on further integrating genomic data into treatment algorithms, facilitating even more personalized care [67, 68]. Artificial neural networks, a form of machine learning, have also been successfully used to predict breast cancer prognosis by considering factors such as age, tumor size, histological type, nuclear pleomorphism, tubule formation, axillary nodal status, mitotic count, and tumor necrosis [69]. Deep learning algorithms, another form of machine learning, have demonstrated better performance than traditional models. For example, the Gail model, which calculates breast cancer risk based on medical and reproductive history, was significantly less effective in malignancy prediction compared to artificial intelligence trained solely on clinical data [70]. The Tyrer-Cuzick model, which calculates the likelihood of carrying BRCA1 and BRCA2 mutations (mutations associated with an increased likelihood of breast cancer), was also outperformed by a hybrid deep learning model [71]. While still in the early stages, these advancements show significant promise for the future of artificial intelligence in predicting breast cancer risk, reducing workload, and predicting potential treatments based on patient DNA analysis.

5.2 How genomic data and clinical factors are used in evolving treatment plans?

Breast cancer treatments are increasingly data-driven, and using genomic information from patients can significantly improve treatment success. NGS, which can sequence DNA and reveal genetic variations associated with diseases, has been employed to better understand patients' tumors. Data gathered from NGS technologies also have the potential to create more personalized care plans for patients [72].

By analyzing a person's genomic data, more effective treatment plans can be tailored to the patient's specific needs. Chromatin immunoprecipitation sequencing (ChIP-seq), a specific form of NGS, has been used to identify changes in protein-DNA interactions among patients [73]. This was achieved using algorithms developed through artificial intelligence. Currently, meta-analyses of data gathered from ChIP-seq have led to the discovery of new protein-DNA binding sites associated with breast cancer [74]. Although NGS is still relatively new, it shows remarkable potential in identifying new treatment avenues for breast cancer. Clinical factors also impact the quality of life during and after treatment. Specifically, using algorithms to investigate drug sensitivity or resistance to previously administered drugs provides physicians with opportunities to more effectively choose treatments if the cancer progresses [75]. Furthermore, exploring clinical factors such as surgical intervention, BMI, and the presence of comorbidities during breast cancer treatment can help correlate with post-treatment quality of life [76]. This suggests that considering clinical factors and genomic data together in algorithms can allow clinicians to plan better for potential treatments, which leads to improved health outcomes.

6. Challenges and limitations of precision medicine

6.1 Major challenges with respect to tumor heterogeneity

The primary goal of precision medicine in breast cancer treatment is to identify specific genome mutations within a patient to match them with the most effective therapy. However, breast cancer is a highly heterogeneous disease, observable through both inter-tumor heterogeneity and intra-tumor heterogeneity [55]. The phenotypes of cells composing a tumor may also be influenced by the normal cells surrounding the area. This complexity is further heightened by the fact that the tumor microenvironment changes as people age, potentially increasing the likelihood of tumor growth [77]. A specific component of the microenvironment in tumor cells, the extracellular matrix (ECM), plays a significant role in inter-cell communication. Breast tissue cells remodel the ECM as the body transitions through different reproductive states. However, deregulation of this remodeling process may lead to ECM-induced signaling that promotes tumor growth [78]. This can result in substantial differences in phenotypes not only within the same individual but also within different regions of the same tumor [79]. Consequently, the wide range of inter-tumor and intra-tumor differences presents a significant challenge that needs further research for precision medicine to be effectively utilized in developing treatment options for patients.

6.2 Major challenges with respect to access to genomic testing

Another challenge precision medicine faces is the limited accessibility of genomic testing for many individuals. For example, communities in rural areas are often underserved and may encounter transportation challenges when trying to reach urban centers that offer genomic testing. In rural Kansas, the introduction of a primary care physician (PCP) clinic with genomic testing significantly shortened the diagnosis time by 5.5 months [80]. This indicates that many rural communities lack access to genomic testing, likely facing long waitlists and delays. Furthermore, this only considers the diagnosis *via* genomic testing and not the availability of the actual treatment.

6.3 Data interpretation issues and other limitations

Data gathered from genomic testing can be difficult to interpret due to the complexity of breast cancer cases. The classification of cancer variants is crucial in determining proper treatment, and incorrect classification may result in either insufficient or excessive therapeutic intervention for the patient [81]. Different variants may also be classified similarly depending on the interpretation method used, making it challenging for physicians to differentiate [82]. Furthermore, differences between the fecal microbiota of healthy women and women with breast cancer have been observed [83]. As discussed earlier, breast cancer heterogeneity depends on the surrounding microenvironment, which includes surrounding bacteria. To properly diagnose breast cancer through genomic testing, more research is needed on how these bacteria influence tumor development and potential treatment avenues [84]. Additionally, more driver mutations for cancer must be identified to fully realize the effectiveness of precision medicine [85]. This presents challenges in treating and interpreting the genomic data of patients with rarer variants of breast cancer. Once these limitations are addressed, precision medicine can significantly impact patient prognosis and personalized treatment.

7. Integration of precision medicine into clinical practice

7.1 Possible strategies to integrate precision medicine into routine care

The integration of precision medicine into routine care involves combining several approaches. First, more reference genomes must be created to better represent different races. Current reference genomes are not typically representative of all populations, such as those of African descent [86]. Furthermore, genomic testing often results in high levels of variants of unknown significance [87]. This is especially true for breast cancer, where the rates of findings with unknown significance in genomic testing are relatively high [88]. One potential solution to these problems is creating a budget allocated specifically for precision medicine. This would help address both technological issues and equitable access. For example, in Belgium, a budget allocation for the reimbursement of NGS has resulted in a greater number of tests being performed [89]. More standardization at both national and international levels is also recommended to increase the integration of precision medicine into routine care. Currently, precision medicine practices vary across hospitals, and it is necessary to examine these differences to identify the most effective practices for proper integration [90]. This is best achieved through collaboration between private, public, and multi-stakeholder sectors, with a focus on growth in the NGS industry [91]. By adopting these strategies, the obstacles preventing the full implementation of precision medicine in healthcare will be removed, and the potential of precision medicine will be fully realized.

7.2 Importance of teamwork, patient education, and shared decision making

In clinics where precision medicine is currently being utilized, fostering collaboration between patients and their healthcare teams can significantly improve health outcomes. Modern guidelines for breast cancer screening highly recommend a stepwise risk assessment that considers personal and family history. Primary care physicians can use this information to determine the most effective screening options for individual patients, thereby enhancing clinical care and shared decision-making [92]. Moreover, assistance from genetic counselors in managing this information increases the efficiency of obtaining the correct diagnosis and treatment by leveraging their expertise in specific cases [93]. Genetic counselors are specifically trained to consider both the results from genome testing and the patient's family and psychological history. The involvement of several trained professionals in data analysis helps reduce the time needed to identify the best screening choices available for the patient. Thus, they play a crucial role in creating shared decision-making opportunities by helping patients navigate their potential options [94]. Finally, creating opportunities for patients to be educated about genome sequencing and how it will help their case can greatly assist in integrating precision medicine into routine care. Patient-organized research summits and other educational events can help patients understand the possibilities and limitations of their treatments [95]. Furthermore, these events can help physicians understand which aspects of treatment are most important to patients. By increasing teamwork and collaboration between patients, primary care physicians, genetic counselors, and other involved parties, the integration of precision medicine into routine care will be smoother and more effective.

8. Future directions and innovations

8.1 New technologies and innovations in the field of precision medicine

Precision medicine represents a revolutionary approach to healthcare, especially in oncology, where an individual's genome can greatly influence which treatment will be most effective. The past decade has seen major advancements in this field, showing great promise in improving health outcomes for breast cancer patients. Currently, one of the most important advancements in precision medicine is its use in determining different treatment options for patients through comprehensive analysis of all genomic mutations [96]. For example, identifying BRCA1 and BRCA2 mutations helps physicians decide which therapies to choose, enabling more effective treatment for patients with BRCA-positive breast cancers. This approach has been implemented and has shown effectiveness so far [97]. Moreover, the challenges presented by subtypes such as triple-negative breast cancer (TNBC)—which accounts for about one-fifth of all breast cancer cases and lacks effective molecular-based therapeutics—underscore the importance of precision medicine [98]. The heterogeneity of TNBC complicates treatment, often relegating patients to traditional and more toxic therapies [99]. Precision medicine can identify biomarkers specific to individual patients, aiding physicians in selecting and optimizing treatment options, including emerging therapies targeting specific subtypes of TNBC [100]. Additionally, precision medicine has been shown to improve endocrine therapy outcomes by reducing the chance of acquiring resistance to drugs from prolonged exposure to therapy. The use of precision medicine in endocrine therapies has led to new innovations in treatment options for hormone receptor-positive breast cancer [101]. Finally, using precision medicine to monitor the progress of treatment through liquid biopsy analysis allows caregivers to track therapy progress in a simple and non-invasive way, while also helping to identify potential new mutations. With proper integration into routine oncology care, these innovations will greatly improve health outcomes for many cancer patients, not just those with breast cancer.

8.2 Current research efforts and potential future breakthroughs

There continues to be ongoing research in the field of precision medicine with many new innovations and technologies still being developed. For example, advancements have been seen in immunotherapy, assisting the patient's immune system to more effectively recognize and eliminate breast cancer tissue. Precision medicine has helped identify drugs that support the immune system in these actions, which is currently undergoing clinical trials with promising results so far [102]. This is particularly important for those with TNBC, who are unresponsive to typical hormonal therapy or HER2-target drugs. Furthermore, developments in NGS are necessary to better account for epigenetic changes, phenotypic plasticity, clonal heterogeneity, and compensatory mutations [103]. Advances in technologies that leverage a patient's epigenome are currently under study. Existing drugs that can modify a person's epigenome for therapeutic effect do not have high specificity for the cancer-causing epigenetic aberrations and may lead to additional toxicity in some patients [104]. Emerging technologies such as CRISPR-based gene editing and new epigenetic therapies offer promising potential. CRISPR holds promise for locus-specific interventions that could target the genetic roots of cancer with high precision. Ongoing research into these technologies will help refine their application in breast cancer treatment, potentially offering cures for previously untreatable cases [105]. Alongside advancements in immunotherapies, these new technologies represent a transformative approach to healthcare. Epigenomics, liquid biopsies, and personalized drug development are revolutionizing the way diseases are diagnosed and treated. As these technologies continue to develop, precision medicine will usher in a new era of cancer therapy.

9. Conclusion

Precision medicine has undeniably transformed the landscape of breast cancer treatment, offering hope for more personalized and effective therapies. The detailed understanding of molecular subtypes and the identification of specific biomarkers have paved the way for targeted therapies that improve patient outcomes. Genomic profiling techniques, such as NGS and FISH, have enhanced our ability to tailor treatments to individual patients, while liquid biopsies and ctDNA provide non-invasive means to monitor disease progression and treatment response. However, the journey toward fully realizing the potential of precision medicine in breast cancer is fraught with challenges. Tumor heterogeneity, treatment resistance, and unequal access to genomic testing remain major obstacles. Tumor heterogeneity, for example, complicates the ability to generalize treatment strategies, requiring a more granular approach that takes into account intra-tumor variations. Data interpretation, especially in genomic sequencing, is also a challenge, as the complexity of the results may hinder clear therapeutic pathways. Integrating precision medicine into routine clinical practice requires concerted efforts in standardization, patient education, and collaboration among healthcare professionals. Standardizing the technologies used in genomic profiling and making them more affordable and accessible will help bridge these gaps. Additionally, patient education about precision medicine and its implications will empower patients to make informed decisions about their treatment. Unequal access to genomic testing, especially in resource-limited settings, exacerbates health disparities in cancer care. Collaborative efforts will be needed to overcome these barriers and ensure equitable access to personalized care. Looking ahead, the continued advancement of technologies and innovations in precision medicine holds great promise for the future. Emerging technologies such as CRISPR-based gene editing, artificial intelligence in predictive modeling, and liquid biopsy innovations offer significant potential for improving treatment outcomes. These advancements, if implemented on a broader scale, could help overcome the current limitations of tumor heterogeneity and resistance mechanisms. By fostering teamwork, enhancing patient education, and promoting shared decision-making, we can further integrate precision medicine into clinical practice, ultimately improving the quality of care and outcomes for breast cancer patients. The field of precision medicine is poised for significant breakthroughs, and with ongoing research and innovation, it has the potential to revolutionize breast cancer treatment.

Conflict of interest

The authors declare no conflict of interest.

Author details

Omer A. Idris[1,2]*, Nicholas Deleon[3], Micah Gustafson[4], Delour Haj[5] and Tiantian Zhang[6]

1 Department of Biological Science, Western Michigan University, Kalamazoo, MI, USA

2 Malate Institute for Medical Research, Malate Inc., Grandville, MI, USA

3 Lyman Briggs College, Michigan State University, Lansing, MI, USA

4 Department of Biological and Health Sciences, Wheaton College, Wheaton, IL, USA

5 Western Michigan University Homer Stryker MD School of Medicine, Kalamazoo, MI, USA

6 Toni Stephenson Lymphoma Center, Department of Hematology and Hematopoietic Stem Cell Transplantation, Bechman Research Institute, City of Hope, Duarte, CA, USA

*Address all correspondence to: omer.a.idris@wmich.edu

References

[1] Efird JT, Jindal C, Biswas T. On the frontiers of breast cancer diagnosis and treatment: Current and future directions in a rapidly changing field. Medicina. 2022;**58**(8):1026. DOI: 10.3390/medicina58081026

[2] Wu H, Chu P. Recent discoveries of macromolecule- and cell-based biomarkers and therapeutic implications in breast cancer. International Journal of Molecular Sciences. 2021;**22**(2):636. DOI: 10.3390/ijms22020636

[3] Aghaei M. Breast cancer, a global health crisis. International Journal of New Findings in Health and Educational Sciences (IJHES). 2023;**1**(2):79-87. DOI: 10.63053/ijhes.23

[4] Jafari SH, Saadatpour Z, Salmaninejad A, Momeni F, Mokhtari M, Nahand JS, et al. Breast cancer diagnosis: Imaging techniques and biochemical markers. Journal of Cellular Physiology. 2018;**233**(7):5200-5213. DOI: 10.1002/jcp.26379

[5] McGuire A, Brown JAL, Kerin MJ. Metastatic breast cancer: The potential of mirna for diagnosis and treatment monitoring. Cancer and Metastasis Reviews. 2015;**34**(1):145-155. DOI: 10.1007/s10555-015-9551-7

[6] Huang Y, Ge H, Zheng M, Cui Y, Fu Z, Wu X, et al. Serum trna-derived fragments (trfs) as potential candidates for diagnosis of nontriple negative breast cancer. Journal of Cellular Physiology. 2019;**235**(3):2809-2824. DOI: 10.1002/jcp.29185

[7] Lee JD, Cai Q, Shu XO, Nechuta S. The role of biomarkers of oxidative stress in breast cancer risk and prognosis: A systematic review of the epidemiologic literature. Journal of Women's Health. 2017;**26**(5):467-482. DOI: 10.1089/jwh.2016.5973

[8] Hai L, Li L, Liu Z, Tong Z, Sun Y. Whole-genome circulating tumor DNA methylation landscape reveals sensitive biomarkers of breast cancer. MedComm. 2022;**3**(3):8-11. DOI: 10.1002/mco2.134

[9] Филиппова ЕА, Бурденный АМ, Лукина СС, Ivanova NA, Пронина ИВ, Казубская ТП, et al. Changes in the methylation level of microrna genes as a factor of breast cancer development and progression. Patologicheskaia Fiziologiia I Eksperimental'naia Terapiia. 2021;**3**:4-11. DOI: 10.25557/0031-2991.2021.03.4-11

[10] Zhang Y, Zhao B, Dong X, Yu M, Wang K, Xie L, et al. tRNA-derived fragments: tRF-gly-ccc-046, trf-tyr-gta-010 and trf-pro-tgg-001 as novel diagnostic biomarkers for breast cancer. Thoracic Cancer. 2021;**12**(17):2314-2323. DOI: 10.1111/1759-7714.14072

[11] Zhao T, Wang M, Chin Y, Gao L, Yang X, Sun S, et al. Identification of mir-25-3p as a tumor biomarker: Regulation of cellular functions via tob1 in breast cancer. Molecular Medicine Reports. 2021;**23**(6):1-10. DOI: 10.3892/mmr.2021.12045

[12] Cao S, Zheng L. Microrna-411 Represents an Innovative Bio-Marker in Breast Cancer Detection. Durham, North Carolina, USA: Research Square; 2020. DOI: 10.21203/rs.3.rs-54155/v1

[13] Adam-Artigues A, Garrido-Cano I, Carbonell-Asíns JA, Lameirinhas A, Simón S, Ortega-Morillo B, et al. Identification of a two-microrna signature in plasma as a novel biomarker

for very early diagnosis of breast cancer. Cancers. 2021;**13**(11):2848. DOI: 10.3390/cancers13112848

[14] Waks AG, Winer EP. Breast cancer treatment: A review. Journal of the American Medical Association. 2019;**321**(3):288-300. DOI: 10.1001/jama.2018.19323

[15] Gao JJ, Swain SM. Luminal A breast cancer and molecular assays: A review. The Oncologist. 2018;**23**(5):556-565. DOI: 10.1634/theoncologist.2017-0535. Epub 2018 Feb 22

[16] Li Z, Wei H, Li S, Wu P, Mao X. The role of progesterone receptors in breast cancer. Drug Design, Development and Therapy. 2022;**16**:305-314. DOI: 10.2147/DDDT.S336643

[17] Ades F, Zardavas D, Bozovic-Spasojevic I, Pugliano L, Fumagalli D, de Azambuja E, et al. Luminal B breast cancer: Molecular characterization, clinical management, and future perspectives. Journal of Clinical Oncology. 2014;**32**(25):2794-2803. DOI: 10.1200/JCO.2013.54.1870. Epub 2014 Jul 21

[18] Kudela E, Samec M, Koklesova L, Liskova A, Kubatka P, Kozubik E, et al. miRNA expression profiles in luminal a breast cancer-implications in biology, prognosis, and prediction of response to hormonal treatment. International Journal of Molecular Sciences. 2020;**21**(20):7691. DOI: 10.3390/ijms21207691

[19] Asif HM, Sultana S, Ahmed S, Akhtar N, Tariq M. HER-2 positive breast cancer—A mini-review. Asian Pacific Journal of Cancer Prevention. 2016;**17**(4):1609-1615. DOI: 10.7314/apjcp.2016.17.4.1609

[20] Escrivá-de-Romaní S, Arumí M, Bellet M, Saura C. HER2-positive breast cancer: Current and new therapeutic strategies. Breast. 2018;**39**:80-88. DOI: 10.1016/j.breast.2018.03.006. Epub 2018 Apr 6

[21] Yin L, Duan JJ, Bian XW, Yu SC. Triple-negative breast cancer molecular subtyping and treatment progress. Breast Cancer Research. 2020;**22**(1):61. DOI: 10.1186/s13058-020-01296-5

[22] Derakhshan F, Reis-Filho JS. Pathogenesis of triple-negative breast cancer. Annual Review of Pathology. 2022;**17**:181-204. DOI: 10.1146/annurev-pathol-042420-093238

[23] Iwamoto T, Kajiwara Y, Zhu Y, Iha S. Biomarkers of neoadjuvant/adjuvant chemotherapy for breast cancer. Chinese Clinical Oncology. 2020;**9**(3):27. DOI: 10.21037/cco.2020.01.06. Epub 2020 Mar 13

[24] Talia KL, Banet N, Buza N. The role of HER2 as a therapeutic biomarker in gynaecological malignancy: Potential for use beyond uterine serous carcinoma. Pathology. 2023;**55**(1):8-18. DOI: 10.1016/j.pathol.2022.11.004. Epub 2022 Nov 23

[25] Božović A, Mandušić V, Todorović L, Krajnović M. Estrogen receptor beta: The promising biomarker and potential target in metastases. International Journal of Molecular Sciences. 2021;**22**(4):1656. DOI: 10.3390/ijms22041656

[26] Hou Y, Peng Y, Li Z. Update on prognostic and predictive biomarkers of breast cancer. Seminars in Diagnostic Pathology. 2022;**39**(5):322-332. DOI: 10.1053/j.semdp.2022.06.015. Epub 2022 Jun 18

[27] Allison KH, Hammond MEH, Dowsett M, McKernin SE, Carey LA, Fitzgibbons PL, et al. Estrogen and progesterone receptor testing in

breast cancer: ASCO/CAP guideline update. Journal of Clinical Oncology. 2020;**38**(12):1346-1366. DOI: 10.1200/JCO.19.02309. Epub 2020 Jan 13

[28] Litton JK, Burstein HJ, Turner NC. Molecular testing in breast cancer. American Society of Clinical Oncology Educational Book. 2019;**39**:e1-e7. DOI: 10.1200/EDBK_237715. Epub 2019 May 17

[29] Kamps R, Brandão RD, Bosch BJ, Paulussen AD, Xanthoulea S, Blok MJ, et al. Next-generation sequencing in oncology: Genetic diagnosis, risk prediction and cancer classification. International Journal of Molecular Sciences. 2017;**18**(2):308. DOI: 10.3390/ijms18020308

[30] Xin R, Gao Y, Gao Y, Wang R, Kadash-Edmondson KE, Liu B, et al. Isocirc catalogs full-length circular rna isoforms in human transcriptomes. Nature Communications. 2021;**12**(1):2-7. DOI: 10.1038/s41467-020-20459-8

[31] Shendure J, Findlay GM, Snyder MW. Genomic medicine–progress, pitfalls, and promise. Cell. 2019;**177**(1):45-57. DOI: 10.1016/j.cell.2019.02.003

[32] Chrzanowska NM, Kowalewski J, Lewandowska MA. Use of fluorescence in situ hybridization (FISH) in diagnosis and tailored therapies in solid tumors. Molecules. 2020;**25**(8):1864. DOI: 10.3390/molecules25081864

[33] Vautrot V, Heckler G, Aigueperse C, Behm-Ansmant I. Fluorescence in situ hybridization of small non-coding RNAs. Methods in Molecular Biology. 2021;**2300**:73-85. DOI: 10.1007/978-1-0716-1386-3_8

[34] Moffitt JR, Zhuang X. RNA imaging with multiplexed error-robust fluorescence In situ hybridization (MERFISH). Methods in Enzymology. 2016;**572**:1-49. DOI: 10.1016/bs.mie.2016.03.020. Epub 2016 Apr 27

[35] Harun A, Liu H, Song S, Asghar S, Wen X, Fang Z, et al. Oligonucleotide fluorescence in situ hybridization: An efficient chromosome painting method in plants. Plants. 2023;**12**(15):2816. DOI: 10.3390/plants12152816

[36] Smith CEP, Prasad V. Targeted cancer therapies. American Family Physician. 2021;**103**(3):155-163

[37] Perou CM, Sørlie T, Eisen MB, van de Rijn M, Jeffrey SS, Rees CA, et al. Molecular portraits of human breast tumours. Nature. 2000;**406**(6797):747-752. DOI: 10.1038/35021093

[38] Chia S, Bramwell V, Tu D, Shepherd LE, Jiang S, Vickery TL, et al. A 50-gene intrinsic subtype classifier for prognosis and prediction of benefit from adjuvant tamoxifen. Clinical Cancer Research. 2012;**18**(16):4465-4472. DOI: 10.1158/1078-0432.ccr-12-0286

[39] Curtis C, Shah SP, Chin S, Turashvili G, Rueda OM, Dunning MJ, et al. The genomic and transcriptomic architecture of 2,000 breast tumours reveals novel subgroups. Nature. 2012;**486**(7403):346-352. DOI: 10.1038/nature10983

[40] Banerji S, Cibulskis K, Rangel-Escareño C, Brown KK, Carter SL, Frederick AM, et al. Sequence analysis of mutations and translocations across breast cancer subtypes. Nature. 2012;**486**(7403):405-409. DOI: 10.1038/nature11154

[41] Ellis MJ, Li D, Shen D, Luo J, Suman VJ, Wallis JW, et al. Whole-genome analysis informs breast cancer response to aromatase inhibition. Nature.

2012;**486**(7403):353-360. DOI: 10.1038/nature11143

[42] Koboldt DC, Fulton RS, McLellan MD, Schmidt H, Kalicki-Veizer J, McMichael JF, et al. Comprehensive molecular portraits of human breast tumours. Nature. 2012;**490**(7418):61-70. DOI: 10.1038/nature11412

[43] Greenwalt I, Zaza N, Das S, Li BD. Precision medicine and targeted therapies in breast cancer. Surgical Oncology Clinics of North America. 2020;**29**(1):51-62. DOI: 10.1016/j.soc.2019.08.004. Epub 2019 Oct 29

[44] Harbeck N, Gnant M. Breast cancer. Lancet. 2017;**389**(10074):1134-1150. DOI: 10.1016/S0140-6736(16)31891-8. Epub 2016 Nov 17

[45] Tarantino P, Viale G, Press MF, Hu X, Penault-Llorca F, Bardia A, et al. ESMO expert consensus statements (ECS) on the definition, diagnosis, and management of HER2-low breast cancer. Annals of Oncology. 2023;**34**(8):645-659. DOI: 10.1016/j.annonc.2023.05.008. Epub 2023 Jun 1

[46] Costa R, Czerniecki BJ. Clinical development of immunotherapies for her2+ breast cancer: A review of her2-directed monoclonal antibodies and beyond. npj Breast Cancer. 2020;**6**(1):2-6. DOI: 10.1038/s41523-020-0153-3

[47] Modi S, Park H, Murthy RK, Iwata H, Tamura K, Tsurutani J, et al. Antitumor activity and safety of trastuzumab deruxtecan in patients with her2-low–expressing advanced breast cancer: Results from a phase ib study. Journal of Clinical Oncology. 2020;**38**(17):1887-1896. DOI: 10.1200/jco.19.02318

[48] Rivas EI, Linares J, Zwick M, Gómez-Llonin A, Guiu M, Labernadie A, et al. Targeted immunotherapy against distinct cancer-associated fibroblasts overcomes treatment resistance in refractory HER2+ breast tumors. Nature Communications. 2022;**13**(1):5310. DOI: 10.1038/s41467-022-32782-3

[49] Slade D. PARP and PARG inhibitors in cancer treatment. Genes & Development. 2020;**34**(5-6):360-394. DOI: 10.1101/gad.334516.119. Epub 2020 Feb 6

[50] Brown JS, O'Carrigan B, Jackson SP, Yap TA. Targeting DNA repair in cancer: Beyond PARP inhibitors. Cancer Discovery. 2017;**7**(1):20-37. DOI: 10.1158/2159-8290.CD-16-0860. Epub 2016 Dec 21

[51] Lord CJ, Ashworth A. PARP inhibitors: Synthetic lethality in the clinic. Science. 2017;**355**(6330):1152-1158. DOI: 10.1126/science.aam7344. Epub 2017 Mar 16

[52] Huang H, Niu J, Wang F, Hu L, Yu Q. A natural compound derivative P-13 inhibits STAT3 signaling by covalently inhibiting Janus kinase 2. Investigational New Drugs. 2019;**37**(3):452-460. DOI: 10.1007/s10637-018-0637-2. Epub 2018 Aug 3

[53] D'Souza A, Spicer D, Lu J. Overcoming endocrine resistance in metastatic hormone receptor-positive breast cancer. Journal of Hematology & Oncology. 2018;**11**(1):80. DOI: 10.1186/s13045-018-0620-6

[54] Tay TKY, Tan PH. Liquid biopsy in breast cancer: A focused review. Archives of Pathology & Laboratory Medicine. 2021;**145**(6):678-686. DOI: 10.5858/arpa.2019-0559-RA

[55] Turashvili G, Brogi E. Tumor heterogeneity in breast cancer. Frontiers in Medicine. 2017;**4**:227. DOI: 10.3389/fmed.2017.00227

[56] Gabriel MT, Knutsen E, Perander M. Current status of circulating tumor cells, circulating tumor dna, and exosomes in breast cancer liquid biopsies. International Journal of Molecular Sciences. 2020;**21**(24):9457. DOI: 10.3390/ijms21249457

[57] Alimirzaie S, Bagherzadeh M, Akbari MR. Liquid biopsy in breast cancer: A comprehensive review. Clinical Genetics. 2019;**95**(6):643-660. DOI: 10.1111/cge.13514. Epub 2019 Feb 27

[58] Noor J, Chaudhry A, Noor R, Batool S. Advancements and applications of liquid biopsies in oncology: A narrative review. Cureus. 2023;**15**:2-5. DOI: 10.7759/cureus.42731

[59] Seale KN, Tkaczuk KHR. Circulating biomarkers in breast cancer. Clinical Breast Cancer. 2022;**22**(3):e319-e331. DOI: 10.1016/j.clbc.2021.09.006. Epub 2021 Sep 22

[60] Barzaman K, Karami J, Zarei Z, Hosseinzadeh A, Kazemi MH, Moradi-Kalbolandi S, et al. Breast cancer: Biology, biomarkers, and treatments. International Immunopharmacology. 2020;**84**:106535. DOI: 10.1016/j.intimp.2020.106535. Epub 2020 Apr 29

[61] Dang DK, Park BH. Circulating tumor DNA: Current challenges for clinical utility. The Journal of Clinical Investigation. 2022;**132**(12):e154941. DOI: 10.1172/JCI154941

[62] Mattos-Arruda LD, Caldas C. Cell-free circulating tumour DNA as a liquid biopsy in breast cancer. Molecular Oncology. 2015;**10**(3):464-474. DOI: 10.1016/j.molonc.2015.12.001

[63] Moding EJ, Nabet BY, Alizadeh AA, Diehn M. Detecting liquid remnants of solid tumors: Circulating tumor DNA minimal residual disease. Cancer Discovery. 2021;**11**(12):2968-2986. DOI: 10.1158/2159-8290.CD-21-0634

[64] Pantel K, Alix-Panabières C. Liquid biopsy and minimal residual disease - latest advances and implications for cure. Nature Reviews. Clinical Oncology. 2019;**16**(7):409-424. DOI: 10.1038/s41571-019-0187-3

[65] Abbosh C, Birkbak NJ, Swanton C. Early stage NSCLC - challenges to implementing ctDNA-based screening and MRD detection. Nature Reviews. Clinical Oncology. 2018;**15**(9):577-586. DOI: 10.1038/s41571-018-0058-3

[66] Moulière F, Chandrananda D, Piskorz A, Moore E, Morris JA, Ahlborn LB, et al. Enhanced detection of circulating tumor dna by fragment size analysis. Science Translational Medicine. 2018;**10**(466):2-7. DOI: 10.1126/scitranslmed.aat4921

[67] Rodriguez-Ruiz A, Lång K, Gubern-Merida A, et al. Can we reduce the workload of mammographic screening by automatic identification of normal exams with artificial intelligence? A feasibility study. European Radiology. 2019;**29**(9):4825-4832. Available from: https://liblynxgateway.com/wmed?url=https://www.proquest.com/scholarly-journals/can-we-reduce-workload-mammographic-screening/docview/2210255965/se-2. DOI: 10.1007/s00330-019-06186-9

[68] Aneja S, Chang E, Omuro A. Applications of artificial intelligence in neuro-oncology. Current Opinion in Neurology. 2019;**32**(6):850-856. DOI: 10.1097/WCO.0000000000000761

[69] Vobugari N, Raja V, Sethi U, Gandhi K, Raja K, Surani SR. Advancements in oncology with artificial intelligence—A review article. Cancers

(Basel). 2022;**14**(5):1349. DOI: 10.3390/cancers14051349

[70] Akselrod-Ballin A, Chorev M, Shoshan Y, Spiro A, Hazan A, Melamed R, et al. Predicting breast cancer by applying deep learning to linked health records and mammograms. Radiology. 2019;**292**:4-8

[71] Yala A, Lehman C, Schuster T, Portnoi T, Barzilay R. A deep learning mammography-based model for improved breast cancer risk prediction. Radiology. 2019;**292**:60-66. DOI: 10.1148/radiol.2019182716

[72] Chekhun S, Bergamino MA, Ferrando Diez A, Arnaldo L, Urbizu A, Quiroga Garcia V, et al. 163P impact of genomic sequencing data on treatment decisions in advanced breast cancer (ABC). ESMO Open. 2023;**8**(1, Supplement 5):102012. ISSN 2059-7029. DOI: 10.1016/j.esmoop.2023.102012

[73] Dzida T, Iqbal M, Charapitsa I, Reid G, Stunnenberg H, Matarese F, et al. Predicting stimulation-dependent enhancer-promoter interactions from ChIP-Seq time course data. PeerJ. 2017;**5**:e3742. DOI: 10.7717/peerj.3742

[74] Piryaei Z, Salehi Z, Ebrahimie E, Ebrahimi M, Kavousi K. Meta-analysis of integrated ChIP-seq and transcriptome data revealed genomic regions affected by estrogen receptor alpha in breast cancer. BMC Medical Genomics. 2023;**16**(1):219. DOI: 10.1186/s12920-023-01655-z

[75] Olow AK, Veer LV, Wolf DM. Toward developing a metastatic breast cancer treatment strategy that incorporates history of response to previous treatments. BMC Cancer. 2021;**21**(1):212. DOI: 10.1186/s12885-021-07912-7

[76] Campos AAL, Bustamante-Teixeira MT, Ervilha RR, et al. Quality of life of women who underwent breast cancer treatment relative to sociodemographic, behavioral, and clinical factors. einstein (Sao Paulo). 2024;**22**:eAO0585. DOI: 10.31744/einstein_journal/2024AO0585

[77] Fane M, Weeraratna AT. How the ageing microenvironment influences tumour progression. Nature Reviews. Cancer. 2020;**20**(2):89-106. DOI: 10.1038/s41568-019-0222-9

[78] Winkler J, Abisoye-Ogunniyan A, Metcalf KJ, Werb Z. Concepts of extracellular matrix remodelling in tumour progression and metastasis. Nature Communications. 2020;**11**(1):5120. DOI: 10.1038/s41467-020-18794-x

[79] Fumagalli C, Barberis M. Breast cancer heterogeneity. Diagnostics (Basel). 2021;**11**(9):1555. DOI: 10.3390/diagnostics11091555

[80] Cohen ASA, Berrios CD, Zion TN, Barrett CM, Moore R, Boillat E, et al. Toward more equitable access to genomic testing for rare diseases in rural populations. The American Journal of Human Genetics. 2024;**111**(5):825-832. DOI: 10.1016/j.ajhg.2024.03.016

[81] Garrett A, Durkie M, Callaway A, CanVIG-UK, et al. Combining evidence for and against pathogenicity for variants in cancer susceptibility genes: CanVIG-UK consensus recommendations. Journal of Medical Genetics. 2021;**58**:297-304. DOI: 10.1136/jmedgenet-2020-107248

[82] De Paolis E, Paris I, Tilocca B, Roncada P, Foca L, Tiberi G, et al. Assessing the pathogenicity of BRCA1/2 variants of unknown significance: Relevance and challenges for Breast Cancer Precision Medicine. Frontiers

in Oncology. 2023;**12**:297-304. DOI: 10.3389/fonc.2022.1053035

[83] Bobin-Dubigeon C, Luu HT, Leuillet S, Lavergne SN, Carton T, Le Vacon F, et al. Faecal microbiota composition varies between patients with breast cancer and healthy women: A comparative case-control study. Nutrients. 2021;**13**(8):2705. DOI: 10.3390/nu13082705

[84] Di Modica M, Arlotta V, Sfondrini L, Tagliabue E, Triulzi T. The link between the microbiota and her2+ breast cancer: The New Challenge of Precision Medicine. Frontiers in Oncology. 2022;**12**:9-11. DOI: 10.3389/fonc.2022.947188

[85] Raza M, Kumar N, Nair U, et al. Current updates on precision therapy for breast cancer associated brain metastasis: Emphasis on combination therapy. Molecular and Cellular Biochemistry. 2021;**476**:3271-3284. DOI: 10.1007/s11010-021-04149-7

[86] Van Der Merwe N, Ramesar R, De Vries J. Whole exome sequencing in South Africa: Stakeholder views on return of individual research results and incidental findings. Frontiers in Genetics. 2022;**13**:3271-3284. DOI: 10.3389/fgene.2022.864822

[87] Christowitz C, Olivier DW, Schneider JW, Kotze MJ, Engelbrecht A-M. Incorporating functional genomics into the pathology-supported genetic testing framework implemented in South Africa: A future view of precision medicine for breast carcinomas. Mutation Research, Reviews in Mutation Research. 2024;**793**:108492. DOI: 10.1016/j.mrrev.2024.108492

[88] Abdel-Razeq H, Tamimi F, Abujamous L, Abdel-Razeq R, Abunasser M, Edaily S, et al. Rates of variants of uncertain significance among patients with breast cancer undergoing genetic testing: Regional perspectives. Frontiers in Oncology. 2022;**12**:673094. DOI: 10.3389/fonc.2022.673094

[89] Delnord M, Van Valckenborgh E, Hebrant A, Antoniou A, Van Hoof W, Waeytens A, et al. Precision cancer medicine: What has translated into clinical use in Belgium? Seminars in Cancer Biology. 2022;**84**:255-262. DOI: 10.1016/j.semcancer.2021.06.010

[90] Baird A-M, Westphalen CB, Blum S, et al. How can we deliver on the promise of precision medicine in oncology and beyond? A practical roadmap for action. Health Science Reports. United States: Wiley; 2023;**6**:e1349. DOI: 10.1002/hsr2.1349

[91] Signé L, Landry Signé SA, Karlin M, Wheeler T, Brahima Sangafowa Coulibaly ZQ, Yaraghi N, Chakravorti B. Advancing Precision Medicine through Agile Governance. 2022

[92] McClintock AH, Golob AL, Laya MB. Breast cancer risk assessment: A step-wise approach for primary care providers on the front lines of shared decision making. Mayo Clinic Proceedings. 2020;**95**(6):1268-1275. Available from: https://liblynxgateway.com/wmed?url=https://www.proquest.com/scholarly-journals/breast-cancer-risk-assessment-step-wise-approach/docview/2409226256/se-2. DOI: 10.1016/j.mayocp.2020.04.017

[93] Conta J, Sternen D, Stasi S, Sarah CC, Wellner M, Dickerson J. An integrated approach to genetic test stewardship: The role of laboratory genetic counselors in test preauthorization and ordering. American Journal of Clinical Pathology. 2019;**suppl. 1, 152**:1268-1275. Available from: https://liblynxgateway.com/

wmed?url=https://www.proquest.com/scholarly-journals/integrated-approach-genetic-test-stewardship-role/docview/2339163557/se-2. DOI: 10.1093/ajcp/aqz130.015

[94] Amendola LM, Golden-Grant K, Scollon S. Scaling genetic counseling in the genomics era. Annual Review of Genomics and Human Genetics. 2021;**22**(1):339-355. DOI: 10.1146/annurev-genom-110320-121752

[95] Goldman L. PL02.06 patient-directed innovation, research and clinical trials. Journal of Thoracic Oncology. 2021;**16**:S64-S65

[96] Paoletti C, Cani AK, Larios JM, Hovelson DH, Aung K, Darga EP, et al. Comprehensive mutation and copy number profiling in archived circulating breast cancer tumor cells documents heterogeneous resistance mechanisms CTC genomic profiling in metastatic breast cancer patients. Cancer Research. 2018;**78**:1110-1122. DOI: 10.1158/0008-5472.CAN-17-2686

[97] Subhan MA, Parveen F, Shah H, Yalamarty SSK, Ataide JA, Torchilin VP. Recent advances with precision medicine treatment for breast cancer including triple-negative sub-type. Cancers (Basel). 2023;**15**(8):2204. DOI: 10.3390/cancers15082204

[98] Monaco ML, Idris OA, Essani K. Triple-negative breast cancer: Basic biology and Immuno-oncolytic viruses. Cancers. 2023;**15**:2393. DOI: 10.3390/cancers15082393

[99] Morash M, Mitchell H, Beltran H, Elemento O, Pathak J. The role of next-generation sequencing in precision medicine: A review of outcomes in oncology. Journal of Personalized Medicine. 2018;**8**:30. DOI: 10.3390/jpm8030030

[100] O'Brien NA, McDermott MSJ, Conklin D, Luo T, Ayala R, Salgar S, et al. Targeting activated PI3K/mTOR signaling overcomes acquired resistance to CDK4/6-based therapies in preclinical models of hormone receptor-positive breast cancer. Breast Cancer Research. 2020;**22**:1-17. DOI: 10.1186/s13058-020-01320-8

[101] Fernández-Lázaro D, García Hernández JL, Caballero GA, Córdova MA, Mielgo-Ayuso J, Cruz-Hernández JJ. Liquid biopsy as novel tool in precision medicine: Origins, properties, identification and clinical perspective of cancer's biomarkers. Diagnostics. 2020;**10**:215. DOI: 10.3390/diagnostics10040215

[102] Howard FM, Villamar D, He G, Pearson AT, Nanda R. The emerging role of immune checkpoint inhibitors for the treatment of breast cancer. Expert Opinion on Investigational Drugs. 2022;**31**(6):531-548. DOI: 10.1080/13543784.2022.1986002

[103] Hossain F, Majumder S, David J, Miele L. Precision medicine and triple-negative breast cancer: Current landscape and future directions. Cancers. 2021;**13**:3739. DOI: 10.3390/cancers13153739

[104] Bennett RL, Licht JD. Targeting epigenetics in cancer. Annual Review of Pharmacology and Toxicology. 2018;**58**:187-207

[105] Sgro A, Blancafort P. Epigenome engineering: New technologies for precision medicine. Nucleic Acids Research. 2020;**48**(22):12453-12482. DOI: 10.1093/nar/gkaa1000

Chapter 5

Recent Breakthroughs in Breast Cancer Endocrinology and Tumor Microenvironmental Interactions

Nicholas Pascuzzi, Mei Li, Reagan Farrell, Sy Bogutski, Falak Sharma, Shakil Khan and KuanHui Ethan Chen

Abstract

Breast cancer remains one of the most prevalent and lethal cancers among women worldwide, accounting for a significant proportion of cancer-related morbidity and mortality. Recent advancements in endocrinology have significantly contributed to understanding the disease's complex mechanisms, leading to more effective treatments and improved patient outcomes. This review highlights the latest breakthroughs in breast cancer endocrinology, focusing on a variety of hormones and their involvement in tumor progression. Additionally, the review explores the effects of hormones in modulating tumor metabolism, including the metabolic reprogramming that cancer cells undergo to support rapid growth and survival. The impact of endocrine factors within the tumor microenvironment is also examined, shedding light on how hormonal signals from surrounding stromal and immune cells can affect tumor behavior and response to treatment. Furthermore, the review delves into potentially new hormone therapies in breast cancer treatments. Innovations in selective estrogen receptor modulators (SERMs), selective estrogen receptor degraders (SERDs), and other hormone-targeting agents have shown promise in overcoming resistance to traditional hormone therapies. These breakthroughs underscore the critical role of endocrinology in the ongoing fight against breast cancer. By elucidating the complex interactions between hormones and breast cancer cells, researchers are paving the way for more targeted and effective therapies.

Keywords: breast cancer, hormone therapy, hormone receptors, tumor metabolism, tumor microenvironment

1. Introduction

Despite significant advancements in breast cancer therapies, the complex biology of breast cancer continues to pose challenges for effective management and prognosis. Breast cancer continues to be one of the most aggressive tumor types in women and is the second leading cause of cancer-related deaths among women [1, 2]. In recent decades, the incidence of breast cancer has been increasing. As reported by the National Cancer Institute in 2024, approximately 310,720 new breast cancer cases and 42,250 related deaths occurred in the United States [3]. Therefore, gaining a deeper understanding of breast tumor development and regulation will aid in shaping future therapeutic strategies for treating breast cancer.

During breast tumor development, heterogeneity in the tumor refers not only to the complex cellular composition, which includes a variety of stromal cells, but also to the presence of various molecules such as hormones, metabolites, and cytokines that collectively influence tumor progression. Among these molecules, hormones stand out as particularly intriguing due to their role in regulating cell growth, survival, differentiation, migration, and other cellular functions. Hormones exert their effects on both tumor and stromal cells, thereby significantly impacting tumor progression. Given that breast cancer predominantly affects women, past research has largely concentrated on female sex hormones or female prevalent hormones such as estrogen, progesterone, and prolactin [4–7]. However, as research on tumor endocrinology has advanced, it has become clear that many other hormones, particularly those linked to obesity, may also play a role in regulating breast tumor development [8–17]. In this context, we aim to discuss recent advances in breast cancer endocrinology, focusing on both sex-related hormones and adipokines.

Another key component of breast tumors is the presence of stromal immune cells. Recent advancements in cancer treatments have highlighted immunotherapies as promising approaches for tumor therapy. This is largely due to the specificity between immune cells and their targets, the ability of immune cells to patrol and seek out tumor cells, and the fact that immune responses represent the body's most natural endogenous defense against tumors, thereby significantly reducing side effects. The role of hormones, particularly sex hormones, in regulating immune functions has been documented [18]. Additionally, breast tumor cells or some breast stromal cells can secrete hormones that act as paracrine signals, further influencing immune cell function [19, 20]. Therefore, we will also explore recent discoveries in endocrine-immune regulation within breast tumors.

In summary, the intricate interplay between hormones and breast cancer encompasses multiple facets, from receptor-mediated signaling and metabolic reprogramming to modulation of the tumor microenvironment and immune response. Continued research in this area holds promise for identifying new biomarkers, understanding mechanisms of resistance, and developing more effective therapeutic strategies to combat breast cancer.

2. Hormones and breast cancer

Breast development is intricately regulated by hormones. As shown in **Table 1**, current research in breast tumor endocrinology has primarily focused on female sex hormones, particularly estrogen and progesterone. Growing interest in other hormones, especially adipokines, has highlighted their important role in breast cancer development. Therefore, we will focus on three categories of hormones: female sex hormones, female-dominant hormones, and adipokines. In this section (Section 2), we will review recent breakthroughs from the past five years concerning well-known female-related hormones while placing greater emphasis on the lesser-studied adipokines in the context of breast cancer progression. In the next section (Section 3), we will examine the relevance of each category to stromal regulation within the tumor microenvironment.

Hormone	# of articles	Hormone	# of articles
Female sex hormones		**Adipokines**	
estrogen	64,895	Leptin	916
progesterone	23,431	Kisspeptin	96
Female dominant hormones		Resistin	99
Prolactin	2035	Adiponectin	509
		Nesfatin	5
		Omentin	12
		Chemerin	15
		Apelin	26
		Visfatin	107

Table 1.
Number of PubMed articles (as of September 2024) on each hormone in breast cancer research.

2.1 Female sex hormones and breast cancers

The well-known classification system of breast cancers into luminal A, luminal B, Her2 overexpression, and triple negative breast cancer (TNBC) subtypes is partly based on the expression of hormone receptors including the estrogen receptor (ER), progesterone receptor (PR), and HER2. Consequently, estrogen and progesterone are the hormones extensively studied in breast cancer.

Upon binding to its receptor, estrogen activates multiple signaling pathways that lead to DNA damage, impaired DNA repair, altered metabolism, and cellular proliferation in breast cancer [21]. Consequently, estrogen receptor (ER) signaling and its integrity play a crucial role in regulating breast cancer development. Recent studies have explored the impact of the estrogen receptor α (ERα) sequence. Hadmi et al. identified three haplotypes within the promoter region of ERα, showing that polymorphisms in this promoter significantly reduce ERα expression and affect downstream cellular functions, such as cell cycle progression and DNA repair [22]. Additionally, Li et al. investigated mutations within the ERα coding region and found that mutations at ERα Y537S and D538G may play significant roles in breast cancer metastasis. These mutations are primarily found in breast cancer cells that have metastasized to distant organs and are less common in primary or localized breast tumors [23]. Moreover, breast cancer cells harboring Y537S and D538G mutations in ERα exhibit enhanced cell–cell adhesion, leading to the formation of compact multi-cellular tumor clusters—a characteristic feature of circulating tumor cells [23].

Like estrogen, progesterone affects breast cancer primarily through its two main isoforms of the progesterone receptor, PR-A and PR-B, enhancing the mitogenic effects of growth factors and regulating cellular heterogeneity [24–26]. A recent study found that progesterone also activates the GPR126/Gi signaling pathway, promoting breast cancer progression [27]. The G protein-coupled receptor GPR126 has been shown to be upregulated in breast cancer tissues and is associated with poor prognosis. Progestin binding to GPR126 has been shown to significantly increase breast cancer cell survival, both *in vitro* and *in vivo*, as demonstrated in a TNBC model using MDA-MB231 cells [27]. However, these growth-promoting effects can be blocked by a mutant form of GPR126 that fails to interact with progestin [27].

One key signaling pathway influenced by estrogen and progesterone is the PI3K/AKT/mTOR pathway, which regulates cellular responses to nutrient availability. Ward et al. found that estrogen targets this pathway, not only enhancing glycolysis in tumors [28] but also upregulating lipogenic enzymes, thereby promoting lipid accumulation [29]. In line with this, Wang et al. demonstrated that estrogen-induced aerobic glycolysis is mediated by the suppression of thioredoxin-interacting protein (TXNIP), a crucial regulator of glucose and lipid metabolism in humans [30]. Progesterone has also been shown to increase the expression of genes involved in fatty acid metabolism, further driving lipogenesis and lipid storage [28]. Notably, the combination of estrogen and progestins synergistically enhances lipid metabolism, contributing to the aggressive nature of hormone receptor-positive breast cancers [28, 31]. Additionally, the PI3K/AKT/mTOR pathway impacts amino acid metabolism [32]. The availability of amino acids like tryptophan, a precursor for serotonin, can affect estrogen synthesis and regulation, thus acting as positive regulators to further enhance estrogen signaling in breast cancer [33].

In summary, while estrogen and progesterone have been extensively studied, recent discoveries reveal novel pathways mediated by these hormones and their role in rewiring tumor metabolism, highlighting potential implications for developing new therapeutic strategies.

2.2 Female-dominant hormone, prolactin, and breast cancers

The peptide hormone prolactin, produced by the anterior pituitary, has been extensively studied for its role in breast cancer development. Elevated serum prolactin levels are positively correlated with breast cancer progression [34–39], and its signaling has been shown to influence breast cancer cell survival, differentiation, migration, and stemness [34, 40–44].

Prolactin exerts its effects through binding to the prolactin receptor (PRLR). In humans, multiple PRLR isoforms exist, with the long isoform being the most abundant and well-characterized, while the intermediate and short forms are less studied. The long isoform is typically associated with Jak2/Stat5 pathway activation, driving cell proliferation, whereas other isoforms may activate different pathways that favor cellular differentiation [45]. Shen et al. identified a novel intermediate PRLR isoform generated through alternative splicing, which adds a unique 13-amino acid tail. Breast cancer cells expressing this isoform exhibit increased proliferation, and its removal reverses the proliferative effect [46].

Given the importance of prolactin/PRLR in breast tumorigenesis, recent efforts have focused on disrupting this interaction to treat breast cancer. Borcherding et al. discovered small molecules, SMI-1 and SMI-6, that block PRLR and suppress breast cancer proliferation [47]. Additionally, a novel antibody-drug conjugate, ABBV-176, demonstrated significant antitumor activity in both *in vitro* and *in vivo* studies [48]. Furthermore, targeting the prolactin receptor with the immunotoxin N8-PE24 was found to restore the sensitivity of breast cancer cells to tamoxifen therapy [49].

Beyond the prolactin/PRLR pathway, Hammer et al. reported that prolactin activates the PAK1 (p21-activated kinase 1) signaling pathway, promoting epithelial-to-mesenchymal transition and enhancing the migratory properties of breast cancer cells [50]. Prolactin has also been suggested to interact with the oxytocin receptor in breast tumor development [51]. Moreover, our recent study revealed that prolactin can redistribute environmental iron via the surface receptor CD44 [52].

Although many studies highlight the tumor-promoting role of prolactin, some reports suggest a protective effect. One research group found that prolactin may play a protective role in breast cancer [53, 54], and a recent clinical trial targeting PRLR did not produce favorable outcomes for cancer patients [55]. Thus, the full scope of prolactin's role and its signaling in breast cancer remains to be fully elucidated.

2.3 Adipokines and breast cancers

Obesity is a well-established risk factor for breast cancer development, but the role of adipokines in breast cancer progression has been less extensively studied, as indicated in **Table 1**. Since many aspects of adipokine biology were uncovered some time ago, **Table 2** provides a brief overview of the previously known actions of adipokines in breast cancers. In this section, we will explore recent discoveries regarding the role of adipokines in breast tumorigenesis.

In **Table 2**, adiponectin stands out as the only adipokine with antitumor effects. Several meta-analyses have confirmed that lower circulating levels of adiponectin are linked to an increased risk of breast cancer development [56]. Adiponectin exhibits anti-inflammatory and antiproliferative properties, indicating a potential protective role against breast cancer [57]. It works by inhibiting cell proliferation, inducing cell cycle arrest, reducing invasiveness, promoting apoptosis and autophagy, lowering cell survival, and counteracting leptin-induced carcinogenesis [58, 59]. Due to its strong antitumor activity, clinical trials have shown that adiponectin levels could serve as predictors for survival rates in breast cancer patients and may help guide the need for more aggressive treatment strategies [60].

Research studies on the role of chemerin and kisspeptin in breast tumors have produced conflicting results. Some studies report that high chemerin expression in breast cancer tissue is linked to poor prognosis and adverse clinical factors, such as larger tumor size, lymph node involvement, and distant metastasis [61, 62]. In contrast, other research suggests that higher expression of chemerin receptors (CMKLR1 and GPR1) in tumor tissue is associated with longer relapse-free survival (RFS), indicating a potential tumor-suppressive function [63]. Similar contradictions are observed with serum chemerin levels. While some studies associate higher serum chemerin with poor prognosis in breast cancer [61, 64], others have found no correlation or even a protective effect [65, 66]. Kisspeptin has been reported to act as both a tumor suppressor and promoter in breast cancer. It has been shown to inhibit breast cancer metastasis by activating eukaryotic translation initiation factor 2α kinase 2 (EIF2AK2) [67]. However, other studies indicate that kisspeptin can reprogram tumor metabolism to promote breast cancer progression [68] and regulate aromatase expression, thereby enhancing estrogen-mediated responses that drive breast tumor growth [69]. Additionally, kisspeptin is linked to genes and proteins involved in cell cycle regulation, proliferation, and cancer cell invasiveness, including matrix

Tumor promoting	Contradictory evidence exist	Tumor suppressive
Leptin; Resistin; Nesfatin; Omentin; Appelin; Visfatin	Kisspeptin; Chemerin	Adiponectin

Table 2.
Summary of current literature on the role of adipokines in breast tumor development.

metalloproteinases [70, 71]. These conflicting findings underscore the need for further research to clarify the clinical significance of both chemerin and kisspeptin in breast cancer.

As shown in **Table 2**, the adipokines leptin, resistin, nesfatin, omentin, apelin, and visfatin have consistently been identified as promoters of breast cancer progression. Among these adipokines, leptin is the most extensively studied, with numerous mechanisms identified for its role in driving breast tumor progression. Recent advances in leptin research have expanded our understanding of its involvement in promoting breast cancer metastasis. A study by Han et al. demonstrated that leptin stimulates vasculogenesis by regulating aquaporin-1 expression [8]. Additionally, leptin has shown significant potential in regulating the epithelial-to-mesenchymal transition in breast cancer stem cells [72].

In addition to leptin, there is growing interest in exploring the effects of resistin and visfatin on breast tumorigenesis. Resistin interacts with four key receptors: ROR1 (Receptor Tyrosine-like Orphan Receptor 1), CAP1 (Cyclase-Associated Protein 1), Decorin, and TLR4 (Toll-like Receptor 4). A recent study by Hasan et al. has demonstrated that resistin promotes breast cancer progression by binding to CAP1, which in turn enhances cAMP, PKA, and NFκB-dependent transcription of inflammatory cytokines, leading to increased invasiveness and proliferation of breast cancer cells [73, 74]. Additionally, although not specifically studied in breast cancer, resistin has been shown to bind to TLR4 in other cancers, triggering pro-inflammatory pathways and promoting lung cancer metastasis [75]. Visfatin activates several signaling pathways that contribute to breast cancer progression. Notably, visfatin promotes breast cancer proliferation through the NF-κB/Notch1 pathway [76]. It has also been shown to enhance breast cancer stemness and tumor angiogenesis [77], both of which are crucial for metastasis. Elevated serum visfatin levels are therefore strongly associated with advanced breast tumors and metastasis [78]. Resistin has been shown to directly affect breast tumor cells, in addition to contributing to an inflammatory microenvironment. At lower concentrations, resistin acts as a potent pro-oxidant, promoting the generation of free radicals that may contribute to tumor heterogeneity [9]. It also enhances breast cancer cell migration, which can lead to bone metastasis [76]. Moreover, resistin treatment reduces let-7 expression, resulting in increased IL-6 and STAT3 expression, which in turn promotes breast cancer stemness and survival [77]. Visfatin, also known as nicotinamide phosphoribosyltransferase, exists in both secreted and intracellular forms. The secreted form functions either as a cytokine that activates TLR4 signaling [78] or as a hormone that stimulates the insulin receptor [79]. Intracellularly, visfatin plays a role in regulating cellular metabolism by influencing nicotinamide adenine dinucleotide (NAD+) metabolism [80]. Due to its roles as a cytokine, hormone, and metabolic regulator, visfatin has been implicated in breast cancer progression by activating various signaling pathways, including the NF-κB/Notch1 pathway [81]. Furthermore, visfatin reshapes breast cancer metabolism by promoting lipogenesis through activation of the EGFR/AKT/GSK3beta pathway, further enhancing cell growth [15]. It has also been linked to increased breast cancer stemness and tumor angiogenesis [82], both key factors in metastasis. Elevated serum levels of visfatin are strongly correlated with advanced breast cancer and metastasis [83]. Given its significant tumor-promoting effects, targeting visfatin with chemical inhibitors or small RNA silencing has shown promising anti-cancer potential [84, 85].

Nesfatin, omentin, and apelin are less well-characterized in terms of their roles in breast cancer. Nesfatin is the least-studied adipokine in breast cancer, with only five publications to date exploring its role. In lung and endometrial cancers, nesfatin has been associated with poor prognosis due to its involvement in promoting epithelial-to-mesenchymal transition [86, 87]. In breast cancer, a recent study by Kmiecik et al. has found that NUCB2/Nesfatin-1 is positively correlated with estrogen receptor (ER) and progesterone receptor (PR) status [88], suggesting that nesfatin may cooperate with ER and PR signaling to regulate breast cancer progression. Omentin-1 is another adipokine that has been minimally studied in breast cancer. As a p53-interacting protein, its role in breast cancer is linked to p53 expression status. Research indicates that serum omentin-1 levels are elevated in breast cancer patients with positive p53 expression, as well as in early-stage breast cancers (stage I) [89]. Omentin-1 also contributes to cancer progression through its pro-angiogenic effects, with studies showing that the omentin-1/Akt pathway promotes angiogenesis via mesenchymal stem cells [90]. Apelin, an endogenous ligand of the G protein-coupled receptor APJ, promotes lymphangiogenesis by activating the ERK and PI3K pathways, facilitating breast cancer micrometastasis to local lymph nodes [91]. This has been further supported by two recent *in vivo* studies, which demonstrated that apelin enhances breast tumor metastasis, and blocking apelin-mediated pathways effectively inhibited breast cancer metastasis [92, 93].

In conclusion, advancements in estrogen and progesterone research in breast cancer have provided important insights for improving current hormonal therapies. Moreover, the growing focus on other hormones, such as prolactin, and the increasing interest in adipokines could offer new treatment possibilities, particularly for hormone receptor-negative breast cancers.

3. Hormonal impact on stromal cells in tumor microenvironment

The tumor microenvironment (TME) refers to the microenvironment surrounding tumors, which includes cellular and non-cellular components that interact with tumor cells and each other [94]. These interactions significantly influence tumor growth, progression, metastasis, and therapeutic efficacy. Previous research has demonstrated that the status of hormones and their receptors significantly impacts stromal cells and tumor-associated immune cells in the TME [95]. In this section, we will review how female sex hormones, female-dominant hormones, and adipokines influence stromal cells within the tumor microenvironment (TME). Our focus will primarily be on non-immune infiltrating cells, including cancer-associated fibroblasts (CAFs), cancer-associated adipocytes (CAAs), and tumor endothelial cells (TECs), as well as tumor-infiltrating immune cells, with an emphasis on tumor-associated macrophages (TAMs) and tumor-infiltrating lymphocytes (TILs).

3.1 Female sex hormones and the stromal cells in the breast TME

3.1.1 Impacts on non-immune stromal cells

Cancer-associated fibroblasts (CAFs) are the most abundant stromal cells in tumors. Estrogen generally promotes fibroblast proliferation and their activation into CAFs [96]. Recent studies have further revealed that estrogen can enhance the tumor-promoting functions of fibroblasts by inducing the secretion of stromal-derived factor-1 (SDF-1α), which recruits myeloid-derived suppressor cells

(MDSCs), fostering immune suppression [97]. Estrogen-stimulated CAFs also release tumor-promoting factors like transforming growth factor-β (TGF-β), vascular endothelial growth factor (VEGF), and interleukin-6 (IL-6), which enhance tumor cell proliferation, angiogenesis, and extracellular matrix (ECM) remodeling [98]. Additionally, estrogen has been shown to alter miRNA expression profiles in CAFs, particularly as breast tumors become more aggressive and metastatic [99]. CAFs also promote stemness in progesterone receptor-positive breast tumors by upregulating CD44 [100].

Breast tissue is composed of many adipocytes, which provide energy for mammary development and maturation. During breast tumor progression, these adipocytes are transformed into cancer-associated adipocytes (CAAs) with proinflammatory characteristics [101]. CAAs contribute to breast tumor growth by producing tumor-promoting metabolites, such as FAM3 metabolism-regulating signaling molecule C (FAM3C) [102]. FAM3C supports the growth of both breast cancer cells and CAAs, and its reduction, through TGFβ neutralization—a key signaling pathway in FAM3C production—has been shown to suppress tumor growth [102]. A recent study by Qureshi et al. revealed that estrogen significantly stimulates adipocytes to secrete C-C motif chemokine ligand 2 (CCL2), IL-6, and IL-8 [103]. CCL2 attracts circulating monocytes, while IL-6 and IL-8 are known to induce inflammation, potentially reshaping the immune environment within breast tumors.

In addition to its indirect role in stimulating angiogenesis through fibroblasts, as previously mentioned, estrogen has been shown to directly enhance endothelial cell (EC) migration and proliferation, as demonstrated in a human umbilical vein EC model since 1995 [104]. Furthermore, VEGF is a known target gene regulated by estrogen receptor signaling due to the presence of an estrogen-responsive element (ERE) within the VEGF gene [105, 106]. While the role of steroid hormones in VEGF production in breast cancer remains debated, recent studies have indicated a positive correlation between estrogen and progesterone levels and VEGF production in ER+ breast cancer cell lines, leading to increased angiogenesis [106, 107]. Estrogen also increases vascular permeability, allowing greater access to nutrients and oxygen, thus promoting tumor growth and metastasis [95].

3.1.2 Impacts on immune stromal cells

Sex hormones are well-known immune modulators, and their roles become increasingly important during tumorigenesis. Estrogen, in particular, has been widely reported to target tumor-associated macrophages (TAMs), driving their polarization toward the tumor-promoting M2 phenotype in the tumor microenvironment (TME) [108]. This M2 phenotype supports tissue remodeling, angiogenesis, and immunosuppression, fostering a tumor-friendly environment. Estrogen, along with progesterone, also sustains macrophage populations and modulates inflammation in the mammary gland, leading to a state of immune tolerance [109]. In breast cancer, TAM infiltration varies according to hormone receptor status. Luminal A breast tumors have less TAM infiltration compared to hormone receptor-negative (HR^-) and luminal B breast tumors [110, 111]. Macrophages exhibit significantly higher expression of M2 phenotype markers when co-cultured with ER^+ breast cancer cells compared to triple-negative breast cancer (TNBC) cells [112]. In ER^+ breast cancer, estrogen enhances TAM recruitment by increasing the secretion of cytokines such as CCL2 and CCL5, promoting tumor cell dissemination [108]. Increased intra-tumoral TAM infiltration is associated with poorer survival outcomes in ER^+/PR^+ tumors, while no such correlation is observed in ER^-/PR^- tumors, suggesting that myeloid cells may mediate pro-tumor effects through estrogen receptor signaling [111].

Tumor-infiltrating lymphocytes (TILs) play a pivotal role in the antitumor response within the tumor microenvironment (TME). Research has demonstrated that the estrogen receptor (ER) pathway is inversely correlated with TIL infiltration in breast cancer, affecting immune cells such as B cells, cytotoxic T lymphocytes (CTLs), helper T cells (Th), and regulatory T cells (Tregs) [113]. Supporting this, a large bioinformatic analysis of 867 node-negative, treatment-naïve breast cancer patients, along with data from 347 additional patients, confirmed that T cell infiltration, particularly $CD8^+$ T cell abundance, is linked to breast cancer progression, with higher levels in basal-like and HER2-positive subtypes and lower levels in luminal A and B subtypes [114]. Consistently, luminal ER^+ breast tumors display greater frequencies of natural killer (NK) cells and neutrophils, whereas ER^- tumors are more enriched in $CD8^+$ CTLs, $CD4^+$ Th1 cells, and B cells [115]. While estrogen receptor status is negatively correlated to T cell infiltration, human and animal models indicate that increased estrogen levels lead to a higher Th2/Th1 ratio among $CD4^+$ TILs [116], contributing to an immunosuppressive TME. Estrogen can also promote the development of an immunosuppressive Th17 phenotype [117]. In relation to CTLs, estrogen indirectly impairs $CD8^+$ TIL function by upregulating Granzyme B proteinase inhibitor-9 (P19), which ultimately diminishes the $CD8^+$ TIL immune response [118]. Estrogen antagonists have been shown to enhance CTL-mediated killing of ER^+ tumors [119]. Additionally, growing evidence suggests that estrogen and progesterone directly regulate the suppressive function of Tregs via FOXP3 [120–122]. Aromatase inhibitors, which block estrogen synthesis, significantly reduce Treg numbers in breast cancer patients [123]. Estrogen increases the expression of programmed death-1 (PD-1) in Tregs [124–126], as well as in endothelial cells and breast cancer cells [127]. PD-1 is an immune checkpoint that delivers an "off" signal, suppressing T cell activity. By inducing PD-1 expression within the tumor microenvironment, estrogen promotes immune evasion by tumor cells. The function of Tregs in breast cancer is strongly linked to the ER expression status of the tumor [128]. Other than T lymphocytes, estrogen has been found to reduce NK cell cytotoxic activity and decrease IL2 and IFN-γ secretion within the TME in both human and animal models, [113]. In contrast to all identified immune-suppressive roles of estrogen above, estrogen promotes B cell survival, increases immunoglobulin production, and enhances the antitumor activity of B cells [95].

3.2 Prolactin and the stromal cells in the breast TME

3.2.1 Impacts on non-immune stromal cells

The impact of prolactin on non-immune stromal cells in tumors has been less explored. However, a recent study by Zheng et al. has demonstrated that stromal fibroblasts can secrete prolactin, which induces tumor cells to produce COX-2, a key molecule involved in inflammation. Treatment of tumor cells with COX-2 inhibitors was shown to reduce tumor development [129]. Furthermore, Tang et al. identified PRLR as a signaling pathway that drives autotaxin expression in fibroblasts and/or leukocytes. Autotaxin supports breast tumor cell growth, and blocking autotaxin with the inhibitor IOA-289 significantly inhibited tumor growth [130].

While prolactin itself does not act directly on endothelial cells, its derivatives do. One such derivative is vasoinhibin, a 16kD peptide produced when prolactin is cleaved by the enzyme cathepsin D. Vasoinhibin exhibits anti-angiogenic properties [131]. However, as cathepsin D is required for vasoinhibin production and is also recognized as a risk factor for tumorigenesis [132], the relationship between prolactin, its derivatives, and cathepsin D warrants further investigation.

3.2.2 Impacts on immune stromal cells

As previously mentioned, prolactin functions by binding to the prolactin receptor (PRLR), which is part of the type I cytokine receptor superfamily. Upon activation, PRLR expression is observed in all immune cells, except for regulatory T cells (Tregs), which express PRLR regardless of their activation status [133]. Since Tregs are known to suppress immune responses, their accumulation is observed in various tumors, including breast cancer [134]. In our recent publication, we demonstrated that prolactin stimulates breast tumor cells to secrete chemokines that recruit Tregs, leading to accumulation of tumor Tregs [135]. Furthermore, systemic knockdown of the long isoform of PRLR significantly reduced Treg infiltration and impaired their ability to drive the epithelial-to-mesenchymal transition in breast tumor cells [135]. In addition to its major effects on Tregs, systemic knockdown of the long isoform of PRLR also resulted in reduced activation of both CD4 and CD8 T cells [43, 135]. This impaired T cell activation is noteworthy because PRLR signaling interacts with Zap70, a critical kinase in the T cell receptor signaling pathway [136]. Therefore, the knockdown of the long isoform of PRLR may directly affect its interaction with Zap70, leading to reduced T cell activation. Alternatively, this may also reflect an indirect effect following Treg accumulation due to prolactin stimulation. Consistent with prolactin's immune-suppressive role in the tumor microenvironment, another recent study from our team has shown that prolactin can redistribute iron from macrophages to breast tumor cells [52]. Since iron release is characteristic of M2 macrophages, further investigation is needed to determine whether the negation of iron maintenance by prolactin is critical for M2 polarization.

In addition to our recent findings, research by Liang et al. has yielded similar conclusions. Their study found that PRLR expression is negatively correlated with breast cancer outcomes, partially due to a reduction in the expression of immune checkpoints [137]. Among the immune checkpoints they examined, PDCD1, CTLA4, TIGIT, and BTLA were associated with better prognosis. However, PRLR expression was inversely correlated with these immune checkpoints, indicating the potential to enhance current breast cancer immunotherapies by targeting the PRLR pathway [137].

3.3 Adipokines and the stromal cells in the breast TME

3.3.1 Impacts on non-immune stromal cells

As research on the role of adipokines in breast cancer is still in its early stages, most studies have focused on leptin. In breast cancer, leptin secreted by cancer-associated fibroblasts (CAFs) enhances the bidirectional interaction between CAFs and breast cancer cells, driving tumor progression [138, 139]. Leptin also exhibits pro-angiogenic properties by promoting endothelial cell proliferation and migration and stimulating the release of pro-angiogenic factors such as VEGF, fibroblast growth factor, platelet-derived growth factor, and IL-8, all of which contribute to tumor growth [140–142]. Additionally, leptin may synergize with estrogen signaling to promote carcinogenesis and tumor angiogenesis [143, 144]. Beyond leptin, both apelin and resistin have been shown to influence tumor stromal cells. Apelin has also been implicated in breast tumor progression by promoting tumor endothelial cell migration, facilitating angiogenesis and metastasis [145]. Resistin stimulates adipose-derived stem cells to secrete the chemokine CXCL5, which activates the ERK signaling pathway and drives breast tumor proliferation [146].

3.3.2 Impacts on immune stromal cells

In addition to estrogen and progesterone, leptin within the breast tumor microenvironment (TME) promotes the polarization of macrophages toward the M2 phenotype [147, 148]. Leptin stimulates tumor-associated macrophages (TAMs) to secrete pro-inflammatory cytokines, such as IL-6, IL-12, and TNF-α, and enhances the expression of pro-angiogenic factors like VEGF, leading to increased tumor angiogenesis [149]. Apelin has been shown to promote breast cancer progression by modulating immune cell infiltration, decreasing the influx of natural killer (NK) T cells, and increasing the presence of polymorphonuclear myeloid-derived suppressor cells (MDSCs), thereby creating an immunosuppressive microenvironment [130]. Chemerin has complex roles in breast cancer. On one hand, it functions as a chemoattractant, drawing immune cells into the tumor microenvironment through its receptors CMKLR1, GPR1, and CCRL2, which can help suppress tumor growth [138]. On the other hand, many of the recruited immune cells, such as macrophages, dendritic cells, and NK cells, may be influenced to adopt a tumor-promoting phenotype. Visfatin also promotes breast cancer progression by inducing inflammatory cytokine production, upregulating co-stimulatory molecules, and enhancing phagocytosis in monocytes [150]. It contributes to the differentiation of monocytes into M2 macrophages, which further suppress immune surveillance and promote malignant behavior in breast cancer [150].

Adiponectin is well known for its anti-inflammatory properties, which help counteract the chronic inflammation in the tumor microenvironment, contributing to its antitumor effects. However, this anti-inflammatory function may also suppress immune responses. For instance, adiponectin has been shown to shift macrophage polarization from the pro-inflammatory M1 subtype to the anti-inflammatory M2 subtype [151] and to influence the antigen-presenting abilities of dendritic cells [152]. In a lymphoma mouse model, dendritic cells overexpressing adiponectin receptors 1 and 2 failed to activate T cells or trigger an antitumor immune response [153]. Despite this, as adiponectin levels are inversely related to breast cancer risk [154], it remains unclear if the absence of an antitumor immune response is due to low adiponectin levels. On the other hand, adiponectin has been shown to positively regulate immune cells in various ways. In the thymus, it accelerates T lymphocyte development and maturation [155], and in colostrum, T cells are more proliferative and active when exposed to adiponectin, while they show reduced proliferation and activation when exposed to leptin [156]. Adiponectin also enhances B cell activation and differentiation [157], and in adiponectin-knockout mice implanted with melanoma and lung cancer cells, reduced macrophage infiltration was observed [158]. Furthermore, tumor-associated regulatory T cells expressing adiponectin exhibit antitumor activity [159]. These conflicting findings on adiponectin's role in immune modulation underscore the need for further research to clarify its complex relationship with immune responses.

In conclusion, tumor heterogeneity is increasingly acknowledged as a critical factor in the development of new cancer therapies. Hormones such as estrogen, prolactin, and adipokines play pivotal roles in influencing the behavior of stromal and immune cells within the breast tumor microenvironment. These hormones not only drive tumor progression but also affect the surrounding cells that contribute to the tumor's growth, survival, and response to treatment. A deeper understanding of how these hormones impact both the tumor and its microenvironment is essential for developing more effective and personalized treatment strategies for breast cancer.

4. Conclusion

Breast cancer, as a leading cause of cancer-related deaths among women, demands a thorough understanding of its underlying mechanisms for improved management and treatment. The intricate interplay of hormones such as estrogen and progesterone with their respective receptors significantly influences the pathogenesis and progression of breast cancer. Additionally, other hormones like prolactin and adipokines also play pivotal roles in reshaping the tumor microenvironment.

Advances in hormonal therapies, including SERMs and aromatase inhibitors, have substantially improved patient outcomes, though challenges like resistance remain. Given the varied effects of hormones on stromal cells within the tumor, the evolving landscape of treatment strategies, especially novel combination therapies, presents significant potential for further advancements. Continued research into the hormonal regulation of breast cancer is essential for uncovering new biomarkers, understanding resistance mechanisms, and developing more effective therapeutic approaches. This ongoing effort is crucial in the fight against breast cancer, aiming to reduce its global burden and improve the quality of life for patients worldwide.

Conflict of interest

The authors declare no conflict of interest.

DOI: http://dx.doi.org/10.5772/intechopen.1007934

Author details

Nicholas Pascuzzi[†], Mei Li[†], Reagan Farrell[†], Sy Bogutski[†], Falak Sharma[†], Shakil Khan[†] and KuanHui Ethan Chen[*†]
Department of Biological Sciences, Texas Tech University, Lubbock, TX, USA

*Address all correspondence to: kuachen@ttu.edu

†All authors contribute equally.

References

[1] Yu L, Chen Y, Luo K. The crosstalk between metabolic reprogramming and epithelial-mesenchymal transition and their synergistic roles in distant metastasis in breast cancer. Medicine (Baltimore). 2024;**103**:e38462

[2] Sung H et al. Global cancer statistics 2020: GLOBOCAN estimates of incidence and mortality worldwide for 36 cancers in 185 countries. CA: a Cancer Journal for Clinicians. 2021;**71**:209-249

[3] SEER*Explorer: An Interactive Website for SEER Cancer Statistics [Internet]. Surveillance Research Program, National Cancer Institute; 2024 Apr 17. [updated: 2024 Jun 27; cited 2024 Oct 12]. Available from: https://seer.cancer.gov/statistics-network/explorer/application.html?site=1&data_type=1&graph_type=2&compareBy=sex&chk_sex_3=3&chk_sex_2=2&rate_type=2&race=1&age_range=1&hdn_stage=101&advopt_precision=1&advopt_show_ci=on&hdn_view=0&advopt_show_apc=on&advopt_display=2#resultsRegion0. Data source(s): U.S. Mortality Data (1969-2022), National Center for Health Statistics, CDC

[4] Key TJ et al. Sex hormones and risk of breast cancer in premenopausal women: A collaborative reanalysis of individual participant data from seven prospective studies. The Lancet Oncology. 2013;**14**:1009-1019

[5] Lu Y et al. Discovery of novel quinoline scaffold selective estrogen receptor degraders (SERDs) for treatment of ER positive breast cancer with enhanced antiproliferative bioactivity through immunogenic cell death (ICD) effects. European Journal of Medicinal Chemistry. 2024;**275**:116534

[6] Lashen AG et al. Nottingham prognostic x (NPx): A risk stratification tool in ER-positive HER2-negative breast cancer: A validation study. Histopathology. Sep 2024;**85**(3):468-477

[7] Singh I, Gupta S, Deshmukh M, Gandhi M, Khopkar-Kale P. Serum prolactin levels as a novel, practical marker for predicting malignant diseases of the breast. Cureus. 2024;**16**:e58375

[8] Han DS, Lee EO. Leptin promotes vasculogenic mimicry in breast cancer cells by regulating aquaporin-1. International Journal of Molecular Sciences. 2024;**25**(10):5215

[9] Pavlova E, Stojchevski R, Avtanski D. The effect of resistin on the redox state of breast cancer cells. Journal of Cancer Research and Clinical Oncology. 2024;**150**:24

[10] Mantzoros C et al. Adiponectin and breast cancer risk. The Journal of Clinical Endocrinology and Metabolism. 2004;**89**:1102-1107

[11] Ning S et al. NUCB2/Nesfatin-1 drives breast cancer metastasis through the up-regulation of cholesterol synthesis via the mTORC1 pathway. Journal of Translational Medicine. 2023;**21**:362

[12] Christodoulatos GS et al. Circulating omentin-1 as a biomarker at the intersection of postmenopausal breast cancer occurrence and cardiometabolic risk: An observational cross-sectional study. Biomolecules. 2021;**11**(11):1609

[13] Shin WJ, Zabel BA, Pachynski RK. Mechanisms and functions of chemerin in cancer: Potential roles in therapeutic intervention. Frontiers in Immunology. 2018;**9**:2772

[14] Hu D et al. Apelin is associated with clinicopathological parameters and prognosis in breast cancer patients. Archives of Gynecology and Obstetrics. 2022;**306**:1185-1195

[15] Rajput PK, Varghese JF, Srivastava AK, Kumar U, Yadav UCS. Visfatin-induced upregulation of lipogenesis via EGFR/AKT/GSK3β pathway promotes breast cancer cell growth. Cellular Signalling. 2023;**107**:110686

[16] Tian J et al. KiSS1 gene as a novel mediator of TGFβ-mediated cell invasion in triple negative breast cancer. Cellular Signalling. 2018;**42**:1-10

[17] Shakya R, Byun MR, Joo SH, Chun KS, Choi JS. Domperidone exerts antitumor activity in triple-negative breast cancer cells by modulating reactive oxygen species and JAK/STAT3 signaling. Biomolecules & Therapeutics (Seoul). 2023;**31**:692-699

[18] Hoffmann JP, Liu JA, Seddu K, Klein SL. Sex hormone signaling and regulation of immune function. Immunity. 2023;**56**:2472-2491

[19] Yaghjyan L, Colditz GA. Estrogens in the breast tissue: A systematic review. Cancer Causes & Control. 2011;**22**:529-540

[20] Clevenger CV, Furth PA, Hankinson SE, Schuler LA. The role of prolactin in mammary carcinoma. Endocrine Reviews. 2003;**24**:1-27

[21] Yedidia-Aryeh L, Goldberg M. The interplay between the cellular response to DNA double-Strand breaks and estrogen. Cells. 2022;**11**(19):3097

[22] Hamdi Y et al. Functional analysis of promoter variants in genes involved in sex steroid action, DNA repair and cell cycle control. Genes (Basel). 2019;**10**(3):186

[23] Li Z et al. Hotspot ESR1 mutations are multimodal and contextual modulators of breast cancer metastasis. Cancer Research. 2022;**82**:1321-1339

[24] Lombardi S et al. Growth hormone is secreted by normal breast epithelium upon progesterone stimulation and increases proliferation of stem/progenitor cells. Stem Cell Reports. 2014;**2**:780-793

[25] Hilton HN et al. Progesterone stimulates progenitor cells in normal human breast and breast cancer cells. Breast Cancer Research and Treatment. 2014;**143**:423-433

[26] Horwitz KB, Sartorius CA. 90 years of progesterone: Progesterone and progesterone receptors in breast cancer: Past, present, future. Journal of Molecular Endocrinology. 2020;**65**:T49-T63

[27] An W et al. Progesterone activates GPR126 to promote breast cancer development via the Gi pathway. Proceedings of the National Academy of Sciences of the United States of America. 2022;**119**:e2117004119

[28] Ward AV et al. Estrogens and progestins cooperatively shift breast cancer cell metabolism. Cancers (Basel). 2022;**14**(7):1776

[29] Hoxhaj G, Manning BD. The PI3K-AKT network at the interface of oncogenic signalling and cancer metabolism. Nature Reviews. Cancer. 2020;**20**:74-88

[30] Wang Y, Chen S. TXNIP links anticipatory unfolded protein response to estrogen reprogramming glucose metabolism in breast cancer cells. Endocrinology. 2022;**163**(1):bqab212

[31] Mahboobifard F et al. Estrogen as a key regulator of energy homeostasis

and metabolic health. Biomedicine & Pharmacotherapy. 2022;**156**:113808

[32] Peng Y, Wang Y, Zhou C, Mei W, Zeng C. PI3K/Akt/mTOR pathway and its role in cancer therapeutics: Are we making headway? Frontiers in Oncology. 2022;**12**:819128

[33] Juhász C et al. Tryptophan metabolism in breast cancers: Molecular imaging and immunohistochemistry studies. Nuclear Medicine and Biology. 2012;**39**:926-932

[34] Clevenger CV, Rui H. Breast cancer and prolactin—New mechanisms and models. Endocrinology. 2022;**163**(10):bqac122

[35] Hankinson SE et al. Plasma prolactin levels and subsequent risk of breast cancer in postmenopausal women. Journal of the National Cancer Institute. 1999;**91**:629-634

[36] Faupel-Badger JM et al. Prolactin serum levels and breast cancer: Relationships with risk factors and tumour characteristics among pre- and postmenopausal women in a population-based case-control study from Poland. British Journal of Cancer. 2010;**103**:1097-1102

[37] Tworoger SS, Hankinson SE. Prolactin and breast cancer etiology: An epidemiologic perspective. Journal of Mammary Gland Biology and Neoplasia. 2008;**13**:41-53

[38] Tworoger SS et al. A 20-year prospective study of plasma prolactin as a risk marker of breast cancer development. Cancer Research. 2013;**73**:4810-4819

[39] Tikk K et al. Circulating prolactin and breast cancer risk among pre- and postmenopausal women in the EPIC cohort. Annals of Oncology. 2014;**25**:1422-1428

[40] Chen KH, Walker AM. Prolactin inhibits a major tumor-suppressive function of wild type BRCA1. Cancer Letters. 2016;**375**:293-302

[41] Sutherland A et al. The role of prolactin in bone metastasis and breast cancer cell-mediated osteoclast differentiation. Journal of the National Cancer Institute. 2016;**108**(3):djv338

[42] O'Leary KA et al. Prolactin synergizes with canonical Wnt signals to drive development of ER+ mammary tumors via activation of the notch pathway. Cancer Letters. 2021;**503**:231-239

[43] Yonezawa T et al. Anti-metastatic outcome of isoform-specific prolactin receptor targeting in breast cancer. Cancer Letters. 2015;**366**:84-92

[44] Radhakrishnan A et al. A pathway map of prolactin signaling. Journal of Cell Communication and Signaling. 2012;**6**:169-173

[45] Huang K, Ueda E, Chen Y, Walker AM. Paradigm-shifters: Phosphorylated prolactin and short prolactin receptors. Journal of Mammary Gland Biology and Neoplasia. 2008;**13**:69-79

[46] Shen S et al. The human intermediate prolactin receptor I-tail contributes breast oncogenesis by targeting Ras/MAPK pathway. Endocrinology. 2024;**165**(6):bqae039

[47] Borcherding DC et al. Suppression of breast cancer by small molecules that block the prolactin receptor. Cancers (Basel). 2021;**13**(11):2662

[48] Anderson MG et al. ABBV-176, a PRLR antibody drug conjugate with a potent DNA-damaging PBD cytotoxin

and enhanced activity with PARP inhibition. BMC Cancer. 2021;**21**:681

[49] Zhang J et al. The immunotoxin targeting PRLR increases tamoxifen sensitivity and enhances the efficacy of chemotherapy in breast cancer. Journal of Experimental & Clinical Cancer Research. 2024;**43**:173

[50] Hammer A, Diakonova M. Prolactin-induced tyrosyl phosphorylation of PAK1 facilitates epithelial-mesenchymal transition. MicroPublication Biology. 2024;**2024**. DOI: 10.17912/micropub.biology.001136

[51] Li D et al. Oxytocin receptor induces mammary tumorigenesis through prolactin/p-STAT5 pathway. Cell Death & Disease. 2021;**12**:588

[52] Farrell R et al. Prolactin drives iron release from macrophages and uptake in mammary cancer cells through CD44. International Journal of Molecular Sciences. 2024;**25**(16):8941

[53] Hachim IY, Hachim MY, Lopez VM, Lebrun JJ, Ali S. Prolactin receptor expression is an independent favorable prognostic marker in human breast cancer. Applied Immunohistochemistry & Molecular Morphology. 2016;**24**:238-245

[54] Hachim IY, Shams A, Lebrun JJ, Ali S. A favorable role of prolactin in human breast cancer reveals novel pathway-based gene signatures indicative of tumor differentiation and favorable patient outcome. Human Pathology. 2016;**53**:142-152

[55] Kelly MP et al. Preclinical activity of the novel anti-prolactin receptor (PRLR) antibody-drug conjugate REGN2878-DM1 in PRLR positive breast cancers. Molecular Cancer Therapeutics. Jul 2017;**16**(7):1299-1311

[56] Gu L et al. Serum adiponectin in breast cancer: A meta-analysis. Medicine (Baltimore). 2018;**97**:e11433

[57] Nehme R, Diab-Assaf M, Decombat C, Delort L, Caldefie-Chezet F. Targeting adiponectin in breast cancer. Biomedicine. 2022;**10**(11):2958

[58] Andò S, Naimo GD, Gelsomino L, Catalano S, Mauro L. Novel insights into adiponectin action in breast cancer: Evidence of its mechanistic effects mediated by ERα expression. Obesity Reviews. 2020;**21**:e13004

[59] Tsankof A, Tziomalos K. Adiponectin: A player in the pathogenesis of hormone-dependent cancers. Frontiers in Endocrinology (Lausanne). 2022;**13**:1018515

[60] Sambiasi D et al. Adipokines in hereditary breast cancer patients and healthy relatives. Oncotarget. 2017;**8**:101255-101261

[61] Song Y, Zhu X, Lin Z, Luo L, Wen D. The potential value of serum chemerin in patients with breast cancer. Scientific Reports. 2021;**11**:6564

[62] Li YQ et al. RARRES2 regulates lipid metabolic reprogramming to mediate the development of brain metastasis in triple negative breast cancer. Military Medical Research. 2023;**10**:34

[63] Kumar JD et al. Chemerin acts via CMKLR1 and GPR1 to stimulate migration and invasion of gastric cancer cells: Putative role of decreased TIMP-1 and TIMP-2. Oncotarget. 2019;**10**:98-112

[64] El-Sagheer G, Gayyed M, Ahmad A, Abd El-Fattah A, Mohamed M. Expression of chemerin correlates with a poor prognosis in female breast cancer patients. Breast Cancer (Dove Med Press). 2018;**10**:169-176

[65] Kim H et al. Chemerin treatment inhibits the growth and bone invasion of breast cancer cells. International Journal of Molecular Sciences. 2020;**21**(8):2871

[66] Pachynski RK et al. Chemerin suppresses breast cancer growth by recruiting immune effector cells into the tumor microenvironment. Frontiers in Immunology. 2019;**10**:983

[67] Kim TH, Cho SG. Kisspeptin inhibits cancer growth and metastasis via activation of EIF2AK2. Molecular Medicine Reports. 2017;**16**:7585-7590

[68] Dragan M et al. G protein-coupled kisspeptin receptor induces metabolic reprograming and tumorigenesis in estrogen receptor-negative breast cancer. Cell Death & Disease. 2020;**11**:106

[69] Yilmaz MB, Oksuz H, Ilgaz NS, Ocal I, Tazehkand MN. The role of kisspeptin on aromatase expression in breast cancer. Bratislavské Lekárske Listy. 2018;**119**:776-780

[70] Guzman S, Brackstone M, Wondisford F, Babwah AV, Bhattacharya M. KISS1/KISS1R and breast cancer: Metastasis promoter. Seminars in Reproductive Medicine. 2019;**37**:197-206

[71] Rasoulzadeh Z et al. Placental kisspeptins differentially modulate vital parameters of estrogen receptor-positive and -negative breast cancer cells. PLoS One. 2016;**11**:e0153684

[72] Bowers LW et al. Leptin signaling mediates obesity-associated CSC enrichment and EMT in preclinical TNBC models. Molecular Cancer Research. 2018;**16**:869-879

[73] Deb A, Deshmukh B, Ramteke P, Bhati FK, Bhat MK. Resistin: A journey from metabolism to cancer. Translational Oncology. 2021;**14**:101178

[74] Hasan R, Zhou GL. The cytoskeletal protein cyclase-associated protein 1 (CAP1) in breast cancer: Context-dependent roles in both the invasiveness and proliferation of cancer cells and underlying cell signals. International Journal of Molecular Sciences. 2019;**20**(11):2653

[75] Gong WJ et al. Resistin facilitates metastasis of lung adenocarcinoma through the TLR4/Src/EGFR/PI3K/NF-κB pathway. Cancer Science. 2018;**109**:2391-2400

[76] Cuachirria-Espinoza RL et al. Analysis of the relationship between resistin with prognosis, cell migration, and p38 and ERK1/2 activation in breast cancer. Biochimie. Oct 2024;**4**:S0300-9084(24)00227-X

[77] Deshmukh SK et al. Resistin induces LIN28A-mediated let-7a repression in breast cancer cells leading to IL-6 and STAT3 upregulation. Cancers (Basel). 2021;**13**(18):4498

[78] Galli U et al. Recent advances in NAMPT inhibitors: A novel immunotherapic strategy. Frontiers in Pharmacology. 2020;**11**:656

[79] Mlyczyńska E et al. In vitro effect of visfatin on endocrine functions of the porcine corpus luteum. Scientific Reports. 2024;**14**:14780

[80] Mogol AN et al. NAD+ metabolism generates a metabolic vulnerability in endocrine-resistant metastatic breast tumors in females. Endocrinology. 2023;**164**(6):bqad073

[81] Park HJ et al. Visfatin promotes cell and tumor growth by upregulating Notch1 in breast cancer. Oncotarget. 2014;**5**:5087-5099

[82] Chiang YF et al. The adipokine visfatin modulates cancer stem cell

properties in triple-negative breast cancer. Biomedicine. 2023;**11**(2):297

[83] Ghaneialvar H et al. Comparison of visfatin levels in patients with breast cancer and endometrial cancer with healthy individuals: A systematic review and meta-analysis. Health Science Reports. 2022;**5**:e895

[84] Ghanem MS et al. Identification of NAPRT inhibitors with anti-cancer properties by In Silico drug discovery. Pharmaceuticals (Basel). 2022;**15**(7):848

[85] Ameli Mojarad M, Pourmahdian A. MicroRNA-26b reduces cell viability by inhibition of nicotinamide phosphoribosyltransferase in breast cancer cells. DNA and Cell Biology. 2022;**41**:735-741

[86] Altan B et al. High expression of nucleobindin 2 is associated with poor prognosis in gastric cancer. Tumour Biology. 2017;**39**:1010428317703817

[87] Takagi K et al. Nucleobindin 2 (NUCB2) in human endometrial carcinoma: A potent prognostic factor associated with cell proliferation and migration. Endocrine Journal. 2016;**63**:287-299

[88] Kmiecik A et al. Expression of NUCB2/NESF-1 in breast cancer cells. International Journal of Molecular Sciences. 2022;**23**(16):9177

[89] Dec P, Poniewierska-Baran A, Modrzejewski A, Pawlik A. The role of omentin-1 in cancers development and progression. Cancers (Basel). 2023;**15**(15):3797

[90] Yin L et al. Omentin-1 effects on mesenchymal stem cells: Proliferation, apoptosis, and angiogenesis in vitro. Stem Cell Research & Therapy. 2017;**8**:224

[91] Baran M, Ozturk F, Canoz O, Onder GO, Yay A. The effects of apoptosis and apelin on lymph node metastasis in invasive breast carcinomas. Clinical and Experimental Medicine. 2020;**20**:507-514

[92] Masoumi J et al. Inhibition of apelin/APJ axis enhances the potential of dendritic cell-based vaccination to modulate TH1 and TH2 cell-related immune responses in an animal model of metastatic breast cancer. Advances in Medical Sciences. 2022;**67**:170-178

[93] Masoumi J et al. Apelin receptor antagonist boosts dendritic cell vaccine efficacy in controlling angiogenic, metastatic and apoptotic-related factors in 4T1 breast tumor-bearing mice. Medical Oncology. 2023;**40**:179

[94] de Visser KE, Joyce JA. The evolving tumor microenvironment: From cancer initiation to metastatic outgrowth. Cancer Cell. 2023;**41**:374-403

[95] Boyle ST. RISING STARS: Hormonal regulation of the breast cancer microenvironment. Journal of Molecular Endocrinology. 2023;**70**(3):e220174

[96] Luo H et al. GPER-mediated proliferation and estradiol production in breast cancer-associated fibroblasts. Endocrine-Related Cancer. 2014;**21**:355-369

[97] Ouyang L et al. Estrogen-induced SDF-1α production promotes the progression of ER-negative breast cancer via the accumulation of MDSCs in the tumor microenvironment. Scientific Reports. 2016;**6**:39541

[98] De Marco P et al. GPER signalling in both cancer-associated fibroblasts and breast cancer cells mediates a feedforward IL1β/IL1R1 response. Scientific Reports. 2016;**6**:24354

[99] Vivacqua A, Muoio MG, Miglietta AM, Maggiolini M. Differential MicroRNA landscape triggered by estrogens in cancer associated fibroblasts (CAFs) of primary and metastatic breast tumors. Cancers (Basel). 2019;**11**(3):412

[100] Diep CH et al. Progesterone receptor signaling promotes cancer associated fibroblast mediated tumorigenicity in ER+ breast cancer. Endocrinology. 2024;**165**(9):bqae092

[101] Na H, Song Y, Lee HW. Emphasis on adipocyte transformation: Anti-inflammatory agents to prevent the development of cancer-associated adipocytes. Cancers (Basel). 2023;**15**(2):502

[102] Kim S et al. FAM3C in cancer-associated adipocytes promotes breast cancer cell survival and metastasis. Cancer Research. 2024;**84**:545-559

[103] Qureshi R et al. The major pre- and postmenopausal estrogens play opposing roles in obesity-driven mammary inflammation and breast cancer development. Cell Metabolism. 2020;**31**:1154-1172.e1159

[104] Morales DE et al. Estrogen promotes angiogenic activity in human umbilical vein endothelial cells in vitro and in a murine model. Circulation. 1995;**91**:755-763

[105] Hyder SM, Nawaz Z, Chiappetta C, Stancel GM. Identification of functional estrogen response elements in the gene coding for the potent angiogenic factor vascular endothelial growth factor. Cancer Research. 2000;**60**:3183-3190

[106] Applanat MP, Buteau-Lozano H, Herve MA, Corpet A. Vascular endothelial growth factor is a target gene for estrogen receptor and contributes to breast cancer progression. Advances in Experimental Medicine and Biology. 2008;**617**:437-444

[107] Takei H, Lee ES, Jordan VC. In vitro regulation of vascular endothelial growth factor by estrogens and antiestrogens in estrogen-receptor positive breast cancer. Breast Cancer. 2002;**9**:39-42

[108] Svensson S et al. CCL2 and CCL5 are novel therapeutic targets for estrogen-dependent breast cancer. Clinical Cancer Research. 2015;**21**:3794-3805

[109] Need EF, Atashgaran V, Ingman WV, Dasari P. Hormonal regulation of the immune microenvironment in the mammary gland. Journal of Mammary Gland Biology and Neoplasia. 2014;**19**:229-239

[110] Campbell MJ et al. Proliferating macrophages associated with high grade, hormone receptor negative breast cancer and poor clinical outcome. Breast Cancer Research and Treatment. 2011;**128**:703-711

[111] Gwak JM, Jang MH, Kim DI, Seo AN, Park SY. Prognostic value of tumor-associated macrophages according to histologic locations and hormone receptor status in breast cancer. PLoS One. 2015;**10**:e0125728

[112] Hollmén M, Roudnicky F, Karaman S, Detmar M. Characterization of macrophage--cancer cell crosstalk in estrogen receptor positive and triple-negative breast cancer. Scientific Reports. 2015;**5**:9188

[113] Smida T, Bruno TC, Stabile LP. Influence of estrogen on the NSCLC microenvironment: A comprehensive picture and clinical implications. Frontiers in Oncology. 2020;**10**:137

[114] Hammerl D et al. Clonality, antigen recognition, and suppression of CD8(+)

T cells differentially affect prognosis of breast cancer subtypes. Clinical Cancer Research. 2020;**26**:505-517

[115] Dannenfelser R et al. Data-driven analysis of immune infiltrate in a large cohort of breast cancer and its association with disease progression, ER activity, and genomic complexity. Oncotarget. 2017;**8**:57121-57133

[116] Khan D, Ansar Ahmed S. The immune system is a natural target for estrogen action: Opposing effects of estrogen in two prototypical autoimmune diseases. Frontiers in Immunology. 2015;**6**:635

[117] Lélu K et al. Estrogen receptor α signaling in T lymphocytes is required for estradiol-mediated inhibition of Th1 and Th17 cell differentiation and protection against experimental autoimmune encephalomyelitis. Journal of Immunology. 2011;**187**:2386-2393

[118] Jiang X, Orr BA, Kranz DM, Shapiro DJ. Estrogen induction of the granzyme B inhibitor, proteinase inhibitor 9, protects cells against apoptosis mediated by cytotoxic T lymphocytes and natural killer cells. Endocrinology. 2006;**147**:1419-1426

[119] Baral E, Nagy E, Kangas L, Berczi I. Combination therapy of the H2712 murine mammary carcinoma with cytotoxic T lymphocytes and anti-estrogens. Anticancer Research. 1997;**17**:3647-3651

[120] Polanczyk MJ et al. Cutting edge: Estrogen drives expansion of the CD4+CD25+ regulatory T cell compartment. Journal of Immunology. 2004;**173**:2227-2230

[121] Prieto GA, Rosenstein Y. Oestradiol potentiates the suppressive function of human CD4 CD25 regulatory T cells by promoting their proliferation. Immunology. 2006;**118**:58-65

[122] Lee JH, Lydon JP, Kim CH. Progesterone suppresses the mTOR pathway and promotes generation of induced regulatory T cells with increased stability. European Journal of Immunology. 2012;**42**:2683-2696

[123] Generali D et al. Immunomodulation of FOXP3+ regulatory T cells by the aromatase inhibitor letrozole in breast cancer patients. Clinical Cancer Research. 2009;**15**:1046-1051

[124] Polanczyk MJ, Hopke C, Vandenbark AA, Offner H. Treg suppressive activity involves estrogen-dependent expression of programmed death-1 (PD-1). International Immunology. 2007;**19**:337-343

[125] Goldberg J et al. The immunology of hormone receptor positive breast cancer. Frontiers in Immunology. 2021;**12**:674192

[126] Rothenberger NJ, Somasundaram A, Stabile LP. The role of the estrogen pathway in the tumor microenvironment. International Journal of Molecular Sciences. 2018;**19**(2):611

[127] Yang L et al. Posttranscriptional control of PD-L1 expression by 17β-estradiol via PI3K/Akt signaling pathway in ERα-positive cancer cell lines. International Journal of Gynecological Cancer. 2017;**27**:196-205

[128] Chung YR, Kim HJ, Jang MH, Park SY. Prognostic value of tumor infiltrating lymphocyte subsets in breast cancer depends on hormone receptor status. Breast Cancer Research and Treatment. 2017;**161**:409-420

[129] Zheng Y et al. COX-2 mediates tumor-stromal prolactin signaling to initiate tumorigenesis. Proceedings of the National Academy of Sciences of the United States of America. 2019;**116**:5223-5232

[130] Tang X, Morris AJ, Deken MA, Brindley DN. Autotaxin inhibition with IOA-289 decreases breast tumor growth in mice whereas knockout of autotaxin in adipocytes does not. Cancers (Basel). 2023;**15**(11):2937

[131] Morohoshi K, Mochinaga R, Watanabe T, Nakajima R, Harigaya T. 16 kDa vasoinhibin binds to integrin alpha5 beta1 on endothelial cells to induce apoptosis. Endocrine Connections. 2018;**7**:630-636

[132] Lee SG et al. Cathepsin D promotes polarization of tumor-associated macrophages and metastasis through TGFBI-CCL20 signaling. Experimental & Molecular Medicine. 2024;**56**:383-394

[133] Legorreta-Haquet MV et al. Prolactin down-regulates CD4+CD25hiCD127low/− regulatory T cell function in humans. Journal of Molecular Endocrinology. 2012;**48**:77-85

[134] Zahran AM et al. Accumulation of regulatory T cells in triple negative breast cancer can boost immune disruption. Cancer Management and Research. 2021;**13**:6019-6029

[135] Chen KHE et al. Translational Oncology. 2021;**14**:101195

[136] Montgomery DW, Krumenacker JS, Buckley AR. Prolactin stimulates phosphorylation of the human T-cell antigen receptor complex and ZAP-70 tyrosine kinase: A potential mechanism for its immunomodulation. Endocrinology. 1998;**139**:811-814

[137] Liang J, Deng Y, Zhang Y, Wu B, Zhou J. PRLR and CACNA2D1 impact the prognosis of breast cancer by regulating tumor immunity. Journal of Personalized Medicine. 2022;**12**(12):2086

[138] Giordano C et al. Activated FXR inhibits leptin signaling and counteracts tumor-promoting activities of cancer-associated fibroblasts in breast malignancy. Scientific Reports. 2016;**6**:21782

[139] Barone I et al. Leptin mediates tumor-stromal interactions that promote the invasive growth of breast cancer cells. Cancer Research. 2012;**72**:1416-1427

[140] Bocian-Jastrzębska A, Malczewska-Herman A, Kos-Kudła B. Role of leptin and adiponectin in carcinogenesis. Cancers (Basel). 2023;**15**(17):4250

[141] Gonzalez-Perez RR, Lanier V, Newman G. Leptin's pro-angiogenic signature in breast cancer. Cancers (Basel). 2013;**5**:1140-1162

[142] Zhou W, Guo S, Gonzalez-Perez RR. Leptin pro-angiogenic signature in breast cancer is linked to IL-1 signalling. British Journal of Cancer. 2011;**104**:128-137

[143] Fusco R et al. Cellular and molecular crosstalk between leptin receptor and estrogen receptor-{alpha} in breast cancer: Molecular basis for a novel therapeutic setting. Endocrine-Related Cancer. 2010;**17**:373-382

[144] Binai NA et al. Expression of estrogen receptor alpha increases leptin-induced STAT3 activity in breast cancer cells. International Journal of Cancer. 2010;**127**:55-66

[145] Uribesalgo I et al. Apelin inhibition prevents resistance and metastasis associated with anti-angiogenic therapy. EMBO Molecular Medicine. 2019;**11**:e9266

[146] Wang YY et al. ADSCs stimulated by resistin promote breast cancer cell malignancy via CXCL5 in a breast cancer coculture model. Scientific Reports. 2022;**12**:15437

[147] Warakomski J, Siemińska L. The role of adipose tissue with particular emphasis on cytokines in the pathogenesis of neoplastic diseases. Wiadomości Lekarskie. 2019;**72**:1551-1558

[148] Afrin S, Ramaiyer M, Begum UAM, Borahay MA. Adipocyte and adipokines promote a uterine leiomyoma friendly microenvironment. Nutrients. 2023;**15**(3):715

[149] Yadav NVS, Barcikowski A, Uehana Y, Jacobs AT, Connelly L. Breast adipocyte co-culture increases the expression of pro-angiogenic factors in macrophages. Frontiers in Oncology. 2020;**10**:454

[150] Wang YY et al. Visfatin enhances breast cancer progression through CXCL1 induction in tumor-associated macrophages. Cancers (Basel). 2020;**12**(12):3526

[151] Luo Y, Liu M. Adiponectin: A versatile player of innate immunity. Journal of Molecular Cell Biology. 2016;**8**:120-128

[152] Tsang JY et al. Novel immunomodulatory effects of adiponectin on dendritic cell functions. International Immunopharmacology. 2011;**11**:604-609

[153] Tan PH et al. Adiponectin receptor signaling on dendritic cells blunts antitumor immunity. Cancer Research. 2014;**74**:5711-5722

[154] Gelsomino L, Naimo GD, Catalano S, Mauro L, Andò S. The emerging role of adiponectin in female malignancies. International Journal of Molecular Sciences. 2019;**20**(9):2127

[155] Zhang Y et al. Adiponectin-expressing Treg facilitate T lymphocyte development in thymic nurse cell complexes. Communications Biology. 2021;**4**:344

[156] Pereira GDAV et al. Leptin, adiponectin, and melatonin modulate colostrum lymphocytes in mothers with obesity. International Journal of Molecular Sciences. 2023;**24**(3):2662

[157] Che N et al. Adiponectin enhances B-cell proliferation and differentiation via activation of Akt1/STAT3 and exacerbates collagen-induced arthritis. Frontiers in Immunology. 2021;**12**:626310

[158] Sun Y, Lodish HF. Adiponectin deficiency promotes tumor growth in mice by reducing macrophage infiltration. PLoS One. 2010;**5**:e11987

[159] Chikaishi W et al. Potential activity of adiponectin-expressing regulatory T cells against triple-negative breast cancer cells through the cell-in-cell phenomenon. Thoracic Cancer. 2023;**14**:1941-1945

Section 2

Innovations in Diagnostic Imaging and Classification

Chapter 6

Screening and Diagnosis Imagery in Breast Cancer: Classical and Emergent Techniques

Georgios Iatrakis, Stefanos Zervoudis, Anastasia Bothou, Eftymios Oikonomou, Konstantinos Nikolettos, Kyriakou Dimitrios, Nalmpanti Athanasia-Theopi, Kritsotaki Nektaria, Kotanidou Sonia, Spanakis Vlasios, Andreou Sotiris, Aise Chatzi Ismail Mouchterem, Kyriaki Chalkia, Christos Damaskos, Nikolaos Garmpis, Nikolaos Nikolettos and Panagiotis Tsikouras

Abstract

In light of the limitations of mammography, ultrasound, and breast MRI, some other breast imaging techniques have recently been investigated to reduce false positive rates and raise breast cancer detection including (1) digital breast tomosynthesis, (2) bilateral contrast-enhanced dual-energy digital mammography, (3) ultrasound elastography, (4) abbreviated breast MRI, (5) magnetic resonance spectroscopy, and (6) ductoscopy and duct cytology. The purpose of this review was to examine the advantages and disadvantages of these six different breast cancer imaging techniques.

Keywords: breast cancer, breast imaging technologies, screening of breast cancer, digital breast tomosynthesis, bilateral contrast-enhanced dual-energy digital mammography, abbreviated breast MRI, magnetic resonance spectroscopy, breast elastography, ductoscopy, duct lavage

1. Introduction

According to the National Cancer Institute, 297,790 new cases and 43,170 anticipated deaths from breast cancer are expected in 2023, making it one of the most common and deadly malignancies for women in the US [1]. The goal of continuously investigating innovations in screening modalities is to create technology that maximizes sensitivity and specificity while minimizing radiation exposure and patient discomfort. According to most international groups, breast cancer screening is suggested with annual or biennial mammography for average-risk women aged 50–74 years [2, 3]. To maximize the benefits of screening mammography and further

IntechOpen

reduce breast cancer mortality, breast cancer screening could start from 45 years of age, according to the American Cancer Society and European screening guidelines [3], or 40 years [4, 5]. However, in high-risk patients, imaging could begin as early as 30 years of age. Despite that mammography remains the gold standard for breast cancer screening [2] (**Figures 1** and **2**), its sensitivity varies from 37% to 71%, while its specificity is approximately 95% [3]. When an abnormality is detected on screening mammography, ultrasonography is frequently utilized for diagnostic follow-up to clarify features of a possible lesion. Although ultrasonography can be used in addition to mammography screening in women with dense breasts (e.g., to spot malignancies not visible on mammography), there is insufficient evidence to support the use of ultrasound alone in screening [3]. With a sensitivity that ranges from 70% to

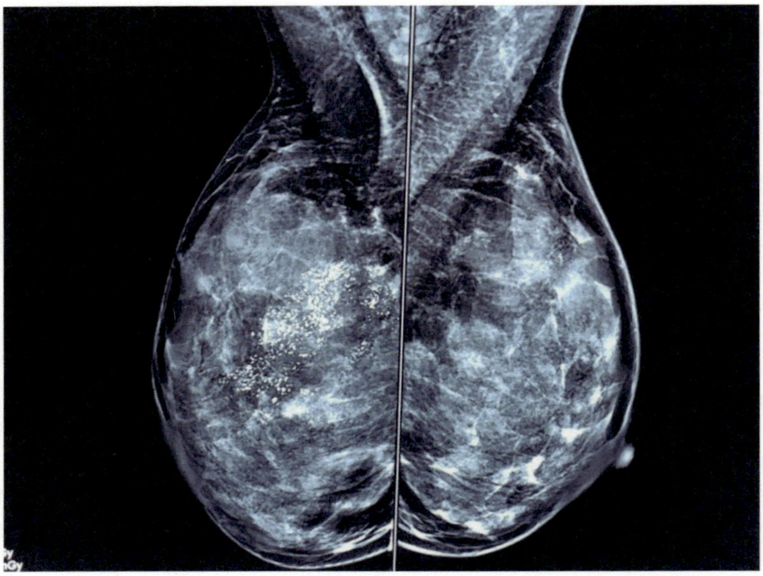

Figure 1.
Early breast cancer (DCIS) in mammography (mediolateral oblique [MLO] view).

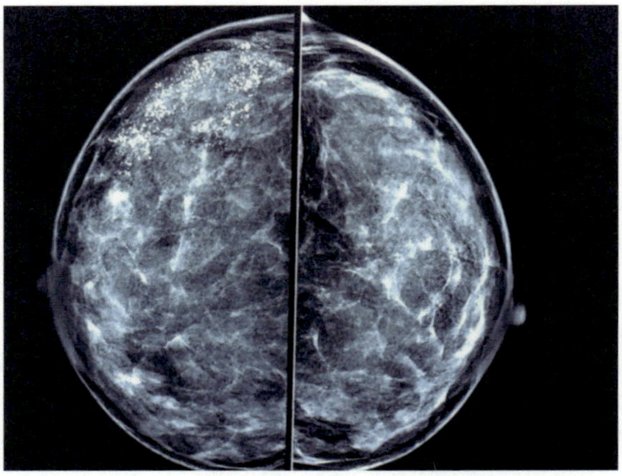

Figure 2.
Early breast cancer (DCIS) in mammography (craniocaudal [CC] view).

100%, breast magnetic resonance imaging (MRI) is thought to be the most sensitive method of breast imaging. However, because of its high cost and limited availability, MRI is typically reserved for high-risk patients and may be regarded as somewhat inaccessible [6].

In light of the limitations of mammography, ultrasound, and breast MRI, some other breast imaging techniques have been investigated including (1) digital breast tomosynthesis, (2) bilateral contrast-enhanced dual-energy spectral mammography, (3) abbreviated breast MRI, (4) magnetic resonance spectroscopy, (5) microwave imaging, (6) ultrasound elastography, (7) PET/CT and PET/MRI, (8) 18F-fluoroestradiol PET, and (9) ductoscopy.

2. Effectiveness of investigated screening techniques

2.1 Digital breast tomosynthesis (DBT)

DBT is an imaging method [7] (**Figure 3**) that was created to be used with digital mammography in order to improve its sensitivity and specificity while lowering the false positive rate. A digital detector and moving X-ray are used in DBT to create a three-dimensional mammography image. Actually, in DBT, individual images are reconstructed into a series of high-resolution slices displayed individually or in a "ciné" mode. DBT can be obtained independently using a synthetic two-dimensional (2D) mammogram that is artificially produced from the 3D picture collection, or it can be used in conjunction with digital mammography [3]. Compared to mammography, DBT provides a more detailed image of the breast that helps clarify any suspicious areas seen on mammograms because it allows decades of images to be taken of the same point in the breast from various angles along an arc. This is because the superimposed benign tissues from a two-dimensional perspective may appear more clinically questionable [8]. Numerous studies have demonstrated the superiority of DBT over standard full-field digital mammography in the detection of breast cancer [9]. Specifically, some prospective clinical trials and retrospective cohort studies

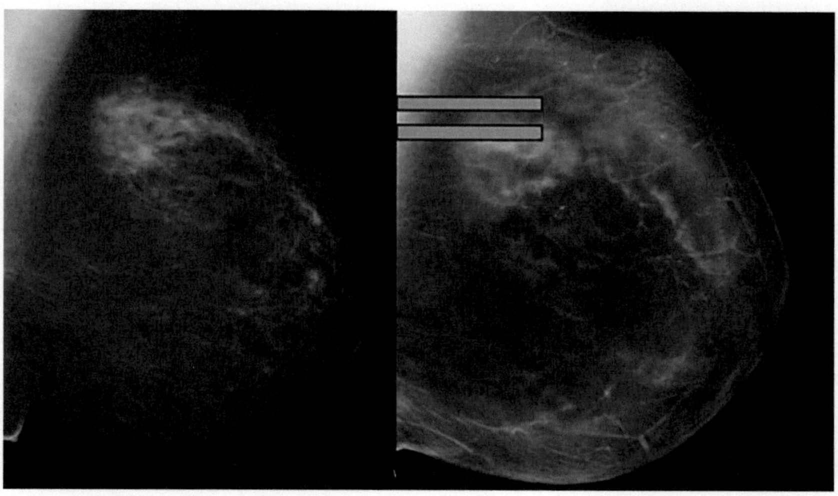

Figure 3.
Digital mammography and tomosynthesis.

indicate that tomosynthesis, as compared to digital mammography, slightly raises the rates of cancer diagnosis and lowers the recall rates for false-positive mammography readings [10–12].

According to a 2018 meta-analysis, DBT increased the incremental cancer detection rate by 1.6 cases per 1000 screens (95% CI 1.1–2.0) compared to digital mammography screening alone [13]. DBT had a poorer recall rate (pooled absolute decrease: −2.2, 95% CI −3.0 to −1.4) than digital mammography alone. The impact of DBT on breast cancer mortality has not been evaluated by any research.

While the patient experience with DBT is not much different from that of mammography, the concern about increased radiation exposure needs to be considered when making this decision. However, because of its better sensitivity and specificity in cancer detection rates when compared to mammography alone, DBT is advised as a cancer screening method, particularly in patients with dense breasts [14].

2.2 Bilateral contrast-enhanced dual-energy spectral mammography (CESM)

Twenty years ago, it was shown that bilateral CESM was a useful diagnostic technique for breast cancer detection [15] (**Figure 4**). CESM combines classic mammography with an iodinated contrast agent to improve diagnostic accuracy. Actually, the method consists of high-energy and low-energy (dual-energy) digital mammography after an intravenous injection of an iodinated contrast liquid. This enables the creation of an "anatomical and functional" image of the breast, with the low-energy component indicating calcifications and the subtracted image showing neovascularization, which represents angiogenesis [16].

Studies indicate that, in 2D digital mammography, CESM can reveal calcifications that would otherwise be undetected. Furthermore, there has not been any research to support the theory that this imaging method is effective in identifying invasive lobular carcinoma (ILC), a type of breast cancer that is known to be challenging to diagnose as it may not manifest as a palpably noticeable mass [16].

Additionally, studies have demonstrated that when combined with mammography, CESM is particularly helpful for detecting breast cancer in women with dense breasts [17]. Moreover, this kind of digital mammography may be a useful alternate technique for patients who cannot undergo a full diagnostic MRI study (e.g., patients

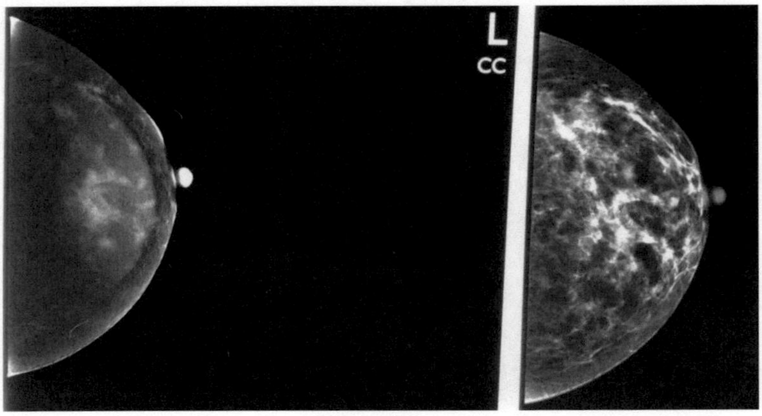

Figure 4.
Angiomammography CESM.

with a pacemaker). It should be mentioned that the use of contrast is not always the best option for patients and is not always effective, particularly in cases of allergy or pathological or drug-induced renal impairment. Interestingly, it should be emphasized that CESM has shown comparable sensitivity with other imaging modalities, including MRI [18]. However, comparing its specificity to the current gold standard for breast cancer screening, it has been discovered to be quite variable [19].

2.3 Abbreviated breast MRI

In contrast to a full diagnostic MRI study, which takes 15–20 minutes, an abbreviated breast MRI (ultrafast) (**Figures 5** and **6**) for breast cancer screening involves a shorter imaging protocol (with fewer sequences) that allows patients to

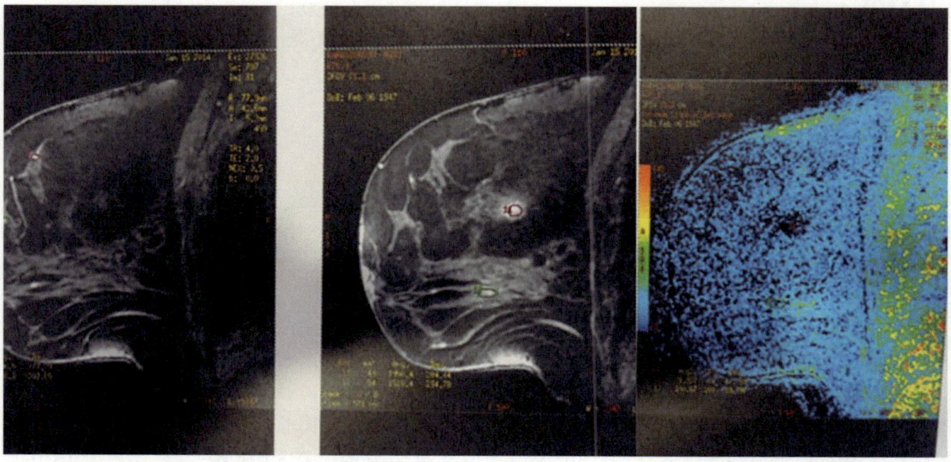

Figure 5.
Breast MRI.

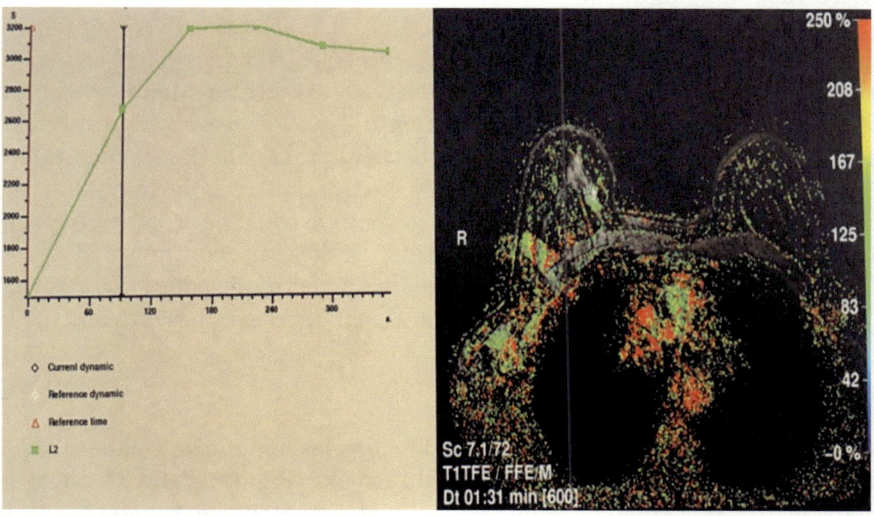

Figure 6.
Breast MRI dynamic study.

spend no more than 5 to 10 minutes within the MRI scanner. Compared to a full MRI, this abbreviated protocol revealed >98% accuracy in the diagnostic setting as well as 100% accuracy in the screening setting [20].

Thus, this technology may be a useful adjunct for patients who cannot undergo a full diagnostic MRI evaluation (e.g., claustrophobic patients). Actually, some recent retrospective studies are showing that the abbreviated MRI protocol has comparable sensitivity with the full diagnostic protocol of MRI [21, 22].

Furthermore, as an example of the reliability of abbreviated MRI imaging, a recent study conducted on women who had previously undergone breast surgery revealed that when an abbreviated MRI imaging was compared to screening mammography and ultrasound, the abbreviated MRI imaging identified all cancers. Thus, it should be emphasized that some cancers detected by abbreviated breast MRI were missed by screening mammography and ultrasound [23]. Similarly, in a recent study, abbreviated MRI discovered breast cancers missed by digital breast tomosynthesis [24].

These findings suggest that abbreviated MRI may be used in screening for breast cancer in women who have low, average, or high risk.

2.4 Magnetic resonance spectroscopy (MRS)

MRS is a specialized an MRI imaging technique allowing the assessment of the chemical composition of breast tissue. In fact, it was observed that malignant tumors have elevated choline levels. Thus, MRS of the breast detects choline and its derivatives in breast tumors [25].

Unfortunately, not all breast cancers express choline, and the method remains investigational due to a substantial number of false negative results.

The method could increase the specificity of the classic breast MRI. Increasing the specificity means fewer false positive findings and, thus, fewer biopsies in many women. In the past, the method showed some promising results in therapy response [26] and could have a future role in predicting outcomes after certain therapies for breast cancer.

2.5 Microwave imaging

The method is based on the difference of certain electric parameters between normal breast tissue and cancer within the microwave spectrum. Microwave imaging does not expose the patient to ionizing radiation and avoids breast compression to achieve best imaging. However, the contrast between malignant tissue, normal fatty, and fibroglandular tissue can be as low as 10%, and, at this level, the resolution is noticeably low resulting in blurred images. The method could be proposed in younger women although further research is necessary as the dielectric contrast in MWI varies greatly at different ages and between individuals. Furthermore, additional research is needed to demonstrate the feasibility of certain techniques to improve the method [27].

2.6 Ultrasound elastography

Breast malignant tumors look larger, and benign lesions appear smaller on the strain elastography compared to a B-mode ultrasound (**Figures** 7 and **8**), an imaging characteristic that could differentiate malignant from benign tumors in certain cases. Furthermore, sharewave elastography is displaying relative stiffness in color differences, distinguishing "harder" malignant tumors from the benign ones [28].

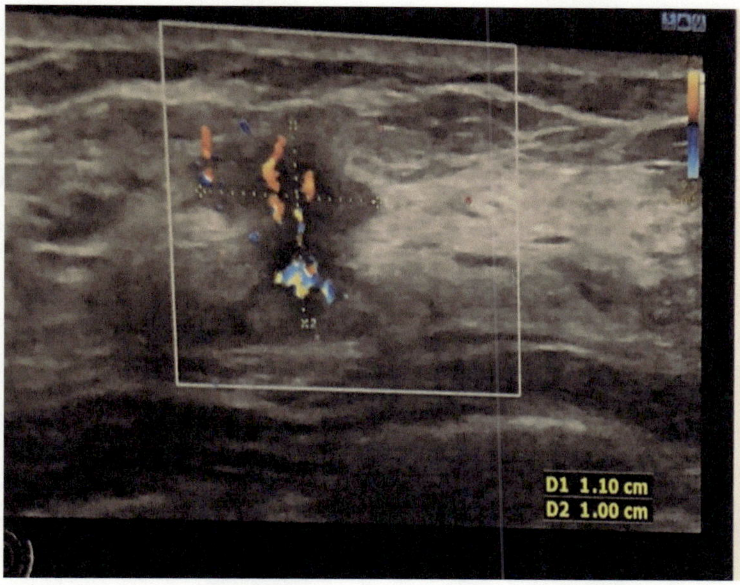

Figure 7.
Breast ultrasound and power Doppler.

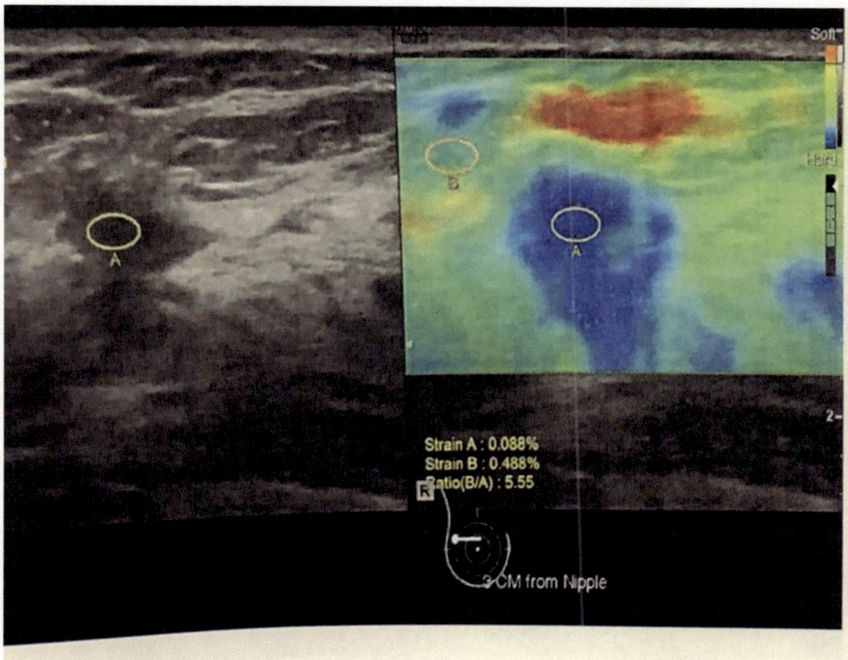

Figure 8.
Breast ultrasound and elastography.

However, size differences and color gradients in the above methods do not provide the information required with high sensitivity, compared to MRI, which is necessary for cancer detection methods. Furthermore, data related to mortality, as in mammography, are missing.

2.7 PET/CT and PET/MRI

For breast cancer imaging, PET/CT (**Figures 9** and **10**) and PET/MRI may be utilized for diagnosis, staging, in cases of probable metastasis at the diagnosis of breast cancer, and evaluation of the treatment response. However, the methods are not proposed for breast cancer screening. Compared to PET/MRI, there is significantly

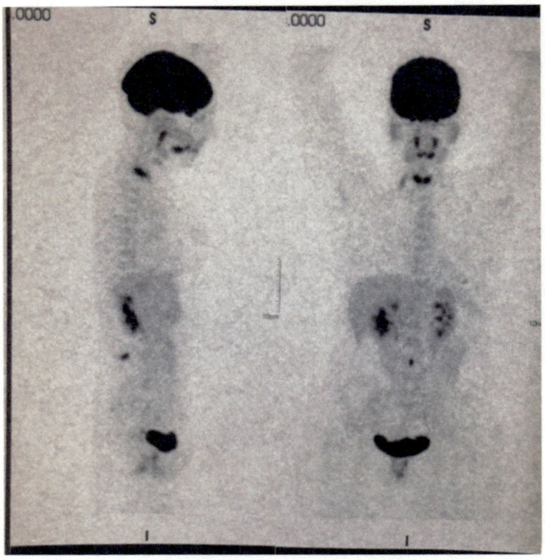

Figure 9.
PET/CT multiple metastasis.

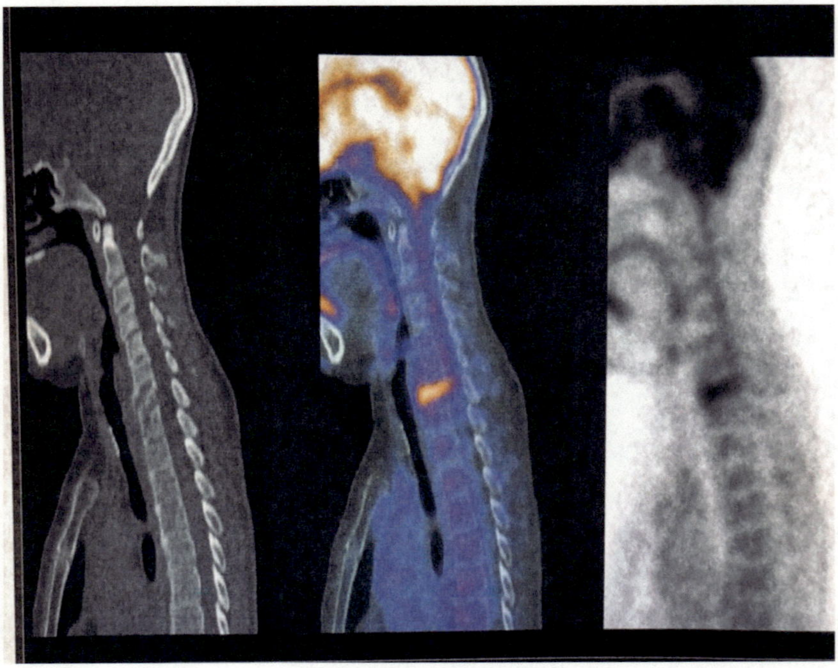

Figure 10.
PET/CT and PET/MRI bone metastasis.

increased radiation exposure to the patient with PET/CT. Furthermore, PET/CT seems inferior to PET/MRI for detecting unsuspected regional or distant diseases [29]. However, compared to PET/MRI scanners, PET/CT scanners are more widely available, and there is a greater experience in their use for distant diseases.

2.8 18F-fluoroestradiol PET (FES-PET)

18F-fluoroestradiol (FES) is a PET tracer with high specificity for estrogen receptor breast cancer. However, the method cannot be used in other cases (as in triple-negative breast cancer), and its usefulness was shown mainly in oligometastatic disease [30].

2.9 Ductoscopy

Ductoscopy is an innovative diagnostic method based on the endoscopic examination of the breast ducts (**Figures 11** and **12**), especially in the case of pathologic nipple discharge. Ductoscopy is performed under local anesthesia or light sedation. The technique is completely painless and takes between 5 and 20 minutes depending on the case. It is a short procedure in which the duct that secretes fluid is dilated, the ductoscope penetrates the duct and the surgeon checks the inside of the duct through the monitor. After the visual examination is completed, saline is injected into the duct, followed by aspiration (duct lavage) for the collection of endothelial cells and

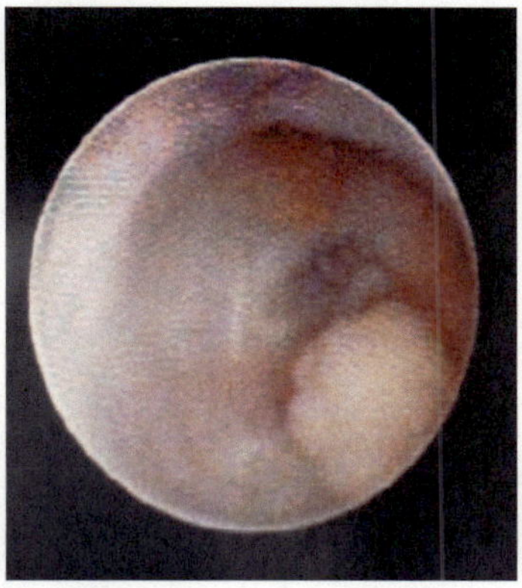

Figure 11.
Breast ductoscopy papilloma.

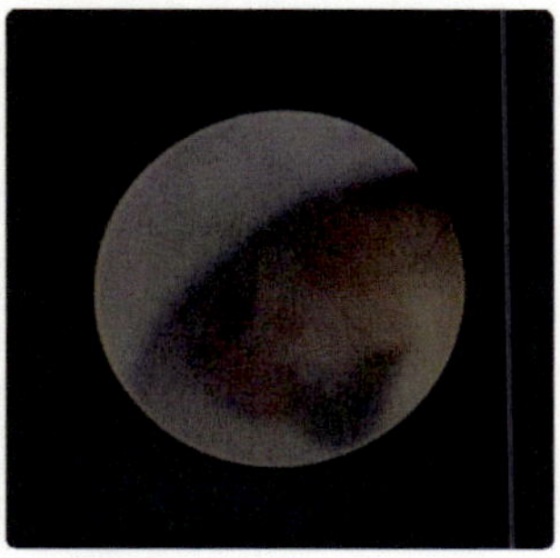

Figure 12.
Breast ductoscopy breast cancer.

cytological examination [31] (**Figure 13**). Recently some specialists have used an additional diagnostic procedure during ductoscopy, the "duct brushing" (**Figure 14**). With a very thin brush, which is inserted into the duct through the ductoscope, the duct walls are scraped to collect more cells (brushing). Then, the cytological examination is performed using the liquid phase technique (ThinPrep), while for greater

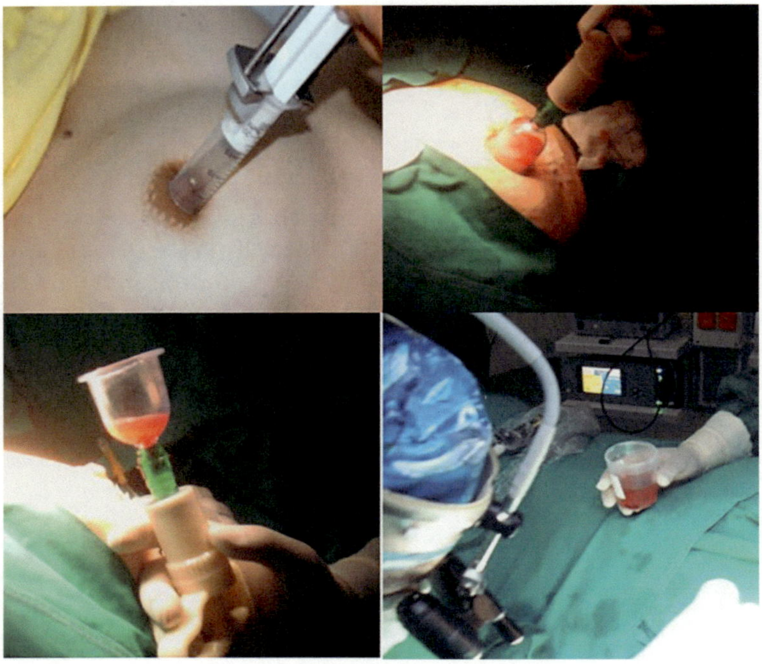

Figure 13.
Zervoudis's mammary pump and duct lavage.

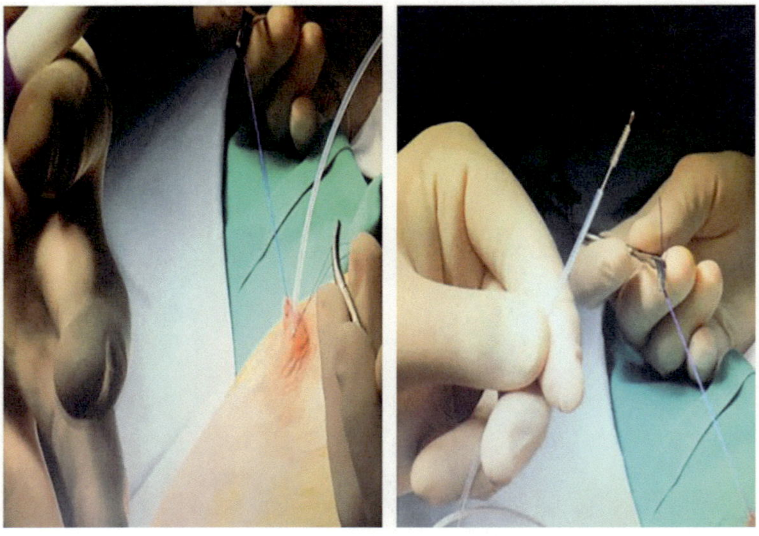

Figure 14.
Duct brushing.

collection of cells for diagnosis, fluid is also taken from the nipple, using a special pump (Zervoudis's mammary pump) [32] (**Figure 13**).

Ductoscopy is an emergent complementary technique of mammography and breast ultrasound used in women with nipple discharge and also to detect breast cancer in patients with very early breast cancer and patients with a heavy family history. Also, if the intraductal tumor needs to be removed, ductoscopy guides the microsurgical procedure of removal (pyramidectomy and microdolicectomy).

Given the diagnostic efficiency of more than 75% and affordable cost, ductoscopy becomes an additional powerful procedure for the surgeon.

The accuracy of the diagnosis is increased when ductoscopy, duct lavage, and duct brushing are combined [33–34]. According to a recent meta-analysis, although liquid cytology has a modest sensitivity, it is a valuable diagnostic tool for the high-specificity detection of breast cancer in patients with pathological nipple discharge [35].

3. Harms of breast cancer screening

In addition to the discomfort and hazards associated with the screening process, false-positive or false-negative results from breast cancer screening can be harmful. Furthermore, an overdiagnosis of breast cancer could be harmful to women. The term "overdiagnosis" describes the diagnosis of illnesses that, had screening not been used, would not have progressed to a clinically important stage. Overdiagnosis results in unneeded testing and therapy, as well as psychological effects and further repercussions from receiving a cancer diagnosis and treatment [3].

3.1 False-positive tests

While test sensitivity and specificity are both significant, false-positive results are frequently the source of greatest concern for patients and physicians. The advice for further testing and procedures if a woman does not have cancer is the clinical consequence. Because breast cancer is less common and the tests are less specific, false-positive findings are more common in younger women [36].

Consequently, even if fewer tumors are discovered, younger women will undergo more follow-up procedures. Interestingly, in a retrospective cohort study of 2400 women, the calculated cumulative risk of a false-positive result following 10 mammograms was 49.1%, and following 10 clinical breast exams (CBEs), it was 22.3% [37].

In a different study, it was estimated that 61.3% of women starting at age 40 who underwent annual mammography would require recall for at least one scan over 10 years, and 7% percent would undergo biopsy in the event of a false-positive reading. For women having biennial (every other year) mammography, the estimated rate of recall was 41.6%, and the rate of biopsy over 10 years was 4.8% [38].

The risk of a false-positive study at the first, and by the ninth, screening mammogram was 98 and 100% in those women with the highest risk variables (young age, prior breast biopsies, a family history of breast cancer, current hormonal therapy, 3 years between screenings, no comparison to prior mammograms, and the tendency of the radiologist to call mammograms abnormal [radiologist's random effect]). On the other hand, the predicted risks for the first and ninth mammograms were 0.7 and 4.6%, respectively, for those with the lowest risk characteristics. The scientists hypothesized that women could have less worry when abnormal mammography was reported if they were aware of their relative risk of a false-positive study based on these characteristics [39].

3.2 Anxiety related to false-positive findings

There is no proof that having false-positive findings will have long-term, persistently unpleasant psychological effects. However, there are short-term, detrimental psychological effects that could last days to weeks [40].

3.3 False-negative tests can delay diagnosis and breast cancer treatment

Screening exams and other medical examinations are not infallible. Sometimes screening mammography results are regarded as negative, yet at the time of the test, the breast does indeed contain cancer. The radiologist may have overlooked these malignancies, or the lesions may not have been obvious on a retrospective imaging examination [41]. A combination of these factors results in the missing diagnosis of about one in eight breast cancers during screening mammography [42]. A false-negative test result is more likely to occur in women who are younger, have dense breasts, have hormone-independent cancer, or have cancer that is proliferating. Consequently, even after a recent negative screening imaging scan, women who exhibit worrying signs or symptoms (e.g., palpable breast lump and new nipple retraction) should have a follow-up evaluation, preferably with a breast surgeon or breast cancer expert.

3.4 Overdiagnosis

The identification of an illness that, had it not been discovered, would not have resulted in morbidity or death is known as overdiagnosis [42]. Certain tumors develop slowly, and some may even go into remission. Overdiagnosis can only be estimated using one of the several methods; it cannot be assessed directly. The percentage of women who receive a false positive for breast cancer ranges from 10% to over 50%, depending on the definition used (e.g., whether ductal carcinoma in situ [DCIS] is included and what age women are studied), as well as the methods used for study design, measurement, and estimation. A perfect screening test would differentiate between malignancies with high or low risk, enabling tailored treatment based on tumor biology [43]. There is not any testing like that accessible. As it is impossible to accurately determine which cancers in a given patient will never progress, treatment is almost always advised.

3.5 Radiation

Although ionizing radiation raises the risk of breast cancer, the majority of cohort studies investigating the issue have included women who were exposed to radiation doses significantly higher than the average glandular dosage for a two-view digital mammography performed at facilities authorized by the American College of Radiology [44]. According to a study conducted in 2015, which supported the adjustment of the US Preventive Services Task Force breast cancer screening guidelines, 16 out of 100,000 women will die from radiation-induced cancer as a result of annual mammography screening throughout their lifetimes [45].

3.6 Ductal carcinoma in situ

DCIS (**Figures 1** and **2**) accounts for about 16% of breast cancer diagnoses in the US. Over 48,000 women in the US received a DCIS diagnosis in 2019 [46]. About 50%

of DCIS cases may not progress to aggressive malignancy, and the natural history of the condition is unclear [47]. It is unknown which cases of DCIS may advance to invasive illness; hence, concerns have been expressed that the discovery of DCIS by mammography may result in overdiagnosis and overtreatment. Typically, the diagnosis leads to surgery and systemic therapy. Suboptimal concordance (84% agreement) across pathologists in identifying DCIS in a breast biopsy sample is another cause for worry. Study pathologists misinterpreted DCIS as invasive breast cancer, and overinterpreted it as benign with or without atypia [48].

3.7 Other possible harms

Another potential harm of breast cancer screening is discomfort, especially during mammography. According to a well-conducted study, patient-controlled breast compression improved the image quality and decreased patient pain [49]. There was a stronger intention to return for another screening assessment when there was less discomfort.

Furthermore, there are more possible risks connected to alternative screening methods. For example, women may not be able to tolerate intravenous gadolinium injection (e.g., because of an allergic response or kidney failure) or may experience claustrophobia, which makes breast MRI unfeasible [50].

3.8 Discussion

Mammography is the gold standard for breast cancer screening [2]. However, its sensitivity is relatively low. Thus, if an abnormality is detected on screening mammography, other imaging techniques are necessary to clarify the initial findings. These techniques include ultrasonography, digital breast tomosynthesis, classic or abbreviated breast MRI, bilateral contrast-enhanced dual-energy spectral mammography, magnetic resonance spectroscopy, microwave imaging, ultrasound elastography, PET/CT, PET/MRI, 18F-fluoroestradiol PET, and ductoscopy. However, it should be emphasized that annual mammography proved beneficial for most women in terms of reduced mortality from breast cancer [51], a finding not yet related to other imaging techniques.

4. Conclusion

The primary key to women's survival from breast cancer is early detection and treatment. As a result, imaging is essential in the diagnosis and management of breast cancer cases. In recent years, DBT, CESM, abbreviated breast MRI, MRS, and breast ductoscopy have become more heavily investigated. Given its potential effects on health and society, research on new breast imaging technologies is crucial. Many patients worry when undergoing breast cancer screening, and any progress made in reducing the financial burden, scan-to-result time, and accuracy will lessen patient anxiety. Although it is clear that no screening technique has yet been created that is more practical or dependable than mammography, advancements in this area are significant enough to warrant further research in the hopes of improving the management of all breast cancer cases.

Author details

Georgios Iatrakis[1], Stefanos Zervoudis[1,2], Anastasia Bothou[1,3], Eftymios Oikonomou[4], Konstantinos Nikolettos[4], Kyriakou Dimitrios[4], Nalmpanti Athanasia-Theopi[4], Kritsotaki Nektaria[4], Kotanidou Sonia[4], Spanakis Vlasios[4], Andreou Sotiris[4], Aise Chatzi Ismail Mouchterem[4], Kyriaki Chalkia[4], Christos Damaskos[5], Nikolaos Garmpis[6], Nikolaos Nikolettos[4] and Panagiotis Tsikouras[4*]

1 University of West Attica, Athens, Greece

2 Rea Maternity Hospital: Breast Unit, Athens, Greece

3 Breast Department of Alexandra General Hospital, Athens, Greece

4 Department of Obstetrics and Gynecology, Democritus University of Thrace, Greece

5 Second Department of Propedeutic Surgery, Laiko General Hospital, Medical School, National and Kapodistrian University of Athens, Athens, Greece

6 Renal Transplatation Unit, Laiko General Hospital, Athens, Greece

*Address all correspondence to: tsikouraspanagiotis@gmail.com

References

[1] Cancer Stat Facts: Female Breast Cancer. 2023. Available from: https://seer.cancer.gov/statfacts/html/breast.html.

[2] Zervoudis S, Iatrakis G, Tomara E, Bothou A, Papadopoulos G, Tsakiris G. Main controversies in breast cancer. World Journal of Clinical Oncology. 2014;**5**(3):359-373. DOI: 10.5306/wjco.v5.i3.359

[3] Elmore JG, Lee CI. Screening for Breast Cancer: Evidence for Effectiveness and Harms. Waltham, MA: UpToDate; 2023

[4] Bastardis-Zakas K, Iatrakis G, Navrozoglou I, Peitsidis P, Salakos N, Malakassis P, et al. Maximizing the benefits of screening mammography for women 40-49 years old. Clinical and Experimental Obstetrics & Gynecology. 2010;**37**(4):278-282

[5] Duffy SW, Vulkan D, Cuckle H, Parmar D, Sheikh S, Smith RA, et al. Effect of mammographic screening from age 40 years on breast cancer mortality (UK age trial): Final results of a randomised, controlled trial. The Lancet Oncology. 2020;**21**(9):1165-1172. DOI: 10.1016/S1470-2045(20)30398-3

[6] Sung J, Lebron L, Keating D, D'Alessio D, Comstock C, Lee C, et al. Performance of dual-energy contrast-enhanced digital mammography for screening women at increased risk of breast cancer. Radiology. 2019;**293**(1):81-88. DOI: 10.1148/radiol.2019182660

[7] Zervoudis S, Iatrakis G, Malakassis P, Tomara E, Bouga A, Grammatikakis I, et al. Tomosynthesis improves breast cancer detection: Our experience. European Journal of Gynaecological Oncology. 2014;**35**(6):666-669

[8] Chong A, Weinstein S, McDonald E, Conant E. Digital breast tomosynthesis: Concepts and clinical practice. Radiology. 2019;**292**(1):1-14. DOI: 10.1148/radiol.2019180760

[9] Nakajima E, Tsunoda H, Ookura M, Ban K, Kawaguchi Y, Inagaki M, et al. Digital breast tomosynthesis complements two-dimensional synthetic mammography for secondary examination of breast cancer. Journal of the Belgian Society of Radiology. 2021;**105**(1):63. DOI: 10.5334/jbsr.2457

[10] Skaane P, Bandos AI, Gullien R, Eben E, Ekseth U, Haakenaasen U, et al. Comparison of digital mammography alone and digital mammography plus tomosynthesis in a population-based screening program. Radiology. 2013;**267**(1):47-56. DOI: 10.1148/radiol.12121373

[11] Ciatto S, Houssami N, Bernardi D, Caumo F, Pellegrini M, Brunelli S, et al. killIntegration of 3D digital mammography with tomosynthesis for population breast-cancer screening (STORM): A prospective comparison study. The Lancet Oncology. 2013;**14**(7):583-589. DOI: 10.1016/S1470-2045(13)70134-7

[12] Friedewald SM, Rafferty EA, Rose SL, Durand M, Plecha D, Greenberg J, et al. Breast cancer screening using tomosynthesis in combination with digital mammography. Journal of the American Medical Association. 2014;**311**(24):2499-2507. DOI: 10.1001/jama.2014.6095

[13] Marinovich M, Hunter K, Macaskill P, Houssami N. Breast cancer screening using tomosynthesis or mammography: A meta-analysis of cancer detection and recall. Journal of the National

Cancer Institute. 2018;**110**(9):942-949. DOI: 10.1093/jnci/djy121

[14] Venkataraman S, Slanetz P, Lee C. Breast Imaging for Cancer Screening: Mammography and Ultrasonography. UpToDate; 2022

[15] Lewin JM, Isaacs PK, Vance V, Larke FJ. Dual-energy contrast-enhanced digital subtraction mammography: Feasibility. Radiology. 2003;**229**(1):261-268. DOI: 10.1148/radiol.2291021276

[16] Sorin V, Sklair-Levy M. Dual-energy contrast-enhanced spectral mammography (CESM) for breast cancer screening. Quantitative Imaging in Medicine and Surgery. 2019;**9**(11):1914-1917. DOI: 10.21037/qims.2019.10.13

[17] Cheung YC, Lin YC, Wan YL, Yeow KM, Huang PC, Lo YF, et al. Diagnostic performance of dual-energy contrast-enhanced subtracted mammography in dense breasts compared to mammography alone: Interobserver blind-reading analysis. European Radiology. 2014;**24**(10):2394-2403. DOI: 10.1007/s00330-014-3271-1

[18] Fallenberg EM, Dromain C, Diekmann F, Engelken F, Krohn M, Singh JM, et al. Contrast-enhanced spectral mammography versus MRI: Initial results in the detection of breast cancer and assessment of tumor size. European Radiology. 2014;**24**(1):256-264. DOI: 10.1007/s00330-013-3007-7

[19] Spick C, Pinker-Domenig K, Rudas M, Helbich T, Baltzer P. MRI-only lesions: Application of diffusion-weighted imaging obviates unnecessary MR-guided breast biopsies. European Radiology. 2014;**24**(6):1204-1210. DOI: 10.1007/s00330-014-3153-6

[20] Ahmadinejad N, Azhdeh S, Arian A, Eslami B, Mehrabinejad MM. Implementation of abbreviated breast MRI in diagnostic and screening settings. Acta Radiologica. 2023;**64**(3):987-992. DOI: 10.1177/02841851221114434

[21] Chen SQ, Huang M, Shen YY, Liu CL, Xu CX. Application of abbreviated protocol of magnetic resonance imaging for breast cancer screening in dense breast tissue. Academic Radiology. 2017;**24**(3):316-320. DOI: 10.1016/j.acra.2016.10.003

[22] Panigrahi B, Mullen L, Falomo E, Panigrahi B, Harvey S. An abbreviated protocol for high-risk screening breast magnetic resonance imaging: Impact on performance metrics and BI-RADS assessment. Academic Radiology. 2017;**24**(9):1132-1138. DOI: 10.1016/j.acra.2017.03.014

[23] Choi BH, Choi N, Kim MY, Yang JH, Yoo YB, Jung HK. Usefulness of abbreviated breast MRI screening for women with a history of breast cancer surgery. Breast Cancer Research and Treatment. 2018;**167**(2):495-502. DOI: 10.1007/s10549-017-4530-z

[24] Weinstein SP, Korhonen K, Cirelli C, Schnall MD, McDonald ES, Pantel AR, et al. Abbreviated breast magnetic resonance imaging for supplemental screening of women with dense breasts and average risk. Journal of Clinical Oncology. 2020;**38**(33):3874-3882. DOI: 10.1200/JCO.19.02198

[25] Sardanelli F, Fausto A, Di Leo G, de Nijs R, Vorbuchner M, Podo F. In vivo proton MR spectroscopy of the breast using the total choline peak integral as a marker of malignancy. American Journal of Roentgenology. 2009;**192**(6):1608-1617. DOI: 10.2214/AJR.07.3521

[26] Tozaki M, Sakamoto M, Oyama Y, O'uchi T, Kawano N, Suzuki T, et al. Monitoring of early response to neoadjuvant chemotherapy in breast

cancer with (1)H MR spectroscopy: Comparison to sequential 2-[18F]-fluorodeoxyglucose positron emission tomography. Journal of Magnetic Resonance Imaging. 2008;**28**(2):420-427. DOI: 10.1002/jmri.21454

[27] Akbari-Chelaresi H, Alsaedi D, Mirjahanmardi SH, El Badawe M, Albishi AM, Nayyeri V, et al. Mammography using low-frequency electromagnetic fields with deep learning. Scientific Reports. 2023;**13**(1):13253. DOI: 10.1038/s41598-023-40494-x

[28] Barr RG. Future of breast elastography. Ultrasonography. 2019;**38**(2):93-105. DOI: 10.14366/usg.18053

[29] Fowler AM, Strigel RM. Clinical advances in PET/MRI for breast cancer. The Lancet Oncology. 2022;**23**(1):e32-e43. DOI: 10.1016/S1470-2045(21)00577-5

[30] Denton M, Taubman K, Sutherland T. 18F-Fluoroestradiol PET in the evaluation of probable oligometastatic breast cancer. Journal of Medical Imaging and Radiation Oncology. 2021;**65**(3):333-334. DOI: 10.1111/1754-9485.13136

[31] Zervoudis S, Tamer V, Iatrakis G, Bothou A, Tokou X, Augoulea A, et al. Improving ductoscopy with duct lavage and duct brushing. European Journal of Gynaecological Oncology. 2014;**35**(5):548-553

[32] Zervoudis S. A simple tool complementary for the diagnosis of breast diseases: The mammary pump. The Breast Journal. 2003;**9**(5):445-447. DOI: 10.1046/j.1524-4741.2003.09524.x

[33] Zervoudis S, Iatrakis G, Daures JP, Bothou A, Aranitis V, Patralexis X, et al. Ductoscopy coupled to duct lavage and duct brushing in pathologic nipple discharge: Our experience. Chirurgia (Bucur). 2020;**115**(3):334-340. DOI: 10.21614/chirurgia.115.3.334

[34] Bothou A, Iatrakis G, Zervoudis S, Tsatsaris G, Lykeridou K, Deuteraiou D, et al. Breast milk suction pumping and a possible relation to breast cancer: A bicentric study. Review Clinical Pharmacology and Pharmacokinetics, International Edition. 2020;**34**(1): 5-8. DOI: https://doi.org/10.5281/zenodo.10040437

[35] Li XQ, Xu F, Lei CQ, Li J, Jiang HC. Accuracy for cytological evaluation in the detection of breast cancer among patients with pathologic nipple discharge: A PRISMA-compliant meta-analysis. Chinese Medical Journal. 2020;**133**:435-443. DOI: 10.1097/CM9.0000000000000643

[36] Lidbrink E, Elfving J, Frisell J, Jonsson E. Neglected aspects of false positive findings of mammography in breast cancer screening: Analysis of false positive cases from the Stockholm trial. BMJ. 1996;**312**(7026):273-276. DOI: 10.1136/bmj.312.7026.273

[37] Elmore J, Barton M, Moceri V, Polk S, Arena P, Fletcher S. Ten-year risk of false positive screening mammograms and clinical breast examinations. The New England Journal of Medicine. 1998;**338**(16):1089-1096. DOI: 10.1056/NEJM199804163381601

[38] Hubbard R, Kerlikowske K, Flowers C, Yankaskas B, Zhu W, Miglioretti D. Cumulative probability of false-positive recall or biopsy recommendation after 10 years of screening mammography: A cohort study. Annals of Internal Medicine. 2011;**155**(8):481-492. DOI: 10.7326/0003-4819-155-8-201110180-00004

[39] Christiansen C, Wang F, Barton M, Kreuter W, Elmore J, Gelfand A, et al. Predicting the cumulative risk of

false-positive mammograms. Journal of the National Cancer Institute. 2000;**92**(20):1657-1666. DOI: 10.1093/jnci/92.20.1657

[40] Tyndel S, Austoker J, Henderson B, Brain K, Bankhead C, Clements A, et al. What is the psychological impact of mammographic screening on younger women with a family history of breast cancer? Findings from a prospective cohort study by the PIMMS Management Group. Journal of Clinical Oncology. 2007;**25**(25):3823-3830. DOI: 10.1200/JCO.2007.11.0437

[41] Lamb L, Mohallem Fonseca M, Verma R, Seely J. Missed breast cancer: Effects of subconscious bias and lesion characteristics. Radiographics. 2020;**40**(4):941-960. DOI: 10.1148/rg.2020190090

[42] Lehman C, Arao R, Sprague B, Lee J, Buist D, Kerlikowske K, et al. National performance benchmarks for modern screening digital mammography: Update from the breast cancer surveillance consortium. Radiology. 2017;**283**(1):49-58. DOI: 10.1148/radiol.2016161174

[43] Esserman L, Shieh Y, Thompson I. Rethinking screening for breast cancer and prostate cancer. Journal of the American Medical Association. 2009;**302**(15):1685-1692. DOI: 10.1001/jama.2009.1498

[44] Ronckers C, Erdmann C, Land C. Radiation and breast cancer: A review of current evidence. Breast Cancer Research. 2005;**7**(1):21-32. DOI: 10.1186/bcr970

[45] Modeling Report: Radiation-Induced Breast Cancer and Breast Cancer Death from Mammography Screening. Supporting document for U.S. Preventive Services Task Force; Breastcancer screening draft recommendations. http://www.uspreventiveservicestaskforce.org/Page/Document/modeling-report-radiation-induced-breast-cancer-and-breast-c/breast-cancer-screening1 [Accessed on June 26, 2015]

[46] American Cancer Society. Breast Cancer Facts & Figures 2019-2020. Available from: https://www.cancer.org/content/dam/cancer-org/research/cancer-facts-and-statistics/breast-cancer-facts-and-figures/breast-cancer-facts-and-figures-2019-2020.pdf [Accessed on November 30, 2020]

[47] Welch H, Woloshin S, Schwartz L. The sea of uncertainty surrounding ductal carcinoma in situ--the price of screening mammography. Journal of the National Cancer Institute. 2008;**100**(4):228-229. DOI: 10.1093/jnci/djn013

[48] Elmore J, Longton G, Carney P, Geller B, Onega T, Tosteson A, et al. Diagnostic concordance among pathologists interpreting breast biopsy specimens. Journal of the American Medical Association. 2015;**313**(11):1122-1132. DOI: 10.1001/jama.2015.1405

[49] Kornguth P, Rimer B, Conaway M, Sullivan D, Catoe K, Stout A, et al. Impact of patient-controlled compression on the mammography experience. Radiology. 1993;**186**(1):99-102. DOI: 10.1148/radiology.186.1.8416595

[50] Monticciolo D. Magnetic resonance imaging of the breast for cancer diagnosis and staging. Seminars in Ultrasound, CT, and MR. 2011;**32**(4):319-330. DOI: 10.1053/j.sult.2011.02.005

[51] Park HL, Chang J, Haridass V, Wang SS, Ziogas A, Anton-Culver H. Mammography screening and mortality by risk status in the California teachers study. BMC Cancer. 2021;**21**(1):1341. DOI: 10.1186/s12885-021-09071-1

Chapter 7

AI-Assisted Breast Imaging

Lulu Wang

Abstract

Artificial intelligence has the potential to improve breast cancer detection and diagnosis. This study aims to explore the latest advances in artificial intelligence-assisted breast imaging technology, with a particular focus on multimodal imaging. By exploring the potential of artificial intelligence in single and multimodal breast imaging, this study aims to contribute to the ongoing efforts to improve breast cancer detection and diagnosis. This study will analyze how artificial intelligence techniques can effectively improve breast cancer detection and diagnosis using single and multimodal imaging techniques. The challenges and future research directions of artificial intelligence assisted breast imaging will be discussed.

Keywords: breast imaging, artificial intelligence, deep learning, breast cancer, automatic classification, early diagnosis

1. Introduction

Breast cancer is the most frequently diagnosed female cancer worldwide [1]. Timely detection and treatment of breast cancer can significantly improve the 5-year survival rate [2]. While mammography, ultrasound, and MRI are commonly used breast imaging methods, each of them has some limitations. Therefore, it is crucial to develop new imaging tools that can enhance the accuracy, efficiency, and reliability of breast cancer diagnosis.

With the rapid development of artificial intelligence (AI) techniques, AI-based diagnostic tools have the potential to revolutionize breast imaging, improving imaging sensitivity, specificity, and accuracy in breast cancer diagnosis [3, 4]. AI algorithms analyze various risk factors to predict an individual's likelihood of developing breast cancer. In addition, AI-assisted diagnosis and decision support tools can help radiologists interpret breast imaging results and choose treatment plans. By exploring the potential of AI in breast imaging, few research groups have reviewed AI-based breast imaging using single modal imaging. Up to date, there is no review report focused on multimodal imaging.

This study aims to explore recent advancements in AI-assisted breast imaging techniques for breast cancer detection, with a particular focus on multimodal imaging. This study will analyze how AI can effectively improve breast cancer detection and diagnosis using single and multimodal imaging techniques. The challenges and future research directions of AI-assisted breast imaging will be discussed.

By exploring the potential of AI in breast imaging, this study contributes to ongoing efforts to improve cancer diagnosis. The ultimate goal is to improve the accuracy and efficiency of breast imaging technology, thereby improving patient prognosis and reducing cancer-related mortality.

2. Breast imaging

Breast mammography is currently gold standard method for breast cancer imaging [5]. However, it also has limitations, such as potential radiation hazards and not being suitable for young women or individuals with dense breasts. Digital breast tomosynthesis (DBT) provides 3D digital images by generating multiple breast images from different angles, making it particularly effective in dense breast tissue and reducing false-positive and false-negative rates [6]. Ultrasound imaging is suitable for imaging dense breast tissue and can guide biopsies, but its interpretations can vary among radiologists and heavily rely on operator expertise [7]. Magnetic resonance imaging (MRI) provides detailed breast images and is typically used for high-risk patients or suspicious findings identified on mammography or ultrasound, but it is expensive and time-consuming, and requires the administration of contrast agents [8]. Microwave imaging (MBI) is emerging as a nonionizing and noninvasive method for breast cancer detection [9, 10]. However, existing MBI systems face imaging speed and resolution limitations that need to be addressed for clinical applications.

In breast imaging, the interpretation of breast lesions can vary due to differences in appearance and the expertise of radiologists. Factors such as fatigue, distractions, and cognitive biases can also impact interpretation, resulting in diagnostic errors. False-positive rates can lead to unnecessary biopsies and interventions, causing patient anxiety and increased costs, while false-negative rates can delay the detection and treatment of cancer.

AI algorithms have received significant attentions in predicting the likelihood of malignancy and assisting radiologists in making accurate diagnoses and treatment decisions in breast imaging [11–15]. AI-based imaging methods offer advantages such as fast processing, consistent and reproducible results, and improved performance over time. By reducing inter-observer variability, AI has the potential to improve patient outcomes and revolutionize breast imaging. Recent studies have demonstrated the potential of AI-based techniques in improving breast cancer detection and classification accuracy and efficiency.

3. AI techniques

Developing an AI-based diagnostic model involves several crucial steps.

1. Collect relevant data such as medical images, patient demographics, clinical history, and pathology reports.

2. The collected data undergoes preprocessing to ensure its quality and compatibility with AI algorithms. This step involves cleaning the data, removing noise, handling missing values, standardizing or normalizing the data, and performing necessary feature extraction or selection.

3. Develop AI model using various machine learning (ML) algorithms, such as logistic regression, support vector machines (SVM), random forests, and deep learning (DL) techniques, such as convolutional neural networks (CNN).

4. Train the proposed AI model using preprocessed data. During training, the model adjusts its internal parameters to minimize prediction errors and maximize accuracy.

5. Evaluate the proposed AI model using the validation data to assess its performance metrics. This step helps to determine the effectiveness of the model and identify areas for improvement. Based on the evaluation results, optimization methods such as hyperparameter tuning, adjusting learning rates, or regularization parameters can improve the performance of the model.

6. Test the proposed AI model using a separate dataset that was not used during training or validation. This step ensures the model's generalizability and ability to predict breast cancer accurately.

7. Once the model has been validated and tested, it can be deployed in clinical settings or integrated into existing imaging systems. This enables real-time prediction and decision support for breast cancer diagnosis and treatment planning, enhancing the overall effectiveness and efficiency of the imaging system.

3.1 Dataset

Breast datasets are crucial in assessing the effectiveness of AI approaches. **Table 1** displays publicly available breast datasets for AI model studies.

Ref.	Dataset	Sample number	Human number	Task
[16]	Digital Database for Screening Mammography (DDSM)	2620	115	Detection
[17]	Mammographic Image Analysis Society (Mini-MIAS)	322	N/A	Classification
[18]	INbreast	410	N/A	Breast cancer detection
[19]	Breast Cancer Digital Repository (BCDR)	1224	N/A	Breast cancer classification
[20]	Curated Breast Imaging Subset of DDSM (CBIS-DDSM)	753	N/A	Detection
[21]	BCDR-F01	362	N/A	Breast cancer classification
[22]	DDSM	2620	N/A	Classification, segmentation
[23]	Mammographic Image Analysis Society (MIAS)	322	N/A	Classification, segmentation

Table 1.
Breast image datasets.

3.2 Performance metrics

Breast screening algorithms that utilize AI have become a common way to identify potential cancer. These algorithms are evaluated based on several performance metrics, including sensitivity, specificity, accuracy, precision, Recall, F1 score, and area under the receiver operating characteristic curve (AUC) [24].

Sensitivity measures the algorithm's ability to correctly identify true positive cases and is essential in minimizing false negatives and avoiding potential cancer cases.

Specificity measures the algorithm's ability to minimize false positives and avoid unnecessary interventions or additional tests for noncancerous cases.

Accuracy is a comprehensive evaluation metric that considers true positive and negative cases.

Precision is a performance metric that measures the proportion of correctly predicted positive cases, assesses the algorithm's ability to avoid false positives, and indicates the reliability of positive predictions made by the system.

Recall measures the proportion of actual positive cases that are predicted correctly by the algorithm, and it helps assess the algorithm's ability to minimize false negatives and avoid missing potential cancer cases.

F1 score provides a balanced measure of the algorithm's performance, considering both false positives and false negatives. It is particularly useful when the dataset is imbalanced, and metrics alone may not provide a complete picture of the algorithm's effectiveness.

AUC, a curve representing the trade-off between sensitivity and specificity for various classification thresholds, provides an aggregate measure of the algorithm's performance. It is commonly used to evaluate classification algorithms' performance.

These metrics comprehensively evaluate the AI algorithm's accuracy, sensitivity, specificity, precision, and overall effectiveness. The following equations are commonly used for numerical representation of metrics mentioned above:

$$\text{Sensitivity} = \text{True Positives} / (\text{True Positives} + \text{False Negatives}) \quad (1)$$

$$\text{Specificity} = \text{True Negatives} / (\text{True Negatives} + \text{False Positives}) \quad (2)$$

$$\text{Accuracy} = (\text{True Positives} + \text{True Negatives}) / (\text{Total Cases}) \quad (3)$$

$$\text{Precision} = \text{True Positives} / (\text{True Positives} + \text{False Positives}) \quad (4)$$

$$\text{Recall} = \text{True Positives} / (\text{True Positives} + \text{False Negatives}) \quad (5)$$

$$\text{F1 Score} = 2^{*} \left(\text{Precision}^{*}\ \text{Recall}\right) / (\text{Precision} + \text{Recall}) \quad (6)$$

4. AI-assisted diagnostic tools

AI architectures, such as machine learning (ML) and deep learning (DL), have been extensively studied to develop AI-assisted diagnosis tools. DL methods, such as convolutional neural networks (CNN), have been mainly studied for breast imaging. For example, Liu et al. [25] proposed grid-based deep feature generation model for breast ultrasonic image classification and obtained accuracy of 97.18% for three classes, namely, malignant, benign, and normal.

Aboutalib et al. [26] investigated the automatic deep learning CNN methods to distinguish recalled-benign images from malignant and negative cases. When the FFDM, DDSM, and combined datasets are selected for training and testing, the AUC values are 0.70–0.81, 0.77–0.96, and 0.76–0.91, respectively. Compared to pre-training on nonmedical datasets alone, the model showed a consistent improvement in AUC with a range of 0.02–0.05 (both $p > 0.05$) when pre-trained on large nonmedical datasets and DDSM dataset. The results demonstrated that the proposed methods may lead to a computerized clinical toolkit to help reduce false recalls.

There are several commercial AI-powered diagnostic tools, including Transpara AI Decision Support System [27], AIDOC [28], and Koios DS [29]. Transpara AI Decision Support System has been extensively used in clinical trials across multiple countries. Aidoc offers a range of AI algorithms for breast imaging to detect and prioritize suspicious findings on mammograms. Koios DS aids radiologists in detecting suspicious lesions in mammograms.

These AI-powered diagnostic tools have enormous potential in improving breast cancer detection and diagnosis accuracy and efficiency. They can help support radiologists in making decisions and improving patient outcomes.

5. Role of AI-assisted tools in breast imaging

5.1 AI for risk assessment

Breast cancer risk is related with breast density [30, 31]. AI-based tools are available for measuring breast density. Traditional methods for measuring breast density focus on the percentage of fibroglandular tissue in total breast tissue without considering the distribution of the tissue. However, studies showed that the distribution of tissue observed in mammograms can correlate with the risk of breast cancer. Further research aims to explore the relationship between the substantial texture found in mammography and the risk of breast cancer.

Recent AI advancements in risk assessment consider tissue distribution and fibroglandular tissue. For instance, Yala et al. [32] developed a DL model that outperformed traditional risk factors. This model was tested and trained on dataset from a single institution. The AI model developed by Lee et al. [33] estimated the short-term risk of screenable breast cancer (sBCa) by analyzing lateral and temporal differences in mammograms. The proposed Radon Cumulative Distribution Transform (RCDT) can highlight subtle signals associated with future sBCa by exploiting lateral and temporal differences in female mammography screening. The authors applied deep convolutional neural network (dCNN) to build a robust classification marker of having sBCa within a year from a negative screening. The final model achieved an AUC of 0.82 and a specificity at a sensitivity of 98% with a 95% confidence interval of 0.40–0.65.

Lauritzen et al. [34] studied whether breast cancer risk assessment improves using the combination model of AI diagnostic system and mammographic texture model. Compared to the diagnostic AI and the texture risk models, the combination model achieved a higher AUC for interval and long-term cancers grouped together. Among women in the 10% of women with the highest combined risk detected by the combined model, 44.1% had interval cancers and 33.7% had long-term cancers. The technique based on AI and mammography texture models can improve risk assessment of interval and long-term cancers and identify people with high risk of breast cancer.

Similar investigations have been conducted with the emergence of AI-based risk estimation for mammograms [35]. Lång et al. [36] investigated the use of AI as a complementary tool for radiologists reading mammograms for breast cancer detection. In this study, participants were randomly assigned to AI-supported screening (intervention group) or standard double reading without AI (control group). Results showed that AI-assisted techniques reduced 44.3% of radiologists' screen-reading workload.

5.2 Integration of AI and medical imaging

AI has garnered considerable attention in breast imaging due to its potential to extract advanced features from medical images automatically. Several DL algorithms are commonly used to detect and classify breast lesions, including convolutional neural networks (CNN), deep belief networks (DBN), recurrent neural networks (RNN), autoencoders, generative adversarial networks (GAN), capsule networks (CN), convolutional recurrent neural networks (CRNN), attention mechanisms, multiscale CNN, and ensemble learning (EL).

CNN classifies the characteristics of images, while DBN detects minor alterations. RNN examines data sequentially, whereas autoencoders learn distinctive features. GAN produces synthetic images, while CN detects and categorizes them. CRNN integrates CNN and RNN, and attention mechanisms concentrate on specific regions. Multiscale CNN examines images at multiple scales, and EL merges deep-learning models to enhance accuracy.

Studies have shown that AI algorithms, such as CNN-based models, have great potential in detecting and classifying breast lesions [37]. Wang studied the recent achievements of DL-based mammography for breast cancer detection and classification [38].

Table 2 lists various AI-based diagnosis models using unimodular medical imaging methods. These findings demonstrate that AI algorithms have the potential to improve breast cancer detection and classification, and enhance the accuracy and efficiency of radiological interpretation.

5.3 Integration of AI and multimodal imaging

Recently, several research groups have applied AI to multimodal imaging for cancer diagnosis. In 2019, Khoshdel et al. [52] developed a model for breast tumor segmentation using microwave and ultrasound breast images. The model was developed using Convolutional Neural Network (CNN)-based U-Net architecture. The researchers' model outperformed CSI and improved breast imaging outcomes.

In 2020, Choi et al. [53] studied the effectiveness of PET/CT and MRI to determine the efficacy of neoadjuvant chemotherapy (NAC) in advanced cancer patients. In this study, the authors applied an ML model to analyze PET/MRI breast images and showed promise in predicting responses to NAC, particularly in the HER2-negative subgroup. The study showed that ML-based PET/MRI has the potential to improve diagnostic capabilities in predicting NAC's efficacy in breast cancer patients.

Huang et al. [54] examined the relationship between breast arterial calcification (BAC) on mammography and CAD-RADS assessed by DL on coronary CT angiography in asymptomatic women over 40. The study found a significant correlation between BAC and CAD-RADS. BAC can serve as an additional diagnostic indicator for predicting CAD severity in women undergoing breast screening mammography.

Ref.	AI model	Imaging method	Goal	Results
[39]	Texture Features with SVM	Mammography	Benign/malignant lesion differentiation	Sensitivity = 94.47%; Specificity = 91.3%
[40]	Texture Features with Decision Tree	Mammography	Benign/malignant lesion differentiation	AUC = 0.995
[30]	Asymmetry Texture Features/ risk-factors with SVM	Mammography	Risk prediction	AUC = 0.725
[41]	Texture Features with Logistic Regression	Mammography	Differentiate contra-lateral healthy images from diseased women from normal cases	AUC = 0.85
[42]	CNN	Mammography	Risk prediction	Sensitivity = 70.3%; Specificity = 60%; AUC = 0.697
[32]	ResNet18	Mammography	Risk prediction	AUC = 0.7
[43]	PGGAN	Mammography	Identifying synthetic samples	Probability ≈ 50%
[44]	GAN	Mammography	Mammogram variation	Accuracy = 89.6%
[45]	GAN	Mammography	Identifying synthetic samples	Probability ≈ 50%
[46]	SSL, GAN, and CNN	Mammography	Lesion detection	Improvements of ≈3 pp on accuracy
[47]	SSL and CNN	Mammography	Normalization, classification and segmentation	Improvements of ≈10–15 pp on AUC scores
[48]	SSL and CNN	Mammography	Cancer detection	Improved 4-fold data efficiency and ≈3 pp on accuracy
[49]	Texture Features/ LBP with SVM	Ultrasound	Benign/malignant lesion differentiation	Sensitivity = 87.04%; Specificity = 87.62%; AUC = 0.9342
[50]	Texture/ Morphology Features with Artificial Neural Network	MRI	Benign/malignant lesion differentiation	AUC = 0.82
[51]	SSL and CNN	Lymph node images, fundus images, and chest X-ray images	Classification and detection	Improvements of ≈2 pp on AUC scores

Table 2.
AI-based models using medical imaging methods.

Yao et al. [55] proposed a model to predict the likelihood of recurrence and metastasis in breast cancer patients. The model achieved an AUC of 0.75. The study helps identify patients with high risk of breast cancer recurrence and who may benefit from additional treatment after surgery.

Misra et al. [56] developed a DL model that combines B-mode ultrasound and elastography ultrasound images to classify breast cancers. They applied a weighted multimodal U-Net (W-MM-U-Net) to identify the location of cancerous lesion and a multimodal fusion framework (MFF) to distinguish benign and malignant lesions. When tested on clinical data, the network performed well with a sensitivity of 100% and specificity of 94.28%.

Kanae et al. [57] evaluated the impact of DL models on improving the accuracy of breast cancer diagnosis. They found that the 4-degree model and radiologist performed better than the 0-degree model in cancer detection, with an AUC of 0.936, indicating higher sensitivity and specificity. Research showed that DL models can improve the accuracy of breast cancer diagnosis.

Tan et al. [58] assessed the performance of AI detection systems to detect breast cancer in females with dense breasts using digital mammography and automated 3D breast ultrasound. When the weights of AI-based digital mammography and AI-based automated 3D breast ultrasound are 0.25 and 0.75, the performance of the multimodal AI systems is significantly better than that of the single-modal system (AUC = 0.865 for AI-Multimodal; AUC = 0.832 for AI-based digital mammography, p = 0.026; AUC = 0.841 for AI-based automated 3D breast ultrasound, p = 0.041). The maximum Youden's index for AI-Multimodal was 0.707 (sensitivity = 79.4%, specificity = 91.2%).

Liu et al. [59] investigated the effectiveness of a DL model using multiple types of medical images to identify the molecular subtype of breast cancer. The researchers found that a combination of DL and multimodal imaging is essential to diagnose breast cancer and select treatment plans.

In 2023, Cruz-Ramos et al. [60] introduced a new Computer-Aided Diagnostic (CAD) system using DL and handcrafted features to classify benign and malignant tumors in ultrasound and mammography images. The new systems were evaluated and compared with recent state-of-the-art systems, obtaining ACC of 97.6%, PRE of 98%, Recall of 98%, F1-Score of 98%, and IBA of 95%.

Yang et al. [61] tested a DL model using ultrasound and mammography images to predict breast lesions in patients with dense breasts. The results showed that the combined performance of the DL model showed AUC values of 0.940 in the test group and 0.906 in the validation group.

Bulut et al. [62] used a combination of PET/CT imaging and DL techniques to analyze images and determine the likelihood of complete recovery from breast cancer in patients who underwent chemotherapy. The deep CNN model could predict complete recovery.

Zhang et al. [63] developed the multimodal DL with intra- and inter-modality attention modules (MDL-IIA) to uncover important connections between mammography and ultrasound. Compared to other cohort models, the proposed MDL-IIA model obtained the highest performance in predicting four-category molecular subtypes, with a Matthews correlation coefficient (MCC) of 0.837 (95% confidence interval [CI]: 0.803, 0.870). Additionally, the proposed model effectively distinguishes between luminal and non-luminal diseases, with an area under the receiver operating characteristic curve of 0.929 (95% CI: 0.903, 0.951).

Han et al. [64] used mammography and ultrasound images to develop a combined ResNet50 model that achieved an AUC of 0.882. Tian et al. [65] developed a model using radiomic and deep features from breast tomosynthesis and ultrasound images to distinguish between benign and malignant tumors with an accuracy of 0.953 and an AUC of 0.959.

6. Challenges and future works

Integrating AI-powered tools in clinical practice holds significant potential, but several limitations must be addressed before successful implementation. One of the primary concerns is algorithm bias, which arises due to AI algorithms' significant dependence on training datasets. Inaccurate recommendations resulting from biased datasets can exacerbate healthcare disparities, highlighting the need to develop diverse and representative datasets that consider age, race, and socioeconomic status variations. Continuous monitoring and auditing of AI-assisted tools should also be conducted to identify and mitigate bias effectively.

Validation of AI-assisted diagnostic tools is critical to ensure their accuracy and safety. Regulatory frameworks must be established to govern the development, deployment, and use of AI tools, emphasizing patient safety, privacy, and ethical considerations. This will enable healthcare professionals and patients to trust the reliability and effectiveness of these tools, improving patient care.

Radiologists play a crucial role in the diagnostic process, and the integration of AI should be viewed as a collaborative effort to improve patient care. Guidelines and training programs should be established to help radiologists understand the capabilities and limitations of AI tools. This will enable them to make informed decisions and provide personalized care based on AI-generated results, ensuring that AI is used appropriately and in the best interest of patients.

Addressing these limitations is crucial to successfully integrating AI-assisted tools in clinical practice. This will help improve diagnostic accuracy, efficiency, and patient outcomes.

7. Conclusion

This research investigates the potential of AI-based imaging tools in improving breast cancer detection, diagnosis, and outcomes. By enhancing the accuracy of breast irregularity identification, hastening interventions, and ultimately saving lives, AI has demonstrated its ability to refine breast cancer diagnosis accuracy, reduce the number of erroneous results, and minimize the occurrence of unnecessary biopsies.

Moreover, AI can transform breast imaging by offering valuable support to radiologists in making informed decisions and tailoring treatment strategies. By analyzing and interpreting extensive datasets, AI algorithms can assist radiologists in identifying subtle patterns and pinpointing potential areas of concern that may have gone unnoticed by human observation.

However, several challenges need to be addressed in integrating AI-supported breast imaging. The most significant challenge is the need for extensive and diverse datasets that accurately reflect the served population. This ensures that AI algorithms are trained on a comprehensive dataset that accurately represents patients, regardless of their age, race, or socioeconomic background. Furthermore, ethical considerations, such as patient confidentiality and responsible AI technology utilization, must be carefully addressed.

Collaborative efforts among researchers, healthcare professionals, and policymakers are essential to promote innovation and ensure the responsible and efficient deployment of AI-supported breast imaging technologies. By adopting a thoughtful approach to these challenges, AI-supported breast imaging has the potential to revolutionize breast imaging and substantially improve breast cancer care.

In conclusion, AI-supported breast imaging has significant potential for enhancing early detection, precise diagnosis, and overall outcomes for breast cancer patients. With a comprehensive and thoughtful approach to challenges and future exploration, AI can transform breast imaging and substantially improve breast cancer care.

Acknowledgements

The author acknowledges the use of Grammarly for language polishing of the manuscript.

Conflict of interest

The authors declare no conflict of interest.

Author details

Lulu Wang[1,2]

1 Department of Engineering, Reykjavík University, Reykjavik, Iceland

2 Department of Physiology and Biomedical Engineering, Mayo Clinic, Rochester, USA

*Address all correspondence to: lwang381@hotmail.com; wang.lulu@mayo.edu

References

[1] Sung H, Ferlay J, Siegel RL, Laversanne M, Soerjomataram I, Jemal A, et al. Global cancer statistics 2020: GLOBOCAN estimates of incidence and mortality worldwide for 36 cancers in 185 countries. CA: A Cancer Journal for Clinicians. 2021;**71**:209-249

[2] Wang L. Early diagnosis of breast cancer. Sensors (Basel). 2017;**17**(7):1572. DOI: 10.3390/s17071572

[3] Negrete NT, Takhtawala R, Shaver M, Kart T, Chang P. Automated breast cancer lesion detection on breast MRI using artificial intelligence. Journal of Clinical Oncology. 2019;**37**(15_suppl):e14612

[4] Abbass HA. An evolutionary artificial neural networks approach for breast cancer diagnosis. Artificial Intelligence in Medicine. 2002;**25**(3):265

[5] Løberg M, Lousdal ML, Bretthauer M, Kalager M. Benefits and harms of mammography screening. Breast Cancer Research. 2015;**17**:1-12

[6] Bian T, Lin Q, et al. Digital breast tomosynthesis: A new diagnostic method for mass-like lesions in dense breasts. The Breast Journal. 2016;**22**(5):535-540

[7] Geisel J, Raghu M, Hooley R. The role of ultrasound in breast cancer screening: The case for and against ultrasound. Seminars in Ultrasound, CT, and MR. 2018;**39**:25-34

[8] Morrow M, Waters J, Morris E. MRI for breast cancer screening, diagnosis, and treatment. Lancet. 2011;**378**:1804-1811

[9] Richard S, Donna W, Briony B, Kabir M, Steven A. Results for the London investigation into dielectric scanning of lesions study of the MARIA M6 breast imaging system. British Journal of Radiology. 2024;**97**(1155):549-552

[10] Wang L. Microwave imaging and sensing techniques for breast cancer detection. Micromachines (Basel). 2023;**14**(7):1462

[11] Stoitsis J, Valavanis I, Mougiakakou SG, Golemati S, Nikita A, Nikita KS. Computer aided diagnosis based on medical image processing and artificial intelligence methods. Nuclear Instruments and Methods in Physics Research Section A: Accelerators, Spectrometers, Detectors and Associated Equipment. 2006;**569**:591-595

[12] Xu F, Sepúlveda MJ, Jiang Z, Wang H, Li J, Yin Y, et al. Artificial intelligence treatment decision support for complex breast cancer among oncologists with varying expertise. JCO Clinical Cancer Informatics. 2019;**3**:1-15. DOI: 10.1200/CCI.18.00159

[13] Hassan NM, Hamad S, Mahar K. Mammogram breast cancer CAD systems for mass detection and classification: A review. Multimedia Tools and Applications. 2022;**81**:20043-20075

[14] Le E, Wang Y, Huang Y, Hickman S, Gilbert F. Artificial intelligence in breast imaging. Clinical Radiology. 2019;**74**:357-366

[15] van de Sande D, Sharabiani M, Bluemink H, Kneepkens E, Bakx N, Hagelaar E, et al. Artificial intelligence based treatment planning of radiotherapy for locally advanced breast cancer. Physics and Imaging in Radiation Oncology. 2021;**20**:111-116

[16] Heath M, Bowyer K, Kopans D, Kegelmeyer P Jr, Moore R, Chang K. Current status of the digital database for screening mammography. In: Digital Mammography. Computational Imaging and Vision. Vol. 11. Dordrecht: Springer; 1998. pp. 457-460

[17] Li B, Ge Y, Zhao Y, Guan E, Yan W. Benign and malignant mammographic image classification based on convolutional neural networks. In: 10th International Conference on Machine Learning and Computing. Beijing, China: Association for Computing Machinery; 2018. pp. 11-15

[18] Inês CM, Igor A, Inês D, António C, Maria JC, Jaime SC. Inbreast: Toward a full-field digital mammographic database. Academic Radiology. 2012;**19**:236-248. DOI: 10.1016/j.acra.2011.09.014

[19] Araújo T, Aresta G, Castro E, Rouco J, Aguiar P, Eloy C, et al. Classification of breast cancer histology images using convolutional neural networks. PLoS ONE. 2017;**12**(6):e0177544

[20] Lee R, Gimenez F, Hoogi A, Miyake K, Gorovoy M, Rubin D. A curated mammography data set for use in computer-aided detection and diagnosis research. Scientific Data. 2017;**4**:170177

[21] Ramos-Pollán R, Guevara-López M, Suárez-Ortega C, Díaz-Herrero G, Franco-Valiente J, Rubio-del-Solar M, et al. Discovering mammography-based machine learning classifiers for breast cancer diagnosis. Journal of Medical Systems. 2011;**1**:11

[22] Heath M, Bowyer K, Kopans D, Moore R, Kegelmeyer WP. Current status of the digital database for screening mammography. In: Digital Mammography. Computational Imaging and Vision. Vol. 13. Netherlands: Springer; 1998. pp. 457-460

[23] Yoon WB, Oh JE, Chae EY, Kim HH, Lee SY, Kim KG. Automatic detection of pectoral muscle region for computer-aided diagnosis using MIAS mammograms. BioMed Research International. 2016;**2016**:5967580

[24] Wang L. Enhanced Holographic Microwave Imaging for MNP Target Tumor Detection. IEEE Access. 2019;**7**:37167-37180. DOI: 10.1109/ACCESS.2019.2905005

[25] Liu H, Cui G, Luo Y, Guo Y, Zhao L, Wang Y, et al. Artificial intelligence-based breast cancer diagnosis using ultrasound images and grid-based deep feature generator. International Journal of General Medicine. 2022;**15**:2271-2282

[26] Aboutalib SS, Mohamed AA, Berg WA, Zuley ML, Sumkin JH, Wu S. Deep learning to distinguish recalled but benign mammography images in breast cancer screening. Clinical Cancer Research. 2018;**24**(23):5902-5909

[27] Transpara ScreenPoint Medical. Available from: https://radiology.healthairegister.com/products/screenpoint-transpara/

[28] AIDOC - Smart Doctor AI Technology Doctor on the Block. Available from: https://www.aidoc.me/

[29] Confident Diagnosis in Seconds. Available from: https://koiosmedical.com/

[30] Tan M, Zheng B, Ramalingam P, Gur D. Prediction of near-term breast cancer risk based on bilateral mammographic feature asymmetry. Academic Radiology. 2013;**20**:1542-1550

[31] Tice JA, Cummings SR, Smith-Bindman R, Ichikawa L, Barlow WE, Kerlikowske K. Using clinical factors and mammographic breast density to

estimate breast cancer risk: Development and validation of a new predictive model. Annals of Internal Medicine. 2008;**148**(5):337-347. DOI: 10.7326/0003-4819-148-5-200803040-00004

[32] Yala A, Lehman C, Schuster T, Portnoi T, Barzilay R. A deep learning mammography-based model for improved breast cancer risk prediction. Radiology. 2019;**292**(1):182716

[33] Lee J, Nishikawa RM, Bandos AI, Zuley ML. Estimating near term breast cancer risk from sequential mammograms using deep learning, radon cumulative distribution transform, and a clinical risk factor: Preliminary analysis. Proc. SPIE 11597, Medical Imaging. 2021: Computer-Aided Diagnosis, 115970Y. DOI: 10.1117/12.2580941

[34] Lauritzen AD, von Euler-Chelpin MC, Lynge E, Vejborg I, Nielsen M, Karssemeijer N, et al. Assessing breast cancer risk by combining AI for lesion detection and mammographic texture. Radiology. 2023;**308**(2):e230227

[35] Sitek A, Wolfe JM. Assessing cancer risk from mammograms: Deep learning is superior to conventional risk models. Radiology. 2019;**292**(1):67-68. DOI: 10.1148/radiol.2019190791. Epub 2019 May 7

[36] Lång K, Josefsson V, Larsson AM, Larsson S, Högberg C, Sartor H, et al. Artificial intelligence-supported screen reading versus standard double reading in the Mammography Screening with Artificial Intelligence trial (MASAI): A clinical safety analysis of a randomised, controlled, non-inferiority, single-blinded, screening accuracy study. The Lancet Oncology. Aug 2023;**24**(8):936-944. DOI: 10.1016/S1470-2045(23)00298-X. PMID: 37541274

[37] Chiao JY, Chen KY, Liao KY, Hsieh PH, Zhang G, Huang TC. Detection and classification the breast tumors using mask R-CNN on sonograms. Medicine (Baltimore). 2019;**98**(19):e15200. DOI: 10.1097/MD.0000000000015200

[38] Zou X, Zhai J, Qian S, Li A, Tian F, Cao X, et al. Improved breast ultrasound tumor classification using dual-input CNN with GAP-guided attention loss. Mathematical Biosciences and Engineering. 2023;**20**(8):15244-15264. DOI: 10.3934/mbe.2023682

[39] Kayode AA, Akande NO, Adegun AA, Adebiyi MO. An automated mammogram classification system using modified support vector machine. Medical Devices (Auckland, N.Z.). 2019;**12**:275-284. DOI: 10.2147/MDER.S206973

[40] Mohanty AK, Senapati MR, Beberta S, Lenka SK. Texture-based features for classification of mammograms using decision tree. Neural Computing and Applications. 2013;**23**:1011-1017

[41] Zheng Y, Keller BM, Ray S, Wang Y, Conant EF, Gee JC, et al. Parenchymal texture analysis in digital mammography: A fully automated pipeline for breast cancer risk assessment. Medical Physics. 2015;**42**:4149-4160

[42] Qiu Y, Wang Y, Yan S, Tan M, Cheng S, Liu H, et al. An initial investigation on developing a new method to predict short-term breast cancer risk based on deep learning technology. In: Medical Imaging 2016: Computer-Aided Diagnosis. Vol. 9785. Bellingham, WA, USA: SPIE; 2016. pp. 517-522

[43] Korkinof D, Harvey H, Heindl A, Karpati E, Williams G, Rijken T, et al. Perceived Realism of High-Resolution Generative Adversarial Network-derived

Synthetic Mammograms. Radiology. Artificial Intelligence. 2021;**32**:e190181

[44] Wu E, Wu K, Cox D, Lotter W. Conditional infilling GANs for data augmentation in mammogram classification. In: Image Analysis for Moving Organ, Breast, and Thoracic Images. Amsterdam, The Netherlands: Springer; 2018. pp. 98-106

[45] Senaras C, Niazi MKK, Sahiner B, Pennell MP, Tozbikian G, Lozanski G, et al. Optimized generation of high-resolution phantom images using cGAN: Application to quantification of Ki67 breast cancer images. PLoS ONE. 2018;**13**:e0196846

[46] Li Z, Cui Z, Wang S, Qi Y, Ouyang X, Chen Q, et al. Domain generalization for mammography detection via multi-style and multi-view contrastive learning. In: Proceedings of the International Conference on Medical Image Computing and Computer-Assisted Intervention; 27 September–1 October 2021; Strasbourg, France. Amsterdam, The Netherlands: Springer; 2021. pp. 98-108

[47] Elkorany AS, Elsharkawy ZF. Efficient breast cancer mammograms diagnosis using three deep neural networks and term variance. Scientific Reports. 2023;**13**:2663. DOI: 10.1038/s41598-023-29875-4

[48] Miller JD, Arasu VA, Pu AX, Margolies LR, Sieh W, Shen L. Self-Supervised Deep Learning to Enhance Breast Cancer Detection on Screening Mammography. arXiv, arXiv:2203.08812. 2022

[49] Wei M, Du Y, Wu X, Zhu J. Automatic classification of benign and malignant breast tumors in ultrasound image with texture and morphological features. In: Proceedings of the 2019 IEEE 13th International Conference on Anti-Counterfeiting, Security, and Identification (ASID); 25-27 October 2019; Xiamen, China. 2019. pp. 126-130. DOI: 10.1109/ICASID.2019.8925194

[50] Nie K, Chen JH, Hon JY, Chu Y, Nalcioglu O, Su MY. Quantitative analysis of lesion morphology and texture features for diagnostic prediction in breast MRI. Academic Radiology. 2008;**15**:1513-1525

[51] Truong T, Mohammadi S, Lenga M. How transferable are self-supervised features in medical image classification tasks? In: Proceedings of the Machine Learning for Health, PMLR, Proceedings of Machine Learning for Health, PMLR 2021;**158**:54-74. arXiv:2108.10048

[52] Khoshdel V, Ashraf A, Lovetri J. Enhancement of multimodal microwave-ultrasound breast imaging using a deep-learning technique. Sensors. 2019;**19**(18):4050

[53] Choi JH, Kim HA, Kim W, Lim I, Lee I, Byun BH, et al. Early prediction of neoadjuvant chemotherapy response for advanced breast cancer using PET/MRI image deep learning. Scientific Reports. 2020;**10**(1):21149. DOI: 10.1038/s41598-020-77875-5

[54] Huang Z, Xiao J, Xie Y, Hu Y, Zhang S, Li X, et al. The correlation of deep learning-based CAD-RADS evaluated by coronary computed tomography angiography with breast arterial calcification on mammography. Scientific Reports. 2020;**10**(1):11532. DOI: 10.1038/s41598-020-68378-4

[55] Yao Y, Lv Y, Tong L, Liang Y, Xi S, Ji B, et al. ICSDA: A multi-modal deep learning model to predict breast cancer recurrence and metastasis risk by integrating pathological, clinical and gene expression data. Briefings in

Bioinformatics. 2022;**23**(6):bbac448. DOI: 10.1093/bib/bbac448

[56] Misra S, Yoon C, Kim KJ, Managuli R, Barr RG, Baek J, et al. Deep learning-based multimodal fusion network for segmentation and classification of breast cancers using B-mode and elastography ultrasound images. Bioengineering & Translational Medicine. 2022;**8**(6):e10480. DOI: 10.1002/btm2.10480

[57] Kanae Y, Endoh D, Yokota H, Taniyama H, Hayashi M. Expression of the PTEN tumor suppressor gene in malignant mammary gland tumors of dogs. American Journal of Veterinary Research. 2006;**67**(1):127-133. DOI: 10.2460/ajvr.67.1.127

[58] Tan T, Rodriguez-Ruiz A, Zhang T, Xu L, Beets-Tan RGH, Shen Y, et al. Multi-modal artificial intelligence for the combination of automated 3D breast ultrasound and mammograms in a population of women with predominantly dense breasts. Insights into Imaging. 2023;**14**(1):10. DOI: 10.1186/s13244-022-01352-y

[59] Liu M, Zhang S, Du Y, Zhang X, Wang D, Ren W, et al. Identification of Luminal A breast cancer by using deep learning analysis based on multi-modal images. Frontiers in Oncology. 2023;**13**:1243126. DOI: 10.3389/fonc.2023.1243126

[60] Cruz-Ramos C, García-Avila O, Almaraz-Damian JA, Ponomaryov V, Reyes-Reyes R, Sadovnychiy S. Benign and malignant breast tumor classification in ultrasound and mammography images via fusion of deep learning and handcraft features. Entropy (Basel). 2023;**25**(7):991. DOI: 10.3390/e25070991

[61] Yang Y, Zhong Y, Li J, Feng J, Gong C, Yu Y, et al. Deep learning combining mammography and ultrasound images to predict the malignancy of BI-RADS US 4A lesions in women with dense breasts: A diagnostic study. International Journal of Surgery. 2024;**110**(5):2604-2613. DOI: 10.1097/JS9.0000000000001186. PMID: 38348891; PMCID: PMC11093459

[62] Bulut G, Atilgan HI, Çınarer G, Kılıç K, Yıkar D, Parlar T. Prediction of pathological complete response to neoadjuvant chemotherapy in locally advanced breast cancer by using a deep learning model with 18F-FDG PET/CT. PLoS ONE. 2023;**18**(9):e0290543. DOI: 10.1371/journal.pone.0290543

[63] Zhang T, Tan T, Han L, Appelman L, Veltman J, Wessels R, et al. Predicting breast cancer types on and beyond molecular level in a multi-modal fashion. npj Breast Cancer. 2023;**9**(1):16. DOI: 10.1038/s41523-023-00517-2

[64] Han J, Hua H, Fei J, Liu J, Guo Y, Ma W, et al. Prediction of disease-free survival in breast cancer using deep learning with ultrasound and mammography: A multicenter study. Clinical Breast Cancer. 2024;**24**:215-226. DOI: 10.1016/j.clbc.2024.01.005. Epub ahead of print

[65] Tian R, Lu G, Zhao N, Qian W, Ma H, Yang W. Constructing the Optimal Classification Model for Benign and Malignant Breast Tumors Based on Multifeature Analysis from Multimodal Images. Journal of Imaging Informatics in Medicine. 2024;**37**. DOI: 10.1007/s10278-024-01036-7. Epub ahead of print. PMID: 38381383

Chapter 8

Advances in Breast Ultrasound Imaging: Enhancing Diagnostic Precision and Clinical Utility

Athar Shams Rana, Javairia Rafique and Hira Riffat

Abstract

Ultrasound imaging is a commonly used modality for breast cancer detection and diagnosis. The diagnostic role of breast ultrasound has been expanded along with the improvement of high-frequency transducers and digital technology. Vascular assessment has progressed enough to depict normal vascular anatomy of the breast and the lymph nodes. Early detection of breast cancer leads to more effective treatment and fewer deaths. Although mammography is mostly used to detect breast cancer, it is spotted that not all cancers can be seen on mammographic images. Accurate ultrasonography (US) investigations facilitate the surgical approach to a very conservative and cosmetic operation. High-resolution sonography can demonstrate the intraductal spread of tumors and their multiple foci more easily than mammography. Pathologic vessels are seen in almost all the tumors, thus improving US sensitivity for nonpalpable carcinomas. New contrast agents will recirculate enough to search for vascular foci during a thorough investigation of both breasts and nodal stations. In this chapter, we summarize advanced breast ultrasound applications for the diagnosis of breast cancer, including ultrasound elastography, contrast-enhanced ultrasound, 3D ultrasound, automatic breast ultrasound, micropure, ultrasound nomograms, and full non-contact laser ultrasound. We have discussed the limitations of our chapter in the "Discussion" section.

Keywords: breast cancer, elastography, micropure, contrast-enhanced ultrasound, high-frequency transducers

1. Introduction

Around the world, breast cancer positions as the most ordinarily analyzed type of malignant growth in females. Yearly, around 1.7 million instances of breast cancer are analyzed around the world, or one new case happens at regular intervals. In United States, about one in eight women is determined to have breast cancer in the course of their life. The 55–64 age range has the most elevated finding rate. Not only is breast cancer more common, but it also stands as the foremost cause of cancer-related fatalities among women worldwide [1].

Dr. Dodd wrote in 1977, "The spatial resolution now a days achieve able in ultrasonograms is inadequate for the detection of subclinical [breast] cancer" [2]. In 1983, Sickles et al. stated: "These data indicate that sonography is not an acceptable substitute for mammography in the detection and diagnosis of breast cancer." Throughout several ages, the core utilization of breast ultrasonography (US) was analyzing difference between cysts and solid masses. Consequently, ultrasound has turned out to be an essential part of the investigative work-up of breast pathologies over the past two eras [3]. Because ultrasonography uses mechanical energy to create a visual depiction of the body's internal structures, radiologists find it particularly interesting. Breast ultrasounds can identify more cancers than mammograms alone, especially in women whose breast parenchyma is dense [1]. Ultrasound (US) utilizes sound waves to scan parenchyma. Ionizing radiation is not used, and there is no need for intravenous contrast. In the 1970s and early 1980s ultrasound was used for abdomen and pelvis scans. Accessible lower-frequency probes were used to try breast ultrasonography, and the possibility of using US for screening was investigated, but the attempt was not successful [4].

When high-frequency transducers were developed in the middle of the 1980s, US could be used to differentiate between solid and cysts in the initial breast cancer phases [5] and then to differentiate between benign and malignant states [4]. Since 1995 when the US was first shown to be able to detect cancers that were missed by mammograms [6]. The usefulness of US as an additional screening for females with dense parenchyma of breast has been demonstrated by multiple single-center studies [4].

Ultrasound may become a primary diagnostic modality when paired with future resolution capabilities of one square millimeter, shifting it from a purely adjunctive category [2].

Ultrasound of the breasts can detect more cancer, especially in women with dense breast, than a mammogram alone [1]. The primary explanation for the US's expanding role is the notable improvement in spatial resolution. The application of tissue harmonics, speckle reduction, and spatial compound imaging improved the clarity of the images [7, 8]. For the most recent US examination of the breast, suitable scanner configurations and refined scanning techniques are also necessary. Modern technological advancements enable a broad range of breast pathologies to be diagnosed, managed, and treated in the US [3].

The objective of this chapter is to investigate recent progress in breast ultrasound imaging methodologies aimed at improving diagnostic accuracy and clinical utility. This chapter clarifies how these developments aid in the more accurate identification, characterization, and surveillance of breast pathologies. It aims to offer insights into the possible influence of improved ultrasound imaging on breast cancer detection, patient management, and overall healthcare outcomes by a thorough evaluation of recent research and practical applications.

2. Breast development and anatomy

2.1 Development of the breast (embryology)

The specialized and altered mammary glands are a kind of sweat gland [9]. The formation of human breast tissue initiates in the embryonic stage around the 5th or 6th week of development. It starts as a single mammary crest and develops into elongated strips of thickened outer germ layer, known as mammary lines, extending from the axilla to the pelvis along the embryo's underside. By the 9th week of gestation, only one set of mammary glands forms in the chest region of the milk line in humans, differing from most mammals, which develop multiple sets of paired glands along this ridge. At this stage, the mammary papilla is formed through the expansion of a cluster of basal cells. Around week 12, surface squamous cells begin to cover the nipple bud. At the same time, mesenchymal cells change into the smooth muscle of the nipple and areola, while epithelial cells reach out descending as mammary conduits, culminating in mammary acini [10]. The ectoderm's ingrowth forms the primary bud, which subsequently results in the formation of each breast. The formation of 15–20 secondary buds, which eventually give rise to milk ducts and their ramifications, is guided by the main bud. Large lactiferous ducts form and empty into a superficial mammary groove, which transforms into nipple during infancy. The nipple is initially recessed at birth and protrudes above the skin as the child grows. A non-occurring elevation results in an inverted nipple. The primary milk ducts form at birth, and mammary glands do not fully develop till puberty. The breast of female does not grow till adolescence, when the production of progesterone and ovarian estrogen causes the breast to enlarge due to the proliferation of connective tissue and epithelial cells. Because of the expansion of mammary glands and a rise in the buildup of adipose tissue, the breast grows during adolescence [9]. The tips of these extensions specialize into lobule-alveolar formations, which are clear, yellowish, and hold colostrum, a viscous liquid. This "witch's milk," activated by placental hormones, is secreted by male and female infants for 4–6 days after birth. The breast's bulk progressively grows in the final weeks of gestation, and the nipple-areola unit (NAU) matures and darkens. Following delivery, the breast begins a process of involution, and colostral secretion ceases due to the withdrawal of placental hormones [10].

The supportive framework of the breast, consisting of connective tissue and adipose tissue, originates from the mesenchyme that spreads across and envelops the epithelial system. Mammary crests in human embryos disappear as the embryo matures, potentially leaving behind a few small segments that may persist in the chest areas. Less than 1% of newborns develop extra breasts (polymastia) or extra nipples (polythelia) laterally with the milk line when the mammary crest fails to regress normally. The most frequent site for supernumerary breasts or extra nipples is between the pubic bone and the regular nipple location (**Figure 1**) [9, 10].

2.2 Pregnancy, lactation, and involution

The ductal system expands and disperses in the adipose tissue during the first trimester in reaction to rising estrogen levels. Moreover, reduced fatty tissue and ductal growth and expansion are induced by elevated estrogen levels. Moreover, estrogen increases the pituitary gland's stimulation, which raises the proportion of prolactin. Mammary glands are developed enough by the 20th week of pregnancy, thanks to prolactin stimulation, to secrete milk components. Elevated levels of progesterone and estrogen inhibit milk production, but colostrum is still secreted during this period. These levels decline during the final trimester and shortly after childbirth, allowing milk production and a final release to aid in breastfeeding. The areola darkens, the breast enlarges, and the Montgomery glands become more prominent during most pregnancies. When lactation ends, a decrease in prolactin causes a phenomenon known as post-lactational involution [11].

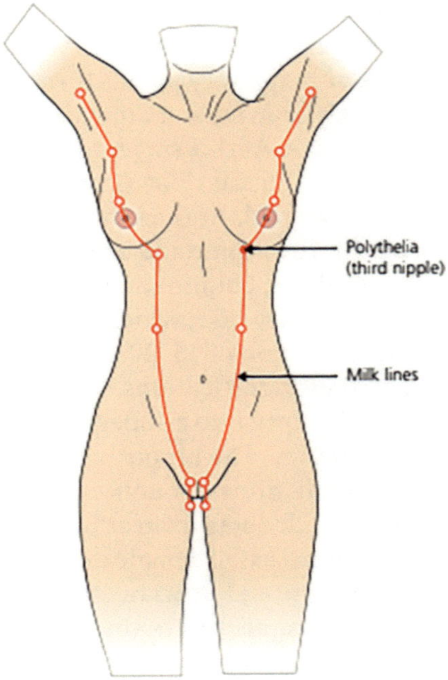

Figure 1.
The mammary ridge stretches from axilla to groin. Abnormal breast, residual nipple, and areola growth may arise at any point along this ridge [10].

2.3 Menopause

The breast recedes during menopause, ductal and glandular elements involute, and the breast becomes mostly composed of stroma and fat. Aging also results in a complete decrease in the quantity of ducts and lobules. Breast shrinkage and loss of contour are caused by a progressive reduction in stromal components and fat over time. Over time, the Cooper suspensory ligaments weaken and eventually cause breast ptosis [9].

2.4 Breast anatomy

With processing of breast milk, human breast achieves its extreme functional potential [12]. The base of the female breast emerges from the front thoracic wall between the second and sixth ribs. The breast's anatomical boundaries run downward from the inframammary fold to the level of the second or third ribs, while its horizontal limit stretches from the outer edge of the sternum inward to mid-axillary line outward. Around two-thirds of the breast is covered by the pectoralis major muscle, with the remaining portion covered by the serratus anterior and the upper part of the abdominal oblique muscle. One spot where breast tissue commonly extends into the axilla is the axillary tail of Spence [9].

The breast comprises glandular and adipose tissue and is safeguarded by Cooper's ligaments, a lax framework of fibrous connective tissue [12].

2.5 The nipple

In nulliparous women, nipple typically resides at the fourth intercostal space level; however, as the breasts become pendulous, its position relative to the intercostal space varies. The nipple receives blood supply from 15 to 20 lactiferous ducts. The areola, housing abundant sebaceous glands often visible to the naked eye, encircles the nipple, along with the Montgomery glands (**Figure 2**) [13].

2.6 Breast density

Breast density is a term used to describe how significantly fat and fibroglandular tissue a woman's breasts contain on a mammography. Compared to imaging of supplementary organs, appearance of normal breast tissue can differ greatly, from low fat and sparse dense tissue to low fat and mostly dense tissue. The American College of Radiology Breast Imaging and Data System (ACR BI-RADS), Fifth Version, divides breast density into four categories. A is practically entirely fatty, B is scattered fibroglandular densities, C is heterogeneously dense, and D is extremely dense. It is believed that types C and D are classified as thick, while types A and B are classified as thin or sparse. Dense breast tissue is typical and normal: About 43% of females at the age of 40 or above have large breasts. Thirty six percent of the density is in Category C, while 7% is in Category D. According to research by Han and others, females with a past of breast carcinoma in their families are more likely than those who do not have dense breasts [4].

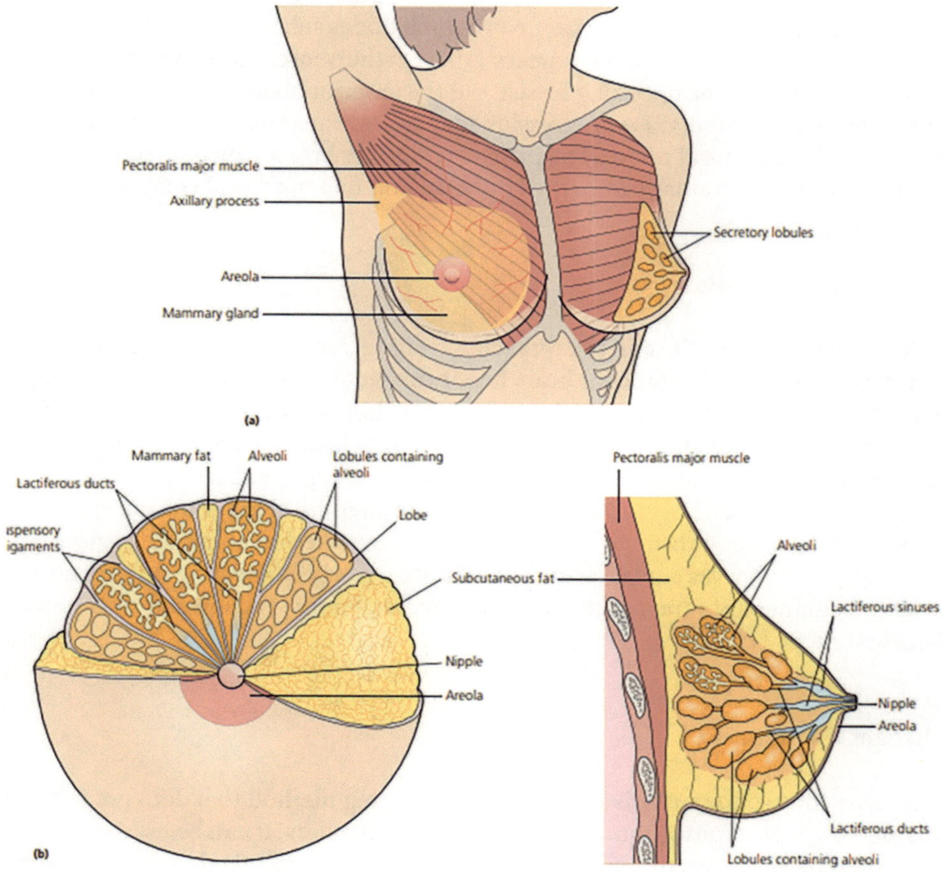

Figure 2.
(a) The breast region's vascular and lymphatic anatomy. (b) Part of the breast: The mammary glands interior structure (left); a breast section displaying milk flow (right) [10].

2.7 Blood supply

Although the internal thoracic artery is the main arterial blood supply to breast, intercostal and lateral thoracic arteries also contribute extra arterial blood flow [14].

2.8 Lymphatic drainage

More than 75% of lymph drainage from the breast goes straight to the axillary lymph nodes [15, 16]. About 20–30 nodes are usually found in the axillary region [17]. The six main groups of axillary lymph nodes that surgeons have identified are the axillary vein group, external mammary group, scapular group, central group, subclavicular group, and interpectoral group—also known as Rotter nodes, located between the pectoralis major and minor muscles [16]. The pectoralis minor muscle serves as the basis for the names of these groupings. Three levels are distinguished between the axillary lymph nodes according to their position in relation to the pectoralis minor muscle. Laterally to the pectoralis minor muscle are level I nodes such as the axillary vein, external mammary, and scapular groups [15]. The pectoralis minor muscle is home to both deep and superficial Level II nodes, which are the central and interpectoral groups. Situated medial to the pectoralis minor muscle is the subclavicular group, also known as Level III nodes. Lymph vessels drain the medial aspect of the breast; they enter the parasternal group of lymph nodes subsequent to the perforating branches of the internal mammary artery [15]. Furthermore, there might be communication between the opposing breast and the anterior abdominal wall's superficial lymphatics. Advanced disease progression may be indicated by supraclavicular drainage or deep cervical nodes. The primary route for breast cancer metastases to spread is lymphatic drainage from the epithelial and mesenchymal components of the tumor [9].

2.9 Sensory innervation

Both the breast and the anterolateral chest wall receive sensory innervation from the anterior and lateral cutaneous branches of the second through sixth intercostal nerves [16, 18]. Furthermore, Blood supply to the skin covering the upper part of the breast comes from the anterior branches of the supraclavicular nerve, which come from the cervical plexus). The nerves that supply the nipple and areola are derived from the plexus formed by the convergence of the lateral and anterior cutaneous divisions of the second through fifth intercostal nerves in the subdermal region. Eventually, these nerves converge in the axilla after freely connecting. In particular, the lateral cutaneous branch of the second intercostal nerve is known as the intercostobrachial nerve [15].

3. Breast ultrasound

Because ultrasonography is a non-invasive imaging method that does not require ionizing radiation exposure and is inexpensive and painless, it can be used often [19].

It would be advantageous if breast ultrasonography were linked to the term "early." Breast cancer detection using ultrasound technology may be highly sensitive and specific. Ultrasound is commonly available, reasonably priced, strong, portable, and low maintenance. Given the rising incidence of breast cancer worldwide and the dearth of prompt imaging-based detection, ultrasound can be a useful primary detection tool and screening technique for breast lesions. Particularly in resource-poor environments without access to mammography, this is valid [19].

3.1 High-frequency transducers used in breast ultrasonography

To successfully visualize anomalies in the mammary tissue and obtain adequate axial and lateral resolution, high-frequency transducers were clearly necessary in the early stages of real-time breast sonography. In textbooks from the past, 7.5 MHz was typically advised. Higher frequencies were utilized, though, as digital broad-band transducers advanced [20].

Schnarkowski et al. [21] discovered in a brief series that a 13 MHz array performed better in terms of breast lesion size and differentiation than a 7.5 MHz array. Schulz-Wendtland et al. conducted a large-scale prospective study [22]. Using sonography imaging at 7.5 MHz, 84% NPV and 83% sensitivity were attained, while at 13 MHz the NPV and sensitivity were 87% and 87%, respectively. With 78% versus 56%, respectively, sensitivity was particularly enhanced for small, invasive cancers (pT1a). In that study, it was also demonstrated that sonography at 13 MHz had a higher accuracy regarding tumor size than sonography at 7.5 MHz [22]. This notion also holds for Doppler scanning, where it is well-known that the ability to detect shallow, sluggish flows is enhanced by the use of higher transmission frequencies. In a study by Rjosk-Dendorfer et al., color Doppler breast sonography was used at 17 MHz instead of 12 points 5 MHz to help distinguish solid masses from cysts, but it had no effect on tumor differentiation [23].

These days, frequencies in the range of 10–15 MHz are typically used for breast sonography. This improves the visibility of lesions against the backdrop of normal breast tissue and enhances the capability to discern subtle variations in gray tones. Moreover, it enables anomalies across the superficial to deep layers of the breasts to be visualized with sufficient spatial resolution, encompassing tissue contrast and axial, and lateral resolution [20].

However, because the ultrasonic (US) beam attenuates when used at a high insonating frequency, penetration is reduced. Transducers with lower frequencies offer superior depth penetration but lower spatial resolution. Higher-frequency transducers, on the other hand, usually offer greater spatial resolution but at the expense of less depth penetration [24].

When used appropriately and with the patient in the supine or supine oblique posture, high-frequency transducers yield the best image quality for the entire breast tissue, as most breasts are only a few centimeters thick. However, having lower-frequency transducers available for deep tissue assessment may be advantageous in cases where patients have disproportionately large breasts. These lower-frequency transducers might be saved for particular situations in order to guarantee sufficient deep-tissue imaging while preserving a respectable level of spatial resolution.

In breast imaging, lower resolution concerns at frequencies below this threshold lead the American College of Radiology practice guidelines to recommend a center frequency of 12 MHz (**Figure 3**) [20].

3.1.1 Nipple and areolar complex abnormalities

Masses in nipple are not common. These consist of melanoma, hemangioma, and adenoma. Due to the nipple's shadowing and image distortion, the retroareolar region

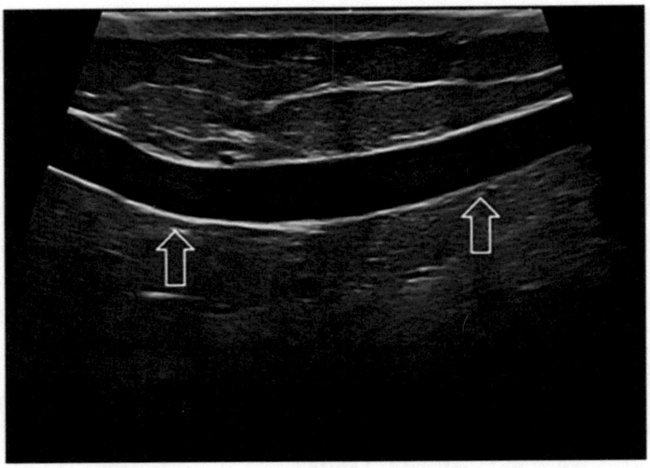

Figure 3.
The breast vein was visualized using a transducer operating at 22 MHz [20].

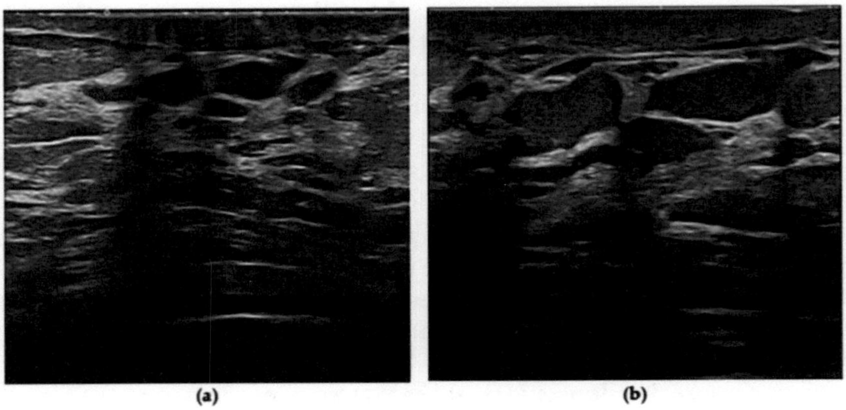

Figure 4.
The ductectasia. Dilated ducts appear at 15 MHz (a) and 22 MHz (b), and are filled with a dense, fluid material [20].

is difficult to scan with sonography. A helpful tip is to compress the para-areolar skin, pull nipple gently without grasping the probe in one hand, and angle the probe toward the retroareolar region [25]. It could be possible to better explore the retroareolar region by using a higher-frequency probe (**Figure 4**) [26].

3.1.2 Male breast on ultrasound

Other than in cases of obvious lipomastia or gynecomastia, the male breast is likewise slender. Although they can appear anywhere, male breast anomalies are typically found in the retroareolar region. The primary task in clinical practice is to distinguish between breast cancer and unilateral, or seemingly unilateral, gynecomastia. The male breast can also have benign tumors, foreign substances, diabetic mastopathy, hematomas, and abscesses as unusual anomalies. High-frequency probes are the best tool for showing all of these changes (**Figure 5**) [24].

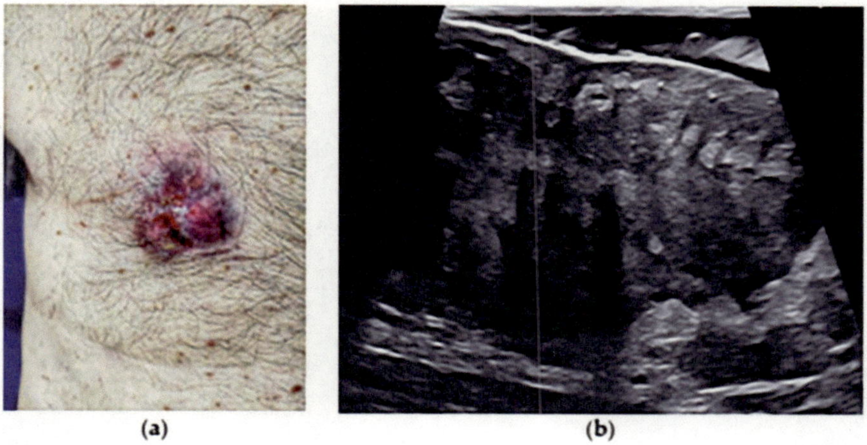

Figure 5.
Localized advanced breast cancer in a man. A high-resolution sonography scan (b) and a clinical picture (a). By using a high-frequency transducer, the nipple-areolar complex can be shown to have tumor tissue infiltrated into it [20].

3.1.3 Dense breast on ultrasound

Mammography has been regarded in the literature as an imperfect and ineffective technology. Even though it reduces the death rate from breast cancer by detecting breast disease, this is especially true in females with dense mammary glands [19]. After high-frequency transducers were developed in the middle of the 1980s, US could be used in the breast, first for benign/malignant differentiation and then for cyst/solid differentiation [5, 27, 28]. A number of single-site studies have confirmed ultrasound's potential as an additional screening tool for women with dense breasts, since the first indications in 1995 that it could identify cancers missed by mammograms [4]. In conclusion, 70% of the tumors were no larger than 1 centimeter, and 94% of the tumors were invasive. Ninety percent of the women whose tumors were detected by sonography had parenchyma that was extremely dense or heterogeneously dense, and 90% of them were in stage 0 or stage I (**Figure 6**) [29].

4. BI-RADS classification

With the intention of standardizing the reporting of mammographic findings, clarifying their interpretation, and improving communication between clinicians, the American College of Radiology (ACR) developed the Breast Imaging Reporting and Data System (BI-RADS) in 1993 [30].

Breast lesions in the ACR BI-RADS US atlas, second edition, are finally categorized based on an analysis of their sonographic properties. In total, there are seven categories. A diagnosis classified as Category 0 requires additional imaging to be added to it. Category 1 refers to the absence of lesions or negative results. A benign lesion without worrisome features is classified as Category 2. Category 3 refers to possible benign conditions with a likelihood of less than 2% for malignancy. A lesion classified as Category 4 is considered suspicious if there is a 2–95% chance that it is malignant and should be biopsied. Category 5 refers to a high possibility of cancer, with a more than 95% probability of malignancy. Knowledge of malignancy or clinical proof of

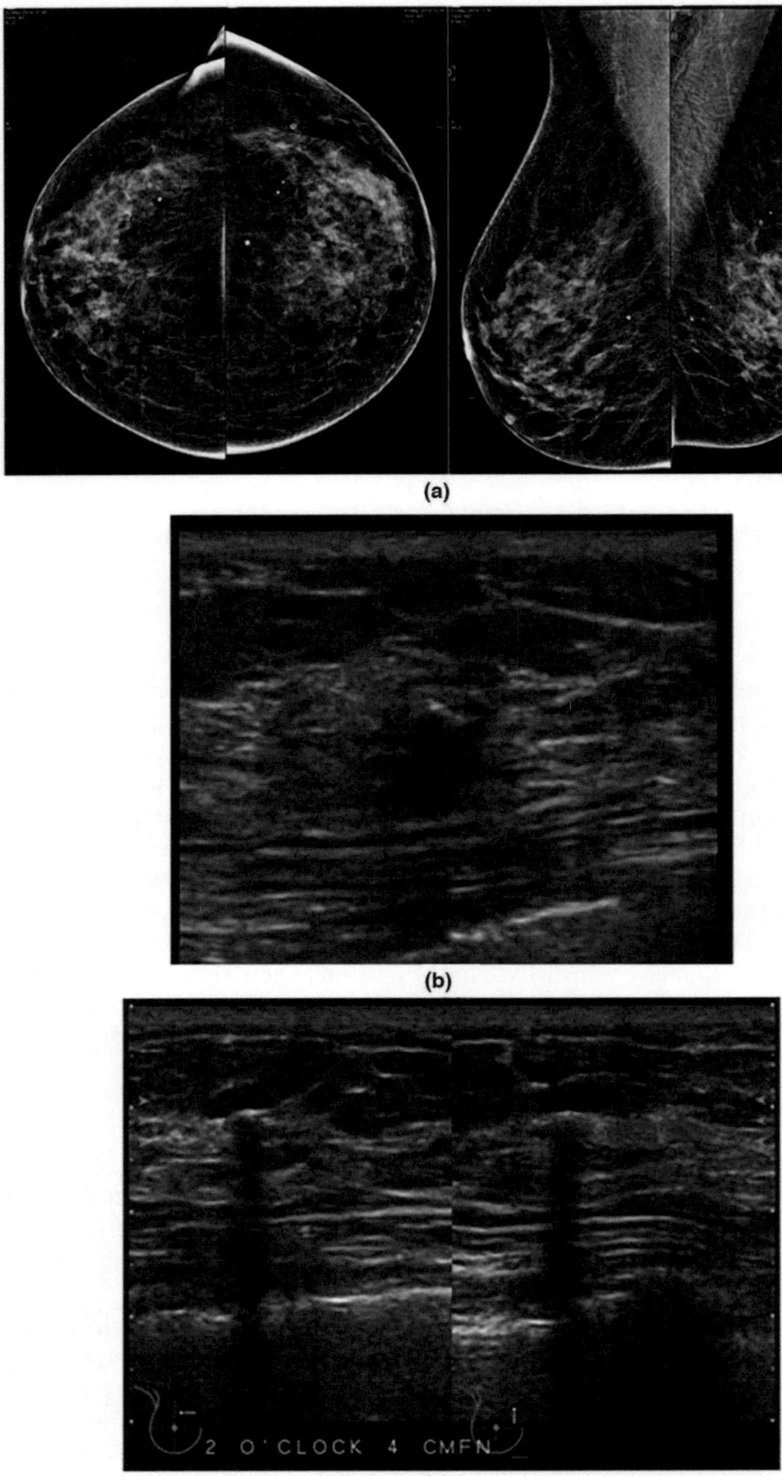

Figure 6.
(A) A woman with category C density who is 73 years old had a negative screening mammography. The screening ultrasound revealed masses in the right (C) and left breasts (B) [4].

malignancy characterize Category 6. Category 4 has three subcategories, 4A, 4B, and 4C, with respective malignance probabilities of 2–10%, 10–50%, and 50–95% due to the large range of malignance probabilities [31].

5. Indications for breast ultrasound

Breast lesions are detected in real time by ultrasonography, which also assesses the physical traits of the lesions, including shape, echogenicity, nodules, and cysts [32].

Common indications for breast ultrasound include the following: [32]

- Detectable lump found during clinical breast examination
- Presence of axillary lymphadenopathy observed on mammogram
- Females under age 40 presenting specific abnormalities during clinical assessment
- Pregnant or lactating individuals
- Identification of suspicious abnormalities on mammography
- Discharge from nipple
- Retractions of skin or nipple inversion
- Visible surgical scars on mammograms
- Gynecomastia
- Suspicion of ruptured implants: used to differentiate between ruptures that occur inside and outside of the capsule
- Percutaneous breast biopsy guided by a needle
- Supervising patients receiving neoadjuvant chemotherapy

5.1 Malignant breast masses detected only by ultrasound

Research on clinical studies has typically determined that when a woman has a negative mammography and is clinically asymptomatic, breast ultrasonography is not helpful in detecting cancer. However, there have been rare reports of tumors found by ultrasonography that were not visible on high-quality mammography or palpable. Using this approach to survey the entire ipsilateral breast in patients in this patient demographic has become more likely to diagnose cancer since high-resolution, real-time handheld sonographic probes have become available [33].

5.2 Benign solid masses

Since fibroadenomas are the most prevalent type of benign breast tumor in women aged 15–35, they are significant. When viewed with real-time sonography, these

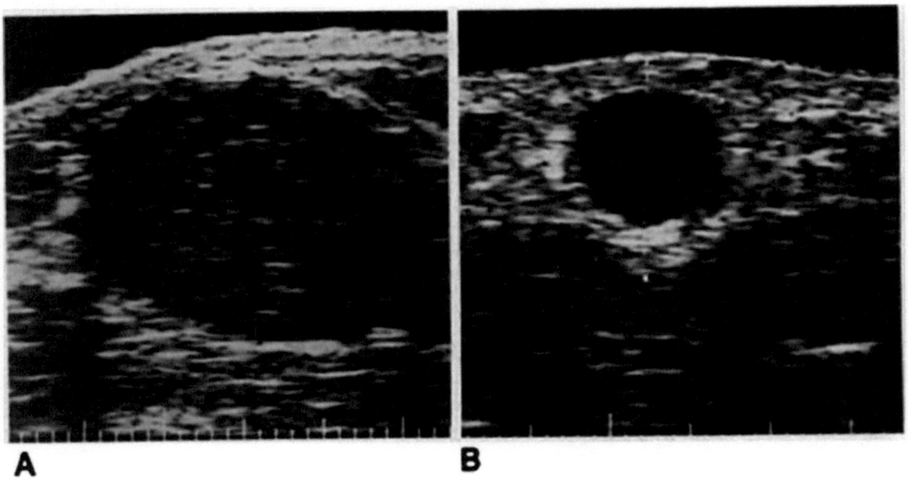

Figure 7.
(A) Fibroadenoma (B) Abscess [6].

lesions usually show a homogenous internal echo pattern and are well-circumscribed. There could be posterior augmentation [6, 33].

Because edema and erythema are the clinical manifestations of inflammatory illness of the breast, it usually presents no problems. The degree of inflammation affects the sonographic appearance.

A well-defined, rounded mass with uniform internal echoes and posterior sound reinforcement can be used to identify an abscess if one has developed. More diffusely inflammatory lesions can destroy normal tissue planes, leaving behind a dominating mass that is poorly defined and unevenly marginated (**Figure 7**) [6, 33].

6. Advances in breast ultrasound

In particular, for women with dense breast parenchyma, adding breast ultrasonography to mammography for supplemental screening can increase the detection rate of breast cancer to 4.2 tumors per 1000 women examined. However, the method is still unavoidably limited due to its low specificity and low positive predictive value (PPV). In addition to interpretation criteria that consider features such as orientation, shape, mass margins, and surrounding effects, other instruments have been developed to characterize breast masses. These include contrast-enhanced harmonic ultrasonography, color Doppler sonography, and sonoelastography. Color Doppler sonography, which evaluates blood vessel presence and shape, has shown 68.0–91.2% sensitivity and 92.7–95.0% specificity in discriminating between benign and malignant breast masses [23].

Furthermore, sonoelastography, an imaging modality that evaluates tissue stiffness, has gained widespread use recently because, in comparison to B-mode sonography alone, it shows a greater specificity in distinguishing between solid breast tumors that are benign and malignant, ranging from 41.0 to 98.5% [34].

Three distinct elastography modalities are presently available. The most common type of sonoelastography is free-hand ultrasonic elastography, which compares signals acquired before and after tissue displacement brought on by manual

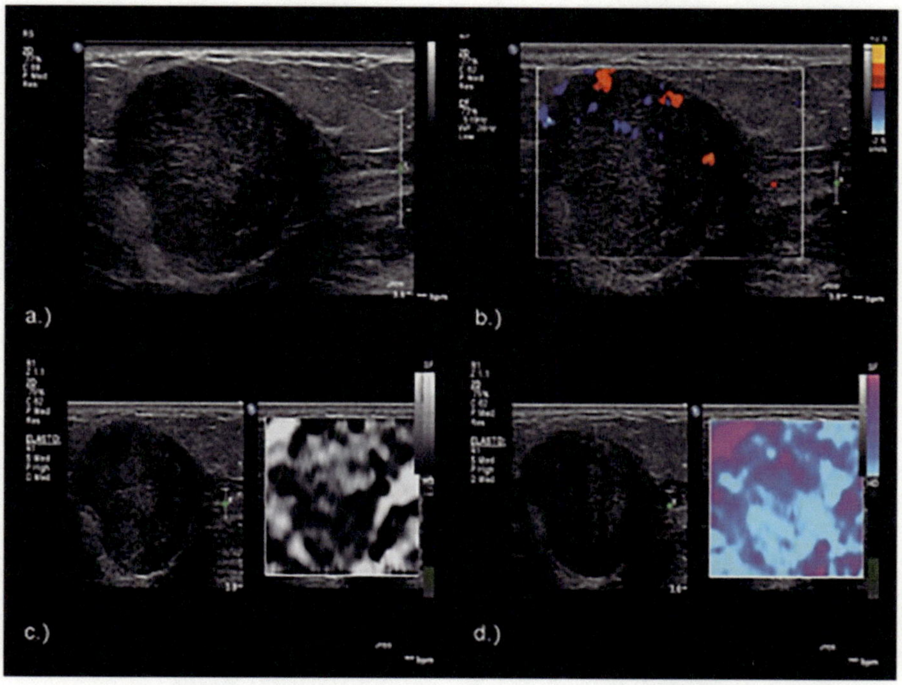

Figure 8.
An ovoid hypoechoic mass is seen on sonography of a 33-year-old female with fibroadenoma, which was histologically confirmed by core needle biopsy (a). (b) Color Doppler sonography reveals an enhanced vascularity, according to the score of 2. (c, d) In sonoelastography a combination of black with white/blue with pink, demonstrating a soft lesion according to Tsukuba-score 2 can be seen [23].

compression. In contrast, quantitative evaluation of tissue elasticity parameters can be done objectively and independently of an operator thanks to shear-wave elasticity (SWE) and acoustic radiation force imaging (ARFI). Furthermore, a number of investigations have demonstrated promise in distinguishing between solid masses and cystic lesions (**Figure 8**) [23].

6.1 Extended field-of-view scanning

The field of view (FOV) of ultrasonography is limited, making it impossible to expose a breast region greater than transducer's footprint in a single scan [8]. Systems with an extended field of view can somewhat overcome this restriction. With no loss of spatial resolution, the program can continually compare the position after the probe is moved in real-time over the skin to build a big 2D image. Large breast lesions can be seen and measured with extended FOV scans. Furthermore, the distance and relationship between a mass and certain anatomic landmark, like nipple or between numerous masses, such as in the case of multifocal/multicentric malignancy, can be shown (**Figure 9**) [35].

6.2 Elastography

US elastography quantifies minute tissue movements brought on by pressure pressures or the viscoelastic characteristics of anomalies in the breast [36]. The existing

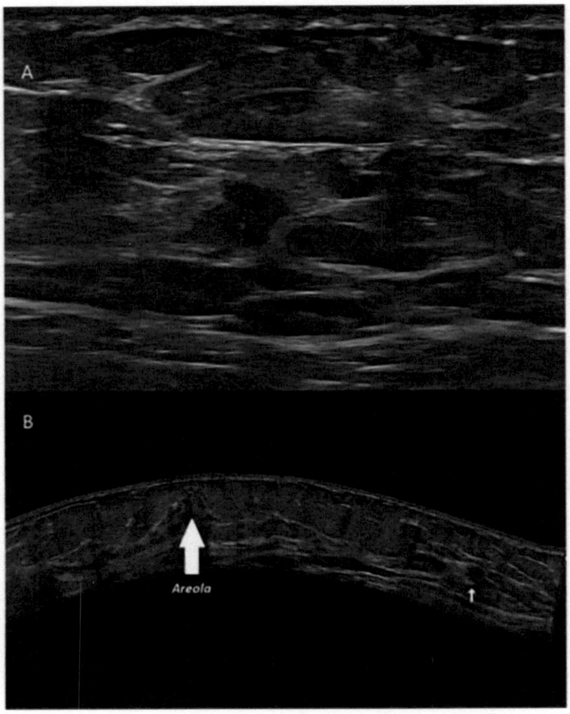

Figure 9.
Breast invasive ductal carcinoma. (A) Axial FOV scan with an arrow pointing to a 4-mm lump and (B) US scan with the lump (arrow) visible throughout the entire breast [3].

methods are strain elastography (which depends on the manual pressure applied by the operator), point shear-wave elastography, acoustic radiation force impulse imaging (ARFI), and 2D/3D shear-wave elastography (which is based on the changes brought about by the concentrated ultrasounds). Numerous techniques (strain-to-fat ratio, subjective scoring, etc.) can be applied to acquire quantitative, semiquantitative, or qualitative data) [3].

Elastography can be used for a variety of purposes, including tumor detection, tumor extent assessment, axillary lymph node status, guidance during percutaneous procedures, and evaluation of tumor response. It has mainly been utilized to characterize breast nodules [3].

Grades of 4 or 5, which are more malleable due to increased strain ratio and shear-wave velocity, are typically categorized as benign. Conversely, harder nodules, which show significant resistance to alteration and have grades of 1 or 2, decreased strain ratio, and decreased shear-wave velocity, are frequently thought to be indicative of malignancy (**Figure 10**) [37].

6.3 Contrast-enhanced ultrasound

The degree of contrast medium enhancement in the Doppler vascular signal is correlated with the grade and malignancy of cancer and provides an indirect measure of the density of tumor microvascular. Originally developed in the 1990s to support low-sensitivity Doppler systems, microbubble contrast media are now utilized for low mechanical-index, grayscale US real-time imaging. Nevertheless, contrast-enhanced

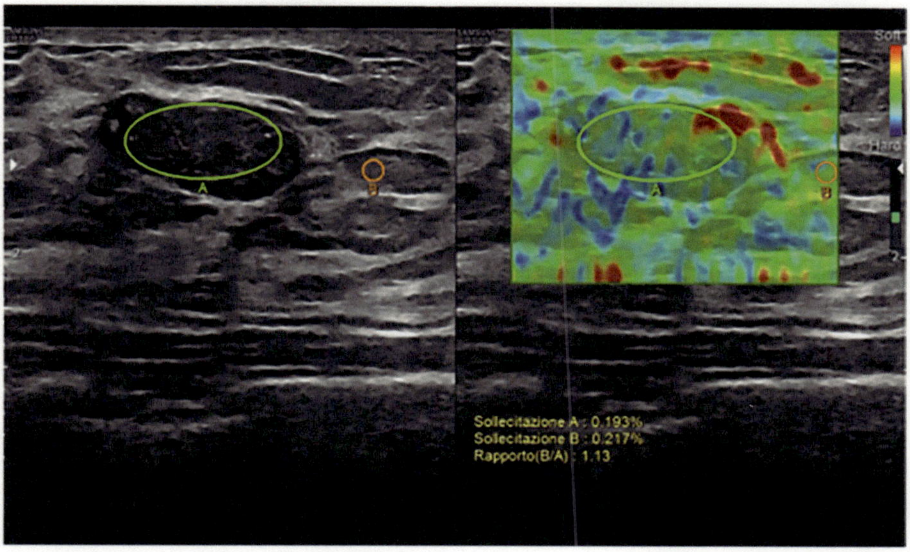

Figure 10.
Breast Fibroadenoma. Assessment of the lesion-to-fat stiffness is possible with the strain ratio [3].

US (CEUS) has not had a major influence on breast imaging despite a large number of publications. This is primarily because the contrast agents that have been on the market up to this point are more effective at lower frequencies used to scan belly than at higher frequencies required to photograph structures that are superficial like breast [38–43].

Breast cancerous nodules exhibit a rapid, intense, but fleeting amplification with varying degrees of variability. Tumors can have radially dispersed, irregular, and tortuous blood arteries surrounding them. CEUS might be a more accurate tumor size measurement than traditional B-mode US [3].

6.4 Three-dimensional ultrasound

For high-resolution 3D breast imaging, there are automated and handheld linear transducers available. Surface renderings of normal and pathological breast structures can be obtained using three-dimensional US, also known as volumetric US. An image that is 3D reconstructed is created in the sagittal, transverse, and coronal planes with only one ultrasonic beam pass, enabling a more precise evaluation of anatomical features and tumor boundaries [8]. Because coronal pictures are parallel to the skin, they offer a special potential made possible by 3D US. It is possible to create a striking image of breast tumors with a retracting, star-shaped outline that powerfully supports malignancy diagnosis (**Figure 11**) [3].

6.5 MicroPure

Clustered microcalcifications are a primary discovery in breast imaging that presents a notable constraint to ultrasound capabilities, as they can be challenging or unfeasible to identify, particularly if they are not linked with a lump [44, 45]. A program called MicroPure™ from Canon (Tokyo, Japan) makes it possible to draw attention to microcalcifications. By utilizing a combination of non-linear imaging and

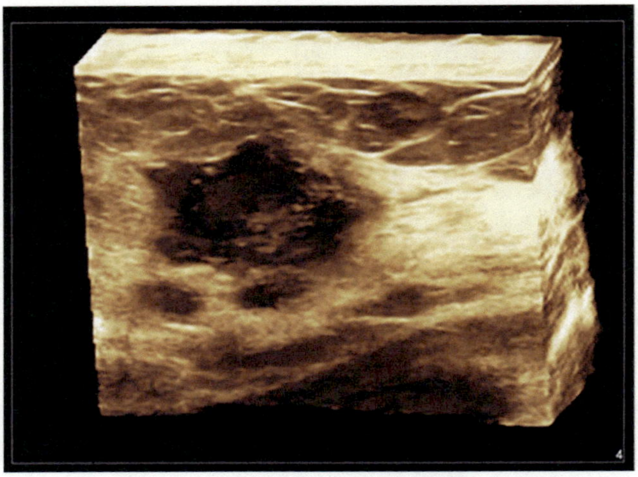

Figure 11.
Breast invasive ductal carcinoma. Coronal 3D visualization of tumor margin infiltration [3].

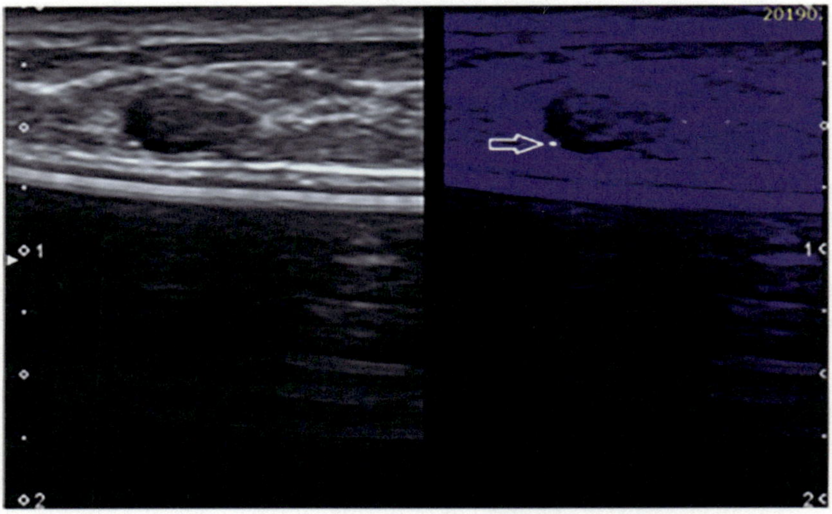

Figure 12.
A patient with a history of augmentation mammography has fibroadenoma. Micropure makes it simple to find a bright dot caused by a tiny amount of calcification [3].

speckle suppression, MicroPure is able to separate calcification from uneven background. Microcalcifications that are Filtered displayed by way of brilliant specks on top of a grayscale US overlaid on a dark blue background (**Figure 12**) [3].

6.6 Automated breast ultrasound

The drawbacks of purported "manual" or "handheld" ultrasound (US) imaging encompass lack of reproducibility, reliance on operator skill, and incapacity to archive volumes and scrutinize extensive breast regions [46]. To get around these restrictions, an automated breast US (ABUS) system—also known as an automated breast volume US—has been developed. Through ABUS, an operator can utilize a substantial, specialized transducer to capture extensive tissue volumes concurrently, ranging from the chest wall to the skin [3].

6.7 Computer-assisted diagnosis—S-detect

Artificial intelligence systems can automatically identify and measure a variety of features from US images thanks to deep learning algorithms. This could make it possible to identify and characterize breast lesions easily and consistently, as well as to predict how patients with locally advanced breast cancer would react to treatment (**Figure 13**) [3].

6.8 Ultrasound nomograms

Using a computer program, Radiomics is able to extract a large number of quantitative features from US pictures [46]. Choosing and extracting well-known US features is the first step in the process of creating a nomogram. Next, a patient cohort for internal and external validation may be consulted during the construction and testing of a model. Quantitative characteristics that are taken using computer algorithms can be used to determine in advance how a breast tumor will respond to treatment, to forecast the prognosis, or to differentiate between different types of breast abnormalities [47].

6.9 Full noncontact laser ultrasound

Complete noncontact laser ultrasound (LUS) imaging offers numerous notable benefits compared to current medical ultrasound (US) technologies. These

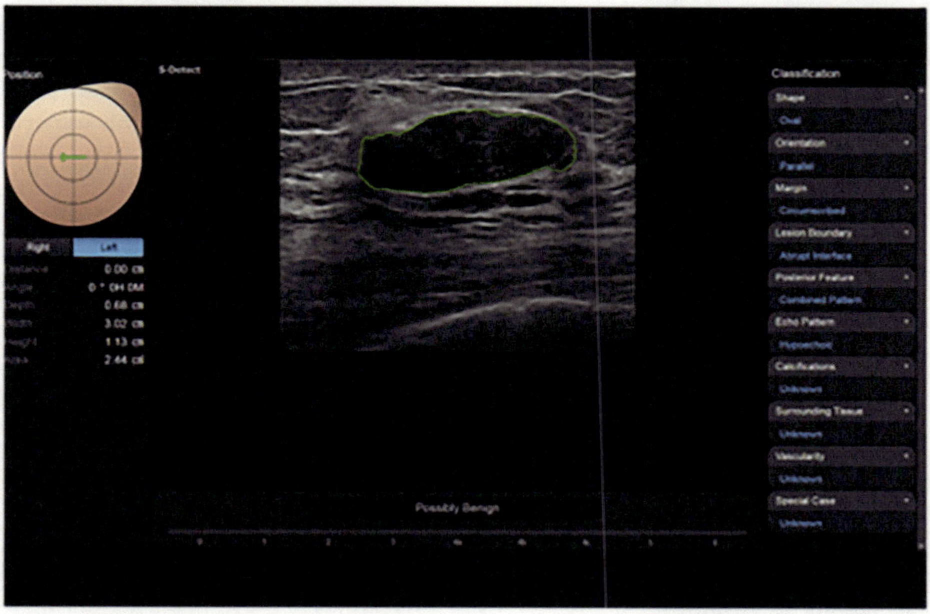

Figure 13.
S-detect automatic BI-RADS descriptor-based measurement and classification of a breast nodule (fibroadenoma) [3].

advantages comprise volumetric imaging, image quality independent of operator skill, enhanced reproducibility, and the absence of coupling agents (gel/water). The design of the LUS system considered here minimizes optical penetration and, more precisely, restricts the conversion of optical energy to acoustic energy at the tissue interface to maximize the amplitude of the generated acoustic signal [48].

7. Discussion

Rongrong Guo et al. conducted a review study in 2017 that comprises the advancement of ultrasound technology as well as the uses of ultrasound in fusion with other modalities. They also include advancements in ultrasound-guided biopsies. According to that review, those techniques are of great importance in diagnosing breast lesions as benign or malignant and can further improve early breast cancer detection. The limitation of that review was that they did not address every aspect of ultrasound imaging for breast cancer in detail.

In this chapter, we provided a wide range of ultrasound imaging techniques that are of great importance in the diagnosis of breast pathologies, whether benign or malignant. We also explain the use of ultrasound technology in diagnosing male breast pathologies. The limitation of this chapter is that we have not provided any ultrasound data in conjunction with other modalities like mammography, MRI, and positron emission tomography (PET) scans.

8. Conclusions

In summary, each ultrasound imaging technology has specific benefits and uses for breast imaging, but taken as a whole, they help to increase diagnostic precision, streamline clinical procedures, and ultimately improve patient care. Future developments in this field of study and technology promise to further enhance breast imaging capabilities and patient outcomes.

Notwithstanding the remarkable progress showcased in this review, it is imperative to draw attention to many persistent constraints and hazards. A big, fatty breast can still cause issues for a US scan; thus, it should never be the primary modality used to assess a situation like this [3].

9. Recommendation

9.1 Elimination of subject dependency

Since ultrasound is operator-dependent, the certainty of missing a tiny lesion in large fatty breasts will be there. To overcome this limitation, we recommend designing a transducer in such a way that the operator only places the transducer on the patient's chest area and that the transducer covers the entire breast and images the breast as a whole. In that way, the chance of missing a tiny obscure lesion in fatty breasts might be reduced.

DOI: http://dx.doi.org/10.5772/intechopen.1005373

Author details

Athar Shams Rana[1*], Javairia Rafique[2] and Hira Riffat[3]

1 Green International University, Lahore, Pakistan

2 Superior University, Lahore, Pakistan

3 The University of Lahore Sargodha Campus, Sargodha, Pakistan

*Address all correspondence to: atharshams44@gmail.com

References

[1] Winters S, Martin C, Murphy D, Navkiran K. Shokar breast cancer epidemiology, prevention, and screening. In: Progress in Molecular Biology and Translational Science. Vol. 151. Pubmed; 10 Oct 2017. ISSN 1877-1173. DOI: 10.1016/bs.pmbts.2017.07.002

[2] Dodd GD. Present status of thermography, ultrasound and mammography in breast cancer detection. Cancer. 1977;**39**(Suppl. 6):2796-2805. DOI: 10.1002/1097-0142(197706)39:6<2796::aid- cncr2820390667>3.0.co;2-0

[3] Catalano O, Fusco R, De Muzio F, Simonetti I, Palumbo P, Bruno F, et al. Recent advances in ultrasound breast imaging: From industry to clinical practice. Diagnostics (Basel). 2023;**13**(5):980. DOI: 10.3390/diagnostics13050980

[4] Gordon PB. The impact of dense breasts on the stage of breast cancer at diagnosis: A review and options for supplemental screening. Current Oncology. 2022;**29**(5):3595-3636. DOI: 10.3390/curroncol29050291

[5] Hilton SV, Leopold GR, Olson LK, Willson SA. Real-time breast sonography: Application in 300 consecutive patients. AJR. American Journal of Roentgenology. 1986;**147**(3):479-486. DOI: 10.2214/ajr.147.3.479

[6] Gordon PB, Goldenberg SL. Malignant breast masses detected only by ultrasound. A retrospective review. Cancer. 1995;**76**:626-630. DOI: 10.1002/1097-0142(19950815)76:4<626::aid-cncr2820760413>3.0.co;2-z

[7] Dempsey PJ. The history of breast ultrasound. Journal of Ultrasound in Medicine. 2004;**23**:887-894. DOI: 10.7863/jum.2004.23.7.887

[8] Hooley RJ, Scoutt LM, Philpotts LE. Breast ultrasonography: State of the art. Radiology. 2013;**268**:642-659. DOI: 10.1148/radiol.13121606

[9] Pandya S, Moore RG. Breast development and anatomy. Clinical Obstetrics and Gynecology. 2011;**54**(1):91-95. DOI: 10.1097/GRF.0b013e318207ffe9

[10] Bistoni G, Farhadi J. Anatomy and physiology of the breast. In: Plastic and Reconstructive Surgery. Approaches and Techniques. 1st ed. Wiley Blackwell; Mar 2015. pp. 479-485. DOI: 10.1002/9781118655412.ch37

[11] Alex A, Bhandary E, McGuire KP. Anatomy and physiology of the breast during pregnancy and lactation. In: Alipour S, Omranipour R, editors. Diseases of the Breast during Pregnancy and Lactation. Advances in Experimental Medicine and Biology. Vol. 1252. Cham: Springer; 2020. pp. 3-7. DOI: 10.1007/978-3-030-41596-9_1

[12] Geddes DT. Inside the lactating breast: The latest anatomy research. Journal of Midwifery & Women's Health. 2007;**52**(6):556-563. DOI: 10.1016/j.jmwh.2007.05.004

[13] Ellis H, Mahadevan V. Anatomy and physiology of the breast. Surgery (Oxford). 2021:1. DOI: 10.1016/J.MPSUR.2012.10.018

[14] Jesinger RA. Breast anatomy for the interventionalist. Techniques in Vascular and Interventional Radiology. 2014;**17**(1):3-9. DOI: 10.1053/j.tvir.2013.12.002

[15] Brunicardi F, Andersen D, Billiar T, et al. Schwartz's Principles of Surgery. 8th ed. New York, NY: The McGraw-Hill Medical Publishing Division; 2004

[16] Bland K, Copeland E. The Breast—Comprehensive Management of Benign and Malignant Diseases. 4th ed. Philadelphia, PA: Saunders; 2009. DOI: 10.1038/sj.bjc.6602192

[17] Drew P, Cawthorn S, Michell M. Interventional Ultrasound of the Breast - Anatomy of the Breast by Menos Lagopoulos. London, UK: Informa Healthcare; 2007. pp. 11-22

[18] Sarhadi N, Shaw-Dunn J, Soutar D. Nerve supply of the breast with special reference to the nipple and areola: Sir Astley Cooper revisited. Clinical Anatomy. 1997;**10**:283-288

[19] Santos R, Ribeiro AR, Marques D. Ultrasound as a method for early diagnosis of breast pathology. Journal of Personalized Medicine. 2023;**13**(7):1156. DOI: 10.3390/jpm13071156

[20] Corvino A, Varelli C, Catalano F, Cocco G, Delli Pizzi A, Boccatonda A, et al. Use of high-frequency transducers in breast sonography. Journal of Personalized Medicine. 2022;**12**(12):1960. DOI: 10.3390/jpm12121960

[21] Schnarkowski P, Schmidt D, Milz P, Kessler M, Reiser MF. Vergleich zwischen herkömmlicher und hochauflösender Sonographie für die Diagnostik von Mammaläsionen [Comparison between current and high resolution ultrasound for diagnosis of breast lesions]. Ultraschall in der Medizin. 1996;**17**(4):190-194. German. DOI: 10.1055/s-2007-1003179

[22] Schulz-Wendtland R, Bock K, Aichinger U, de Waal J, Bader W, Albert US, et al. Mamma-Sonographie mit 7.5 MHz versus 13 MHz: Ist eine Verbesserung der diagnostischen Sicherheit im Rahmen der komplementären Mammadiagnostik möglich? [Ultrasound examination of the breast with 7.5 MHz and 13 MHz-transducers: Scope for improving diagnostic accuracy in complementary breast diagnostics?]. Ultraschall in der Medizin. 2005;**26**(3):209-215. German. DOI: 10.1055/s-2005-857897

[23] Rjosk-Dendorfer D, Gürtler VM, Sommer WH, Reiser M, Clevert DA. Value of high resolution compression elastography and color doppler sonography in characterisation of breast lesions: Comparison of different high-frequency transducers. Clinical Hemorheology and Microcirculation. 2014;**57**(2):129-135. DOI: 10.3233/CH-141824

[24] Carpentier B, Hayward J, Strachowski L. Enhancing your acoustics: Ultrasound image optimization of breast lesions. Journal of Ultrasound in Medicine. 2017;**36**(7):1479-1485. DOI: 10.7863/ultra.16.09018

[25] Dylke ES, Benincasa Nakagawa H, Lin L, Clarke JL, Kilbreath SL. Reliability and diagnostic thresholds for ultrasound measurements of dermal thickness in breast lymphedema. Lymphatic Research and Biology. 2018;**16**(3):258-262. DOI: 10.1089/lrb.2016.0067

[26] Yoon JH, Yoon H, Kim EK, Moon HJ, Park YV, Kim MJ. Ultrasonographic evaluation of women with pathologic nipple discharge. Ultrasonography. 2017;**36**(4):310-320. DOI: 10.14366/usg.17013

[27] Harper AP, Kelly-Fry E, Noe JS, Bies JR, Jackson VP. Ultrasound in the evaluation of solid breast masses. Radiology. 1983;**146**(3):731-736. DOI: 10.1148/radiology.146.3.6298858

[28] Stavros AT, Thickman D, Rapp CL, Dennis MA, Parker SH, Sisney GA. Solid breast nodules: Use of sonography to distinguish between benign and malignant lesions. Radiology. 1995;**196**(1):123-134. DOI: 10.1148/radiology.196.1.7784555

[29] Berg WA. Supplemental screening sonography in dense breasts. Radiologic Clinics of North America. 2004;**42**(5):845-851, vi. DOI: 10.1016/j.rcl.2004.04.003

[30] Heinig J, Witteler R, Schmitz R, Kiesel L, Steinhard J. Accuracy of classification of breast ultrasound findings based on criteria used for BI-RADS. Ultrasound in Obstetrics and Gynecology. Sep 2008;**32**(4):573-578. DOI: 10.1002/uog.5191. PMID: 18421795

[31] Luo WQ, Huang QX, Huang XW, Hu HT, Zeng FQ, Wang W. Predicting breast cancer in breast imaging reporting and data system (BI-RADS) ultrasound category 4 or 5 lesions: A nomogram combining radiomics and BI-RADS. Scientific Reports. 2019;**9**(1):11921. DOI: 10.1038/s41598-019-48488-4

[32] Malherbe K, Tafti D. Breast ultrasound. In: StatPearls [Internet]. Treasure Island (FL): StatPearls Publishing; 2024

[33] Berg WA, Blume JD, Cormack JB, Mendelson EB, Lehrer D, Böhm-Vélez M, et al. ACRIN 6666 investigators. Combined screening with ultrasound and mammography vs mammography alone in women at elevated risk of breast cancer. JAMA. 2008;**299**(18):2151-2163. DOI: 10.1001/jama.299.18.2151

[34] Prantl L, Englbrecht MA, Schoeneich M, Kuehlmann B, Jung EM, Kubale R. Semiquantitative measurements of capsular contracture with elastography--First results in correlation to baker score. Clinical Hemorheology and Microcirculation. 2014;**58**(4):521-528. DOI: 10.3233/CH-141812

[35] Catalano O, Wortsman X. Dermatology ultrasound. Imaging technique, tips and tricks, high-resolution anatomy. Ultrasound Quarterly. 2020;**36**(4):321-327. DOI: 10.1097/RUQ.0000000000000520

[36] Sivakumaran L, Alturkistani H, Lerouge S, Bertrand-Grenier A, Zehtabi F, Thérasse É, et al. Strain ultrasound elastography of aneurysm sac content after randomized endoleak embolization with sclerosing vs. non-sclerosing chitosan-based hydrogels in a canine model. Journal of Vascular and Interventional Radiology. 2022;**33**(5):495-504.e3. DOI: 10.1016/j.jvir.2022.02.003

[37] Lee SH, Chang JM, Cho N, Koo HR, Yi A, Kim SJ, et al. Practice guideline for the performance of breast ultrasound elastography. Ultrasonography. 2014;**33**(1):3-10. DOI: 10.14366/usg.13012

[38] De Muzio F, Grassi F, Dell'Aversana F, Fusco R, Danti G, Flammia F, et al. A narrative review on LI-RADS algorithm in liver tumors: Prospects and pitfalls. Diagnostics (Basel). 2022;**12**(7):1655. DOI: 10.3390/diagnostics12071655

[39] Catalano O, Sandomenico F, Vallone P, Setola SV, Granata V, Fusco R, et al. Contrast-enhanced ultrasound in the assessment of patients with indeterminate abdominal findings at positron emission tomography imaging. Ultrasound in Medicine & Biology. 2016;**42**(11):2717-2723. DOI: 10.1016/j.ultrasmedbio.2016.06.023

[40] Granata V, Grassi R, Fusco R, Setola SV, Belli A, Piccirillo M, et al.

Abbreviated MRI protocol for the assessment of ablated area in HCC patients. International Journal of Environmental Research and Public Health. 2021;**18**(7):3598. DOI: 10.3390/ijerph18073598

[41] Barretta ML, Catalano O, Setola SV, Granata V, Marone U, D'Errico GA. Gallbladder metastasis: Spectrum of imaging findings. Abdominal Imaging. 2011;**36**(6):729-734. DOI: 10.1007/s00261-011-9696-y

[42] Granata V, Fusco R, Catalano O, Avallone A, Palaia R, Botti G, et al. Diagnostic accuracy of magnetic resonance, computed tomography and contrast enhanced ultrasound in radiological multimodality assessment of peribiliary liver metastases. PLoS One. 2017;**12**(6):e0179951. DOI: 10.1371/journal.pone.0179951

[43] Granata V, de Lutio di Castelguidone E, Fusco R, Catalano O, Piccirillo M, Palaia R, et al. Irreversible electroporation of hepatocellular carcinoma: Preliminary report on the diagnostic accuracy of magnetic resonance, computer tomography, and contrast-enhanced ultrasound in evaluation of the ablated area. La Radiologia Medica. 2016;**121**(2):122-131. DOI: 10.1007/s11547-015-0582-5

[44] Park AY, Seo BK, Cho KR, Woo OH. The utility of MicroPure™ ultrasound technique in assessing grouped microcalcifications without a mass on mammography. Journal of Breast Cancer. 2016;**19**(1):83-86. DOI: 10.4048/jbc.2016.19.1.83

[45] Guo R, Lu G, Qin B, Fei B. Ultrasound imaging technologies for breast cancer detection and management: A review. Ultrasound in Medicine & Biology. 2018;**44**(1):37-70. DOI: 10.1016/j.ultrasmedbio.2017.09.012

[46] Chiao JY, Chen KY, Liao KY, Hsieh PH, Zhang G, Huang TC. Detection and classification the breast tumors using mask R-CNN on sonograms. Medicine (Baltimore). 2019;**98**(19):e15200. DOI: 10.1097/MD.0000000000015200

[47] Gao Y, Luo Y, Zhao C, Xiao M, Ma L, Li W, et al. Nomogram based on radiomics analysis of primary breast cancer ultrasound images: Prediction of axillary lymph node tumor burden in patients. European Radiology. 2021;**31**(2):928-937. DOI: 10.1007/s00330-020-07181-1

[48] Zhang X, Fincke JR, Wynn CM, Johnson MR, Haupt RW, Anthony BW. Full noncontact laser ultrasound: First human data. Light: Science & Applications. 2019;**8**:119. DOI: 10.1038/s41377-019-0229-8

Chapter 9

Application of Magnetic Resonance Imaging in Breast Cancer Patients

Yue Zhang and Ying Qian

Abstract

The advantage of the multi-parametric method for breast cancer is the different contributions of diverse parameters in the magnetic resonance image (MRI). T1-weighted imaging (T1WI) detects the signal intensity differences in tissue according to different longitudinal relaxation times. Dynamic contrast-enhanced magnetic resonance imaging (DCE-MRI) can estimate the vascularity and permeability of the lesion by semiquantitative and quantitative parameters. The ultrafast DCE-MRI presents the new kinetic parameters. Diffusion-weighted imaging (DWI) provides information related to tumor cell density, and advanced diffusion-weighted imaging techniques, such as diffusion kurtosis imaging, intravoxel incoherent motion, and time-dependent diffusion MRI, exhibit new perspectives of microscale tissue assessment. Moreover, T2-weighted imaging is important for the measurement of the water content of the tissue. Magnetic resonance spectroscopy (MRS) can detect choline levels and choline metabolites in the tissue. Magnetic resonance elastography (MRE) can provide quantitative mechanical properties of breast tissue, including stiffness, elasticity, and viscosity, to improve the specificity for breast lesion characterization. In this chapter, we provide a technical and theoretical background for these parameters and reveal the application of multi-parameter imaging in breast cancer.

Keywords: MRI, multi-parametric, T1-weighted imaging, T2-weighted imaging, DCE-MRI, diffusion-weighted imaging, MRS, MRE

1. Introduction

Breast cancer is the most commonly diagnosed cancer for women in the world. The incidence of breast cancer has increased in recent decades and has become a major burden on women's health worldwide [1]. The five-year breast cancer survival rate has steadily improved in most developed countries [2], while early detection, accurate diagnostic, and therapeutic management are still necessary measures to reduce mortality. The concept of Breast Imaging Reporting and Data System has been proposed, and tumor classification and grading are evaluated according to imaging characteristics. This classification still has limitations because it depends largely on the experience of the doctors. A biopsy is advised before surgery for patients with suspected breast lesions to confirm the nature of the tumor. However, the gold standard can be provided by biopsy for the suspicious lesions, while the biopsy is invasive, which may provide uncertain lesion information for the too large tumor, and the heterogeneity of the whole tumor cannot be reflected [3].

Image technology can measure the size, morphology, and imaging characteristics of the tumor and has been applied in the prognosis evaluation, diagnosis, and treatment of tumors as a most convenient and direct tool. New technologies based on different imaging modalities have emerged for precision medicine and individualized treatment of cancer patients [4]. The workflow of MRI image processing included image acquisition and reconstruction, lesion segmentation, feature extraction, and data analysis. The segmentation process should be reliable, reproducible, and accurate. Manual drawing by experienced radiologists is considered the standard method, while it is time-consuming and not suitable for large databases [5]. The semiautomatic and automatic methods perform well under a big difference between lesions and background intensity, and both have been developed in recent decades to improve accuracy [6]. The features extracted from images include shape, intensity, texture, gradient, wavelet features, fractal dimension, etc. [7]. Some extracted features of regions of interest (ROI) seem redundant for a particular task, so it is important to use machine algorithms to select useful information. Machine learning algorithms include support vector machines, decision trees, deep neural networks, random forests, etc. [6]. Features with reproductive, informative, and nonredundant features are then selected to assess associations with clinical outcomes.

For the diagnosis of malignant tumors, tumor subtypes, metabolism, angiogenesis, and the tumor microenvironment (TME) are important. The intrinsic subtypes, which are initially determined by gene expression profiling, are connected with the biological characteristics of breast cancer [8]. The intrinsic subtypes, based on human epidermal growth factor 2 (HER 2), estrogen receptor (ER), Ki-67 index, and progesterone receptor, are widely verified in clinical [9]. Although these immunohistochemical subtypes are confirmed by histopathological sampling, the image techniques especially the multi-parametric approaches are still used to predict different subtypes [10–12]. Metabolism and angiogenesis are two biomarkers of cancer and can be estimated by contrast-enhanced MRI [13]. Proliferation can be evaluated by DWI [14], and increased preproliferative metabolism becomes an early signal of tumor growth. The TME including tumor-infiltrating lymphocytes (TIL) and cancer-associated fibroblasts (CAF) are important for tumor formation and development. TIL is a predictor of response to cancer immunotherapy, including predictors concerned with atezolizumab and pembrolizumab. CAF decreases cell apoptosis and improves the viability of cancer cells, migration, and proliferation [15]. CAF can cause poor prognosis for HER2-negative or node-negative hormone receptor-positive breast cancer patients [16]. The irregular tumor-associated vascular network yields inefficient perfusion and causes hypoxia [17].

Magnetic resonance imaging (MRI) is a noninvasive imaging technique with great potential to obtain scalable data and assess the entire tumor characteristics of imaging. The information acquired by dynamic contrast-enhanced (DCE), diffusion-weighted imaging (DWI), T2-weighted imaging (T2WI), MR spectroscopy (MRS), T1-weighted imaging (T1WI), magnetic resonance elastography (MRE), etc. can be used to establish clinical prognosis prediction models and provide a noninvasive method for tumor genotyping [18]. In clinical practice, MRI is expected to be an imaging biomarker for different kinds of tumors. Magnetic resonance imaging of the breast is widely used for screening, staging, evaluating efficacy, and monitoring recurrence, especially to provide supplementary information for mammography and ultrasonography [3]. In this study, we aim to provide a comprehensive review focusing on basic information, main features, and applications of individual MRI parameters and multi-parametric approaches for breast cancer.

2. Mechanisms of cancer imaging

2.1 T1-weighted imaging

T1-weighted imaging (T1WI) indicates the signal intensities reflecting the differences among tissue longitudinal relaxation time in the magnetic resonance image. Intravenous access is usually required for the T1-weighted sequence in the detection of breast lesions [19]. T1-weighted imaging can be executed without or with fat suppression. Images often are obtained in the axial plane, which has a higher speed than in the sagittal plane and produces a better contour of both breasts. Since the morphological assessment requires more details, the in-plane pixel size of T1-weighted imaging should be 1 * 1 mm or smaller [20–22]. By using modern MRI techniques and breast coils, it is easy to obtain a higher resolution (1 mm isotropic and lower) without a prolonged acquisition time of more than 90 seconds per volume. This permits reconstruction in any plane and is helpful for evaluating lesions, especially for non-mass lesions. The T1-weighted imaging was often used to measure the size and texture of breast lesions [23, 24]. Compared to the pure ductal carcinoma *in situ* (DCIS) group, the DCIS with invasion group had a higher nuclear grade, larger mean lesion size, and coarser, more complex, and heterogeneous texture, higher maximum gray-level intensity, and a greater concentration of high gray-level intensity [24]. **Figure 1** shows the images of T1WI for breast cancer patients.

T1-weighted images should be obtained before contrast agent administration first. After contrast injection, T1-weighted acquisition was repeated to depict enhancing abnormalities. Considering most breast cancers get peak enhancement about 60–90 seconds after injection of contrast, the time point of acquiring the images is crucial. The posterior contrast images are mainly used to detect lesions. Subtraction images between the images obtained before and after the contrast are needed to be created for images without fat suppression [25]. Subtracted images also contribute to the acquisition of fat suppression, as they can help distinguish truly enhanced structures from lesions with native high signal intensity at T1 [26]. The maximum intensity projection images generated from these subtracted images assist rapid lesion detection [27, 28], while poor fat suppression, chemical shift artifacts, and motion artifacts could blur the small lesions in projection images.

The two T1-weighted acquisitions, before and nearly 90 seconds after contrast injection, are generally adequate for lesion detection according to the success of the abbreviated protocols for breast MRI [29]. A previous study revealed no significant difference in the ratios of tumor length diameter measured by 1.5-T gadolinium-enhanced T1-weighted (Gd-T1WI) and DWI compared to pathology [30]. A previous retrospective study enrolled 281 patients and used machine learning classifiers to create predictive models for pathological complete response (pCR) in breast cancer after neoadjuvant therapy (NAT). The models based on T1-weighted images before contrast and the first-phase T1-weighted images after contrast were evaluated. The classifiers of random forest (RF) (area under the curve [AUC]: 0.914, accuracy 87.0%, sensitivity 85.2%, specificity 88.1%) and light gradient boosting machine (LightGBM) (AUC 0.836, accuracy 78.6%, sensitivity 68.2%, specificity 90.0%) showed promising

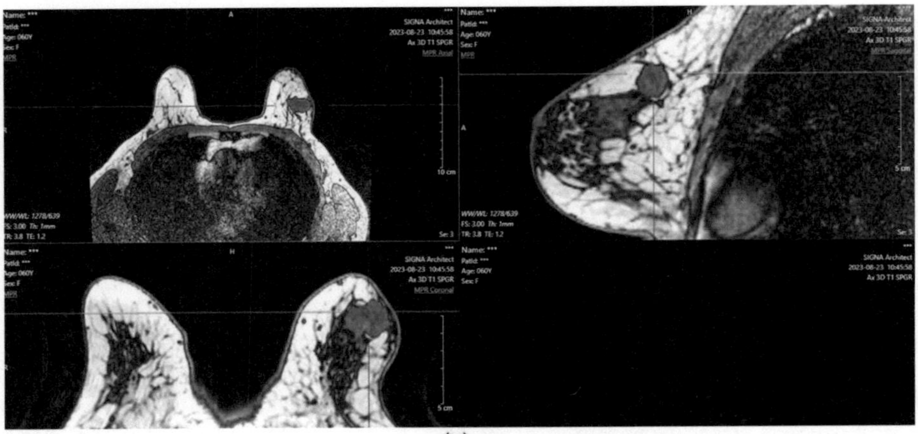

(a)

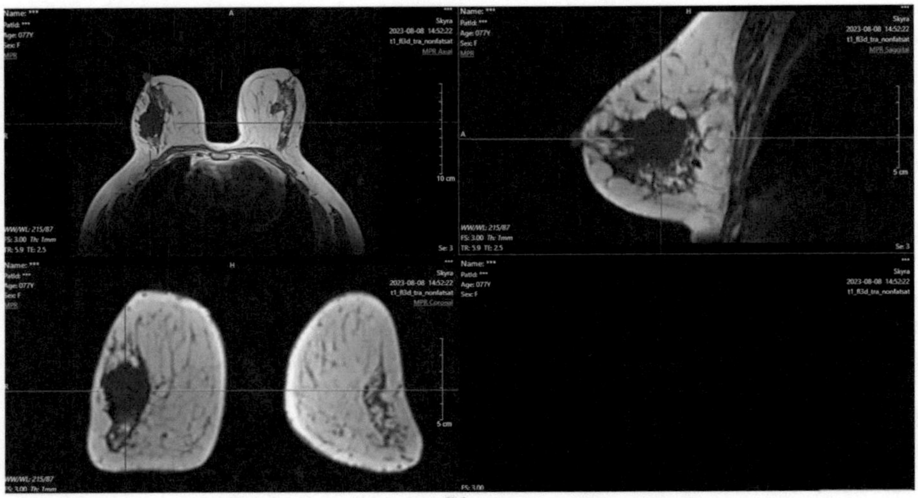

(b)

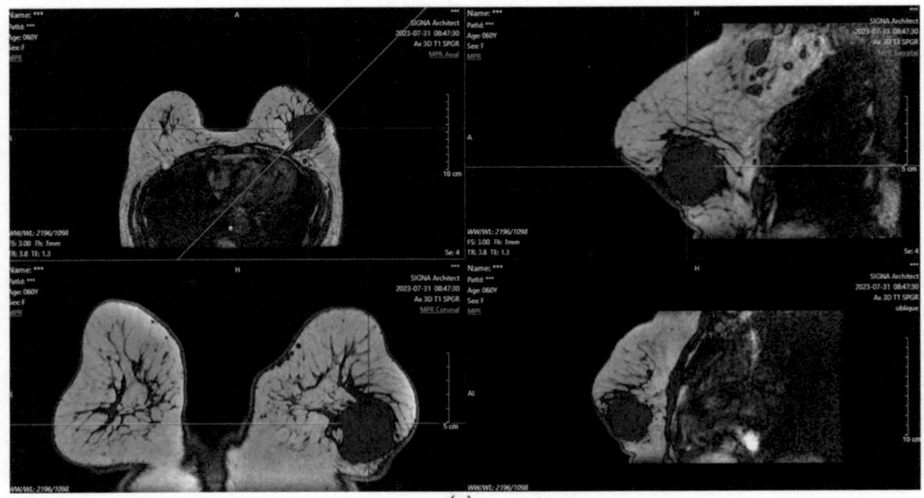

(c)

Figure 1.
The images of T1WI for three breast cancer patients. (a)–(c) indicate the images for the first patient with left breast cancer, the second patient with right breast cancer, and the third patient with left breast cancer respectively.

results for luminal and triple-negative breast cancers, respectively [31]. All other sequences improve the differentiation of breast lesions with the aim of preventing false-positive and false-negative classifications.

2.2 Dynamic contrast-enhanced magnetic resonance imaging

Dynamic contrast-enhanced (DCE) MRI is an imaging tool to assess vascular status by intravenous injection of gadolinium-based contrast agents. Enhanced information at least three time points is required to plot time-intensity curves and perform qualitative analysis [32]. In order to get suitable spatial resolution (about 1 mm pixel size) of the image, the temporal resolution of the DCE is usually 1–2 minutes [33]. Initially rapid enhancement and delayed clearance are the most typical kinetic patterns for malignancy [4]. The DCE-MRI possesses good temporal resolution, can detect the real-time blood supply for tumors, and is important in grading breast lesions [34–36]. A recent systematic review and meta-analysis including 13 studies on machine learning (ML) applied the DCE MRI images to predict axillary lymph node metastases for 1618 breast cancer patients, described a pooled diagnostic odds ratio, sensitivity, specificity, and AUC of 21.56, 0.82, 0.83, and 0.89, respectively [37]. The tumor-associated blood vessels that are activated to proliferate by angiogenic factors could have irregular or thick shapes for the breast cancer. When the contrast medium arrives at the tumor capillaries, it begins to leak into the contiguous tissue. The contrast agents will accumulate in the tumor due to this kind of leakage, which may cause different DCE-MRI signal patterns for the breast cancer. **Figure 2** shows the images of DCE MRI for the breast cancer patients.

The Tofts model following first-order kinetics was presented in 1999 [38]. This model assumes that contrast agents can be exchanged between plasma and interstitial fluid compartments of the tissue. The Tofts model could provide key parameters of tissue perfusion and permeability according to the concentration of contrast medium in the tissue over time. The transfer constant K_{trans} is the most commonly used, which represents the rate of contrast transfer from plasma to extravascular extracellular space (EES). In other words, it is the rate at which the contrast agent enters into the EES. The K_{trans} is the product of the permeability surface area and tissue blood flow, which is related to the perfusion and permeability [39]. Previous studies demonstrated that K_{trans} was connected with tumor size and microvessel density [40]. Kep represents the rate at which the contrast medium is returned from the EES to the plasma. The value of Ve is the EES volume divided by the tissue and interstitial volume, which denotes the accumulated space after the contrast agent crosses the endothelial barrier [41]. The malignant breast lesions showed significantly higher K_{trans}, Kep values compared to the benign breast lesions. K_{trans} had a negative correlation with ER expression. Kep was negatively correlated with PR expression and positively correlated with the Ki-67 index. Tumor diameter was correlated with the Kep [23]. It is noteworthy that the estimation of parameters with the Tofts model requires detailed time-intensity information over 5 minutes, which is rarely clinically feasible.

2.3 Ultrafast DCE-MRI

The ultrafast DCE-MRI (UF-DCE-MRI) of the breast proposed in 2014 is a novel method to evaluate the vascularity of breast cancer [42]. With rapid acquisition techniques (including view-sharing and compressed sensing (CS)), UF-DCE-MRI

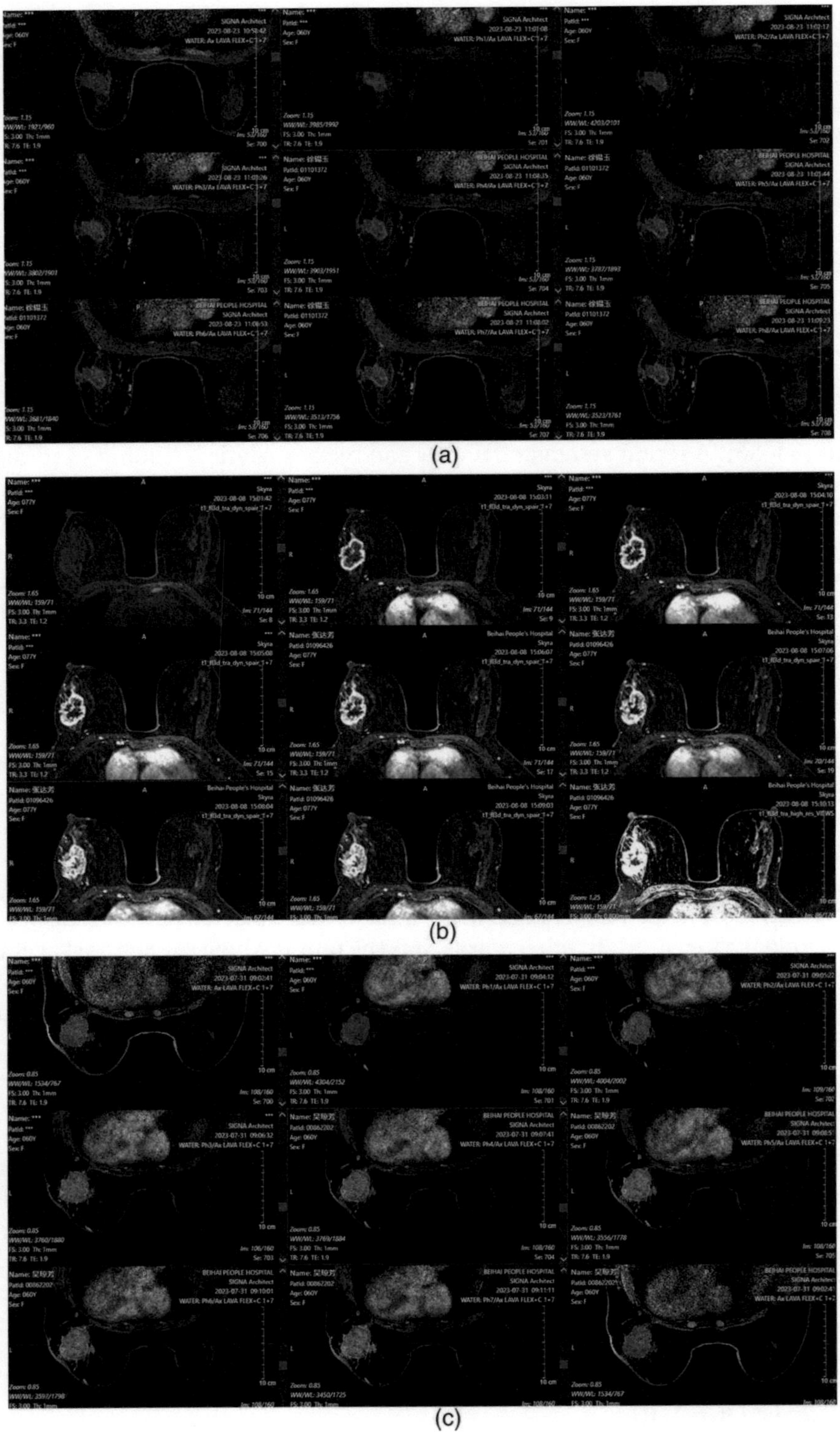

Figure 2.
The images of DCE MRI for three breast cancer patients. (a)–(c) indicate images of different time points for the first patient with left breast cancer, the second patient with right breast cancer, and the third patient with left breast cancer respectively.

focuses on the early phase after contrast application with a temporal resolution of several seconds [43, 44]. The fastest enhancing hypervascular lesions can be easily identified and differentiated from more slowly enhancing lesions with the detailed temporal resolution. Considering the enhancement of malignant breast lesions comes earlier than background parenchymal enhancement (BPE), UF-DCE MRI is especially useful for the patients with significant BPE [45, 46]. In time series reconstruction, view-sharing shares phase-encoded views from one image to the next. The centrality of k-space associated with contrast is frequently sampled to update faster. It can recover the sparse representation images by randomly undersampled k-space data using the nonlinear recovery protocol for CS technology [47]. View-sharing is more general than CS, although it may be blurred.

The kinetic parameters of UF-DCE-MRI have been widely investigated for diagnosis [12, 43, 48–50]. The kinetic parameters of UF-DCE-MRI involve the maximum slope (MS), representing the upslope steep of the time-intensity curve, and bolus arrival time (BAT) and time to enhancement (TTE), which indicate the beginning enhanced time of breast lesions. MS values of breast cancer are larger than benign lesions, while TTE and BAT are shorter. The intraclass correlation coefficients are 0.94–0.99 and 0.85–0.88 for MS and TTE, showing good inter-reader agreement for these two parameters [12, 48, 51]. These kinetic parameters show comparable diagnostic power in the differentiation of benign and malignant breast lesions with high consistency, suggesting that they may replace kinetic parameters obtained from conventional DCE-MRI with much shorter scan times (dozens of seconds after contrast agent injection) [43].

In addition to distinguishing benign and malignant breast lesions, these novel kinetic parameters are associated with receptor status, intrinsic subtypes, and other breast cancer prognostic markers. Invasive breast cancer showed larger MS and shorter TTE or BAT than cancer *in situ* [43, 50], and shorter TTE was shown to involve from upgrade in situ to aggressive cancer [52, 53]. Some studies have found that escalation to invasive cancer was significantly associated with higher MS or shorter TTE as revealed by preoperative UF-DCE MRI in patients with biopsy-confirmed ductal carcinomas *in situ* (DCIS) [52, 54]. Compared to the pure ductal carcinoma *in situ* (DCIS) group, the DCIS with invasion group had a higher nuclear grade ($P < 0.001$) and larger mean MS ($P = 0.002$) [24]. Cancers with aggressive features including high Ki-67 labeling index, large tumor diameter, or high histological or nuclear grade are joint with abundant vascularity, resulting in higher MS as well as shorter TTE and BAT [49, 50, 55, 56]. Some studies have shown a correlation between parameters derived from UF-DCE MRI and histopathological microvascular density [57, 58]. The accuracy of pathological complete response (pCR) prediction may be improved by kinetic parameters of UF-DCE MRI, and UF-DCE MRI may contribute to the accurate detection of residual invasive cancer and the potential usefulness in neoadjuvant systemic therapy (NST) [59]. Different aspects of breast cancer biology could be demonstrated by specific information of UF-DCE MRI on the early part of perfusion and blood volume [41].

2.4 Diffusion-weighted imaging

Diffusion-weighted imaging (DWI) MRI quantifies the random movement of water molecules in tissue without using an exogenous contrast agent, which is influenced by tissue microstructure and cell density [60]. Since cancer lesions produce abnormal water movement patterns, this movement is quantified for tumor visualization [61]. This quantitative water diffusion is expressed by the apparent diffusion coefficient (ADC) or ADC map. The ADC values of the breast lesions were deemed as quantitative parameters for proliferation, diagnosis, treatment response, and predicting subtypes [60]. The ADC values in malignant breast cancer are low for the limited flow of water and can distinguish normal breast tissue, benign tumors, and invasive cancer [61, 62]. The differences in ADC among invasive carcinoma, carcinoma *in situ*, and benign tumors before and after contrast were significant [63]. ADC is associated with cell density, and ADC values are lower in breast malignancies because of increased cellularity in breast malignancies. Ki-67 is a common index to reflect the cell proliferation rate, and ADC showed a higher power to predict Ki-67 level with a pooled AUC of 0.969 compared to 0.944 of DCE for breast cancer patients [64]. Although studies are limited, there is already evidence that DWI can show a distinction between benign and malignant lesions that could otherwise not be visualized using mammography or tomosynthesis. Previous studies caused a 34.5% reduction in unnecessary and invasive MRI-guided biopsy without additional negative predictive value [61]. The DWI has the potential to reduce more than 30% costs by reducing unnecessary procedures [61]. **Figure 3** illustrates the DWI images of the breast cancer patients.

More advanced models and parameters such as diffusion tensor imaging (DTI), intravoxel incoherent motion (IVIM), and diffusion kurtosis imaging (DKI) [65–68] are proposed for assessing breast cancer property. The IVIM MRI using multi-b-value signals reflects the true diffusion coefficient D, microcapillary perfusion, and blood volume fraction (f or f_{IVIM}). Lower D ($<1.5 * 10^{-3}$ m m^2/s) and higher f (about 10%) were found for malignant breast tumors compared with nonmalignant tumors [69]. D and f values were correlated with the pathological grade. Tumor diameter was correlated with the D and f values ($r = -0.278, 0.293$) [23]. Instead, the diffusion kurtosis quantifies the deviation of the Gaussian diffusion of the high b-values [66, 67]. The mean kurtosis (MK) of malignant lesions was significantly higher than that of benign lesions. The area under the curve was above 0.85 for MK. The sensitivity and specificity of MK for diagnosing malignant tumors were 83.3 and 87.0%, respectively [62]. High kurtosis values (bigger than 0.7) are usually detected for malignant breast lesions because of the increased microstructural complexity in cancer tissue. The IVIM and diffusion kurtosis can be used to differentiate malignant from benign, correlate with prognostic factors, and predict response to treatment in breast lesions [69]. Diffusion tensor imaging can detect tissue anisotropy and distinguish malignant and benign breast lesions with high sensitivity and specificity [69, 70].

Overall, the advantages of DWI are evident; however, the disadvantages precluding the use of diffusion-weighted imaging as a major form of breast cancer screening still exist. The imaging methods often require multiple b-values or multi-directional image acquisition, which may lead to longer scanning time than that of routine MRI. There is a large degree of overlap between morphological and microstructural elements in benign and malignant breast lesions, implying a similar overlap in ADC values. Thus, DWI has not a clear and consistent ADC cut-off value [71, 72]. Also, the exponential fit stability of IVIM seems not enough high because of the lower SNR of DWI images, especially for those high b-value images [18]. DWI as a supplement to MRI is considered particularly useful during surgery and may contribute to the localization of some tumors or the localization of the most aggressive points within the tumor. Standardizing and optimizing the breast DWI protocol is a key strategy with the aim of establishing a parameter range that can be universally implemented in a variety of clinical scanners [73].

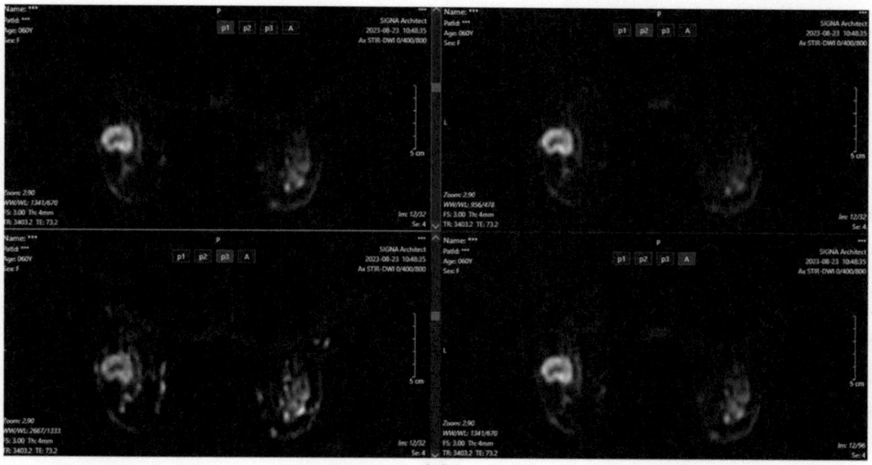

(a)

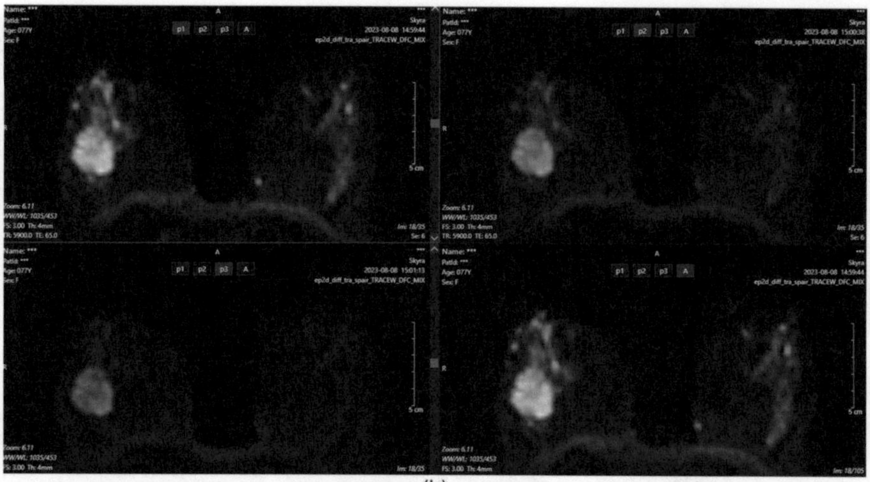

(b)

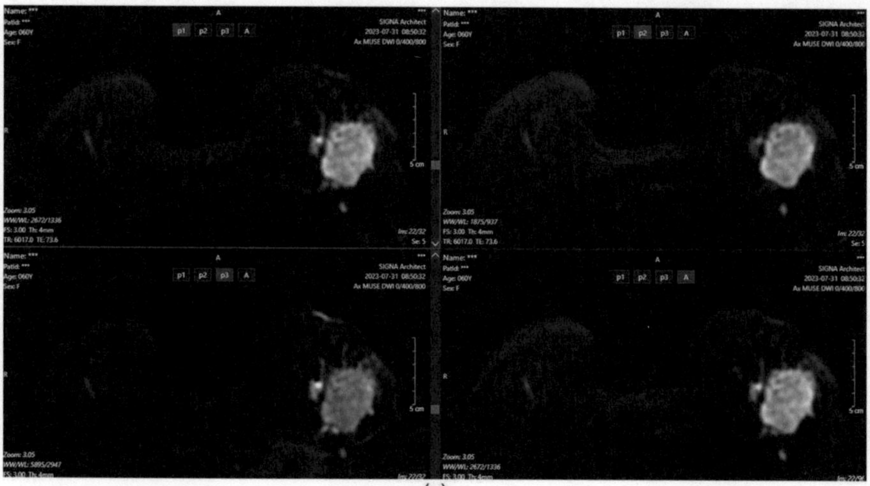

(c)

Figure 3.
The DWI images of three breast cancer patients. (a)–(c) indicate the images for the first patient with left breast cancer, the second patient with right breast cancer, and the third patient with left breast cancer respectively.

2.5 T2-weighted imaging

T2-weighted imaging (T2WI) is a routine MRI sequence that reflects the water content of the tissue. T2-weighted imaging can delineate the morphology of the lesions without fat suppression and detect the cyst easily with fat suppression. Most masses presenting high signal intensity of T2-weighted imaging are benign such as lymph nodes, fat necrosis, cysts, and apocrine metaplasia [74]. Most cancers do not display high signal intensity relevant to the parenchyma for low water content and high cellularity in T2-weighted imaging, while breast lesions including cysts, fibroadenomas, phyllodes tumors, and mucinous carcinomas have higher signal intensities on T2-weighted images [21]. Quantitative values and standard deviation of T2-weighted imaging (T2WI) after the contrast injection were valuable for the classification of benign and malignant breast lesions [75]. The texture-volume model on the high-resolution 3D T2WI effectively differentiated negative and positive lymph

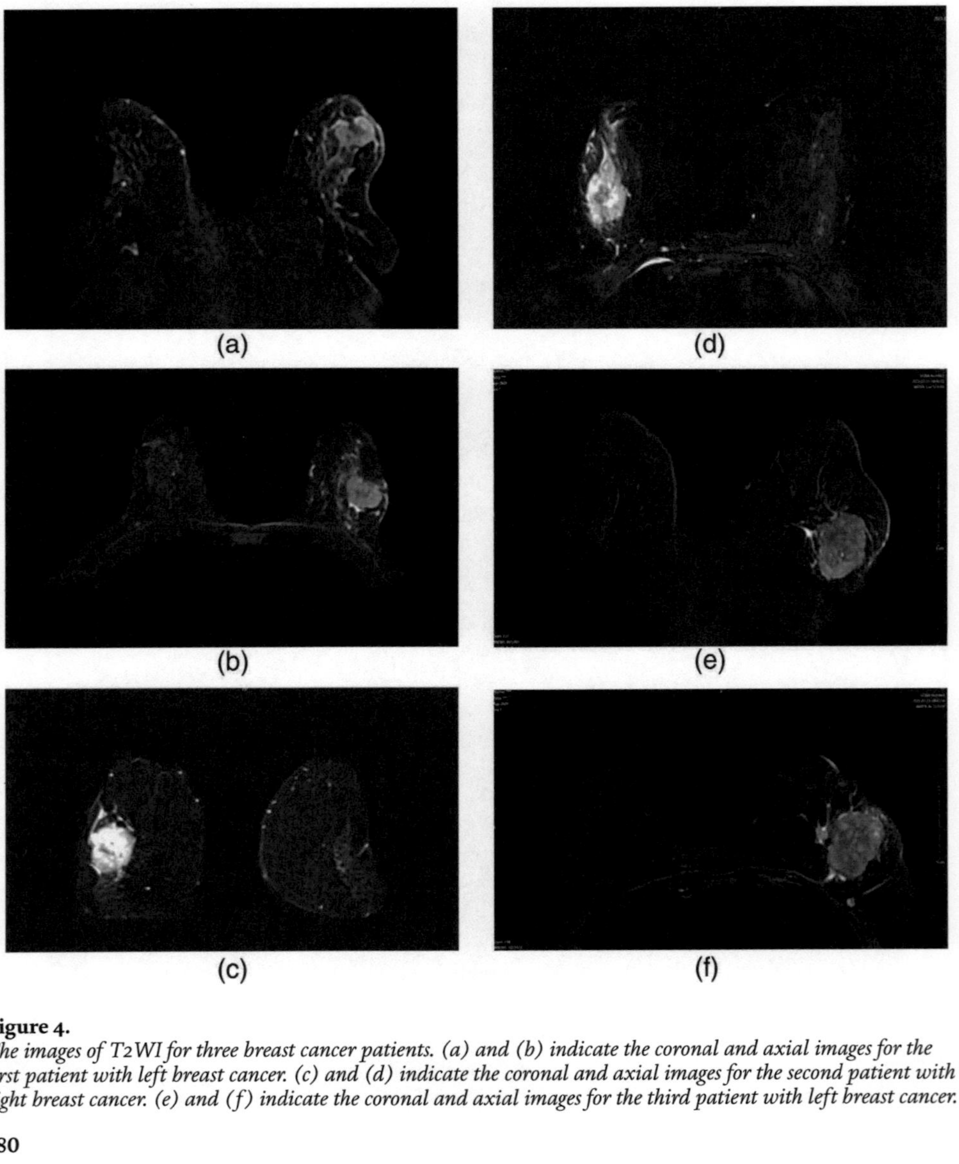

Figure 4.
The images of T2WI for three breast cancer patients. (a) and (b) indicate the coronal and axial images for the first patient with left breast cancer. (c) and (d) indicate the coronal and axial images for the second patient with right breast cancer. (e) and (f) indicate the coronal and axial images for the third patient with left breast cancer.

node (LN) metastasis for node-negative breast cancer patients. The area under the curves (AUCs) of the texture-volume model in the validation cohort was 0.8129. The positive predictive value, negative predictive value, sensitivity, specificity of the texture-volume model were 49, 96, 90, and 69% respectively [76]. Furthermore, focal breast edema shows the high signal intensity of T2-weighted MRI and has a poor prognosis and aggressive histology [77, 78]. Breast edema is divided into four grade scores: (1), no edema; (2), peritumoral edema; (3), prepectoral edema and (4), subcutaneous edema [79]. Breast edema was an independent risk factor of sentinel lymph node (SLN) metastasis according to the logistic regression analysis. The model combined with breast edema score (BES) had remarkably improved the predictive performance for SLN metastasis in contrast to the clinicopathological model alone (AUC, 0.77 vs. 0.71; $p = 0.005$). The BES also had significantly positive correlations with the histologic grade, tumor diameter, non-luminal subtypes, and Ki-67 index. A higher grade of breast edema could cause breast cancer aggressiveness and improve the risk of SLN metastasis. The BES is helpful to predict SLN metastasis in T2-weighted imaging [80]. Due to the long scan time required for T2 lonely, synthetic MRI including T1 and T2 maps in a few minutes may be helpful to obtain information on T2 [81]. **Figure 4** shows the images of T2WI for the breast cancer patients.

2.6 Proton magnetic resonance spectroscopy (^{1}H-MRS)

Proton magnetic resonance spectroscopy (^{1}H-MRS) is a noninvasive technique without radiation and has recently been studied for breast cancer diagnosis [72]. ^{1}H-MRS can decompose the chemical components of the tissue *in vivo* studies [82]. This means that the technique is able to distinguish benign from malignant lesions by detecting choline levels and choline metabolites increasing in invasive cancers owing to increased cell metabolism process rates and turnover [61]. The choline metabolite is reliable for displaying a single spectral peak. Elevated tCho in the neoplastic tissue can capture altered intracellular metabolic and become a signal for increased cellular proliferation [83]. The tCho peak becomes a marker of malignancy for it is reduced earlier before morphological changes during chemotherapy [83, 84]. A systematic review included eight eligible studies involving 632 females and 687 breast lesions indicated DWI and MRS had comparable sensitivity and specificity in differentiating benign and malignant breast lesions. The pooled specificity and sensitivity of DWI were 88 and 92%, respectively. The pooled specificity and sensitivity of MRS were 85 and 85%, respectively. No significant difference was found in the specificity and sensitivity between DWI and MRS [85]. Previous studies also found a positive predictive value of 88% for MRS [82]. In order to locate suspicious breast tissue, the ^{1}H-MRS must be paired with other imaging modalities. This imaging counterpart is almost entirely exclusive in existing studies for redundancy. Another obvious caveat of using ^{1}H-MRS is the source of false negatives because not all cancers have high levels of choline and may even be completely choline-negative. Less aggressive cancers are unlikely to have steady high spectroscopic peaks [82]. The k21 value that indicates the contrast exchange rate between extravascular and intravascular spaces could be used to minimize this shortcoming for the height of the choline peak usually corresponding to the amplitude of the k21 value [82]. However, the use of ^{1}H-MRS is limited to studies due to the need for specially designed sequences, difficulties in standardizing and quantification, common low-quality spectra, and comparatively long acquisition times [86]. The multi-parametric MRI including MRS is helpful to reduce the grade

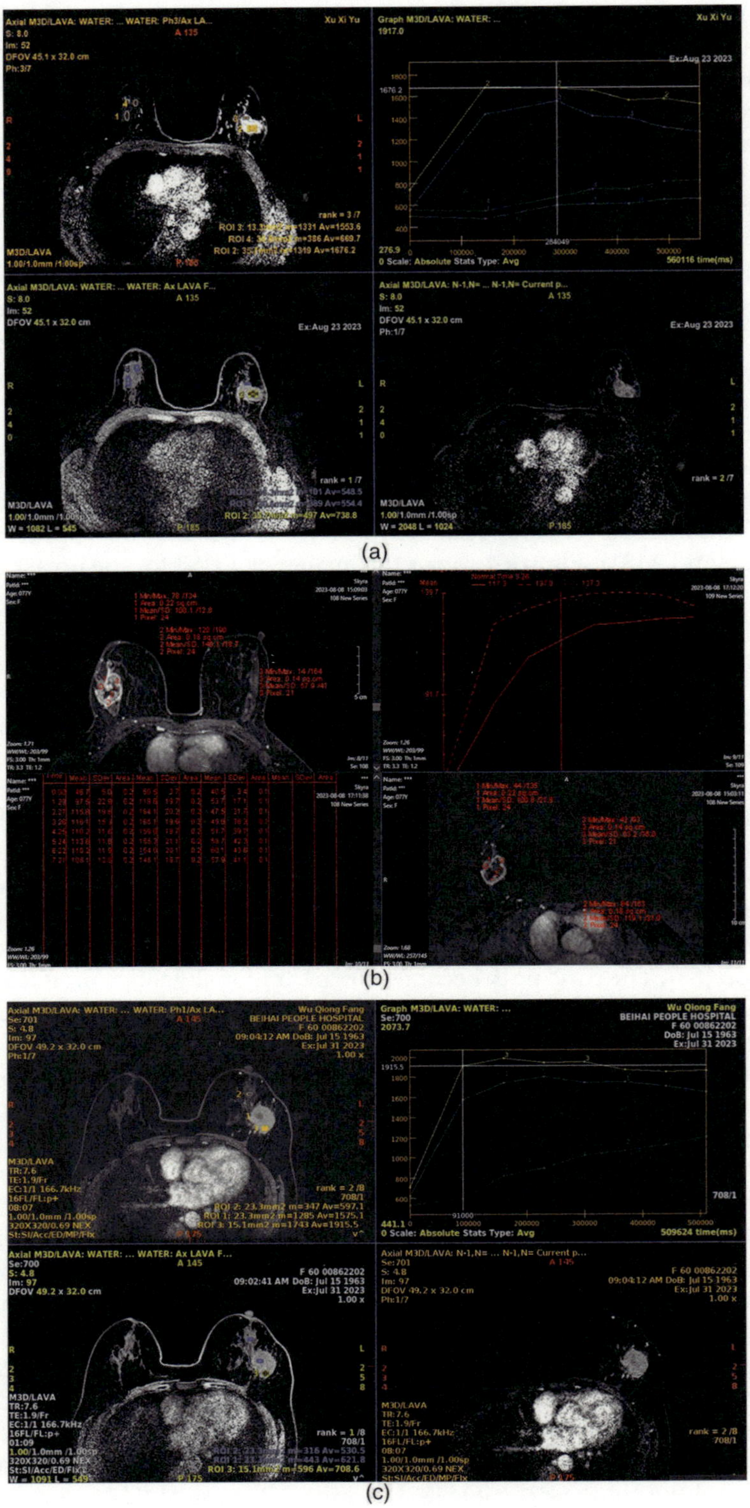

Figure 5.
The images of MRS for three breast cancer patients. (a)–(c) indicate the images for the first patient with left breast cancer, the second patient with right breast cancer, and the third patient with left breast cancer respectively.

of suspicious lesions, promote diagnostic accuracy, and grade the risk of lymph node metastasis [87, 88]. **Figure 5** shows the images of MRS for the breast cancer patients.

2.7 Magnetic resonance elastography (MRE)

Magnetic resonance elastography (MRE) acquires images of quantitative tissue stiffness by converting images of propagating shear waves into maps of shear modulus. As a nonionizing, noninvasive, cross-sectional MR imaging technique, breast MRE has provided insight into quantitative mechanical properties of breast tissue, such as elasticity, stiffness, and viscosity. These parameters of mechanical properties are beneficial for improving diagnostic performance or histological characterization for breast cancer. Previous MRE studies have investigated prognostic factors that can add diagnostic information for patient treatment including desmoplasia associated with breast cancer, stiffening of the surrounding stroma, and necrosis [27, 89]. Breast carcinomas had a high stiffness compared with surrounding benign tissues [90]. A previous study including 22 healthy volunteers demonstrated that dense breasts, including heterogeneous dense and extremely dense breasts, had a significantly higher mean stiffness value compared with fatty and scattered fibroglandular breasts [91]. A study including 50 average-risk and 86 high-risk patients with dense breasts showed significantly higher mean elasticity, stiffness, and viscosity in high-risk patients compared with those in average-risk patients. Stiffness was a significant predictor of risk status [92]. Previous study with 35 patients found higher median elasticity for malignant lesions compared to the benign lesions [93]. Malignant lesions were also found to be stiffer than fibroadenoma, fibrocystic changes, and overall breast tissue excluding the lesion [94]. Previous studies of larger patient populations have denoted more liquid-like behavior has been exhibited for the malignant lesions with more aggressive features or certain subtypes, suggesting that viscosity or frequency-dependent power-law behavior of tissue may be indicator to improve discrimination between benign and malignant lesions [95–97]. A previous study with 1380 breast cancer patients proved that cancer cell unjamming significantly increased distant metastatic risk [98]. Thus, increased fluidity associated with unjamming and measured by MRE is a good prognostic parameter for tumor progression [99]. Some studies found that the addition of MRE can increase specificity or diagnostic accuracy for breast lesion characterization [95, 97, 100]. A study with animal models demonstrated MRE could provide sensitive imaging biomarkers of tumor collagen deposition and its therapeutic modulation [101]. Considering collagen can increase tumor stuffiness, regulate tumor immunity, and promote metastases [102], MRE may be helpful to understand the pathophysiologic functions of collagen in breast cancer. The scan time and spatial resolution for MRE are still needed to be improved. More work is needed to improve the capacity of diagnostic performance, predicting the prognostic features of breast malignancy and monitoring treatment with neoadjuvant chemotherapy for MRE [103]. Research and techniques of MRE are still developing currently [89].

3. Multi-parametric approaches

In the field of breast cancer, multi-parametric imaging describes combined multiple imaging parameter patterns to overcome limitations in specificity and improve diagnosis, preoperative assessment, and treatment monitoring [104–107].

Multi-parametric MRI usually concerns combining information from different types of sequences, such as T2WI, T1WI, DWI, DCE-MRI, MRS, MRE. This combination depends on the target of the imaging and the scanning anatomical site. Multiple parameters can be quantitatively combined to build the model or data of different imaging sequences and modalities can be combined for visual evaluation. Techniques like non-rigid image registration are helpful for image shift or distortion [108].

Different parameters jointly could frequently provide complementary information and increase the cognition of breast cancer biology. A small malignancy may become noticeable on DWI with the correlation of DCE-MR images because of the lower spatial resolution of DWI. DWI with the assistance of DCE imaging could improve specificity while maintaining similar sensitivity [109]. The multi-parametric approach was initially used to identify the benign and malignant breast lesions. IVIM and DCE-MRI could differentiate benign and malignant breast lesions, and their combination showed significantly better diagnostic efficiency. The AUC values of DCE, IVIM, and DCE + IVIM were 0.828, 0.882, and 0.901 respectively [23]. A multi-parametric MRI analysis, including a total of 341 lesions (161 malignant and 180 benign), comprising MRI features (root sign, time-intensity curves, internal enhancement, margins, and presence of edema), patient age and quantitative ADC value denoted improved diagnostic performance (AUC above 0.95) and might have avoided more unnecessary biopsies in comparison with the Kaiser score (KS) [110]. Ninety-five breast cancer patients were investigated by T2WI, T1WI, DCE, DWI, and ADC multi-modality MRI. The area under the curves (AUCs) of plain scan + enhanced + diffuse for diagnosing breast cancer were 0.927 [111]. However, multi-parametric data are now also used to predict subtypes [4]. Multi-parametric MRI is superior to semantic models to effectively predict the molecular subtypes of breast cancer. SHapley Additive exPlanations (SHAP) analysis demonstrated that higher kurtosis, lower iAUC, lower kurtosis, and lower D* were particular features for luminal B, luminal A, HER2-enriched subtypes, and triple-negative breast cancer respectively [112]. A study including 198 patients investigated the effectiveness of diverse radiomics models for preoperatively differentiating lymphovascular invasion (LVI) in clinically node-negative breast cancer (BC). Radiomics features came from T1WI, T2WI, DCE, DWI, and ADC sequences. AUC value of 0.936 in the training dataset and an AUC value of 0.876 in the validation dataset were required [113]. A study including 161 patients with invasive ductal carcinoma (non-special type) of breast cancer predicted the low expression state of HER2. The area under the ROC curve (AUC) values for the verification set of positive, negative, and low HER2 expression were 0.66, 0.73, and 0.84 for the joint sequence model including DCE-T1WI and T2WI, respectively [114]. Multi-parametric MRI is used to predict the response after neoadjuvant therapy. Excellent predictions with AUC above 0.9 were obtained [115, 116], although they would be lower for an external test set [116]. The multi-parametric method may be useful to assess the status related to TME [117, 118].

The most popular imaging combinations include DCE, DWI (ADC values), and T2WI [119, 120]. A previous study including 329 female patients (138 malignant, 191 benign) found the model comprising DCE, DWI, and T2WI achieved the highest performance in the test set (AUC = 0.888) and was the optimized choice for breast lesion classification with high sensitivity (bigger than 98%) in radiomics [119]. The patients were investigated by diffusion-weighted images (DWI), T2WI, and kinetic features of dynamic contrast-enhanced (DCE) based on Breast Imaging Reporting and Data Systems. Breast cancer with high stroma had spiculated margins, lower Short Tau Inversion Recovery (STIR) signal intensity, and a heterogeneous pattern of enhancement. The margin of mass, STIR signal intensity, and enhancement pattern of breast cancer were significantly correlated with the tumor stroma ratio (TSR) [120]. Recently, deep learning and machine learning have been prevalent for better image quality or prediction models. Application of the deep learning (DL) resulted in higher average signal-to-noise ratio (SNR) (1.2–2.8 times), contrast-to-noise ratio (CNR) (1.0–1.8 times), and image sharpness (1.2–1.7 times). Overall, the DL reconstruction demonstrated improved T2-weighted image quality in clinical breast MRI [121]. The 90% accuracy on the validation set for discriminating HR +(presence of the hormone receptor) versus HR -(not presence of the hormone receptor) breast cancers was acquired by a decision tree and nine predictors on T2-weighted subtraction images. The combination of artificial intelligence techniques and radiomics analysis could be used to predict breast cancer histological outcomes [122]. An unenhanced model containing T2WI and DWI was relatively accurate compared to the model using the gadolinium agent for distinguishing between benign and malignant breast lesions. The unenhanced radiomics model also acquired favorable predictions for testing cohorts (AUCs, 0.818–0.840). There are no statistical differences between the AUCs of the unenhanced radiomics model and those of the two radiologists [123]. Furthermore, most of the multi-parametric imaging studies were retrospective. Considering the diagnosis of cancer is typically based on the history of symptoms, physical examination, and characteristic abnormalities found in MRI, the longitudinal evaluation for cancer patients is important [124]. A study including 100 patients assessed early neoadjuvant systemic therapy (NAST) response for triple-negative breast cancer (TNBC) by functional tumor volumes (FTVs) estimated from DCE MRI. FTVs at two cycles and at four cycles of NAST can potentially predict treatment response with the AUC was 0.82 and 0.84 respectively in TNBC patients [125], while the longitudinal MRI studies on breast cancer seems too few.

Quantification of multi-parametric imaging parameters can be used to describe pathophysiological and physiological processes by standardized approach. Owing to the large number of imaging features, AI techniques including feature extraction, feature selection, classifier/regression/time-to-event, and evaluation are increasingly being applied to develop machine learning (ML) algorithms for specific diagnostic targets. Integrated complementary parameters at the molecular, functional, morphological, and metabolic levels can provide important information for the disease process and tissue changes in breast cancer. The pattern recognition approaches for semiautomatic or automatic detection of target regions become more prevalent. These advances will result in the broader application of imaging features into clinical practice in the future [126].

4. Conclusions

Multi-parametric imaging including various and complementary information improves histological characterization, diagnostic performance, or prognostic prediction. T1WI detects the breast lesions according to particular-longitudinal relaxation time. The kinetic parameters of UF-DCE-MRI and DCE-MRI observe the perfusion and vascularity of the breast lesions. The parameters from advanced DWI and ADC values reflect tissue architecture, tumor cellularity, and microperfusion. The T2-weighted imaging obtains information of the tissue surrounding the breast tumor. MRS can detect choline levels and choline metabolites in the tissue. MRE provides quantitative mechanical properties of breast tissue. It is very important to understand the technical and theoretical background of these parameters and their clinical significance. Along with the increasing application of AI techniques, the precise identification, exact location, and quantitative characteristics of multi-parametric imaging will be broadly used to improve diagnosis, pathological assessment, treatment monitoring, and nursing care for the breast cancer patients.

Acknowledgements

This work is supported by the Basic Scientific Research Capacity Improvement Program for young and middle-aged college teachers in Guangxi, 2023, 2023KY1491, “Classification of skin cancer based on image fractal dimension” [107]. The images in this study are supported by Beihai people’s hospital. The authors have declared that no competing interests exist in the writing of this publication.

Author details

Yue Zhang[1,2,3]* and Ying Qian[4]

1 Department of Electronic and Information Engineering, Beihai Vocational College, Beihai Open University, Beihai, China

2 Department of Mechanical and Electrical Engineering, Beihai Vocational College, Beihai Open University, Beihai, China

3 Department of General Education, Beihai Vocational College, Beihai Open University, Beihai, China

4 Computer Teaching and Research Office, Iron Man Middle School, Daqing, China

*Address all correspondence to: zhangyue_three@163.com

References

[1] Bray F, Ferlay J, Soerjomataram I, Siegel RL, Torre LA, Jemal A. Global cancer statistics 2018: GLOBOCAN estimates of incidence and mortality worldwide for 36 cancers in 185 countries. CA: a Cancer Journal for Clinicians. 2018;**68**(6):394-424

[2] Allemani C, Weir HK, Carreira H, et al. Global surveillance of cancer survival 1995-2009: Analysis of individual data for 25,676,887 patients from 279 population-based registries in 67 countries (CONCORD-2). Lancet. 2015;**385**(9972):977-1010

[3] Dong-Man Ye MD, Hao-Tian Wang BS, Tao Y. The application of Radiomics in breast MRI: A review. Technology in Cancer Research & Treatment. 2020;**19**:1-16

[4] Kataoka M, Iima M, Miyake KK, Honda M. Multiparametric approach to breast cancer with emphasis on magnetic resonance imaging in the era of personalized breast cancer treatment. Investigative Radiology. 2024;**59**:26-37

[5] Chen B, Zhang R, Gan Y, et al. Development and clinical application of radiomics in lung cancer. Radiation Oncology. 2017;**12**(1):154-154

[6] Limkin EJ, Sun R, Dercle L, et al. Promises and challenges for the implementation of computational medical imaging (radiomics) in oncology. Annals of Oncology. 2017;**28**(6):1191-1206

[7] Zhang Y, Chen M, Man L, Lin G, Qian Y. Study on skin cancer classification based on image fractal dimension. In: 2024 International Conference on Energy and Electrical Engineering (EEE), Nanchang, China. Nanchang, China: EEE; 2024. pp. 1-3. DOI: 10.1109/EEE59956.2024.10709720. Available from: https://ieeexplore.ieee.org/document/10709720

[8] Perou CM, Sorlie T, Eisen MB, et al. Molecular portraits of human breast tumours. Nature. 2000;**406**:747-752

[9] Goldhirsch A, Wood WC, Coates AS, et al. Strategies for subtypes—Dealing with the diversity of breast cancer: Highlights of the St. Gallen international expert consensus on the primary therapy of early breast cancer 2011. Annals of Oncology. 2011;**22**:1736-1747

[10] Zhang L, Zhou XX, Liu L, et al. Comparison of dynamic contrast-enhanced MRI and non–mono-exponential model-based diffusion-weighted imaging for the prediction of prognostic biomarkers and molecular subtypes of breast cancer based on radiomics. Journal of Magnetic Resonance Imaging. 2023;**58**(5):1590-1602

[11] Szep M, Pintican R, Boca B, et al. Multiparametric MRI features of breast cancer molecular subtypes. Medicina (Kaunas, Lithuania). 2022;**58**:1716

[12] Ohashi A, Kataoka M, Iima M, et al. A multiparametric approach to predict triple-negative breast cancer including parameters derived from ultrafast dynamic contrast-enhanced MRI. European Radiology. 2023;**33**(11):8132-8141

[13] Hanahan D, Weinberg RA. Hallmarks of cancer: The next generation. Cell. 2011;**144**:646-674

[14] Romeo V, Helbich TH, Pinker K. Breast PET/MRI hybrid imaging and

targeted tracers. Journal of Magnetic Resonance Imaging. 2023;**57**:370-386

[15] Baghban R, Roshangar L, Jahanban-Esfahlan R, et al. Tumor microenvironment complexity and therapeutic implications at a glance. Cell Communication and Signaling: CCS. 2020;**18**:59

[16] Tanaka Y, Ohno T, Kadonaga T, et al. Podoplanin expression in cancer-associated fibroblasts predicts unfavorable prognosis in node-negative breast cancer patients with hormone receptor-positive/HER2-negative subtype. Breast Cancer. 2021;**28**:822-828

[17] Schaaf MB, Garg AD, Agostinis P. Defining the role of the tumor vasculature in antitumor immunity and immunotherapy. Cell Death & Disease. 2018;**9**:115

[18] Zhang Y. Editorial for "multiparametric magnetic resonance imaging of the kidneys: Effects of regional, side, and hydration variations on functional quantifications". Journal of Magnetic Resonance Imaging. 2023;**58**(1):234-235

[19] Mann RM, Cho N, Moy L. Breast MRI: State of the art. Radiology. 2019;**292**:520-536

[20] Mann RM, Kuhl CK, Kinkel K, Boetes C. Breast MRI: Guidelines from the European Society of Breast Imaging. European Radiology. 2008;**18**(7):1307-1318

[21] Sardanelli F, Boetes C, Borisch B, et al. Magnetic resonance imaging of the breast: Recommendations from the EUSOMA working group. European Journal of Cancer. 2010;**46**(8):1296-1316

[22] Newell MS, Giess CS, Argus AD, et al. ACR Practice Parameter for the Performance of Contrastenhanced Magnetic Resonance Imaging (MRI) of the Breast. Reston, VA: American College of Radiology; 2018

[23] Zhang J, Zheng Y, Li L, Wang R, Jiang W, Ai K, et al. Combination of IVIM with DCE-MRI for diagnostic and prognostic evaluation of breast cancer. Magnetic Resonance Imaging. 2024;**113**:110204

[24] Kim MY, Yoen H, Ji H, Park SJ, Kim SM, Han W, et al. Ultrafast MRI and T1 and T2 Radiomics for predicting invasive components in ductal carcinoma in situ diagnosed with percutaneous needle biopsy. Korean Journal of Radiology. 2023;**24**(12):1190-1199

[25] Flanagan FL, Murray JG, Gilligan P, Stack JP, Ennis JT. Digital subtraction in Gd-DTPA enhanced imaging of the breast. Clinical Radiology. 1995;**50**(12):848-854

[26] Cheung HS, Tse GM, Lai SY, Yeung DK. Relationship between lesion size and signal enhancement on subtraction fat-suppressed MR imaging of the breast. Magnetic Resonance Imaging. 2004;**22**(9):1259-1264

[27] Mango VL, Morris EA, David Dershaw D, et al. Abbreviated protocol for breast MRI: Are multiple sequences needed for cancer detection? European Journal of Radiology. 2015;**84**(1):65-70

[28] Kuhl CK, Schrading S, Strobel K, Schild HH, Hilgers RD, Bieling HB. Abbreviated breast magnetic resonance imaging (MRI): First postcontrast subtracted images and maximum-intensity projection-a novel approach to breast cancer screening with MRI. Journal of Clinical Oncology. 2014;**32**(22):2304-2310

[29] Leithner D, Moy L, Morris EA, Marino MA, Helbich TH, Pinker K. Abbreviated MRI of the breast: Does it provide value? Journal of Magnetic Resonance Imaging. 2019;**49**(7):e85-e100

[30] Yamamoto S, Okada Y, Yoshida N, et al. An investigation into the effect of different static magnetic fields of 1.5-T and 3.0-T MRI on the measurement of tumor diameters in breast cancer. Cureus. 2024;**16**(1):e52838

[31] Li X, Li C, Wang H, Jiang L, Chen M. Comparison of radiomics-based machine-learning classifiers for the pretreatment prediction of pathologic complete response to neoadjuvant therapy in breast cancer. PeerJ. 2024;**12**:e17683

[32] Morris EA, Comstock CE, Lee CH. ACR BI-RADS® Magnetic Resonance Imaging. Reston, VA: American College of Radiology; 2013

[33] Mann RM, Kuhl CK, Moy L. Contrast-enhanced MRI for breast cancer screening. Journal of Magnetic Resonance Imaging. 2019;**50**:377-390

[34] Chikarmane SA, Birdwell RL, Poole PS, Sippo DA, Giess CS. Characteristics, malignancy rate, and follow-up of BI-RADS category 3 lesions identified at breast MR imaging: Implications for MR image interpretation and management. Radiology. 2016;**280**(3):707-715

[35] Strobel K, Schrading S, Hansen NL, Barabasch A, Kuhl CK. Assessment of BI-RADS category 4 lesions detected with screening mammography and screening US: Utility of MR imaging. Radiology. 2015;**274**(2):343-351

[36] Mahoney MC, Gatsonis C, Hanna L, Demartini WB, Lehman C. Positive predictive value of BI-RADS MR imaging. Radiology. 2012;**264**(1):51-58

[37] Zhang J, Li L, Zhe X, Tang M, Zhang X, Lei X, et al. The diagnostic performance of machine learning-based Radiomics of DCE-MRI in predicting axillary lymph node metastasis in breast cancer: A meta-analysis. Frontiers in Oncology. 2022;**12**:1-10. DOI: 10.3389/fonc.2022.799209

[38] Tofts PS, Brix G, Buckley DL, et al. Estimating kinetic parameters from dynamic contrast-enhanced T(1)-weighted MRI of a diffusable tracer: Standardized quantities and symbols. Journal of Magnetic Resonance Imaging. 1999;**10**:223-232

[39] Sourbron SP, Buckley DL. On the scope and interpretation of the Tofts models for DCE-MRI. Magnetic Resonance in Medicine. 2011;**66**:735-745

[40] Kim SH, Lee HS, Kang BJ, et al. Dynamic contrast-enhanced MRI perfusion parameters as imaging biomarkers of angiogenesis. PLoS One. 2016;**11**:e0168632

[41] Cuenod CA, Balvay D. Perfusion and vascular permeability: Basic concepts and measurement in DCE-CT and DCE-MRI. Diagnostic and Interventional Imaging. 2013;**94**:1187-1204

[42] Mann RM, Mus RD, van Zelst J, et al. A novel approach to contrast-enhanced breast magnetic resonance imaging for screening: High-resolution ultrafast dynamic imaging. Investigative Radiology. 2014;**49**:579-585

[43] Kataoka M, Honda M, Ohashi A, et al. Ultrafast dynamic contrast-enhanced MRI of the breast: How is it used? Magnetic Resonance in Medical Sciences. 2022;**21**:83-94

[44] Kataoka M, Iima M, Miyake KK, Matsumoto Y. Multiparametric imaging of breast cancer: An update of current applications. Diagnostic and Interventional Imaging. 2022;**103**:574-583

[45] Honda M, Kataoka M, Iima M, Miyake KK, Ohashi A, Kishimoto AO, et al. Background parenchymal enhancement and its effect on lesion detectability in ultrafast dynamic contrast-enhanced MRI. European Journal of Radiology. 2020;**129**:108984

[46] Kim SY, Cho N, Choi Y, Shin SU, Kim ES, Lee SH, et al. Ultrafast dynamic contrast enhanced breast MRI: Lesion conspicuity and size assessment according to background parenchymal enhancement. Korean Journal of Radiology. 2020;**21**:561-571

[47] Lustig M, Donoho D, Pauly JM. Sparse MRI: The application of compressed sensing for rapid MR imaging. Magnetic Resonance in Medicine. 2007;**58**:1182-1195

[48] Honda M, Kataoka M, Onishi N, et al. New parameters of ultrafast dynamic contrast-enhanced breast MRI using compressed sensing. Journal of Magnetic Resonance Imaging. 2020;**51**:164-174

[49] Onishi N, Sadinski M, Hughes MC, et al. Ultrafast dynamic contrast-enhanced breast MRI may generate prognostic imaging markers of breast cancer. Breast Cancer Research. 2020;**22**:58

[50] Yamaguchi K, Nakazono T, Egashira R, et al. Maximum slope of ultrafast dynamic contrast-enhanced MRI of the breast: Comparisons with prognostic factors of breast cancer. Japanese Journal of Radiology. 2021;**39**:246-253

[51] Ohashi A, Kataoka M, Iima M, et al. A multiparametric approach to diagnosing breast lesions using diffusion-weighted imaging and ultrafast dynamic contrast-enhanced MRI. Magnetic Resonance Imaging. 2020;**71**:154-160

[52] Miceli R, Gao Y, Qian K, et al. Predicting upgrade of ductal carcinoma in situ to invasive breast cancer at surgery with ultrafast imaging. AJR. American Journal of Roentgenology. 2023;**221**:34-43

[53] Onishi N, Kataoka M, Kanao S, et al. Ultrafast dynamic contrast-enhanced MRI of the breast using compressed sensing: Breast cancer diagnosis based on separate visualization of breast arteries and veins. Journal of Magnetic Resonance Imaging. 2018;**47**:97-104

[54] Heo S, Park AY, Jung HK, Ko KH, Kim Y, Koh J. The usefulness of ultrafast MRI evaluation for predicting histologic upgrade of ductal carcinoma in situ. European Journal of Radiology. 2021;**136**:109519

[55] Ohashi A, Kataoka M, Iima M, et al. Prediction of Ki-67 expression of breast cancer with a multi-parametric model using MRI parameters from ultrafast DCE-MRI and DWI. In: Proc. SPIE 12286, 16th International Workshop on Breast Imaging (IWBI2022), 122860B (13 July 2022), Leuven, Belgium. 2022. DOI: 10.1117/12.2625747

[56] Shin SU, Cho N, Kim SY, Lee SH, Chang JM, Moon WK. Time-to-enhancement at ultrafast breast DCE-MRI: Potential imaging biomarker of tumour aggressiveness. European Radiology. 2020;**30**(7):4058-4068

[57] Mori N, Abe H, Mugikura S, et al. Ultrafast dynamic contrast-enhanced breast MRI: Kinetic curve assessment

using empirical mathematical model validated with histological microvessel density. Academic Radiology. 2019;**26**(7):e141-e149

[58] Xiao J, Rahbar H, Hippe DS, et al. Dynamic contrast-enhanced breast MRI features correlate with invasive breast cancer angiogenesis. npj Breast Cancer. 2021;7(1):42

[59] Kataoka M, Honda M, Sagawa H, Ohashi A, Sakaguchi R, Hashimoto H, et al. Ultrafast dynamic contrast-enhanced MRI of the breast: From theory to practice. Journal of Magnetic Resonance Imaging. 2024;**60**(2):401-416

[60] Iima M, Honda M, Sigmund EE, et al. Diffusion MRI of the breast: Current status and future directions. Journal of Magnetic Resonance Imaging. 2020;**52**:70-90

[61] Jochelson MS, Dershaw DD, Sung JS, et al. Bilateral contrast-enhanced dual-energy digital mammography: Feasibility and comparison with conventional digital mammography and MR imaging in women with known breast carcinoma. Radiology. 2013;**266**:743-751. DOI: 10.1148/radiol.12121084

[62] Gao Y, Wang Y, Zhang H, Li X, Han L. The outstanding diagnostic value of DKI in multimodal magnetic resonance imaging for benign and malignant breast tumors a diagnostic accuracy study. Medicine. 2023;**102**:40

[63] Li X, Ao Y, Lan M, Wang C, Zhao J, Chen H, et al. Effect of contrast agent on T2-weighted fat-suppressed imaging and diffusion-weighted imaging in the diagnosis of breast tumors. Quantitative Imaging in Medicine and Surgery. 2024;**14**(5):3655-3664

[64] Wang M, Mei T, You Ling GONG. The quality and clinical translation of radiomics studies based on MRI for predicting Ki-67 levels in patients with breast cancer. The British Journal of Radiology. 2023;**96**(1150):20230172

[65] Yamaguchi K, Nakazono T, Egashira R, et al. Diagnostic performance of diffusion tensor imaging with readout-segmented echo-planar imaging for invasive breast cancer: Correlation of ADC and FA with pathological prognostic markers. Magnetic Resonance in Medical Sciences. 2017;**16**:245-252

[66] Iima M, Yano K, Kataoka M, et al. Quantitative non-Gaussian diffusion and intravoxel incoherent motion magnetic resonance imaging: Differentiation of malignant and benign breast lesions. Investigative Radiology. 2015;**50**:205-211

[67] Honda M, Le Bihan D, Kataoka M, et al. Diffusion kurtosis imaging as a biomarker of breast cancer. BJR Open. 2023;**5**:20220038

[68] Iima M, Kataoka M, Kanao S, et al. Intravoxel incoherent motion and quantitative non-Gaussian diffusion MR imaging: Evaluation of the diagnostic and prognostic value of several markers of malignant and benign breast lesions. Radiology. 2018;**287**:432-441

[69] Iima M, Thakur S, Jerome NP, et al. IVIM and non-Gaussian DWI of the breast. Iima M, Partridge SC, Le Bihan D. Diffusion MRI of the Breast. Philadelphia, PA: Elsevier; 2023: 116-125

[70] Luo J, Hippe DS, Rahbar H, et al. Diffusion tensori maging for characterizing tumor microstructure and improving diagnostic performance on breast MRI: A prospective observational study. Breast Cancer Research. 2019;**21**:102

[71] Sorin V, Sklair-Levy M. Dual-energy contrast-enhanced spectral

mammography (CESM) for breast cancer screening. Quantitative Imaging in Medicine and Surgery. 2019;**9**:1914-1917. DOI: 10.21037/qims.2019.10.13

[72] Grigoryants NF, Sass S, Alexander J. Novel Technologies in Breast Imaging: A scoping review. Cureus. 2023;**15**(8):e44061

[73] Malyarenko D, Wilmes LJ, Chenevert TL. Multiplatform standardization of breast DWI protocols: Quality control and test objects. Iima M, Partridge SC, Le Bihan D. Diffusion MRI of the Breast. Philadelphia, PA: Elsevier; 2022: 220-243

[74] Westra C, Dialani V, Mehta TS, Eisenberg RL. Using T2-weighted sequences to more accurately characterize breast masses seen on MRI. AJR. American Journal of Roentgenology. 2014;**202**(3):W183-W190

[75] Li X, Fan Z, Jiang H, Niu J, Bian W, Wang C, et al. Synthetic MRI in breast cancer: Differentiating benign from malignant lesions and predicting immunohistochemical expression status. Scientific Reports. 2023;**13**(1):17978

[76] Shimizu H, Mori N, Mugikura S, Maekawa Y, Miyashita M, Nagasaka T, et al. Application of texture and volume model analysis to dedicated axillary high-resolution 3D T2-weighted MR imaging: A novel method for diagnosing lymph node metastasis in patients with clinically node-negative breast cancer. Magnetic Resonance in Medical Sciences. 2024;**23**(2):161-170

[77] Uematsu T. Focal breast edema associated with malignancy on T2-weighted images of breast MRI: Peritumoral edema, prepectoral edema, and subcutaneous edema. Breast Cancer. 2015;**22**:66-70

[78] Bae MS, Shin SU, Ryu HS, et al. Pretreatment MR imaging features of triple-negative breast cancer: Association with response to neoadjuvant chemotherapy and recurrence-free survival. Radiology. 2016;**281**:392-400

[79] Harada TL, Uematsu T, Nakashima K, et al. Evaluation of breast edema findings at T2-weighted breast MRI is useful for diagnosing occult inflammatory breast cancer and can predict prognosis after neoadjuvant chemotherapy. Radiology. 2021;**299**:53-62

[80] Xie S, Tang W, Zhang C, Wang J, Wang M, Zhou Y. Classification of breast edema on T2-weighted imaging for predicting sentinel lymph node metastasis and biological behavior in breast cancer. Clinical Radiology. 2024;**79**(8):e1003-e1009. DOI: 10.1016/j.crad.2024.04.014. Epub 2024 Apr 27

[81] Meng T, He N, He H, et al. The diagnostic performance of quantitative mapping in breast cancer patients: A preliminary study using synthetic MRI. Cancer Imaging. 2020;**20**:88

[82] Geraghty P, van den Bosch M, Spielman DM, et al. MRI and (1)H MRS of the breast: Presence of a choline peak as malignancy marker is related to K21 value of the tumor in patients with invasive ductal carcinoma. The Breast Journal. 2008;**14**:574-580

[83] Bolan PJ, Nelson MT, Yee D, et al. Imaging in breast cancer: Magnetic resonance spectroscopy. Breast Cancer Research. 2005;7:149-152

[84] Tozaki M, Sakamoto M, Oyama Y, et al. Predicting pathological response to neoadjuvant chemotherapy in breast cancer with quantitative ^{1}H MR spectroscopy using the external standard method. Journal of Magnetic Resonance Imaging. 2010;**31**:895-902

[85] Billy CA, Darmiati S, Prihartono J. Diagnostic accuracy of diffusion weighted imaging compared to magnetic resonance spectroscopy in differentiation of benign and malignant breast lesions: A systematic review and meta-analysis. European Journal of Radiology. 2023;**168**:111124

[86] Sardanelli F, Carbonaro LA, Montemezzi S, et al. Clinical breast MR using MRS or DWI: Who is the winner? Frontiers in Oncology. 2016;**6**:217

[87] Pinker K, Bogner W, Baltzer P, et al. Improved diagnostic accuracy with multiparametric magnetic resonance imaging of the breast using dynamic contrast-enhanced magnetic resonance imaging, diffusion-weighted imaging, and 3-dimensional proton magnetic resonance spectroscopic imaging. Investigative Radiology. 2014;**49**:421-430

[88] Sodano C, Clauser P, Dietzel M, et al. Clinical relevance of total choline (tCho) quantification in suspicious lesions on multiparametric breast MRI. European Radiology. 2020;**30**:3371-3382

[89] Harvey SC, Di Carlo PA, Lee B, Obadina E, Sippo D, Mullen L. An abbreviated protocol for high-risk screening breast MRI saves time and resources. Journal of the American College of Radiology. 2016;**13**(11):R74-R80

[90] Sarvazyan AP, Skovoroda AR, Emelianov SY, et al. Biophysical bases of elasticity imaging. In: Jones JP, editor. Acoustical Imaging. Boston, MA: Springer US; 1995. pp. 223-240

[91] Hawley JR, Kalra P, Mo X, Raterman B, Yee LD, Kolipaka A. Quantification of breast stiffness using MR elastography at 3 tesla with a soft sternal driver: A reproducibility study. Journal of Magnetic Resonance Imaging. 2017;**45**:1379-1384

[92] Patel BK, Pepin K, Brandt KR, Mazza GL, Pockaj BA, Chen J, et al. Association of breast cancer risk, density, and stiffness: Global tissue stiffness on breast MR elastography (MRE). Breast Cancer Research and Treatment. 2022;**194**(1):79-89

[93] Lorenzen J, Sinkus R, Lorenzen M, et al. MR elastography of the breast: Preliminary clinical results. Rofo. 2002;**174**:830-834

[94] Xydeas T, Siegmann K, Sinkus R, Krainick-Strobel U, Miller S, Claussen CD. Magnetic resonance elastography of the breast: Correlation of signal intensity data with viscoelastic properties. Investigative Radiology. 2005;**40**:412-420

[95] Sinkus R, Siegmann K, Xydeas T, Tanter M, Claussen C, Fink M. MR elastography of breast lesions: Understanding the solid/liquid duality can improve the specificity of contrast-enhanced MR mammography. Magnetic Resonance in Medicine. 2007;**58**:1135-1144

[96] Bohte AE, Nelissen JL, Runge JH, et al. Breast magnetic resonance elastography: A review of clinical work and future perspectives. NMR in Biomedicine. 2018;**31**:e3932

[97] Siegmann KC, Xydeas T, Sinkus R, Kraemer B, Vogel U, Claussen CD. Diagnostic value of MR elastography in addition to contrast-enhanced MR imaging of the breast-initial clinical results. European Radiology. 2010;**20**:318-325

[98] Gottheil P, Lippoldt J, Grosser S, Renner F, Saibah M, Tschodu D, et al. State of cell unjamming correlates with distant metastasis in cancer patients. Physical Review X. 2023;**13**(3):031003

[99] Sauer F, Grosser S, Shahryari M, Hayn A, Guo J, Braun J, et al. Changes in tissue fluidity predict tumor aggressiveness In vivo. Advancement of Science. 2023;**10**:2303523

[100] Balleyguier C, Ben Lakhdar A, Dunant A, Mathieu MC, Delaloge S, Sinkus R. Value of whole breast magnetic resonance elastography added to MRI for lesion characterization. NMR in Biomedicine. 2018;**31**:e3795

[101] Li J, Zormpas-Petridis K, Boult JKR, Reeves EL, Heindl A, Vinci M, et al. Investigating the contribution of collagen to the tumor biomechanical phenotype with noninvasive magnetic resonance Elastography. Cancer Research. 2019;**79**(22):5874-5883

[102] Xu S, Xu H, Wang W, et al. The role of collagen in cancer: From bench to bedside. Journal of Translational Medicine. 2019;**17**:309

[103] Patel BK, Samreen N, Zhou Y, Chen J, Brandt K, Ehman R, et al. MR Elastography of the breast: Evolution of technique, case examples, and future directions. Clinical Breast Cancer. 2021;**21**(1):e102-e111

[104] Marino MA, Helbich T, Baltzer P, Pinker-Domenig K. Multiparametric MRI of the breast: A review. Journal of Magnetic Resonance Imaging. 2018;**47**(2):301-315

[105] Pinker K, Helbich TH, Morris EA. The potential of multiparametric MRI of the breast. The British Journal of Radiology. 2017;**90**(1069):20160715

[106] Zhu CR, Chen KY, Li P, Xia ZY, Wang B. Accuracy of multiparametric MRI in distinguishing the breast malignant lesions from benign lesions: A meta-analysis. Acta Radiologica. 2021;**62**(10):1290-1297

[107] Zhang Y. Editorial for "effect of physical exercise on MRI-assessed brain perfusion in chemotherapy-treated breast cancer patients: A randomized controlled trial". Journal of Magnetic Resonance Imaging. 2024;**59**(5):1681-1682

[108] Takatsu Y, Sagawa H, Nakamura M, et al. Novel distortion correction method for diffusion-weighted imaging based on non-rigid image registration between low b value image and anatomical image. Magnetic Resonance Imaging. 2019;**57**:277-284

[109] Yadav P, Chauhan S. Effectivity of combined diffusion-weighted imaging and contrast-enhanced MRI in malignant and benign breast lesions. Polish Journal of Radiology. 2018;**83**:e82-e93

[110] Meng L, Zhao X, Guo J, Lin L, Cheng M, Xing Q, et al. Improved differential diagnosis based on BI-RADS descriptors and apparent diffusion coefficient for breast lesions: A multiparametric MRI analysis as compared to Kaiser score. Academic Radiology. 2023;**30**(Suppl. 2):S93-S103

[111] Zhang Z, Lan H, Zhao S. Analysis of the value of quantitative features in multimodal MRI images to construct a radio-omics model for breast cancer diagnosis. Breast Cancer: Targets and Therapy. 2024;**16**:305-318

[112] Huang Y, Wang X, Cao Y, Li M, Li L, Chen H, et al. Multiparametric MRI model to predict molecular subtypes of breast cancer using Shapley additive explanations interpretability analysis. Diagnostic and Interventional Imaging. 2024;**105**(5):191-205

[113] Jiang Y, Zeng Y, Zuo Z, Yang X, Liu H, Zhou Y, et al. Leveraging multimodal MRI-based radiomics analysis with diverse machine learning models to evaluate lymphovascular

invasion in clinically node-negative breast cancer. Heliyon. 2024;**10**:e23916

[114] Li H, Hou Y, Xue L-Y, Fan W-L, Gao B-L, Yin X-P. Use of MRI Radiomics models in evaluating the low HER2 expression in breast cancer. Current Medical Imaging. 2024;**20**:e15734056234429

[115] Fan M, Wu X, Yu J, et al. Multiparametric MRI radiomics fusion for predicting the response and shrinkage pattern to neoadjuvant chemotherapy in breast cancer. Frontiers in Oncology. 2023;**13**:1057841

[116] Zhou Z, Adrada BE, Candelaria RP, et al. Prediction of pathologic complete response to neoadjuvant systemic therapy in triple negative breast cancer using deep learning on multiparametric MRI. Scientific Reports. 2023;**13**:1171

[117] Yamaguchi K, Hara Y, Kitano I, et al. Relationship between MRI findings and invasive breast cancer with podoplanin-positive cancer-associated fibroblasts. Breast Cancer. 2021;**28**:572-580

[118] Bian T, Wu Z, Lin Q, et al. Evaluating tumor-infiltrating lymphocytes in breast cancer using preoperative MRI-based radiomics. Journal of Magnetic Resonance Imaging. 2022;**55**:772-784

[119] Wang G, Guo Q, Shi D, Zhai H, Luo W, Zhang H, et al. Clinical breast MRI-based Radiomics for distinguishing benign and malignant lesions: An analysis of sequences and enhanced phases. Journal of Magnetic Resonance Imaging. 2024;**60**(3):1178-1189

[120] Mumin NA, Hamid MTR, Hamid SA, Chiew S-F, Saman MSA, Rahmat K. Magnetic resonance imaging features of invasive breast cancer association with the tumour stromal ratio. PLoS One. 2023;**18**(8):e0290772

[121] Allen TJ, Henze Bancroft LC, Unal O, Estkowski LD, Cashen TA, Korosec F, et al. Evaluation of a deep learning reconstruction for high-quality T2-weighted breast magnetic resonance imaging. Tomography. 2023;**9**(5):1949-1964

[122] Petrillo A, Fusco R, Barretta ML, Granata V, Raso MM, Porto A, et al. Radiomics and artificial intelligence analysis by T2-weighted imaging and dynamic contrast-enhanced magnetic resonance imaging to predict breast cancer histological outcome. La Radiologia Medica. 2023;**128**(11):1347-1371

[123] Liu Y, Jia X, Zhao J, Peng Y, Yao X, Xuege H, et al. A machine learning-based unenhanced Radiomics approach to distinguishing between benign and malignant breast lesions using T2-weighted and diffusion-weighted MRI. Journal of Magnetic Resonance Imaging. 2024;**60**(2):600-612

[124] Zhang Y. Editorial for longitudinal multi-parametric quantitative MRI evaluation of acute and chronic multiple sclerosis paramagnetic rim lesions. Journal of Magnetic Resonance Imaging. 2024. DOI: 10.1002/jmri.29585. Online ahead of print. Available from: https://pubmed.ncbi.nlm.nih.gov/39269287/

[125] Panthi B, Adrada BE, Candelaria RP, et al. Assessment of response to Neoadjuvant systemic treatment in triple-negative breast cancer using functional tumor volumes from longitudinal dynamic contrast-enhanced MRI. Cancers (Basel). 2023;**15**(4):1025

[126] Bäuerle T, Dietzel M, Pinker K, Bonekamp D, Zhang KS, Schlemmer H-P, et al. Identification of impactful imaging biomarker: Clinical applications for breast and prostate carcinoma. Fortschr Röntgenstr. 2024;**196**:354-362

Chapter 10

BCNet: A Novel Deep Learning Model for Enhanced Breast Cancer Classification Using Histopathological Images

Mikiyas Amare Getu, Chao Lu, Yumeng Liu, Anam Mehmood, Zoya Iqbal and Xianbin Zhang

Abstract

Breast cancer is the most commonly diagnosed cancer among women and a leading cause of cancer-related deaths globally, necessitating accurate and timely diagnosis for effective treatment. Histopathological examination of breast tissue samples is the gold standard for diagnosing breast cancer, but this process is subjective, time-consuming, and reliant on the level of the pathologist's expertise. This study introduces a new deep learning model, Breast Cancer Network (BCNet), specifically designed to detect and classify breast cancer. BCNet, a 22-layer convolutional neural network (CNN), aims to enhance diagnostic accuracy by capturing high-level discriminative features tailored to breast tissue images. The BCNet model was evaluated against established CNN models, demonstrating superior performance, achieving an accuracy of up to 99.8% for binary classification and 99.6% for multi-class classification at different magnifications. These results highlight BCNet's robustness and potential to reduce diagnostic errors and assist pathologists. Future research should explore the generalizability of BCNet across larger datasets and its integration into clinical workflows to provide real-time, AI-assisted diagnostic support.

Keywords: breast cancer, BCNet, convolutional neural network, deep learning, histopathological images

1. Introduction

Breast cancer ranked as the second leading cause of global cancer incidence in 2022, with an estimated 2.3 million new cases, accounting for 11.6% of all cancer cases. Among women, breast cancer is the most commonly diagnosed cancer and remains the leading cause of cancer-related deaths globally [1]. This emphasizes a critical need for accurate and timely diagnosis to ensure effective treatment and improved patient outcomes.

Histopathological analysis of breast tissue samples remains the gold standard for diagnosing breast cancer. This method involves the microscopic examination of tissue lesions through tissue sections stained with hematoxylin and eosin to distinguish between benign and malignant tumors [2]. However, the accuracy of this model heavily depends on the expertise of pathologists, making it subject to variability, potential diagnostic errors, and time-consuming procedures [3]. Additionally, there is a global shortage of experienced histopathologists, particularly in underdeveloped countries and small hospitals [4]. The diagnosis by histopathologists is inherently subjective, lacking an objective evaluation basis. Therefore, there is an urgent need for an efficient and objective breast cancer diagnostic method to alleviate the workload of histopathologists [5].

Advancements in artificial intelligence, particularly deep learning, offer a promising solution by providing accurate and consistent diagnostic tools, potentially transforming breast cancer diagnosis [6]. Convolutional Neural Networks (CNNs), a class of deep learning models, have demonstrated exceptional performance in various image classification tasks, including medical image analysis [7]. Using CNNs for breast cancer detection and classification can potentially reduce diagnostic errors, expedite the diagnostic process, and assist pathologists by providing reliable second opinions [8].

Several studies have compared different CNN models for classifying benign and malignant breast cancer images. For example, one study compared models such as VGG16, VGG19, InceptionV3, and ResNet50 [9]. Another study combined a CNN model with Long Short-Term Memory (LSTM) networks to classify benign and malignant tumors [10]. Additional research has adapted the InceptionV3 and Inception_ResNetV2 architectures to address both binary and multi-class breast cancer classification issues [11]. Furthermore, a study on breast cancer detection and classification using pre-trained models, including Xception, InceptionV3, ResNet50, VGG16, and MobileNet, along with a proposed model called BCCNN, found that BCCNN achieved the highest accuracy [12]. However, these studies have primarily relied on pre-trained models through transfer learning. While transfer learning leverages the power of existing state-of-the-art CNNs, it often faces limitations such as the dependency on the source domain's features, which may not capture the intricate patterns of histopathological images [13]. These models may also suffer from decreased performance due to domain mismatch and the risk of overfitting when fine-tuned on relatively small histopathological datasets [14].

In this study, we aim to develop a new deep learning CNN model called BCNet (Breast Cancer Network) specifically designed to detect and classify breast cancer using histopathological images from the Breast Cancer Histopathological Image Classification (BreakHis) dataset [15]. BCNet addresses the limitations of pre-trained models by incorporating architecture and training strategies tailored to the unique characteristics of breast tissue images, potentially enhancing accuracy. Although BCNet shares foundational components with pre-existing CNN models, it introduces a novelty that optimizes it specifically for breast cancer histopathology. BCNet includes custom feature extraction layers designed to capture the unique features and morphology of breast tissue images, which differentiates it from models like ResNet [16] and VGG [17] which are designed for general-purpose image classification. Additionally, BCNet integrates domain-specific modifications such as customized layers, batch normalization, and dropout techniques tailored to unique requirements for breast tissue images.

The novelty of BCNet's model lies in focusing on domain-specific features rather than a generalized CNN architecture. Unlike general CNN models like DenseNet [18] or ResNet [16], BCNet includes domain-specific optimizations such as tailored magnification handling and advanced data augmentation techniques to enhance its ability to capture fine-grained histological features, improving its diagnostic accuracy. Furthermore, BCNet is specially designed to address the challenges of breast cancer histopathology, such as the variety of image magnifications, including 40X, 100X, 200X, and 400X, and class imbalances between benign and malignant samples [15].

Our proposed BCNet model aimed to enhance the diagnostic accuracy of histopathological image classification by learning complex patterns within the images. We compared the performance of BCNet with existing state-of-the-art CNN models, including VGGNet [17], AlexNet [19], DenseNet [18], and ResNet [16], to demonstrate its effectiveness and superiority in breast cancer diagnosis. Through the use of CNN, we aim to address the challenges in breast cancer histopathology, ultimately contributing to improved diagnostic precision and patient care.

2. Methods

Figure 1 illustrates the process of inputting data for both binary and multi-class classification, combining the features from these classifications, pre-processing, BCNet model development, and the comparison of its performance with existing models.

2.1 Dataset

The Breast Cancer Histopathological Image Classification (BreakHis) is a large-scale dataset composed of 7909 microscopic images of breast tumor tissue collected from 82 patients. BreaKHis is divided into benign and malignant breast tumors with

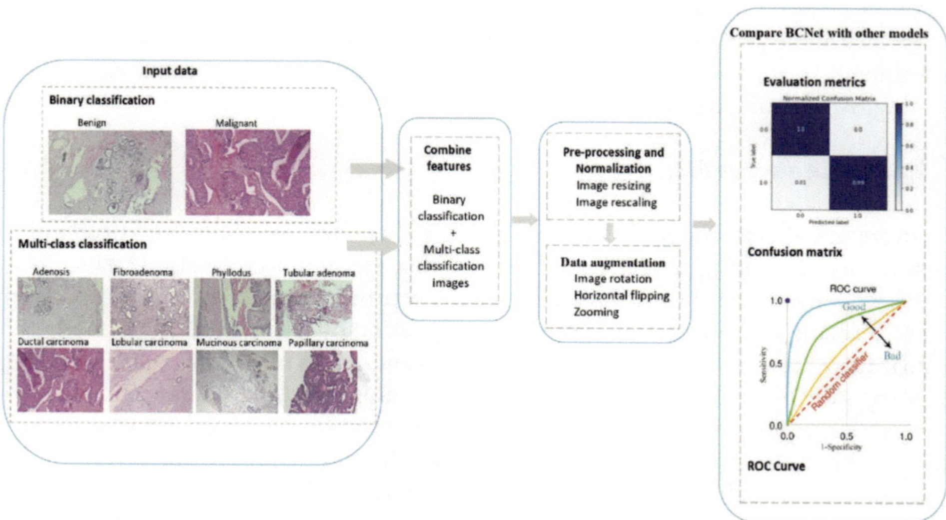

Figure 1.
Study flow.

Tumor subtypes		Magnification factors			
	Number of patients	40x	100x	200x	400x
Benign					
Adenosis	4	114	113	111	106
Fibroadenoma	10	253	260	264	237
Tubular adenoma	3	109	121	108	115
Phyllodes adenoma	7	149	150	140	130
Malignant					
Ductal carcinoma	38	864	903	896	788
Lobular carcinoma	5	156	170	163	137
Mucinous carcinoma	9	205	222	196	169
Papillary carcinoma	6	145	142	135	138
Total	82	1995	2081	2013	1820

Table 1.
Benign and malignant tumor classification with respect to magnification factors.

four magnification factors: 40X, 100X, 200X, and 400X. Both benign and malignant breast tumors are classified into distinct subtypes. The benign breast tumor is classified into adenosis, fibroadenoma, phyllodes tumor, and tubular adenoma. Whereas the malignant breast tumor is classified into ductal carcinoma, lobular carcinoma, mucinous carcinoma, and papillary carcinoma. The classification and size of the BreakHis is described in **Table 1**. The dataset used in this study was published by Spanhol et al. [20] and it can be accessed through the following link https://web.inf.ufpr.br/vri/databases/breast-cancer-histopathological-database-breakhis/.

2.1.1 Splitting dataset

To ensure the generalizability of the experimental outcomes in the classification assignment, the datasets with four magnification levels were randomly divided into training, validation, and testing sets at a ratio of 0.7:0.15:0.15.

2.2 Image pre-processing

Image pre-processing plays a crucial role in enhancing the quality and utility of breast cancer histology images for subsequent analysis and classification tasks. The pre-processing steps typically involve several key procedures aimed at standardizing and optimizing the images for accurate interpretation by machine learning models. It significantly affects the detection and classification results of breast cancer. Firstly, the images are resized to 256*256 pixels to ensure uniformity in dimensions, facilitating efficient processing and comparison across samples. This step is particularly important because the images were captured at different magnification levels.

Secondly, normalization techniques such as rescaling 1./255 were applied to adjust the intensity values across the images. This process enhances the contrast and visibility of important features within the tissue samples, aiding in the detection of relevant patterns by classification algorithms. Additionally, color normalization was done based on RGB channels to standardize the color distribution across images, reducing variability due to differences in staining protocols or imaging conditions. This step ensures consistency in the appearance of tissue features, facilitating more robust and reliable classification outcomes.

2.3 Data augmentation

To address issues such as overfitting and imbalanced class distributions, we performed data augmentation techniques on the dataset. This was achieved using the ImageDataGenerator function within Keras, allowing us to apply image rotations of up to ±20 degrees, horizontal flipping, as well as shifts in width and height (set at 0.2), shearing (0.2), and zooming (0.2). The classes within the breast tumor dataset exhibited an imbalance, particularly with a significant number of ductal carcinoma instances in malignant tumors and fibroadenoma instances in benign tumors, resulting in a Gaussian distribution pattern [21]. We implemented an oversampling method using the aforementioned data augmentation strategies to balance the number of images across each class of breast cancer histopathology.

2.4 Breast cancer network (BCNet) model development

Breast Cancer Network (BCNet) is a proposed model consisting of 22 layers with an input shape of (256 x 256 x 3). BCNet is a newly developed CNN model for detecting and classifying breast cancer. The output of the model is classified into 8 classes, which include adenosis, fibroadenoma, phyllodes tumor, tubular adenoma, ductal carcinoma, lobular carcinoma, mucinous carcinoma, and papillary carcinoma. The proposed model contains input, convolutional, pooling, and dense layers, and a fully connected layer including a SoftMax activation function.

2.4.1 BCNet model architecture and training parameters

Table 2 summarizes the architecture and parameters of our newly developed deep learning model for classifying benign and malignant subtypes of breast cancer histopathology images. The input layer of the model processes images with dimensions of 256 x 256 x 3, accommodating the RGB channels. The model employs a Conv2D layer with 32 filters of size 3x3 for feature extraction. This is helpful for capturing fine-grained details in histopathological images for identifying different cancer subtypes. A filter size of 3*3 facilitates the model learning process. Following the convolutional layer, a MaxPooling2D layer with a 2x2 pool size is used to reduce the spatial dimensions of the feature maps [7, 22]. MaxPooling is important in the downsampling of the feature maps, reducing the number of parameters and computation to retain important tumor features. Batch normalization is applied to stabilize and accelerate the training process, particularly in complex tasks such as histopathological analysis. The Rectified Linear Unit (ReLU) activation function [23] is used to introduce non-linearity, allowing the model to learn complex representations. The model is trained using the categorical cross-entropy loss function, suitable for multi-class classification tasks.

The architecture includes a batch size of 32 and a SoftMax activation function in the output layer to classify the images into one of the eight predefined classes. The SoftMax function converts raw model predictions into probabilities, which improves model interpretability. The Adam optimizer, with a learning rate of 0.001, is employed to adjust the weights during training. A dropout rate of 0.5 is incorporated

Model parameters	Values
Input layer	256 x 256 x 3
Channels	3(RGB)
Convolutional	Conv2D (32 (3, 3))
Pooling	Maxpooling2D (2, 2)
Batch Normalization	Yes
Activation	ReLU
Loss	Categorical_crossentropy
Batch size	32
Activation function	SoftMax
Class	8
Optimizer	Adam
Learning rate	0.001
Drop out	0.5
Metrics	Accuracy
Number of epochs	20

Table 2.
Parameters and hyperparameters used for BCNet model development.

to prevent overfitting by randomly dropping neurons during training. This dropout technique helps to ensure that the model is not dependent on a single neuron, which might affect the generalizability of the model to new data, which is particularly useful for clinical applications where the consequence of overfitting is significant. The model's performance is evaluated using accuracy as the primary metric, and training is conducted over 20 epochs to ensure sufficient learning while avoiding the risk of overfitting. This configuration aims to achieve a robust and accurate classification of breast cancer histopathology images.

This model has a complex architecture used to learn the intricate or complex patterns of the histology images, and it has approximately 6.7×10^7 parameters.

BCNet was a deep learning CNN model used to perform binary and multi-class classification of histopathological images of breast cancer.

2.5 Model performance evaluation metrics

Evaluation metrics play a crucial role in assessing the performance of deep learning models, particularly in the context of medical image analysis such as breast cancer detection [24]. The following evaluation metrics include accuracy [24, 25]; recall (sensitivity), specificity [26, 27]; precision [28–30]; ROC, and area under the curve (AUC) [31].

2.5.1 Confusion matrix

A confusion matrix is a valuable tool used to evaluate the performance of a classification model by comparing the predicted and actual class labels of a dataset.

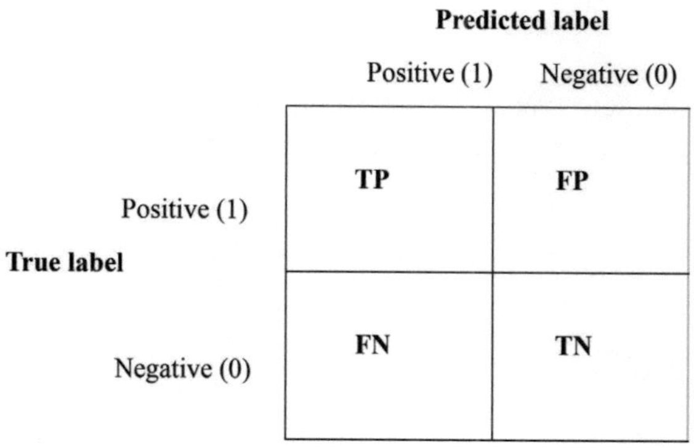

Figure 2.
Confusion matrix for classification report.

It provides a clear summary of true positives (TP), true negatives (TN), false positives (FP), and false negatives (FN) predicted by the model. **Figure 2** illustrates a sample confusion matrix, presenting predictions based on their accuracy. This matrix serves as a basis for calculating metrics like ROC curve, recall, specificity, accuracy, and others, offering insights into the model's classification capabilities [31].

2.5.2 Accuracy

Accuracy measures how much the model correctly predicts the outcome.

$$Accuracy = \frac{TP + FP}{TP + FN + FP + TN}$$

2.5.3 Precision

Precision is an evaluation metric that quantifies the ratio of correctly predicted positive cases to all predicted positive cases, emphasizing the model's ability to avoid false positives.

$$Precision = \frac{TP}{TP + FP}$$

2.5.4 Sensitivity

Sensitivity, also referred to as true positive rate (TPR), is a performance metric in classification that gauges the model's accuracy in identifying positive cases correctly. It is calculated as the ratio of true positives (P1) to the total of actual positive cases (P1 + N1), represented as a percentage or a decimal ranging from 0 to 1. Sensitivity is mathematically expressed as:

$$Sensitivity = \frac{TP}{TP + TN}$$

2.5.5 Specificity

Specificity complements recall by measuring the model's ability to correctly identify negative cases out of all actual negative cases.

$$Specificity = \frac{TN}{TN + FP}$$

2.5.6 ROC curve and AUC

The ROC curve serves as a visual representation of a binary classification (benign and malignant) model's performance across various classification thresholds, comparing the true positive rate (TPR) to the false positive rate (FPR). A superior model exhibits a higher TPR and a lower FPR. The curve showcases the TPR-FPR balance, with the area under the curve (AUC) reflecting overall performance; a perfect model has an AUC of 1.0, while a random model scores 0.5. Moving toward the top-left corner in the ROC space signifies an improved classifier accuracy, with a higher TPR and lower FPR, thus enhancing positive case identification while minimizing false positives.

3. Results

We employed our newly developed BCNet model for both binary and multi-class classification of histopathological breast cancer images, comparing its performance with existing state-of-the-art CNN models. After pre-processing the data, we applied data augmentation techniques, including rotation, horizontal flipping, shearing, zooming, scaling, and color normalization. Additionally, we resized the images to ensure uniform dimensions.

During the training process, the neural network model was iteratively refined until the loss converged to $1e^{-02}$, optimizing the weights to improve accuracy.

Current studies on histopathological images of breast cancer predominantly focus on binary classification. However, multi-class classification is crucial for accurate treatment and prognosis. Therefore, we conducted a multi-class classification study using BCNet. The experimental results of our model improved the diagnostic accuracy of using histopathological breast cancer images.

3.1 Model prediction

Evaluation metrics are essential for assessing the performance of deep learning models, especially in medical image analysis, such as breast cancer detection [24]. To evaluate the classification of benign and malignant cancer images, we utilized metrics including accuracy, sensitivity, specificity, ROC, and AUC curves for both binary and multi-class classifiers. These metrics were derived from the confusion matrix, considering true positives (TP), false positives (FP), true negatives (TN), and false negatives (FN).

Our proposed BCNet model's binary classifier achieved remarkable accuracy for images at different magnifications: 99.6% for 40X, 99.8% for 100X, 99.7% for 200X, and 99.1% for 400X (see **Table 3**). These results demonstrate the model's high efficacy in distinguishing between benign and malignant breast cancer images.

Type of classification	Magnification factor	Accuracy (%)	Sensitivity (%)	Specificity (%)
Binary classifier	40X	99.6	98.1	99.6
	100X	99.8	97.3	99.9
	200X	99.7	98.9	99.6
	400X	99.1	97.3	98.2
Multi-class classifier	40X	99.1	98.1	97.6
	100X	98.3	96.5	98.9
	200X	99.6	98.7	98.6
	400X	98.9	96.3	98.2

Table 3.
BCNet model performance metrics for binary and multi-class classification of breast cancer.

The proposed BCNet model multi-class classifier for 40×, 100×, 200×, and 400× images showed an accuracy of 99.1, 98.3, 99.6, and 98.9%, respectively, as shown in **Table 3**.

The BCNet model outperformed the existing CNN models for both the binary and the multi-class classifiers, as reported in **Table 4**.

3.1.1 Confusion matrix for a binary classifier

The confusion matrix of the binary classifier for the BCNet model, as depicted in **Figure 3**, demonstrates that our proposed model correctly classified 626 out of 628 samples, 897 out of 903 samples, 777 out of 780 samples, and 595 out of 600 samples.

Study	Classifier	Dataset	Accuracy (%)			
			40x	100x	200x	400x
Binary classification [32]	ResNet152	Breakhis	98.6	97.9	98.3	97.6
[33]	NDCNN	Breakhis	94.4	95.9	97.2	96.0
[34]	GoogleNet	Breakhis	94.8	94.4	94.7	93.5
[35]	NDCNN	Breakhis	95.8	96.9	96.7	94.9
[36]	VGGnet	Breakhis	91.2	91.4	88.5	84.5
[37]	AlexNet	Breakhis	90.6	90.5	91.3	91.3
[38]	DenseNet	Breakhis	94.7	95.9	96.7	89.1
Proposed model	BCNet	Breakhis	99.6	99.8	99.7	99.1
Multi-class classification [32]	ResNet152	Breakhis	95.6	94.8	95.6	94.6
[35]	NDCNN	Breakhis	92.8	93.9	93.7	92.9
[39]	NDCNN	Breakhis	88.2	84.6	83.1	83.9
[10]	CNN-RNN hybrid	Breakhis	96.5	92.6	88.9	92.5
Proposed model	BCNet	Breakhis	99.1	98.3	99.6	98.9

Table 4.
Binary and multi-class classification models comparison with existing state-of-the-art models.

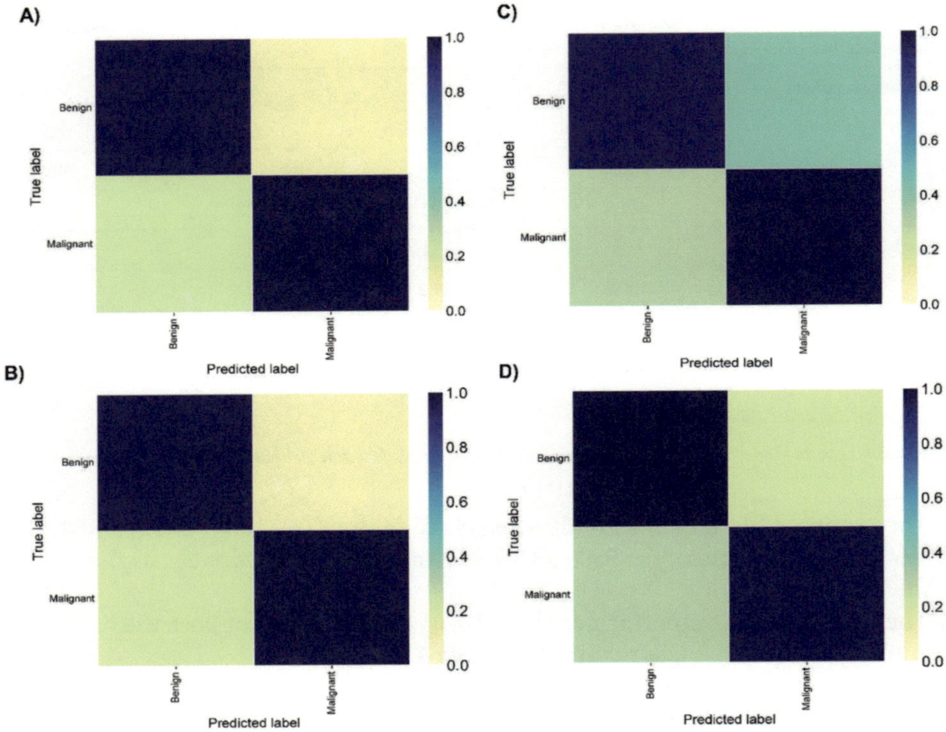

Figure 3.
BCNet model binary classifier confusion matrix at different magnification levels: 40× (A), 100× (B), 200× (C), and 400× (D).

3.1.2 ROC-AUC curve analysis for the BCNet model in binary classification

The ROC-AUC curves for the proposed BCNet model in binary classification at different magnifications, as shown in **Figure 4**, illustrated the model's exceptional performance in distinguishing between benign and malignant histopathology images. The model achieved an impressive ROC-AUC value of 0.996 at 40× magnification, demonstrating near-perfect classification accuracy at this lower magnification level. At 100× magnification, the model attained a flawless ROC-AUC value of 1.000, indicating perfect classification performance, where the model correctly identified all instances without error. For 200× magnification images, the model maintained a high level of accuracy with an ROC-AUC value of 0.972, showcasing its robustness and ability to handle increased image complexity. Finally, at 400× magnification, the ROC-AUC value was 0.994, reaffirming the model's high accuracy even at the highest magnification level. These consistently high ROC-AUC values across different magnifications underscore the BCNet model's reliability and effectiveness in the binary classification of breast cancer histopathology images, regardless of the magnification factor.

3.1.3 Confusion matrix for multi-class classifier

The confusion matrix for the BCNet model's multi-class classifier, as illustrated in **Figure 5**, provides a detailed breakdown of correctly classified samples across

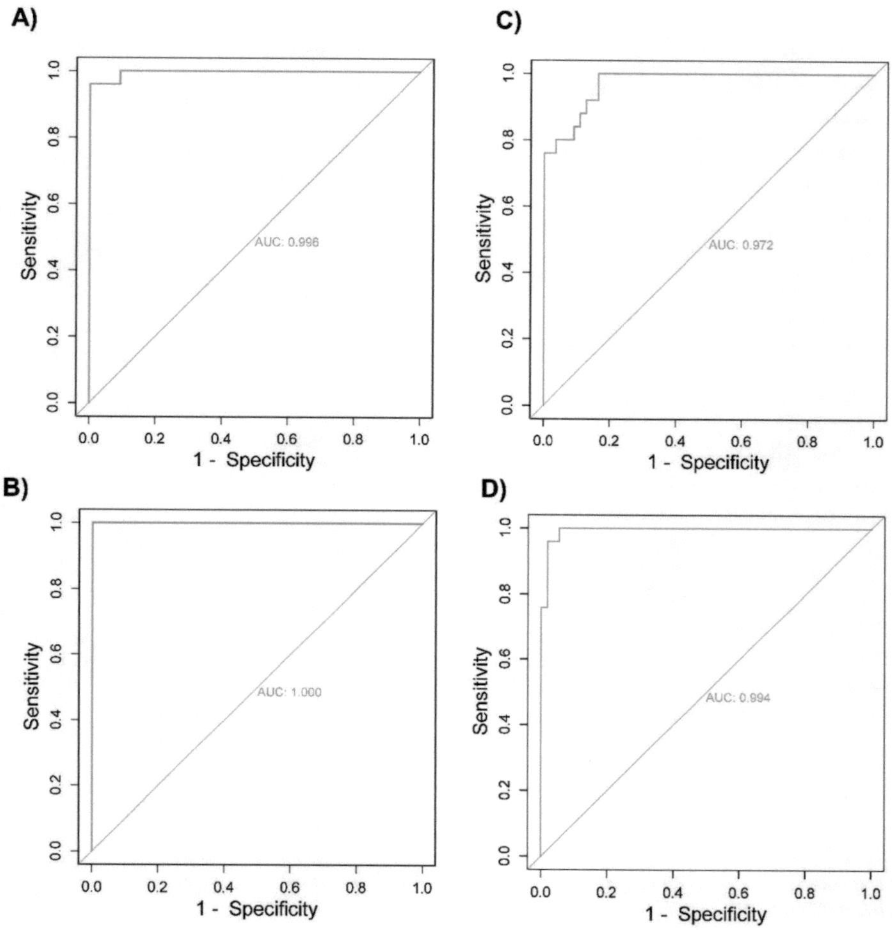

Figure 4.
ROC-AUC curves of the BCNet model for binary classification at different magnifications. The results are presented for histopathology images with magnification factors of 40× (A), 100× (B), 200× (C), and 400× (D).

different magnification levels. Specifically, the model correctly classified 614 out of 628 samples at 40× magnification, 878 out of 903 samples at 100× magnification, 765 out of 780 samples at 200× magnification, and 572 out of 600 samples at 400× magnification. These results highlight the model's high accuracy in distinguishing between the different classes in the dataset.

3.1.4 ROC-AUC curve analysis for the BCNet model in multi-class classification

The ROC-AUC curves for the BCNet model's multi-class classifier at different magnifications are illustrated in **Figure 6**. The performance of the model is assessed across four magnification levels: 40×, 100×, 200×, and 400×. Overall, the ROC-AUC curves across all magnifications illustrate the proposed model's excellent capability in multi-class classification, with consistently high AUC values that confirm the reliability and robustness of the classifier in distinguishing between various breast cancer histopathology image classes.

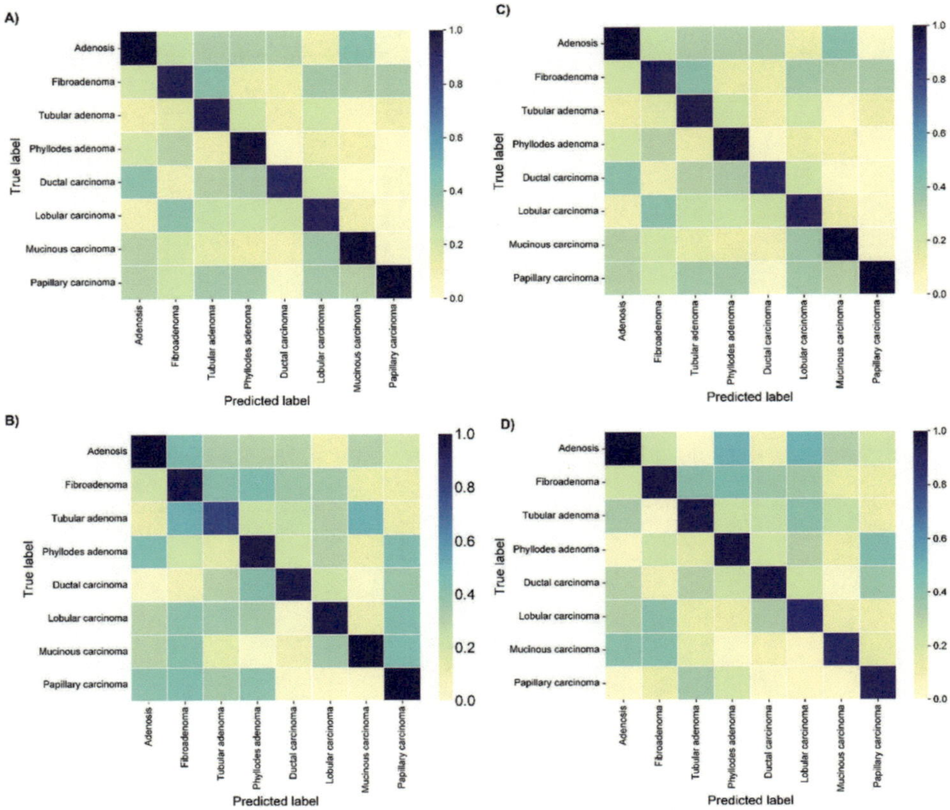

Figure 5.
Confusion matrix for the BCNet model's multi-class classifier at different magnification levels: 40× (A), 100× (B), 200× (C), and 400× (D).

4. Discussion

The findings from our study demonstrated the potential of our proposed BCNet model to enhance the accuracy and reliability of breast cancer detection and classification using histopathological images. BCNet has shown promising results by using CNN specifically tailored for the unique characteristics of breast tissue histopathology and surpassing the performance of existing state-of-the-art models in both binary and multi-class classification tasks. We expand on the integration of BCNet into clinical workflows, focusing on its role in assisting pathologists with decision-making to improve diagnostic accuracy and reduce workload.

The main contribution of this study is the development of BCNet, a 22-layer CNN model designed to manage the complexities of histopathological images, which often exhibit high variability due to differences in staining, magnification levels, and tissue morphology [20]. The architecture of BCNet, including its use of batch normalization, dropout, and Adam optimizer, has proven effective in reducing overfitting [40] and improving generalization across different magnification levels and tumor subtypes.

Our results indicate that BCNet achieves superior accuracy compared to pre-trained models such as VGG16 [20], VGG19 [20], Inception-V3 [11], DenseNet [38], and ResNet152 [32], which have traditionally been used through transfer learning.

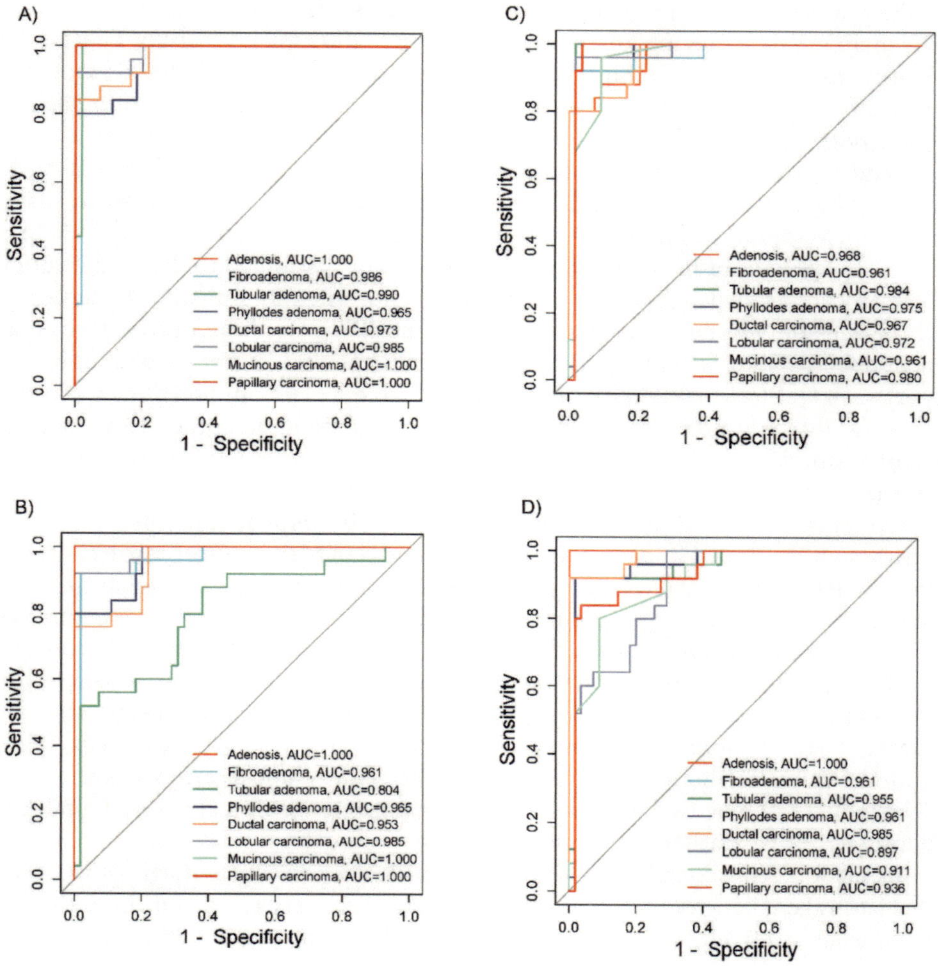

Figure 6.
ROC-AUC curves of the BCNet model in a multi-class classifier at different magnifications. The ROC-AUC results are shown for histopathology images with magnification factors of 40× (A), 100× (B), 200× (C), and 400× (D).

Despite transfer learning providing a strong starting point, it often suffers from limitations due to domain mismatch between the source domain of the pre-trained model and the target domain of histopathological images. In addition, our model also performed better than other combined models, such as the combination of ResNet50 and Inception module [41], and the CNN model with LSTM networks [10]. While transfer learning can provide a strong starting point, it often suffers from limitations due to domain mismatch between the pre-trained model's source domain and histopathological images [14]. In contrast, BCNet was designed and trained from scratch on the BreakHis dataset, allowing it to better capture the domain-specific features relevant to breast cancer histopathology.

In binary classification, BCNet achieved an accuracy of up to 99.8% at 100x magnification, demonstrating its robustness in distinguishing between benign and malignant tumors. This high level of accuracy is crucial for clinical applications, where early and precise diagnosis can significantly impact treatment decisions and patient outcomes, including the patient's recovery and survival [42]. For multi-class classification, BCNet outperformed existing models such as a novel 6B-Net deep CNN model [43], achieving up to 99.6% accuracy at 200x magnification. This model performance is particularly important for pathologists, as it contributes to identifying specific subtypes of breast cancer, each of which may require different treatment approaches.

In addition to high accuracy metrics, the practical application of BCNet can be enhanced by integrating explainable AI techniques such as Gradient-weighted Class Activation Mapping (Grad-CAM) [44], which provides a heatmap visualization to indicate the regions of histopathological images that contributed to the model's interpretability and transparency. This transparency allows health professionals to verify and trust the model's decisions, facilitating the model's integration into routine breast cancer diagnostics, particularly in settings with high pathologist workloads or limited expertise [44]. BCNet could be considered a valuable second opinion during routine screenings for early detection, ultimately improving patient outcomes. However, careful evaluation is necessary to integrate with existing clinical infrastructure. Potential challenges include compatibility with existing systems, clinicians' training requirements, and workflow adjustments for successful implementation.

Although the BreakHis dataset is widely accepted in breast cancer research, we acknowledge the potential risk of overfitting despite robust data augmentation techniques and the need for larger and more diverse datasets to address the concerns about the broader generalizability of our findings. To improve the BCNet generalizability, we performed data augmentation to artificially increase the size of the dataset using different techniques such as rotations, horizontal flipping, width and height shifts, shearing, zooming, and color normalization [45, 46]. Additionally, we plan to extend our model validation across multiple datasets and larger clinical samples. Although BCNet is currently focused on breast cancer diagnosis, its architecture is adaptable for other types of histopathological analysis.

Despite its future contributions, integrating BCNet into cancer diagnostics experienced several challenges, including ethical and legal concerns that must be addressed for responsible implementation. The ethical and legal concerns include: (1) Data privacy: The AI system's dependency on large datasets is exposed to patient data security and privacy-related risks. Our study utilized a dataset that is anonymized and secured to handle patient information through encryption to keep confidentiality and comply with data protection regulations such as the General Data Protection Regulation (GDPR) and Health Insurance Portability and Accountability Act (HIPAA) [15]. (2) Algorithmic bias: AI models trained on biased datasets may exacerbate existing healthcare disparities. If trained predominantly on data from specific demographic groups, there is a risk of misdiagnosis or lower accuracy for minority populations, thus widening health inequalities and inequities [47]. We ensured that the BreakHis dataset was representative and bias mitigation strategies were applied throughout the development process [20]. Additionally, it covers a wide range of breast cancer subtypes through its huge collection of histopathological images [15]. (3) Diagnostic errors and accountability: Misdiagnoses or incorrect model predictions could have a detrimental effect on cancer care. It is necessary to establish a regulatory framework to ensure accountability in AI deployment in the healthcare system, including promoting transparency in decision-making processes using explainable AI (XAI) techniques [48, 49]. Furthermore, healthcare providers should supervise the use of BCNet, enhancing decision-making instead of replacing clinician decision-making [50]. Healthcare institutions should obtain informed consent from the patients to integrate the BCNet model into patient care. The other potential challenges might be overcoming resistance from clinicians who are not familiar with AI and the potential for diagnostic errors if the model is not properly calibrated for varying clinical scenarios. The continual validation of the model is critical to ensure generalizability. Therefore, healthcare professionals should be trained on how to interpret and utilize AI results effectively [50].

While BCNet addresses some of the limitations of transfer learning, further research could explore hybrid approaches that combine transfer learning with domain-specific training to enhance model performance. Future research should also focus on clinical validation of BCNet across diverse clinical environments to facilitate integration into clinical workflows. Although this study focused on experimental validation using histopathological images, we are actively working toward collaborations with health institutions to test BCNet in real clinical settings. These efforts will help to evaluate its practicality, reliability, and adaptability, ensuring its performance is robust in real-world scenarios. The integration of BCNet into clinical workflows involves developing user-friendly interfaces and tools compatible with existing pathology systems, providing real-time, AI-assisted diagnostic support for pathologists. Additionally, the interpretability of the model's predictions remains an important area for future research. Finally, while our study focuses on breast cancer histopathology, the methodologies, and insights gained from developing BCNet could be adapted to other cancers and histopathological image analysis. This broader application has the potential to revolutionize cancer diagnostics and pave the way for more accurate, efficient, and accessible diagnostic tools across various medical domains.

5. Conclusion

Our newly developed BCNet represents a significant advancement in the field of breast cancer diagnostics. The BCNet model, specifically designed for breast cancer classification, demonstrated superior performance compared to existing state-of-the-art CNN models in both binary and multi-class classification tasks. These findings suggest that BCNet could significantly enhance diagnostic precision, reduce the burden on pathologists, and improve patient outcomes. Future studies should focus on validating BCNet across larger, more diverse datasets and integrating it into clinical practice to fully realize its potential in improving breast cancer diagnostics.

Conflict of interest

The authors declare no conflict of interest.

Author details

Mikiyas Amare Getu[1*], Chao Lu[2], Yumeng Liu[2], Anam Mehmood[3], Zoya Iqbal[4,5] and Xianbin Zhang[6]

1 College of Health Science, Woldia University, Woldia, Ethiopia

2 Department of Radiology of Shenzhen University General Hospital, Shenzhen, China

3 School of Biomedical Engineering, Shenzhen University, China

4 College of Medicine, Shantou University, Shantou, China

5 The University of Lahore, Lahore, Pakistan

6 Department of General Surgery and Institute of Precision Diagnosis and Treatment of Digestive System Tumors, Carson International Cancer Center, Shenzhen University General Hospital, Shenzhen University, Shenzhen, China

*Address all correspondence to: makmiky86@gmail.com

References

[1] Bray F et al. Global cancer statistics 2022: GLOBOCAN estimates of incidence and mortality worldwide for 36 cancers in 185 countries. CA: a Cancer Journal for Clinicians. 2024;**74**(3):229-263. DOI: 10.3322/caac.21834

[2] Zeiser FA, da Costa CA, Roehe AV, da Righi R, Marques NMC. Breast cancer intelligent analysis of histopathological data: A systematic review. Applied Soft Computing. 2021;**113**:107886

[3] Elmore JG et al. Diagnostic concordance among pathologists interpreting breast biopsy specimens. JAMA. 2015;**313**:1122-1132

[4] Fleming KA et al. An essential pathology package for low- and middle-income countries. American Journal of Clinical Pathology. 2017;**147**:15-32

[5] Rashmi R, Prasad K, Udupa CBK. Breast histopathological image analysis using image processing techniques for diagnostic puposes: A methodological review. Journal of Medical Systems. 2021;**46**:7

[6] Carriero A, Groenhoff L, Vologina E, Basile P, Albera M. Deep Learning in Breast Cancer Imaging: State of the Art and Recent Advancements in Early 2024. Vol. 14. Basel, Switzerland: Diagnostics; 2024

[7] Yu H, Yang LT, Zhang Q, Armstrong D, Deen MJ. Convolutional neural networks for medical image analysis: State-of-the-art, comparisons, improvement and perspectives. Neurocomputing. 2021;**444**:92-110

[8] Zhao Y et al. Application of deep learning in histopathology images of breast cancer: A review. Micromachines. 2022;**13**(12):2197

[9] Zhang H, Han L, Chen K, Peng Y, Lin J. Diagnostic efficiency of the breast ultrasound computer-aided prediction model based on convolutional neural network in breast cancer. Journal of Digital Imaging. 2020;**33**:1218-1223

[10] Srikantamurthy MM, Rallabandi VPS, Dudekula DB, Natarajan S, Park J. Classification of benign and malignant subtypes of breast cancer histopathology imaging using hybrid CNN-LSTM based transfer learning. BMC Medical Imaging. 2023;**23**:19

[11] Xie J, Liu R, Luttrell J 4th, Zhang C. Deep learning based analysis of histopathological images of breast cancer. Frontiers in Genetics. 2019;**10**:80

[12] Abunasser BS, Al-Hiealy MRJ, Zaqout IS, Abu-Naser SS. Convolution neural network for breast cancer detection and classification using deep learning. Asian Pacific Journal of Cancer Prevention. 2023;**24**:531-544

[13] Kim HE et al. Transfer learning for medical image classification: A literature review. BMC Medical Imaging. 2022;**22**:69

[14] Zhao Z, Alzubaidi L, Zhang J, Duan Y, Gu Y. A comparison review of transfer learning and self-supervised learning: Definitions, applications, advantages and limitations. Expert Systems with Applications. 2024;**242**:122807

[15] Spanhol FA, Oliveira LS, Petitjean C, Heutte L. A dataset for breast cancer histopathological image classification. IEEE Transactions on Biomedical Engineering. 2016;**63**:1455-1462

[16] He K, Zhang X, Ren S, Sun J. Deep residual learning for image recognition. In: 2016 IEEE Conference on Computer Vision and Pattern Recognition (CVPR). Piscataway, NJ: IEEE; 2016. pp. 770-778. DOI: 10.1109/CVPR.2016.90

[17] Simonyan K, Zisserman A. Very deep convolutional networks for large-scale image recognition. In: 3rd International Conference on Learning Representations (ICLR 2015). San Diego, CA: Computational and Biological Learning Society; 2015. pp. 1-14

[18] Huang G, Liu Z, Van Der Maaten L, Weinberger KQ. Densely connected convolutional networks. In: Proceedings - 30th IEEE Conference on Computer Vision and Pattern Recognition, CVPR 2017 Vols 2017-January 2261-2269. Piscataway, NJ, USA: IEEE; 2017

[19] Krizhevsky A, Sutskever I, Hinton GE. Imagenet classification with deep convolutional neural networks. Advances in Neural Information Processing Systems. 2012;**25**:1-9

[20] Spanhol FA, Oliveira LS, Petitjean C, Heutte L. Breast cancer histopathological image classification using convolutional neural networks. In: International Joint Conference on Neural Networks (IJCNN). Vancouver, BC, Canada: IEEE; 2016. pp. 2560-2567. DOI: 10.1109/IJCNN.2016.7727519

[21] Bengio Y, Goodfellow I, Courville A. Deep learning. MIT Press. 2016;**29**:1-73

[22] Pacal I, Karaboga D, Basturk A, Akay B, Nalbantoglu U. A comprehensive review of deep learning in colon cancer. Computers in Biology and Medicine. 2020;**126**:104003

[23] Alom MZ, et al. The History Began from AlexNet: A Comprehensive Survey on Deep Learning Approaches. arXiv; 2018

[24] Kaushal C, Bhat S, Koundal D, Singla A. Recent trends in computer assisted diagnosis (CAD) system for breast cancer diagnosis using histopathological images. IRBM. 2019;**40**:211-227

[25] Anwar F, Attallah O, Ghanem N, Ismail MA. Automatic breast cancer classification from histopathological images. In: 2019 International Conference on Advances in the Emerging Computing Technologies (AECT). Piscataway, NJ: IEEE; 2020. pp. 1-6. DOI: 10.1109/AECT47998.2020.9194194

[26] Roy SD, Das S, Kar D, Schwenker F, Sarkar R. Computer aided breast cancer detection using Ensembling of texture and statistical image features. Sensors. 2021;**21**:3628

[27] Budak Ü, Cömert Z, Rashid ZN, Şengür A, Çıbuk M. Computer-aided diagnosis system combining FCN and Bi-LSTM model for efficient breast cancer detection from histopathological images. Applied Soft Computing. 2019;**85**:105765

[28] Yan R et al. Breast cancer histopathological image classification using a hybrid deep neural network. Methods. 2020;**173**:52-60

[29] Cireşan DC, Giusti A, Gambardella LM, Schmidhuber J. Mitosis detection in breast cancer histology images with deep neural networks. MICCAI: International Conference on Medical Image Computing and Computer Assisted Intervention. 2013;**16**:411-418

[30] Gour M, Jain S, Sunil Kumar T. Residual learning based CNN for breast cancer histopathological image

classification. International Journal of Imaging Systems and Technology. 2020;**30**:621-635

[31] Narayanan BN, Krishnaraja V, Ali R. Convolutional neural network for classification of histopathology images for breast cancer detection. In: 2019 IEEE National Aerospace and Electronics Conference (NAECON). Dayton, OH, USA: IEEE; 2019. pp. 291-295. DOI: 10.1109/NAECON46414.2019.9058279

[32] Gandomkar Z, Brennan PC, Mello-Thoms C. MuDeRN: Multi-category classification of breast histopathological image using deep residual networks. Artificial Intelligence in Medicine. 2018;**88**:14-24

[33] Nahid A-A, Kong Y. Histopathological breast-image classification using local and frequency domains by convolutional neural network. Information. 2018;**9**(1):19

[34] Das K, Karri SPK, Guha Roy A, Chatterjee J, Sheet D. Classifying histopathology whole-slides using fusion of decisions from deep convolutional network on a collection of random multi-views at multi-magnification. In: 2017 IEEE 14th International Symposium on Biomedical Imaging (ISBI 2017). Piscataway, NJ: IEEE; 2017. pp. 1024-1027. DOI: 10.1109/ISBI.2017.7950690

[35] Han Z et al. Breast cancer multi-classification from histopathological images with structured deep learning model. Scientific Reports. 2017;**7**:4172

[36] Zhi W et al. Using transfer learning with convolutional neural networks to diagnose breast cancer from histopathological images. In: Liu D, Xie S, Li Y, Zhao D, El-Alfy E-SM, editors. Neural Information Processing. Cham: Springer International Publishing; 2017. pp. 669-676

[37] Deniz E et al. Transfer learning based histopathologic image classification for breast cancer detection. Health Information Science and Systems. 2018;**6**:18

[38] Gupta V, Bhavsar A. Sequential modeling of deep features for breast cancer histopathological image classification. In: Proceedings of the IEEE Computer Society Conference on Computer Vision and Pattern Recognition Workshops (CVPRW). Los Alamitos, CA: IEEE Computer Society; 2018. pp. 2335-2342

[39] Bardou D, Zhang K, Ahmad SM. Classification of breast cancer based on histology images using convolutional neural networks. IEEE Access. 2018;**6**:24680-24693

[40] Li H et al. Keeping Deep Learning Models in Check: A History-Based Approach to Mitigate Overfitting. IEEE Access. IEEE; 2024

[41] Ashraf FB, Alam SMM, Sakib SM. Enhancing breast cancer classification via histopathological image analysis: Leveraging self-supervised contrastive learning and transfer learning. Heliyon. 2024;**10**:e24094

[42] Ghorbian M, Ghorbian S. Usefulness of machine learning and deep learning approaches in screening and early detection of breast cancer. Heliyon. 2023;**9**:e22427

[43] Umer MJ, Sharif M, Kadry S, Alharbi A. Multi-class classification of breast cancer using 6B-net with deep feature fusion and selection method. Journal of Personalized Medicine. 2022;**12**(5):683

[44] Selvaraju RR et al. Grad-cam: Visual explanations from deep networks via gradient-based localization. In:

Proceedings of the IEEE International Conference on Computer Vision. Piscataway, NJ: IEEE; 2017. pp. 618-626

[45] Deng L, Yu D. Deep learning: methods and applications. Foundations and Trends® in Signal Processing. 2014;**7**(3-4):197-387. DOI: 10.1561/2000000039

[46] Mikołajczyk A, Grochowski M. Data augmentation for improving deep learning in image classification problem. In: 2018 International Interdisciplinary PhD Workshop (IIPhDW). New York: IEEE; 2018. pp. 117-122. DOI: 10.1109/IIPHDW.2018.8388338

[47] Esteva A et al. A guide to deep learning in healthcare. Nature Medicine. 2019;**25**:24-29

[48] Tang L, Li J, Fantus S. Medical artificial intelligence ethics: A systematic review of empirical studies. Digital Health. 2023;**9**:20552076231186064

[49] Aggarwal R et al. Diagnostic accuracy of deep learning in medical imaging: A systematic review and meta-analysis. NPJ Digital Medicine. 2021;**4**:65

[50] Alowais SA et al. Revolutionizing healthcare: The role of artificial intelligence in clinical practice. BMC Medical Education. 2023;**23**:689

Section 3

Targeted Therapies and Molecular Strategies

Chapter 11

Neuropilin-1: A Promising Therapeutic Target for Triple-Negative Breast Cancer

Noura Al-Zeheimi and Sirin A. Adham

Abstract

Despite the advanced methods to treat breast cancer, triple-negative breast cancer (TNBC) remains challenging to manage due to the lack of specific targeted therapy. Research findings in the past two decades focused on providing evidence that the Neuropilin-1 (NRP-1) protein enhances the progression and metastasis of breast cancer with more emphasis on TNBC; however, there are limited clinical trials to date to state its availability and validity as a biomarker or drug target for future clinical use. In this chapter, we summarized and discussed the available biomarkers for breast cancer and the different targeted therapies used. We also focused on NRP-1 and all the associated molecules that can be new targets for diagnosis and treatments, particularly for TNBC. This up-to-date chapter might spark the start of employing all the *in vitro* and *in vivo* findings to functionalize more serious clinical NRP-1 research and use.

Keywords: breast cancer, TNBC, NRP-1, therapeutic targets, biomarker, survival, EMT, metastasis

1. Introduction

Locally advanced breast cancer (LABC) patients are usually presented with stage III disease, according to the American Joint Committee on Cancer TNM (Tumor size, Node status, metastasis) [1]. Patients with LABC are receiving neoadjuvant chemotherapy combined with targeted therapy depending on the molecular subtype [2]. Neoadjuvant chemotherapy showed variable outcomes with regard to local recurrence and survival due to the heterogeneity of breast tumors depending on clinical and pathological assessments in terms of TNM staging, molecular subtypes, tumor microenvironment, and immunophenotype [3]. Although neoadjuvant chemotherapy showed an increased survival rate among LABC patients, patients are still at higher risk of local recurrence and distant metastasis when compared to patients with operable breast tumors [4].

Recent studies showed that, although LABC patients might share the same histopathological features, they have heterogeneous molecular profiles. These profiles influence the response to treatment and thus subject patients to varying degrees of chemoresistance, cancer recurrence, and metastasis [5]. Each patient's molecular signature provides a better understanding of the disease and improves the prediction of the treatment outcome [6, 7]. Consequently, there is a desperate need to utilize Omics-Based techniques such as genomics, transcriptomics, proteomics, metabolomics, and epigenomics to accurately build a treatment strategy and predict patients' response and survival [8]. All Omics-based data will eventually provide insight into tailored treatment based on their molecular signature.

Investigating the molecular fingerprint of breast cancer might lead to finding new targeted therapies for patients with advanced disease and metastasis. There is a significant demand to find new targeted therapies for patients with aggressive disease. In breast cancer, the triple-negative subtype, which usually presents in younger patients and exhibits an aggressive nature, is an urgent necessity for new targeted therapies to reduce the risk of recurrence and metastasis, especially in those diagnosed at the advanced stage of the disease [9].

2. Current targeted biomarkers and therapies used in breast cancer diagnosis and treatment

Recently, extensive progress in biomarkers has been made in the diagnosis, molecular subtyping, and treatment of breast cancer to enhance therapy and increase patients' survival. The immunohistochemistry (IHC) status of the three biomarkers, estrogen receptor (ER), progesterone receptor (PR), and human epidermal receptor 2 (HER2), is routinely evaluated to determine the molecular subtypes of breast cancer [10]. The proliferation marker Ki67% was also used in the classification of molecular subtypes of breast cancer as a predictive marker of response to neoadjuvant chemotherapy [11, 12]. Androgen receptor, which is a steroid receptor expressed in 70% of breast cancer patients, showed a better prognosis among ER+ cases [13, 14].

According to the expression of different receptors, breast cancer patients are classified into distinct molecular subtypes: luminal A and luminal B (both are hormone positive), triple-positive (Hormone and HER2 positive), HER2-type (Hormone negative and HER2 positive), and triple-negative (ER, PR and HER2 are negative) [15]. Further clinicopathological parameters such as tumor size, grade, nodal status, and distant metastasis are used to determine the treatment selection and predict outcome and survival [16].

Breast cancer has many FDA-approved targeted therapies against the well-established prognostic markers ER and HER2. Several ER-targeted therapies have been used to treat hormone receptor-positive breast cancer. Tamoxifen is a selective estrogen receptor modulator that acts as an antiestrogen by inhibiting estrogen binding to its receptor [17, 18]. Toremifene is another selective estrogen receptor blocker that has been used in hormone receptor-positive (HR+) breast cancer in early and late-stage disease [19]. Elacestrant is an ER antagonist for the treatment of estrogen receptor (ER)-positive, HER2-negative (HER2-) in locally advanced and/or metastatic breast cancer [20]. Exemestane is a steroidal third-generation aromatase inhibitor (AI) endocrine therapy with high tolerability for early and advanced HR+ breast cancer [21]. Fulvestrant is an estrogen receptor inhibitor for advanced and metastatic HR+ breast cancer [22, 23]. Letrozole is a third-generation aromatase inhibitor (AI inhibitor) with greater potency than other AIs, including Anastrozole, exemestane, formestane, and aminoglutethimide [24, 25]. Ribociclib is an endocrine therapy for HR+/HER2- breast cancer and, when combined with letrozole, improves overall survival [26]. Anastrozole is a nonsteroidal aromatase inhibitor that impedes the transformation of adrenal androgens (e.g., testosterone) to estrogen, which is better than Tamoxifen for advanced breast cancer in postmenopausal women as shown from a randomized trial multicenter in North America [27].

Additional targeted therapies were used to treat HR+ breast cancer to reduce cell proliferation. Abemaciclib (Verzenios) is a cyclin-dependent kinase 4 and 6 inhibitor for HR+/HER2- breast cancer cases as single-agent therapy and in combination with an aromatase inhibitor or fulvestrant [28]. Palbociclib is also a cyclin-dependent kinase 4 and 6 (CDK4 and CDK6) inhibitor used to treat advanced and metastatic HR+/HER2- metastatic breast cancer [29]. Capivasertib is a small-molecule inhibitor of all three AKT forms that, when combined with fulvestrant, the progression-free survival was significantly longer in advanced breast cancer with HR+/HER2- [30]. Alpelisib is used to treat *PIK3CA*-mutated breast cancer and shows better outcomes relative to other PI3K inhibitors for treating postmenopausal women with HR+/HER2- advanced breast cancer [31]. Everolimus is a mammalian rapamycin (mTOR) target, which helps to stop or arrest cancer growth and is used to treat HR+/HER2- metastatic breast cancer [32].

Moreover, many targeted therapies were used to treat HER2-positive (HER2+) breast cancer patients. Trastuzumab is a monoclonal antibody against HER2 and a type of tyrosine kinase inhibitor (TKI) [33] showed a reduction in cancer recurrence in the HER2+ subtype of breast cancer [34]. Lapatinib is a dual receptor tyrosine kinase inhibitor that selectively targets ErbB-1 (EGFR) and ErbB-2 (HER2) in advanced and metastatic HER+ breast tumors [35–37]. Enhertu (Fam-trastuzumab-deruxtecan-nxki) is another tailored therapy for HER2+ or HER2-low (with an IHC score between 1+ and 2+) breast cancer combined with a topoisomerase inhibitor (deruxtecan) [38]. Margetuximab is an anti-HER2 with prospective immunoregulation action for metastatic HER2+ breast cancer [39]. Neratinib, along with Capecitabine, is used in treating advanced or metastatic HER2+ breast cancer. It is an irreversible TKI with strong effectiveness against trastuzumab-resistant breast cancer [40]. Pertuzumab is an anti-HER2 that binds to the extracellular domain of HER2. Both pertuzumab and trastuzumab are used in the treatment of HER2+ breast cancer as they bind to different domains and function as dual inhibitors for metastatic or locally advanced HER2+ breast cancer [41]. Tucatinib is another tyrosine kinase inhibitor and highly selective for HER2 tyrosine kinase. Combining Tucatinib with trastuzumab and capecitabine improved progression-free survival and overall survival in HER+ breast cancer patients [42]. Further biomarkers used for routine assessment of breast cancer are the serine protease urokinase plasminogen activator (uPA), a trypsin-like protease, and its inhibitor PAI-1. They are considered vital molecules involving local invasion and degradation of the extracellular matrix (ECM) [43, 44]. Both uPA and PAI-1 were stronger predictors of outcome than tumor size, grade, hormone receptor status, or patient age in patients with node-negative or node-positive tumors [45]. The prognostic effect of uPA and PAI-1 was mainly observed in HER2+ tumors [46].

All the mentioned targeted therapies, biomarkers, or tests mainly concern ER-positive or HER2-positive breast cancer. Unfortunately, limited targeted therapies were FDA-approved for triple-negative breast cancer (TNBC) tumors with ER-negative/HER2-negative, and chemotherapy remains the primary systemic therapy [47]. Pembrolizumab is a type of immunotherapy, an anti-programmed death receptor ligand 1 (PD-1) monoclonal antibody [48]. PD-1 is a cell-surface protein expressed by various immune cells, including T-cells; it is activated by its ligands

PDL1 and PDL2. This molecule is expressed by tumor cells, especially basal-like (TNBC), to inhibit immune response. PD1/PDL1 inhibitors were used in TNBC and showed better survival and response to chemotherapy [49]. Olaparib is a poly-ADP ribose polymerase (PARP) inhibitor; PARPs are a group of enzymes activated by the DNA damage process. Inhibition of PARPs leads to cell apoptosis. Olaparib is used for the treatment of patients with metastatic HER2- and BRCA1 or BRCA2 mutated breast cancer tumors [50]. A substantial proportion of TNBC patients are carriers of a BRCA1 or BRCA2 gene mutation [51]. Talazoparib is another PARP inhibitor used to treat BRCA-positive breast cancer [52, 53]. Sacituzumab govitecan is an anti-trophoblast cell-surface antigen 2 (Trop-2) linked with SN-38, the active metabolite of irinotecan and an inhibitor for topoisomerase I [54]. Sacituzumab Govitecan significantly improves overall survival of metastatic TNBC [55]. TOP2A is a type II topoisomerase enzyme that plays a crucial role in relaxing the DNA double helix and has also been used as a marker for breast cancer. A study showed that cryptolepine (not FDA-approved yet), an inhibitor of TOP2A, reduces chemoresistance by targeting the proliferation of breast cancer cells [56].

Multigene signatures such as OncotypeDX, Prosigna, and MammaPrint are crucial prognostic and predictive assays that classify the risk of recurrence in the early stages of ER-positive breast cancer treated with adjuvant therapy. OncotypeDX is a multigene test with a 21-gene signature that predicts cancer recurrence and the benefits of chemotherapy in ER+ breast cancer patients [57, 58]. Prosigna is another test with 50 gene signatures that adds prognostic data by assessing the distant recurrence in ER-positive breast cancer [58]. Additionally, MammaPrint is a 70-gene signature assay to categorize ER-positive primary breast cancer into low/high risk of relapse [57].

3. Neuropilin-1 as a potential biomarker for breast cancer supported by clinical, *in vitro* and *in vitro* studies

Neuropilin-1 (NRP-1) is a 130- to 135-kDa transmembrane glycoprotein and was discovered as part of the gene family encoding proteins differentially expressed in mammalian nervous systems involved explicitly in axon guidance [59, 60]. NRP-1 has three domains: the largest domain is the extracellular part with two complement binding domains (CUB (c1 and c2)), two coagulation factor domains (b1 and b2), and one MAM domain (c), one transmembrane domain and a short intracellular/cytoplasmic domain with 39 amino acids [60]. NRP-1 was first identified to bind to semaphorin III (Sema III) and affect the neuronal cells' development [59]. NRP-1 with SEMA3A was shown to guide and organize the neural crest cells [61].

Since NRP-1 has many domains, it's a co-receptor for SEMA3A, which functions in axon guidance, and a co-receptor for vascular endothelial growth factor (VEGF), a member of the angiogenesis family [62]. The role of NRP-1 in promoting cancer was initially identified through its involvement in the process of forming blood vessels from pre-existing ones, "angiogenesis," by binding to VEGF, which is a crucial process in cancer growth. In addition, NRP-1 was found to be expressed in endothelial cells along with the VEGF family, and NRP-1 alone was shown to enhance VEGF, mediating endothelial cell migration, suggesting its role in the epithelial-to-mesenchymal transition (EMT) pathway [63]. Thus, the targeted therapy anti-VEGF, a monoclonal antibody, bevacizumab, was FDA-approved in 2008 to reduce/block tumor angiogenesis in different cancers, including metastatic colorectal, lung, and breast cancer [64].

Although bevacizumab showed an increased response rate, it failed to demonstrate overall survival (OS) benefit in breast cancer [65]. Consequently, the approval of bevacizumab was reversed in 2010 as no overall survival improvement data was shown in breast cancer clinical trials [66]. These data suggest that NRP-1 promotes breast cancer not necessarily through VEGF and angiogenesis but instead through proliferation, survival, and EMT-related pathways.

NRP-1 is expressed in invasive breast tumors, specifically the triple-negative subtype [67–71]. NRP-1 exists in two forms: the transmembrane protein and the circulating/soluble form. The increased expression of both was shown to be associated with poor prognosis breast cancer [67, 68, 72].

Assessing the expression of NRP-1 in breast cancer tissues and other cancers has gained significant interest [67, 68, 73–79]. Remarkably, NRP-1 expression in breast cancer tissues was associated with a worse prognosis. In breast cancer tissues, the expression of NRP-1 was upregulated in patients with triple-negative subtype, advanced nodal disease (N3), and metastatic patients [80]. Additionally, the co-receptor of NRP-1, placental growth factor (PLGF), was overexpressed in the triple-negative patients' tissues [67, 81]. Besides, tissue NRP-1 was found to increase post-neoadjuvant chemotherapy in relapsed cases. Patients with low immunoreactive score (IRS) tissue NRP-1 post-neoadjuvant chemotherapy showed improved overall survival [68].

Although soluble NRP-1 (sNRP-) levels did not differentiate normal from breast cancer patients, there were increased sNRP-1 levels in patients with advanced stage [67]. Additionally, the increased levels of soluble NRP-1 after neoadjuvant chemotherapy in LABC were observed in patients who showed partial response (pPR) to the treatment compared to patients who showed complete response (pCR) [68]. A recent study showed that low soluble NRP-1 levels in patients exhibited a better survival rate [72].

Previous studies showed that patients with high NRP-1 levels were correlated with low survival rates. An online survival analysis tool (Kaplan–Meier Plotter) that collects GEO, EGA, and TCGA data and links gene expression with clinical analysis splits patients into high/low expressions according to the median value [82]. Selecting Affymetrix ID/Gene symbol: 210510 (**Figure 1A**), the survival analysis was done on 4929 breast cancer patients and showed that high NRP-1 expression is associated with low survival. Additionally, when RNA-seq data were selected instead of mRNA, the results were done on 2976 breast cancer patients (**Figure 1B**), and the findings were aligned with the mRNA, in which high NRP-1 levels are linked to low survival rates. Another interactive platform, UALCAN, analyzed cancer OMICS data from the TCGA database and showed that NRP-1 expression at the mRNA (**Figure 1C**) or protein (**Figure 1D**) levels increased with stage 3 breast cancer patients. Furthermore, UALCAN was utilized to analyze the expression data of NRP-1 based on ERBB2 (HER2) expression in metastatic cases, which again showed an increase in the NRP1 levels in metastatic patients overexpressing ERBB2 (**Figure 1E**). Moreover, NRP-1 expression showed a notable increase in patients with advanced nodal disease (**Figure 1F**).

Overexpression of NRP-1 in the triple-positive breast cancer cells BT-474 cells, which generally express low levels of NRP-1, activates the Tenascin C/integrin β3 axis; both molecules are part of the extracellular matrix (ECM) and involved in ECM remodeling resulting in triggering the survival pathway through focal adhesion kinase (FAK) and the proliferation and survival markers Akt and NF-κB p_{65} respectively [83]. Furthermore, NRP-1 silencing in MCF-7 and SK-BR-3 cells exhibited an increased

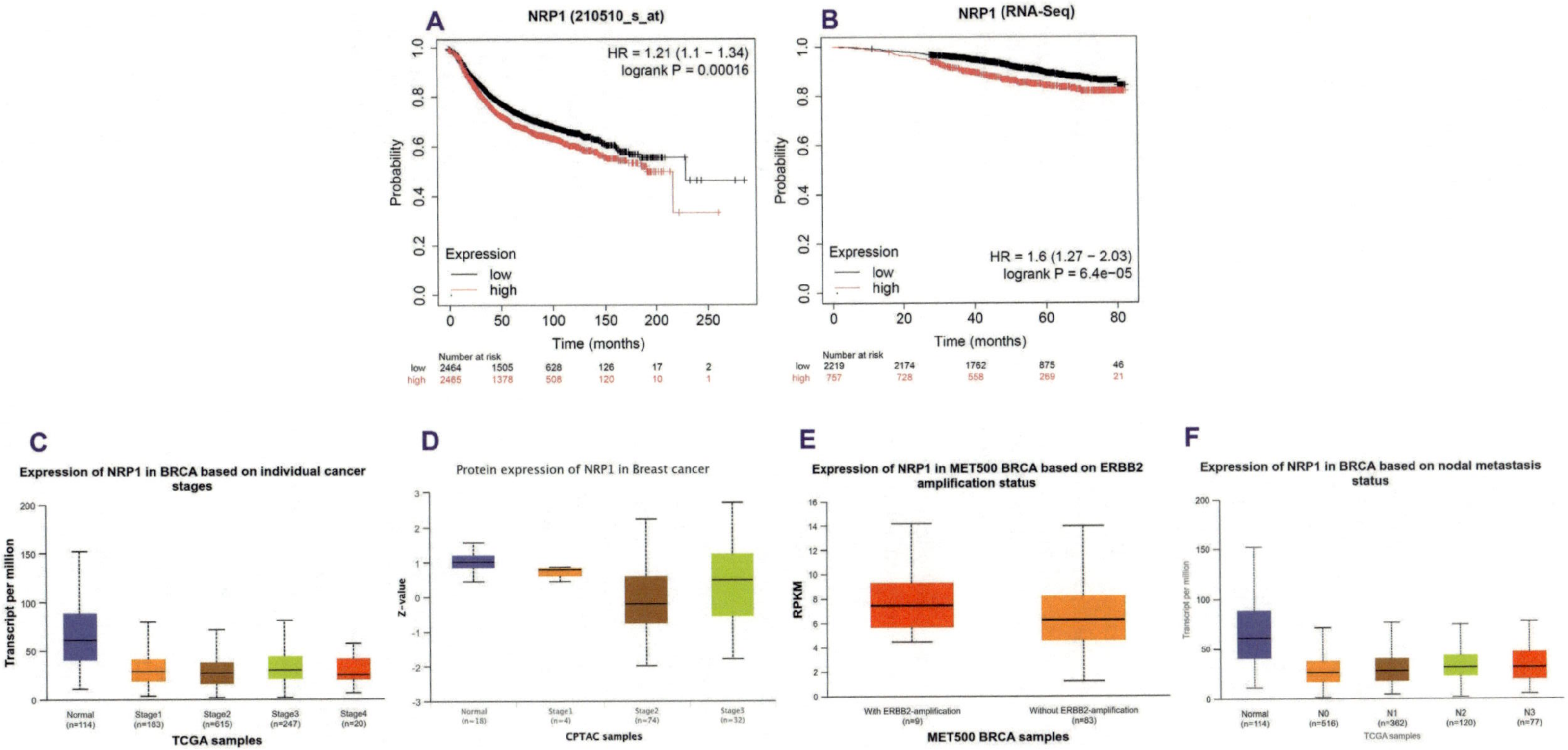

Figure 1.

High NRP-1 levels are associated with lower survival rates. The Kaplan–Meier curves were created using the Kaplan–Meier Plotter (https://kmplot.com/analysis/index.php?p=service&cancer=breast). The survival curves were generated using mRNA (A) and RNA-seq (B) data. Increased levels of NRP-1 were observed in stage 3 at the mRNA (C) and protein (D) levels. Higher expression of NRP-1 was also noticed in metastatic patients who overexpress ERBB2 (E) and in cases of advanced nodal disease (F).

apoptosis rate [84]. NRP-1 knockdown in claudin-low cells reduces cell proliferation *in vitro* and *in vivo*. Proliferation and invasion are inhibited due to the reduction in phosphorylation of mitogen-activated protein kinases MAPK p42 and p44, the critical molecules of signal transduction from the cell surface to the nucleus and EMT mediators ZEB1 and ITG6A, respectively [85].

In an *in vitro* study, a Tranilast drug was used to suppress cancer stem cells (CSCs) in three breast cancer cell lines: MDA-MB-231, MCF7, and BT-474. The results showed reduced mammosphere formation, downregulation of NRP-1, and inhibition of NF-κB survival axis. Furthermore, using an anti-NRP-1 antibody or siRNA to inhibit NRP-1 reduced mammosphere formation and NF-κB survival axis. Additionally, the proliferation axis phospho-AKT and ERK1/2 were decreased slightly. These results suggest that NRP-1 is critical in CSC formation and is directly linked to NF-κB survival axis activation [86]. Additionally, the VEGF-A/NRP-1 axis promotes cancer stem cells by activating the Wnt/β-catenin pathway, contributing to cell-cell interactions and self-renewal in MCF7 cells [87].

Further *in vitro* study showed that the expression of miR-376a, a type of non-coding RNA, is positively correlated with OS in breast cancer patients. Upregulation of miR-376a suppresses breast cancer cell proliferation and induces apoptosis when tested in MCF7, MDA-MB-231, and MDA-MB- 453 cells. Vimentin, an EMT mediator, was downregulated by miR-376a, suggesting that miR-376a attenuates EMT and invasion pathways. Interestingly, the suppressive effect of miR-376 s is related to NRP-1 expression and downstream signaling of Wnt/β-catenin [88].

An *in vivo* study showed that VEGF-A/NRP-1 plays a role in inducing breast cancer metastasis and reducing FOXO3a expression. FOXO3a promotes the expression of miR-29b-2 and miR-338. miR-29b-2 suppresses VEGF-A, while miR-338 block NRP-1. The overexpression of miR-29b-2 and miR-338 facilitates FOXO3a to suppress the VEGF-A/NRP1 axis and, consequently, breast cancer invasion and metastasis [89]. Another *in vivo* study used the shRNA-NRP1 on the xenograft model to test the function of NRP-1 in radiotherapy sensitivity. NRP-1 Knockout inhibited the growth of xenograft tumors. They found that NRP-1 promotes CSC by reducing the expression of apoptotic marker Bcl-2 through methyltransferase WTAP in an m6A-dependent way [90].

Collectively, clinical, *in vitro*, and *in vivo* studies confirmed the critical role of NRP-1 in breast cancer development, proliferation, invasion (EMT), metastasis, survival, and chemoresistance. As a consequence, NRP-1 can be a potential therapeutic target for aggressive types and metastatic breast cancer.

4. NRP-1 as a biomarker and drug target in triple-negative breast cancer (TNBC)

Triple-negative breast cancer (TNBC) is a subtype that represents 15% of all breast cancer patients and mainly occurs in young patients under 40 years old of all breast cancer cases [47]. Patients with TNBC have shorter relapse-free survival and show worse overall survival (OS) and propensity toward metastasis [91]. Patients with this subtype have been restricted with few treatment modalities, chemotherapy, surgery, radiation, and few approved targeted therapies compared to other breast cancer subtypes. Thus, more attention is required to find new targeted therapies and personalized treatments for this subtype.

Remarkably, NRP-1 is highly expressed in TNBC compared to other subtypes, as proven by *in vitro* and clinical studies. A study on vasculogenic mimicry, which means the development of vascular components by cancer cells, used public TNBC transcriptome data and showed that NRP-1 is one of the biomarkers identified to regulate vasculogenic mimicry in TNBC [92].

An additional study on TNBC cells illustrated that NRP-1 plays a role in cancer stemness via activating RAS signaling that functions in malignant transformation [93]. This confirms the role of NRP-1 in TNBC cell stemness. In another study on MDA-MB-231 and MDA-MB-468, TNBC cells showed that inhibition of VEGF-A reduces the binding of VEGF-A to NRP-1, thus lowering the migration ability of TNBC cells, suggesting the role of NRP-1 in TNBC migration [93]. Moreover, angiogenesis is a crucial process for breast cancer development. As previously mentioned, the approval of bevacizumab, the antiangiogenic targeted therapy for breast cancer, was reversed due to increased hypoxia and stem cell enrichment. Thus, a new study by Wang et al., 2020 suggested the use of NRP-1 targeted delivery of nucleus accumbens-associated protein-1 (NAC-1), which induces hypoxia and stem cells in breast cancer; therefore, NAC-1 siRNA (siNAC-1) facilitated by tLyP-1 peptide-functionalized chimeric polymersomes (tLyP-1-Ps) increased the sensitivity of antiangiogenic therapy (bevacizumab) in TNBC model *in vivo* [94].

In an *in vitro* study of TNBC cells, MDA-MB-231 showed activation of the proliferation and invasion of cells exhibiting high levels of VEGF and NRP-1. The study showed that silencing NRP-1 or VEGF inhibits cell growth and invasion by attenuating the EMT pathway and NF-κBp_{65} phosphorylation [73]. Another study illustrates the role of VEGF-A in inducing NRP-1 and associated downstream signaling, GAPVD1 (GTPase regulator)/Wnt/β-catenin, to regulate tumor-associated macrophages in TNBC, enhancing cancer stemness [70]. A functional study on NRP-1 in cells displayed that NRP-1 binds with transforming growth factor (TGF)-β to trigger the TGF-β pathway, a key player in cell differentiation and migration, thus stimulating molecules involved in the EMT pathway [95].

Another study demonstrating the role of NRP-1 in TNBC cells showed that silencing NRP-1 through siRNA decreased the effects of HS3ST3B (heparan sulfate 3-O-sulfotransferases), which is known to promote the proliferation and reduce the pro-apoptosis of TNBC cells [96], suggesting that the tumor induction effect mediated by HS3ST3B is regulated by NRP-1 expression.

In clinical studies, NRP-1 overexpression was observed in the tissues [67, 97] and blood [67] of TNBC, compared to other subtypes. In addition, NRP-1 functions as an independent prognostic factor, as patients with high NRP-1 levels exhibited shorter OS [68, 97]. Furthermore, Blocking NRP-1 in TNBC cells enhances the chemosensitivity of paclitaxel by reducing cell proliferation and migration and increasing apoptosis [97]. Meanwhile, NRP-1 knockdown TNBC cells showed a reduced ability of cells to form colonies and increase paclitaxel chemosensitivity [68]. Clinical analysis of breast cancer in TCGA and METABRIC showed that NRP-1 is highly expressed in the TNBC subtype [98]. The observation from the same study showed that 60% of TNBC cases showed high expression of VEGF-A (angiogenic marker and a ligand for NRP-1) and low expression of semaphorin (an antiangiogenic and anti-lymphangiogenic molecule, which is also a ligand for NRP-1). This explains why the TNBC subtype showed an aggressive nature and high metastatic ability [98]. Moreover, a study on TNBC showed that high levels of RNA-binding protein (PUM2) were observed in the tissues of TNBC, which was negatively associated with OS and relapse-free survival but positively correlated with distance metastasis. *In vitro* experiments showed that high levels of PUM2 mediate the stemness of the cancer cells. Interestingly, via bioinformatic analysis, PUM2 binds to NRP-1 3′UTR, promotes its expression, and enhances TNBC stemness competing with miR-376a [99].

Existing literature supports the role of NRP-1 in TNCB by inhibiting apoptosis, reducing survival, and inducing stemness, EMT, chemoresistance, and metastasis. Consequently, NRP-1 can be the future potential therapeutic target for TNBC to enhance the patient's prognosis.

5. The role of NRP-1 and associated molecules in triggering the aggressive nature of breast cancer

NRP-1 is a multifunctional molecule that acts as a co-receptor for many molecules involved in tumor proliferation and metastasis. In an *in vitro* study, we showed that NRP-1 expression increased significantly in TNBC cells resistant to chemotherapy by activating the TNC/integrin β3/FAK/NF-κBp_{65} axis. In addition, EMT mediators ZEB1 and vimentin showed a significant increase in the chemotherapy-resistant cells [100]. Using CRISPR-Cas9, NRP-1 knockout in TNBC cells, MDA-MB-231 showed decreased metastasis regulators integrin-β3 and TNC levels. Additionally, an *in vivo* experiment showed a reduction in metastatic lesions in the lung of xenograft models injected with NRP-1 Knockout cells (NRP-1 KO); this might be due to a downregulation of fibronectin-1 FN1 and ECM remodeling-related molecules, supported by RNA-seq data that shows ECM is one of the most enriched pathways due to NRP-1 knockdown [69, 101]. Since NRP-1 KO cells exhibited fewer metastatic lesions in the lung, this proposes the role of NRP-1 in the EMT pathway promoting the metastatic features in breast cancer, specifically in TNBC. RNA sequencing of the NRP-1 KO cells offered further insight into the NRP-1-associated molecules, such as Integrinβ3, TNC, FN1, OPN, COL6A3, GPX3, CCL20, ACVRL1, and ERBB2 [69], which might promote the metastatic ability of NRP-1.

5.1 NRP-1 and Integrinβ3

Functional studies showed that NRP-1 and Integrinβ3 demonstrated synchronized upregulation or downregulation. NRP-1 overexpression in triple-positive cells, BT-474 showed a simultaneous increase in the level of Integrinβ3 [83]. Moreover, NRP-1 KO showed a concurrent downregulation of Integrinβ3 [69]. Additionally, increased levels of NRP-1 due to chemoresistance in TNBC cells were associated with a parallel increase of Integrinβ3 [100]. Moreover, in the coimmunoprecipitation experiment to prove the interaction between NRP-1 and HER2, Integrinβ3 interacted with both HER2 and NRP-1, suggesting a binding between NRP-1 and Integrinβ3 [100]. Another molecule from the integrin family, ITGA6, was shown to work with NRP-1 to enhance mammary stem cell function [85]. Goel and Mercurio discussed how the binding of NRP1 to integrin-α5β1 regulates the function of integrin independently from the VEGF165/Sema3A axis. In contrast, the VEGF/NRP-1 axis regulates other integrins to promote their binding to ECM ligands [102]. Another study showed that downregulating integrin-β3, integrin-α5, and neuropilin-1 in endothelial cells reduces angiogenesis and consequently decreases cell growth [103]. Collectively, inhibiting both Integrinβ3 and NRP-1 may boost the therapeutic ability of NRP-1 in breast cancer.

5.2 NRP-1 and ECM-related molecules *TNC*, *FN1*, *OPN*, and COL6A3

Tenascin C (TNC), a glycoprotein in the extracellular matrix (ECM), is overexpressed in TNBC and activates cell proliferation and invasion. TNC knockdown by siRNA reduces cell growth and invasion significantly [104]. Moreover, TNC was shown to bind to different adhesion molecules, activate the oncogenic factor NOTCH, and promote breast cancer metastasis to the lung [105]. Additionally, immunofluorescent showed that NRP-1 KO cells exhibit a joint downregulation of NRP-1 and TNC, and these cells showed fewer metastatic lesions to the lung compared to control cells that express high levels of both NRP-1 and TNC [69]. These data suggest that both NRP-1 and TNC work synergically to boost metastasis. The studies that showed NRP-1 upregulation due to chemoresistance show a co-overexpression of TNC [83, 100]. TNC cofunctions with Integrin $\alpha v\beta 1$ and activates the TGFβ1, an EMT mediator in breast cancer cells [106]. Targeting TNC with PL3 peptide showed that this peptide also interacts with NRP-1 in tumor xenografts, enhancing tumor detection and imaging [107]. Furthermore, a peptide to target TNC, PL3, could also be internalized by NRP-1, improving the delivery efficiency when tested in breast cancer cells [108].

Fibronectin 1 (FN1) is a glycoprotein present in two forms: at the cell surface in the ECM and as a soluble protein in the plasma. It functions as EMC remodeling. Meta-analysis of 597 breast cancer samples and 409 adjacent normal samples showed that FN1 expression is high in breast tumors and associated with poor prognosis and shorter overall survival. Targeting FN1 *in vitro* using miR-429 inhibits TNBC cell proliferation and invasion by affecting the Wnt/β-catenin signaling pathway [109]. A study on nasopharyngeal carcinoma showed that NRP-1 inhibition reduced FN1 levels, attenuating cell invasion. This suggests a joint function of NRP-1 and FN1 in cancer cell invasion [110]. Another study in an advanced gastric cancer showed that NRP-1 interacted with FN1 to coordinate EMT, and NRP-1 inhibition decreases cell proliferation and invasion [111]. FN1 is identified as a key mediator for breast cancer invasion and metastasis [112]. This gives insight into its role in NRP-1 KO cells, which exhibited less metastatic lesions to the lung due to the downregulation of FN1 [69]. The expression of both molecules, NRP-1 and FN1, was shown to be positively correlated in mesothelioma [113]. High NRP-1 levels are well known in Claudin-low breast cancer, TNBC, and these cells were identified to express high levels of EMT markers such as ZEB1, vimentin, and N-cadherin in addition to FN1 [114].

Osteopontin (OPN) is a glycoprotein in the ECM associated with many functions, including intracellular interaction, and plays a role in the immune system by binding to integrins and CD44, respectively. Additionally, OPN plays a role in tumor development by promoting cancer proliferation, angiogenesis, and metastasis [115]. OPN plays a role in malignancy due to its interaction with many molecules, such as integrins, CD44, EGFR, TGFα, MMP (matrix metalloproteinases), and uPA [116]. A study showed that elevated levels of OPN and VEGF are correlated with the levels of NRP-1 and NF-κB in breast cancer. An *in vitro* study on the TNBC MDA-MB-231 illustrates that OPN might mediate the interaction between NRP-1 and VEGF to promote cancer cell motility. Inhibiting VEGF or blocking OPN and NRP-1 arrest tumor growth and angiogenesis [117]. Another *in vitro* study on MDA-MB-231 showed that curcumin, in combination with anti-VEGF/NRP-1, can significantly inhibit cell motility induced by OPN [118]. Moreover, OPN was downregulated in NRP-1 KO cells, indicating that the two molecules exhibit joint function in enhancing cell motility through ECM remodeling [69].

COL6A3 is a collagen type VI alpha 3 chain and plays a critical role with other collagen proteins from the same family in breast cancer brain metastasis [119].

Additionally, COL6A3 was shown to induce cancer stem cells and enhance lung metastasis in breast cancer when connected with the stem cell marker ANTXR1 [120]. NRP-1 KO cells, which exhibited restricted metastasis to the lung, showed an increase in expression levels of COL6A3, which might indicate that COL6A3 induces cancer metastasis via coordination with proteins from the collagen family and other stem cell mediators [69].

5.3 NRP-1 and CCL20

CCL20 is a C-C motif chemokine ligand 20 involved in immune regulation and inflammation pathways. Taxane, a chemotherapeutic agent used to treat breast cancer patients, was observed to induce CCL20 expression. The expression of CCL20 enhances breast cancer stem cells via MAPK or protein kinase Cζ (PKCζ), which promotes the induction of NF-κB survival axis, as shown in TNBC cells *in vitro* [121]. CCL20 is a potential therapeutic target in breast cancer as it modulates distinct tumor development pathways, including EMT, invasion, angiogenesis, chemoresistance, and immunosuppression [122]. NRP-1 and CCL20 were identified to induce similar pathways involving angiogenesis and metastasis in breast cancer [123]. Thus, when NRP1 was knocked out, CCL20 expression was significantly reduced [69]. In hypoxic conditions, CCL20 and NRP-1 were induced by tumor-associated macrophages (TAM) to promote tumor development. Using anti-NRP-1 might help to inhibit TAM from entering hypoxic areas [124]. Dual overexpression of NRP-1 and CCL20 drives tumorigeneses.

5.4 NRP-1 and ACVRL1

ACVRL1 is an activin A receptor like type 1 and is a protein-coding gene member of the TGFβ receptor family. High levels of ACVRL1 were observed in TAM, driving resistance to PD-1 therapy in clinical trials of breast cancer. ACVRL1 regulates immunomodulating and angiogenesis in breast cancer [125]. NRP-1 and ACVRL1 interact with each other, and NRP-1 deletion was associated with a reduction in ACVRL1 levels in TNBC cells and smooth muscle cells [69, 126]. Both NRP-1 and ACVRL1 (ALK1) interact to regulate angiogenesis, as proven by functional studies [127].

5.5 NRP-1 and HER2 (ERBB2)

HER2 is a transmembrane human epidermal growth factor receptor overexpressed in approximately 30% of breast cancers. HER2 has three domains: an extracellular domain (ECD), a single transmembrane domain, and an intracellular domain (ICD). Breast cancer patients with HER2+ are linked to poor prognosis, high risk of metastasis, and resistance to therapies [128]. Its anti-apoptotic function leads to resistance to Taxol treatment [129]. Surprisingly, dual expression of NRP-1 and HER2 was observed in resistant breast cancer cells to chemotherapy. Overexpression of HER2 using Gateway cloning in TNBC, MDA-MB-231, and luminal A, MCF7 cells exhibit simultaneous overexpression of NRP-1. Coimmunoprecipitation proves the binding of HER2 to NRP-1 [100]. Furthermore, NRP-1 KO showed a reduction in the intracellular HER2 (ICD) of the TNBC cells [69], which was reported previously that some basel-like tumors expressed IDC HER2 and showed the same features as HER2+ Cells [130]. Co-expression of NRP-1 and HER2 indicates their role in promoting breast cancer metastasis and resistance.

5.6 NRP-1 and GPX3

GPX3 is a glutathione peroxidase X3 and is identified as one member of the anti-oxidant enzymes that protect cells from DNA oxidation, which usually leads to mutation and, consequently, cancer development [131]. GPX3 is a tumor suppressor and is downregulated in breast tumor tissues; therefore, *in vitro* overexpression of GPX3 in breast cancer cells suppresses cancer proliferation, migration, and colony formation [132]. The same study demonstrates that the clinical analysis using the survival data and receiver operating characteristic (ROC) of breast cancer showed that overexpression of GPX3 is associated with a better prognosis. A clinical study in breast cancer showed that GPX3 is significantly reduced in patients with lymph node metastasis [133]. In contrast, hypermethylation of GPX3 promotor was significantly detected in inflammatory breast cancer [134]. Low expression of GPX was associated with breast cancer development and recurrence [135, 136]. Limited studies tested the correlation between NRP-1 and GPX3 expression; however, RNA-seq analysis on NRP-1 KO cells showed that these cells showed lower metastatic ability and high expression of the tumor suppressor GPX3 [69].

Current studies highlighted the significant role of NRP-1 and associated molecules in promoting breast cancer proliferation, survival, angiogenesis, stemness, EMT, chemoresistance, and Metastasis (**Figure 2**). Therefore, NRP-1 can potentially be the target for breast cancer cells, improving the patient's outcomes.

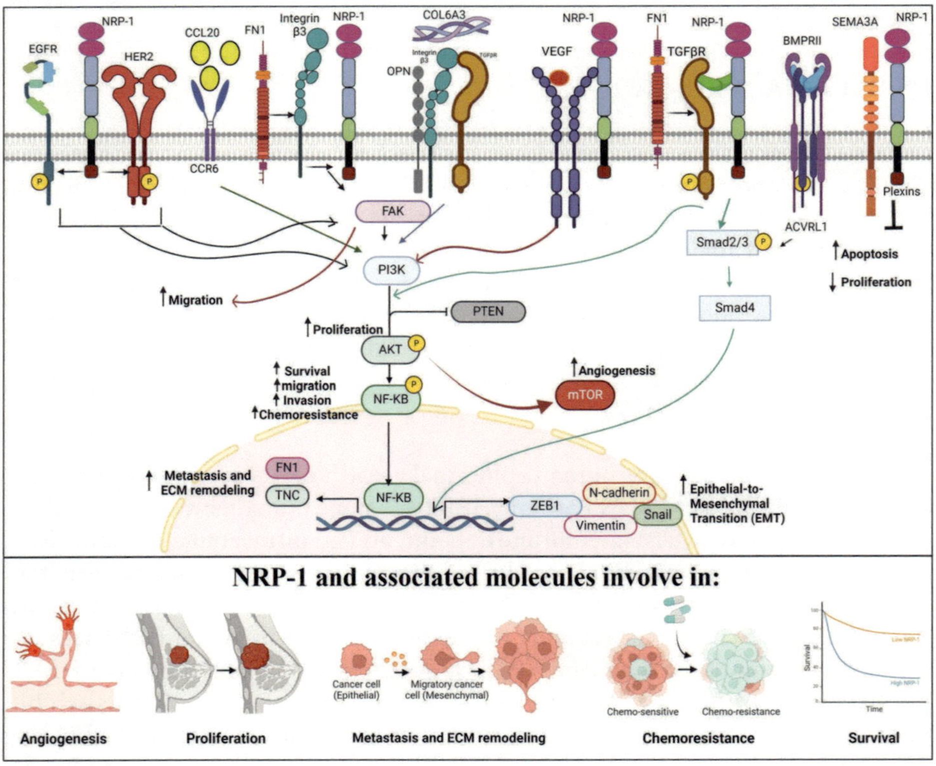

Figure 2.
NRP-1 and associated molecules, VEGF, Integrinβ3, HER2, EGFR, CCL20, COL6A3, OPN, ACVRL1, TGFβ, and FN1, activate the FAK, AKT, NF-κB, Smad, mTOR, and EMT pathways. These pathways promote angiogenesis, tumor proliferation, ECM remodeling, metastasis, chemoresistance, and cancer cell survival. (The figure was created using BioRender).

A summary of RNA sequencing analysis on NRP-1 knockout in TNBC cells (MDA-MB-231-KO) revealed that the ECM-receptor interaction, focal adhesion, and cell adhesion molecules are the most affected pathways [69]. These pathways play crucial roles in remodeling breast cancer cells, promoting motility, inducing the transition from epithelial to mesenchymal form, enhancing stemness, developing chemoresistance, and preparing cells for invasion and metastasis. Thus, they highlight the role of NRP-1 in TNBC metastasis and invasion. Additionally, they showed that the PI3K-AKT signaling pathway and other pathways in cancer are also influenced by NRP-1 knockout, explaining why cells overexpressing NRP-1 exhibit high proliferation and drive breast cancer progression.

6. NRP-1-targeted therapies tested *in vitro* and in vivo

NRP-1 was identified to express in many pathways, including angiogenesis, EMT, PI3K/AKT, and NF-κB survival axis, and chemoresistance-related pathways. Additionally, functional studies inhibiting NRP-1 showed promising results in interfering with tumor growth and slowing its progression. Thus, targeting NRP-1 with anti-NRP-1 therapy might yield promising results in clinical practice by enhancing prognosis, reducing metastasis burden, and increasing survival rate.

Genentech, in 2007, produced two monoclonal antibodies against NRP-1. One antibody blocked the SMA3A binding site (a1 & a2), and the other blocked the VEGF binding site (b1 & b2). Using the antibodies in combination with anti-VEGF therapy reduces tumor growth significantly [137]. In 2014, a cost-effective small VEGF-A_{165}/NRP-1 antagonist was tested *in vitro* and *in vivo*. This organic compound contains phenylbenzimidazole and benzodioxane moieties connected by a stablecarboxy-thiourea spacer. In *vivo*, the antagonist reduced the tumor growth in MDA-MB-231-xenografted mice and consequently improved mouse survival. This antagonist showed antiangiogenic activity and reduced vessel development [138]. A breast cancer-targeting peptide CLKADKAKC (CK3) that enhances its binding to NRP-1 was tested in 2014 in xenograft tumors and showed no penetration into lungs and heart *in vivo*, making this peptide a promising targeted therapy against NRP-1 [139]. A monoclonal antibody (mAb) was also tested in MCF-7 breast cancer cells, and the study illustrates that anti-NRP-1 mAb suppressed fibronectin and the formation of NRP-1-$\alpha5\beta1$ integrin complexes and, consequently, blocked focal adhesion kinase (FAK) signaling [140]. NRPa-308 is another antagonist against NRP-1, which was tested *in vitro* in MDA-MB-231 cells and showed an antiangiogenic and anti-proliferative effect. *In vivo*, in MDA-MB-231 xenografted models, this antagonist reduced the tumor growth and attenuated new vessel development, thus increasing the median survival of treated mice [141]. Dual targeting antibody IDB0076 against VEGF-A and NRP-1 showed no adverse effect when the toxicity assessment was done in cynomolgus monkeys. This antibody blocks pathways related to pro-angiogenesis and growth-related regulators [142]. Another mAb targeting NRP-1 was designed to have a high affinity for the NRP-1 receptor (A22p) linked with the C-terminus of Fc of human immunoglobulin G1 via a 15-residue $(G_4S)_3$ linker to produce Fc-A22p, Fc was added to enhance the penetration of the mAb to the tumor vessels and tissues and binds with NRP-1 in human umbilical vein endothelial (HUVEC) xenograft model. Additionally, the administration of anti-EGF receptor mAb cetuximab and the anti-HER2 mAb trastuzumab with NRP-1mAb (mAb-A22p) antibodies effectively improved the penetration to the extravascular tumor and enhanced ani-tumor efficacy [143].

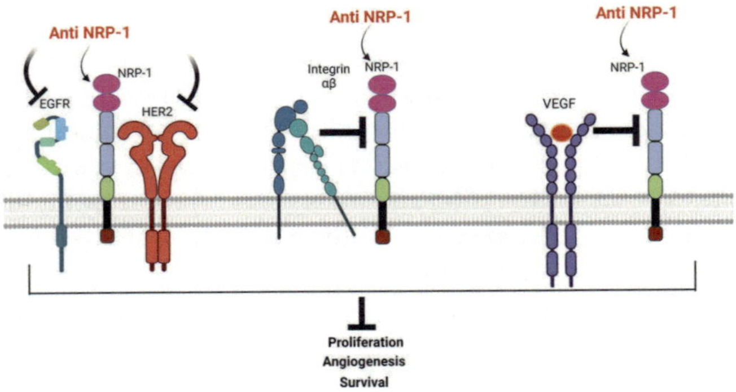

Figure 3.
Targeting NRP-1 by blocking the binding site for VEGF or Integrinαβ inhibits angiogenesis and cancer cell survival. Dual targeting of the NRP-1 and HER/EGFR axis would constrain cancer cell proliferation and survival. (The figure was created using BioRender).

The anti-NRP-1 suggested targeted therapies tested *in vitro* and *in vivo* in combination with other therapies showed promising results and thus encouraged further clinical trials to improve survival and reduce cellular proliferation and angiogenesis in TNBC (**Figure 3**).

7. NRP-1-targeted therapy in clinical trials

Although many antagonists, peptide-based and monoclonal antibodies against NRP-1 tested *in vitro* and *in vivo*, none reached the clinical trials except the monoclonal antibody MNRP1685A. MNRP1685A is a monoclonal antibody that was the first anti-NRP-1 to reach phase I clinical trials. A blood-based analysis was done when MNRP1685A was used in combination with bevacizumab to optimize the drug dose. The data showed that MNRP1685A suppresses the VEGF pathway and improves the blockage of the VEGF pathway mediated by bevacizumab, as proven by increased levels of plasma PLGF [144]. A phase Ia study of MNRP1685A showed that patients experience adverse side effects related to drug infusion with primary symptoms of pruritus, rash, and transient platelet count decreases and was controlled by premedication with dexamethasone [145, 146]. In the phase 1b trials, when MNRP1685A was tested with bevacizumab, high proteinuria was observed, discouraging further evaluation of MNRP1685A [147].

Since then, more antagonists, peptide-based and monoclonal antibodies, have been developed and shown promising *in vitro* and *in vivo* results, thus advocating for continued clinical trials to enhance patient survival, perhaps focusing on more personalized treatment fashion with the modern mode of drug delivery system will reduce the side effects seen in the past study. With the new research data showing NRP-1 is not acting only as a co-receptor for VEGFR2 but rather with HER-2 in the context of breast cancer, it is worth repeating the clinical trial precisely with patients that show high NRP-1 in resected tumors.

8. Challenges in translating anti-NRP-1 therapy to clinical trials

One of the main obstacles to targeting NRP-1 is that NRP-1 acts as a co-receptor for many molecules. NRP1 signals on multiple signaling pathways such as proliferation, metastasis, cell cycle progression, angiogenesis, and ECM remodeling [86, 148–151]. Therefore, targeting one region/site in the NRP-1 gene might affect specific pathways and show promising *in vitro* and *in vivo* results. Still, it might not show the expected outcomes when moved to clinical trials. This might be due to the limited *in vitro*/*in vivo* analysis to check the efficacy of the anti-NRP-1 therapy in different pathways. In addition, differences in the biology and tumor microenvironment between 2D culture, animal models, and humans might also have reduced the efficiency of targeting NRP-1 [152]. Furthermore, NRP-1 was also known to induce cell growth and resistance to therapy by evading the immune system [153], making it challenging to produce a safe and effective anti-NRP-1 therapy. Additionally, NRP-1 is involved in various pathways for normal endothelial cell development and axonal guidance [154]; thus, using NRP-1-interfering molecules might lead to side effects in clinical trials.

To address the challenges, targeting multiple molecules, including NRP-1 and associated molecules, could help decrease the rate of failed clinical trials. Combining NRP-1 inhibitors with specific nano-drug delivery systems may produce accurate outcomes and promising results and reduce side effects in clinical trials.

9. Conclusion

The chapter discussed the importance of NRP-1 as a potential drug target for TNBC and all the other associated molecules from the new data obtained from the next-generation sequencing and data analysis. New targets were developed to target NRP-1, ranging from small-molecule inhibitors, traditional monoclonal antibodies, and peptide-based monoclonal antibodies. Only a few clinical trials investigated the efficacy of targeting NRP-1, and the daily research shows evidence of the importance of NRP-1 and all the associated molecules and pathways in enhancing the metastatic ability of breast cancer cells and shutting this route will significantly reduce the burden of the tumor development and metastasis.

10. Future research recommendations

There is a demand for serious consideration of the data obtained and utilization in a clinical setting as a future outlook and based on the significant advancement in the methods of drug delivery systems that can be used to efficiently and specifically target the cells overexpressing NRP-1, such as the use of either cell-based, nanoparticles or combined therapies that can carry one of the binding ligands of NRP-1 and encapsulate the drugs targeting NRP-1 overexpressing cells precisely without interacting with the adjacent normal cells. Since Phase I clinical trials with targeted therapies showed much higher patient response rates and even faster FDA approvals compared with Phase I trials with chemotherapies, the best step forward regarding the compounds targeting NRP-1 and the associated cellular pathways is to start clinical trials that should be dependent on specialist's team decision that includes medical oncologists, research, and pharmaceutical companies. To tailor the trial, patients' histopathology, staging, and individualized treatment plans based on pharmacogenomics profiles should be the main determinants of the inclusion of patients. With that all, targeting NRP-1 based on patients' histopathology and disease status should benefit without the side effects seen with the usual drug delivery system used in the past.

Author details

Noura Al-Zeheimi[1*] and Sirin A. Adham[2]

1 Applied Biology Section, College of Applied Science and Pharmacy, University of Technology and Applied Sciences, Oman

2 Department of Biology, College of Science, Sultan Qaboos University, Muscat, Oman

*Address all correspondence to: noura.alzeheimi@utas.edu.om

References

[1] Kalli S et al. American joint committee on cancer's staging system for breast cancer: What the radiologist needs to know. Radiographics. 2018;**38**(7):1921-1933

[2] Giordano SH. Update on locally advanced breast cancer. The Oncologist. 2003;**8**(6):521-530

[3] Wang X et al. Radiomics predicts the prognosis of patients with locally advanced breast cancer by reflecting the heterogeneity of tumor cells and the tumor microenvironment. Breast Cancer Research. 2022;**24**(1):20

[4] Mathew J et al. Neoadjuvant chemotherapy for locally advanced breast cancer: A review of the literature and future directions. European Journal of Surgical Oncology (EJSO). 2009;**35**(2):113-122

[5] Rivenbark AG, O'Connor SM, Coleman WB. Molecular and cellular heterogeneity in breast cancer: Challenges for personalized medicine. The American Journal of Pathology. 2013;**183**(4):1113-1124

[6] Guo L et al. Breast cancer heterogeneity and its implication in personalized precision therapy. Experimental Hematology & Oncology. 2023;**12**(1):3

[7] Baird RD, Caldas C. Genetic heterogeneity in breast cancer: The road to personalized medicine? BMC Medicine. 2013;**11**:1-5

[8] Micheel CM, Nass SJ, Omenn GS. Omics-based clinical discovery: Science, technology, and applications. In: Evolution of Translational Omics: Lessons Learned and the Path Forward. Washington, DC: National Academies Press (US); 2012. PMID: 24872966. DOI: 10.17226/13297

[9] Marra A et al. Practical classification of triple-negative breast cancer: Intratumoral heterogeneity, mechanisms of drug resistance, and novel therapies. npj Breast Cancer. 2020;**6**(1):54

[10] Prat A et al. Clinical implications of the intrinsic molecular subtypes of breast cancer. The Breast. 2015;**24**:S26-S35

[11] Miglietta L et al. Clinical and pathological response to primary chemotherapy in patients with locally advanced breast cancer grouped according to hormonal receptors, Her2 status, grading and Ki-67 proliferation index. Anticancer Research. 2009;**29**(5):1621-1625

[12] Ellis MJ et al. Outcome prediction for estrogen receptor–positive breast cancer based on postneoadjuvant endocrine therapy tumor characteristics. Journal of the National Cancer Institute. 2008;**100**(19):1380-1388

[13] Hu R et al. Androgen receptor expression and breast cancer survival in postmenopausal women. Clinical Cancer Research. 2011;**17**(7):1867-1874

[14] Giovannelli P et al. The androgen receptor in breast cancer. Frontiers in Endocrinology. 2018;**9**:492

[15] Orrantia-Borunda E et al. Subtypes of breast cancer. Chapter 3, Breast Cancer [Internet]. 2022. PMID: 36122153. DOI: 10.36255/exon-publications-breast-cancer-subtypes

[16] Dai X et al. Cancer hallmarks, biomarkers and breast cancer molecular subtypes. Journal of Cancer. 2016;7(10):1281

[17] Group, E.B.C.T.C. Tamoxifen for early breast cancer: An overview of the randomised trials. The Lancet. 1998;**351**(9114):1451-1467

[18] Osborne CK. Tamoxifen in the treatment of breast cancer. New England Journal of Medicine. 1998;**339**(22):1609-1618

[19] Mustonen MV, Pyrhönen S, Kellokumpu-Lehtinen P-L. Toremifene in the treatment of breast cancer. World Journal of Clinical Oncology. 2014;**5**(3):393

[20] Hoy SM. Elacestrant: First approval. Drugs. 2023;**83**(6):555-561

[21] Zucchini G et al. Clinical utility of exemestane in the treatment of breast cancer. International Journal of Women's Health. 2015;**7**:551-563. DOI: 10.2147/IJWH.S69475

[22] Nathan MR, Schmid P. A review of fulvestrant in breast cancer. Oncology and Therapy. 2017;**5**:17-29

[23] Boér K. Fulvestrant in advanced breast cancer: Evidence to date and place in therapy. Therapeutic Advances in Medical Oncology. 2017;**9**(7):465-479

[24] Bhatnagar AS. The discovery and mechanism of action of letrozole. Breast Cancer Research and Treatment. 2007;**105**(Suppl. 1):7-17

[25] He D-X, Ma X. Clinical utility of letrozole in the treatment of breast cancer: A Chinese perspective. Oncotargets and Therapy. 2016;**9**:1077-1084. DOI: 10.2147/OTT.S81087. eCollection 2016

[26] Hortobagyi GN et al. Overall survival with ribociclib plus letrozole in advanced breast cancer. New England Journal of Medicine. 2022;**386**(10):942-950

[27] Nabholtz J et al. Anastrozole is superior to tamoxifen as first-line therapy for advanced breast cancer in postmenopausal women: Results of a North American multicenter randomized trial. Journal of Clinical Oncology. 2000;**18**(22):3758-3767

[28] Fala L. Verzenio (Abemaciclib) a New CDK4/CDK6 Inhibitor Approved for HR-Positive, HER2-Negative Advanced or Metastatic Breast Cancer. USA: Oncology Guide to FDA Approvals; 2018

[29] Serra F et al. Palbociclib in metastatic breast cancer: Current evidence and real-life data. Drugs in Context. 2019;**8**:212579. DOI: 10.7573/dic.212579. eCollection 2019

[30] Turner NC et al. Capivasertib in hormone receptor–positive advanced breast cancer. New England Journal of Medicine. 2023;**388**(22):2058-2070

[31] Chang D-Y, Ma W-L, Lu Y-S. Role of alpelisib in the treatment of PIK3CA-mutated breast cancer: Patient selection and clinical perspectives. Therapeutics and Clinical Risk Management. 2021;**17**:193-207. DOI: 10.2147/TCRM.S251668. eCollection 2021

[32] Royce ME, Osman D. Everolimus in the treatment of metastatic breast cancer. Breast Cancer: Basic and Clinical Research. 2015;**9**:BCBCR. S29268

[33] Zheng Y et al. Ado-tratuzumab emtansine beyond breast cancer: Therapeutic role of targeting other HER2-positive cancers. Frontiers in Molecular Biosciences. 2023;**10**:1165781

[34] Bradley R et al. Trastuzumab for early-stage, HER2-positive breast cancer: A meta-analysis of 13 864 women in seven randomised trials. The Lancet Oncology. 2021;**22**(8):1139-1150

[35] Hall PS, Bhosle J, Cameron DA. Lapatinib in the management of breast cancer. Clinical Practice. 2009;**6**(4):553

[36] Nelson MH, Dolder CR. A review of lapatinib ditosylate in the treatment of refractory or advanced breast cancer. Therapeutics and Clinical Risk Management. 2007;**3**(4):665-673

[37] Riera R et al. Lapatinib for treatment of advanced or metastasized breast cancer: Systematic review. Sao Paulo Medical Journal. 2009;**127**:295-301

[38] Siddiqui T et al. Enhertu (fam-trastuzumab-deruxtecan-nxki)–revolutionizing treatment paradigm for HER2-low breast cancer. Annals of Medicine and Surgery. 2022;**82**:104665. DOI: 10.1016/j.amsu.2022.104665

[39] Alasmari MM. A review of margetuximab-based therapies in patients with HER2-positive metastatic breast cancer. Cancers. 2022;**15**(1):38

[40] Chila G et al. The clinical efficacy and safety of neratinib in combination with capecitabine for the treatment of adult patients with advanced or metastatic HER2-positive breast cancer. Drug Design, Development and Therapy. 2021;**15**:2711-2720. DOI: 10.2147/DDDT.S281599. eCollection 2021

[41] Ishii K, Morii N, Yamashiro H. Pertuzumab in the treatment of HER2-positive breast cancer: An evidence-based review of its safety, efficacy, and place in therapy. Core Evidence. 2019;**14**:51-70. DOI: 10.2147/CE.S217848. eCollection 2019

[42] Murthy RK et al. Tucatinib, trastuzumab, and capecitabine for HER2-positive metastatic breast cancer. New England Journal of Medicine. 2020;**382**(7):597-609

[43] Ferroni P et al. Plasma plasminogen activator inhibitor-1 (PAI-1) levels in breast cancer–relationship with clinical outcome. Anticancer Research. 2014;**34**(3):1153-1161

[44] Gouri A et al. Plasminogen activator system and breast cancer: Potential role in therapy decision making and precision medicine. Biomarker Insights. 2016;**11**:105-111

[45] Duffy MJ. Urokinase plasminogen activator and its inhibitor, PAI-1, as prognostic markers in breast cancer: From pilot to level 1 evidence studies. Clinical Chemistry. 2002;**48**(8):1194-1197

[46] Witzel I et al. Role of urokinase plasminogen activator and plasminogen activator inhibitor mRNA expression as prognostic factors in molecular subtypes of breast cancer. Oncotargets and Therapy. 2014;7:2205-2213. DOI: 10.2147/OTT.S65344. eCollection 2014

[47] Lee J. Current treatment landscape for early triple-negative breast cancer (TNBC). Journal of Clinical Medicine. 2023;**12**(4):1524

[48] Schmid P et al. Pembrolizumab for early triple-negative breast cancer. New England Journal of Medicine. 2020;**382**(9):810-821

[49] Sabatier R et al. Prognostic and predictive value of PDL1 expression in breast cancer. Oncotarget. 2015;**6**(7):5449

[50] Caulfield SE, Davis CC, Byers KF. Olaparib: A novel therapy for metastatic breast cancer in patients with a BRCA1/2 mutation. Journal of the Advanced Practitioner in Oncology. 2019;**10**(2):167

[51] Dent RA et al. Phase I trial of the oral PARP inhibitor olaparib in combination

with paclitaxel for first-or second-line treatment of patients with metastatic triple-negative breast cancer. Breast Cancer Research. 2013;**15**:1-8

[52] Wang M, Chen S, Ao D. Targeting DNA repair pathway in cancer: Mechanisms and clinical application. MedComm. 2021;**2**(4):654-691

[53] Odunsi K, Pejovic T. Immune checkpoint and poly (ADP–ribose) polymerase inhibition for recurrent platinum-resistant ovarian and metastatic triple-negative breast cancers. JAMA Oncology. 2019;**5**(8):1103-1105

[54] de Nonneville A et al. Sacituzumab govitecan in triple-negative breast cancer. Annals of Translational Medicine. 2022;**10**(11):647, 1-6. DOI: 10.21037/atm-22-813

[55] Bardia A et al. Sacituzumab govitecan in metastatic triple-negative breast cancer. New England Journal of Medicine. 2021;**384**(16):1529-1541

[56] Mehraj U et al. Cryptolepine targets TOP2A and inhibits tumor cell proliferation in breast cancer cells-an in vitro and in silico study. Anti-Cancer Agents in Medicinal Chemistry (Formerly Current Medicinal Chemistry-Anti-Cancer Agents). 2022;**22**(17):3025-3037

[57] Vieira AF, Schmitt F. An update on breast cancer multigene prognostic tests—Emergent clinical biomarkers. Frontiers in Medicine. 2018;**5**:248

[58] Abdelhakam DA, Hanna H, Nassar A. Oncotype DX and Prosigna in breast cancer patients: A comparison study. Cancer Treatment and Research Communications. 2021;**26**:100306

[59] Kolodkin AL et al. Neuropilin is a semaphorin III receptor. Cell. 1997;**90**(4):753-762

[60] He Z, Tessier-Lavigne M. Neuropilin is a receptor for the axonal chemorepellent Semaphorin III. Cell. 1997;**90**(4):739-751

[61] Schwarz Q, et al. Neuropilin-Mediated Neural Crest Cell Guidance Is Essential to Organise Sensory Neurons into Segmented Dorsal Root Ganglia. Development. Jun 2009;**136**(11):1785-1789. DOI: 10.1242/dev.034322. Epub 2009 Apr 22

[62] Pellet-Many C et al. Neuropilins: Structure, function and role in disease. Biochemical Journal. 2008;**411**(2):211-226

[63] Wang L et al. Neuropilin-1-mediated vascular permeability factor/vascular endothelial growth factor-dependent endothelial cell migration. Journal of Biological Chemistry. 2003;**278**(49):48848-48860

[64] Van Meter ME, Kim ES. Bevacizumab: Current updates in treatment. Current Opinion in Oncology. 2010;**22**(6):586-591

[65] Kümler I, Christiansen OG, Nielsen DL. A systematic review of bevacizumab efficacy in breast cancer. Cancer Treatment Reviews. 2014;**40**(8):960-973

[66] Varella L, Abraham J, Kruse M. Revisiting the role of bevacizumab in the treatment of breast cancer. In: Seminars in Oncology. Seminars in Oncology. Aug 2017;**44**(4):273-285. DOI: 10.1053/j.seminoncol.2017.10.010. Epub 2017 Oct 24

[67] Naik A et al. Neuropilin-1 associated molecules in the blood distinguish poor prognosis breast cancer: A cross-sectional study. Scientific Reports. 2017;**7**(1):3301

[68] Al-Zeheimi N et al. Neoadjuvant chemotherapy alters neuropilin-1, PlGF,

and SNAI1 expression levels and predicts breast cancer patients response. Frontiers in Oncology. 2019;**9**:323

[69] Al-Zeheimi N et al. Neuropilin-1 knockout and rescue confirms its role to promote metastasis in MDA-MB-231 breast cancer cells. International Journal of Molecular Sciences. 2023;**24**(9):7792

[70] Wang L et al. VEGFA/NRP-1/GAPVD1 axis promotes progression and cancer stemness of triple-negative breast cancer by enhancing tumor cell-macrophage crosstalk. International Journal of Biological Sciences. 2024;**20**(2):446

[71] Ma X et al. Bioinformatics analysis and clinical significance of NRP-1 in triple-negative breast cancer. Heliyon. 2024;**10**(5):e27368. DOI: 10.1016/j.heliyon.2024.e27368. eCollection 2024 Mar 15

[72] Rachner TD et al. Soluble Neuropilin-1 is an independent marker of poor prognosis in early breast cancer. Journal of Cancer Research and Clinical Oncology. 2021;**147**:2233-2238

[73] Luo M et al. VEGF/NRP-1axis promotes progression of breast cancer via enhancement of epithelial-mesenchymal transition and activation of NF-κB and β-catenin. Cancer Letters. 2016;**373**(1):1-11

[74] Cheng W et al. NRP-1 expression in bladder cancer and its implications for tumor progression. Tumor Biology. 2014;**35**:6089-6094

[75] Oplawski M et al. Expression of NRP-1 and NRP-2 in endometrial cancer. Current Pharmaceutical Biotechnology. 2019;**20**(3):254-260

[76] Jubb AM et al. Neuropilin-1 expression in cancer and development. The Journal of Pathology. 2012;**226**(1):50-60

[77] Kamiya T et al. The preserved expression of neuropilin (NRP) 1 contributes to a better prognosis in colon cancer. Oncology Reports. 2006;**15**(2):369-373

[78] Okon IS et al. Aberrant NRP-1 expression serves as predicator of metastatic endometrial and lung cancers. Oncotarget. 2016;**7**(7):7970

[79] Wu Y-N et al. NRP1 is a prognostic factor and promotes the growth and migration of cells in intrahepatic cholangiocarcinoma. Cancer Management and Research. 2020;**12**:7021-7032. DOI: 10.2147/CMAR.S260091. eCollection 2020

[80] Seifi-Alan M et al. Neuropilin-1 expression is associated with lymph node metastasis in breast cancer tissues. Cancer Management and Research. 2018;**10**:1969-1974. DOI: 10.2147/CMAR.S169533. eCollection 2018

[81] Ferrario C et al. Expression of neuropilin-1 and related proteins in breast cancer. Cancer Research. 2006;**66**(Supplement 8):1182-1182

[82] Györffy B et al. An online survival analysis tool to rapidly assess the effect of 22,277 genes on breast cancer prognosis using microarray data of 1,809 patients. Breast Cancer Research and Treatment. 2010;**123**:725-731

[83] Naik A et al. Neuropilin-1 promotes the oncogenic tenascin-C/integrin β3 pathway and modulates chemoresistance in breast cancer cells. BMC Cancer. 2018;**18**:1-14

[84] Han Z et al. Effects of RNA interference-mediated NRP-1 silencing on the proliferation and apoptosis of

breast cancer cells. Molecular Medicine Reports. 2015;**12**(1):513-519

[85] Tang YH et al. Neuropilin-1 is over-expressed in claudin-low breast cancer and promotes tumor progression through acquisition of stem cell characteristics and RAS/MAPK pathway activation. Breast Cancer Research. 2022;**24**(1):8

[86] Glinka Y et al. Neuropilin-1 is expressed by breast cancer stem-like cells and is linked to NF-κB activation and tumor sphere formation. Biochemical and Biophysical Research Communications. 2012;**425**(4):775-780

[87] Zhang L et al. VEGF-A/neuropilin 1 pathway confers cancer stemness via activating Wnt/β-catenin axis in breast cancer cells. Cellular Physiology and Biochemistry. 2017;**44**(3):1251-1262

[88] Zhang L et al. miR-376a inhibits breast cancer cell progression by targeting neuropilin-1 NR. Oncotargets and Therapy. 2018;**11**:5293-5302. DOI: 10.2147/OTT.S173416. eCollection 2018

[89] Song Y et al. FOXO3a-driven miRNA signatures suppresses VEGF-A/NRP1 signaling and breast cancer metastasis. Oncogene. 2021;**40**(4):777-790

[90] Wang Y et al. NRP1 contributes to stemness and potentiates radioresistance via WTAP-mediated m6A methylation of Bcl-2 mRNA in breast cancer. Apoptosis. 2023;**28**(1):233-246

[91] Rodríguez-Pinilla SM et al. Prognostic significance of basal-like phenotype and fascin expression in node-negative invasive breast carcinomas. Clinical Cancer Research. 2006;**12**(5):1533-1539

[92] Ren Y et al. Constructing a novel prognostic model for triple-negative breast cancer based on genes associated with vasculogenic mimicry. Aging (Albany NY). 2024;**16**(9):8086

[93] Wagner K-U. Know thy cells: Commonly used triple-negative human breast cancer cell lines carry mutations in RAS and effectors. Breast Cancer Research. 2022;**24**(1):44

[94] Wang H et al. Systemic delivery of NAC-1 siRNA by neuropilin-targeted polymersomes sensitizes antiangiogenic therapy of metastatic triple-negative breast cancer. Biomacromolecules. 2020;**21**(12):5119-5127

[95] Zhang J et al. The miR-124-3p/neuropilin-1 axis contributes to the proliferation and metastasis of triple-negative breast cancer cells and co-activates the TGF-β pathway. Frontiers in Oncology. 2021;**11**:654672

[96] Hellec C et al. The pro-tumoral activity of heparan sulfate 3-O-sulfotransferase 3B (HS3ST3B) in breast cancer MDA-MB-231 cells is dependent on the expression of neuropilin-1. Molecules. 2018;**23**(10):2718

[97] Wang H et al. Neuropilin1, a novel independent prognostic factor and therapeutic target in triple-negative breast cancer. Neoplasma. 2020;**67**(6):1335-1342. DOI: 10.4149/neo_2020_191127N1223. Epub 2020 Jul 13

[98] Fertig EJ et al. Analysis of gene expression of secreted factors associated with breast cancer metastases in breast cancer subtypes. Scientific Reports. 2015;**5**(1):12133

[99] Zhang L et al. RNA binding protein PUM2 promotes the stemness of breast cancer cells via competitively binding to neuropilin-1 (NRP-1) mRNA with miR-376a. Biomedicine & Pharmacotherapy. 2019;**114**:108772

[100] Al-Zeheimi N, Adham SA. Modeling Neoadjuvant chemotherapy resistance in vitro increased NRP-1 and HER2 expression and converted MCF7 breast cancer subtype. British Journal of Pharmacology. 2020;**177**(9):2024-2041

[101] Maric G et al. GPNMB cooperates with neuropilin-1 to promote mammary tumor growth and engages integrin α5β1 for efficient breast cancer metastasis. Oncogene. 2015;**34**(43):5494-5504

[102] Goel HL, Mercurio AM. Enhancing integrin function by VEGF/neuropilin signaling: Implications for tumor biology. Cell Adhesion & Migration. 2012;**6**(6):554-560

[103] Fowler W. Defining the Roles of Endothelial Adhesion Receptors during Mammary Gland Development, Functional Differentiation, and Cancer. Norwich, UK: University of East Anglia; 2020

[104] Alharth AS, WA A. Tenascin-C (TNC) promotes breast cancer cell invasion and proliferation: Functional effects of TNC knockdown in highly invasive breast cancer cell lines. American Journal of Medical and Biological Research. 2015;**3**(2):55-61

[105] Oskarsson T et al. Breast cancer cells produce tenascin C as a metastatic niche component to colonize the lungs. Nature Medicine. 2011;**17**(7):867-874

[106] Katoh D et al. Tenascin-C induces phenotypic changes in fibroblasts to myofibroblasts with high contractility through the integrin αvβ1/transforming growth factor β/SMAD signaling axis in human breast cancer. The American Journal of Pathology. 2020;**190**(10):2123-2135

[107] Lingasamy P et al. Tumor-penetrating peptide for systemic targeting of tenascin-C. Scientific Reports. 2020;**10**(1):5809

[108] Lee YE, Hwang BH. Tumor homing peptides as fusion partners of therapeutic proteins for efficient delivery to cancer cells. Biotechnology and Bioprocess Engineering. 2023;**28**(3):483-490

[109] Zhang L et al. MiR-429 suppresses proliferation and invasion of breast cancer via inhibiting the Wnt/β-catenin signaling pathway. Thoracic Cancer. 2020;**11**(11):3126-3138

[110] Ma X-M. NRP-1 gene expression in nasopharyngeal carcinoma tissue and regulating effect of targeted inhibition of gene expression on cell function. Journal of Hainan Medical University. 2016;**22**(13):5-8

[111] Wu C et al. Neuropilin-1 interacts with fibronectin-1 to promote epithelial–mesenchymal transition progress in gastric cancer. Oncotargets and Therapy. 2020;**13**:10677-10687. DOI: 10.2147/OTT.S275327. eCollection 2020

[112] Wang Y et al. Systematic identification of the key candidate genes in breast cancer stroma. Cellular & Molecular Biology Letters. 2018;**23**:1-15

[113] Xie D et al. Four immune-related genes (FN1, UGCG, CHPF2 and THBS2) as potential diagnostic and prognostic biomarkers for carbon nanotube-induced mesothelioma. International Journal of General Medicine. 2021;**14**:4987-5003. DOI: 10.2147/IJGM.S324365. eCollection 2021

[114] Lynam L-R. Characterising the Role of Neuropilin-1 in Claudin-Low Breast Cancer. Australia: Queensland University of Technology; 2023

[115] Zhao H et al. The role of osteopontin in the progression of solid organ tumour. Cell Death & Disease. 2018;**9**(3):1-15

[116] Tuck AB, Chambers AF, Allan AL. Osteopontin overexpression in breast cancer: Knowledge gained and possible implications for clinical management. Journal of Cellular Biochemistry. 2007;**102**(4):859-868

[117] Chakraborty G, Jain S, Kundu GC. Osteopontin promotes vascular endothelial growth factor–dependent breast tumor growth and angiogenesis via autocrine and paracrine mechanisms. Cancer Research. 2008;**68**(1):152-161

[118] Chakraborty G et al. Curcumin suppresses breast tumor angiogenesis by abrogating osteopontin-induced VEGF expression. Molecular Medicine Reports. 2008;**1**(5):641-646

[119] Zhang L et al. Identification of potential genes related to breast cancer brain metastasis in breast cancer patients. Bioscience Reports. 2021;**41**(10):BSR20211615

[120] Chen D et al. ANTXR1, a stem cell-enriched functional biomarker, connects collagen signaling to cancer stem-like cells and metastasis in breast cancer. Cancer Research. 2013;**73**(18):5821-5833

[121] Chen W et al. CCL20 triggered by chemotherapy hinders the therapeutic efficacy of breast cancer. PLoS Biology. 2018;**16**(7):e2005869

[122] Kwantwi LB et al. Multifaceted roles of CCL20 (CC motif chemokine ligand 20): Mechanisms and communication networks in breast cancer progression. Bioengineered. 2021;**12**(1):6923-6934

[123] Méndez-García LA et al. Breast cancer metastasis: Are cytokines important players during its development and progression? Journal of Interferon & Cytokine Research. 2019;**39**(1):39-55

[124] Van Overmeire E et al. Mechanisms driving macrophage diversity and specialization in distinct tumor microenvironments and parallelisms with other tissues. Frontiers in Immunology. 2014;**5**:127

[125] Talkhoncheh MS et al. Abstract P2-20-08: Expression of ACVRL1 in a subset of recruited tumor-associated macrophages drives resistance to PD-1 therapy in human breast cancer. Cancer Research. 2023;**83**(Supplement 5):P2-20-08-P2-20-08

[126] Kilari S et al. Neuropilin-1 deficiency in vascular smooth muscle cells is associated with hereditary hemorrhagic telangiectasia arteriovenous malformations. JCI Insight. 2022;**7**(9):e155565. DOI: 10.1172/jci.insight.155565

[127] Aspalter IM et al. Alk1 and Alk5 inhibition by Nrp1 controls vascular sprouting downstream of Notch. Nature Communications. 2015;**6**(1):7264

[128] Eccles SA. The role of c-erbB-2/HER2/neu in breast cancer progression and metastasis. Journal of Mammary Gland Biology and Neoplasia. 2001;**6**:393-406

[129] Yu D, Hung MC. Role of erbB2 in breast cancer chemosensitivity. BioEssays. 2000;**22**(7):673-680

[130] Panis C et al. The positive is inside the negative: HER2-negative tumors can express the HER2 intracellular domain and present a HER2-positive phenotype. Cancer Letters. 2015;**357**(1):186-195

[131] Chang C et al. Extracellular glutathione peroxidase GPx3 and its role in cancer. Cancers. 2020;**12**(8):2197

[132] Lou W et al. Overexpression of GPX3, a potential biomarker for

diagnosis and prognosis of breast cancer, inhibits progression of breast cancer cells in vitro. Cancer Cell International. 2020;**20**:1-15

[133] Saelee P, Pongtheerat T, Sophonnithiprasert T. Reduced expression of GPX3 in breast cancer patients in correlation with clinical significance. Global Medical Genetics. 2020;7(03):087-091

[134] Mohamed MM et al. Promoter hypermethylation and suppression of glutathione peroxidase 3 are associated with inflammatory breast carcinogenesis. Oxidative Medicine and Cellular Longevity. 2014;**2014**(1):787195

[135] Demircan K et al. Serum selenium, selenoprotein P and glutathione peroxidase 3 as predictors of mortality and recurrence following breast cancer diagnosis: A multicentre cohort study. Redox Biology. 2021;**47**:102145

[136] Zhang M-L et al. Involvement of glutathione peroxidases in the occurrence and development of breast cancers. Journal of Translational Medicine. 2020;**18**:1-11

[137] Pan Q et al. Blocking neuropilin-1 function has an additive effect with anti-VEGF to inhibit tumor growth. Cancer Cell. 2007;**11**(1):53-67

[138] Borriello L et al. Structure-based discovery of a small non-peptidic Neuropilins antagonist exerting in vitro and in vivo anti-tumor activity on breast cancer model. Cancer Letters. 2014;**349**(2):120-127

[139] Feng G-K et al. SPECT and near-infrared fluorescence imaging of breast cancer with a neuropilin-1-targeting peptide. Journal of Controlled Release. 2014;**192**:236-242

[140] Zeng F et al. A monoclonal antibody targeting neuropilin-1 inhibits adhesion of MCF7 breast cancer cells to fibronectin by suppressing the FAK/p130cas signaling pathway. Anti-Cancer Drugs. 2014;**25**(6):663-672

[141] Liu W-Q et al. NRPa-308, a new neuropilin-1 antagonist, exerts in vitro anti-angiogenic and anti-proliferative effects and in vivo anti-cancer effects in a mouse xenograft model. Cancer Letters. 2018;**414**:88-98

[142] Ko J-H et al. Preclinical efficacy and safety of an anti-human VEGFA and anti-human NRP1 dual-targeting bispecific antibody (IDB0076). Biomolecules. 2020;**10**(6):919

[143] Shin T-H et al. Enhancement of the tumor penetration of monoclonal antibody by fusion of a neuropilin-targeting peptide improves the antitumor efficacy. Molecular Cancer Therapeutics. 2014;**13**(3):651-661

[144] Xin Y et al. Pharmacokinetic and pharmacodynamic analysis of circulating biomarkers of anti-NRP1, a novel antiangiogenesis agent, in two phase I trials in patients with advanced solid tumors. Clinical Cancer Research. 2012;**18**(21):6040-6048

[145] Weekes CD et al. A phase I study of the human monoclonal anti-NRP1 antibody MNRP1685A in patients with advanced solid tumors. Investigational New Drugs. 2014;**32**:653-660

[146] Weekes C et al. A first-in-human phase I study to evaluate the fully human monoclonal antibody MNRP1685A (anti-NRP1) administered intravenously every three weeks in patients with advanced solid tumors. Journal of Clinical Oncology. 2010;**28**(Suppl. 15):3014-3014

[147] Patnaik A et al. A phase Ib study evaluating MNRP1685A, a fully human

anti-NRP1 monoclonal antibody, in combination with bevacizumab and paclitaxel in patients with advanced solid tumors. Cancer Chemotherapy and Pharmacology. 2014;**73**:951-960

[148] Niland S, Eble JA. Neuropilins in the context of tumor vasculature. International Journal of Molecular Sciences. 2019;**20**(3):639

[149] Raimondi C. Neuropilin-1 enforces extracellular matrix signalling via ABL1 to promote angiogenesis. Biochemical Society Transactions. 2014;**42**(5):1429-1434

[150] Yaqoob U et al. Neuropilin-1 stimulates tumor growth by increasing fibronectin fibril assembly in the tumor microenvironment. Cancer Research. 2012;**72**(16):4047-4059

[151] Kiso M et al. Long isoform of VEGF stimulates cell migration of breast cancer by filopodia formation via NRP1/ARHGAP17/Cdc42 regulatory network. International Journal of Cancer. 2018;**143**(11):2905-2918

[152] Rizzolio S et al. Neuropilin-1 upregulation elicits adaptive resistance to oncogene-targeted therapies. The Journal of Clinical Investigation. 2018;**128**(9):3976-3990

[153] Chuckran CA et al. Neuropilin-1: A checkpoint target with unique implications for cancer immunology and immunotherapy. Journal for Immunotherapy of Cancer. 2020;**8**(2):e000967. DOI: 10.1136/jitc-2020-000967

[154] Gerhardt H et al. Neuropilin-1 is required for endothelial tip cell guidance in the developing central nervous system. Developmental Dynamics: An Official Publication of the American Association of Anatomists. 2004;**231**(3):503-509

Chapter 12

miRNA-Based Therapeutic Strategy and Its Application in Breast Cancer

Sema Misir, Serap Ozer Yaman, Osman Akidan, Ceylan Hepokur and Yuksel Aliyazicioglu

Abstract

Currently, microRNAs (miRNAs) have become a research hotspot in cancer and molecular biology. It is essential to reveal the biological effects of miRNAs on cancer development and progression, as well as their potential diagnostic and prognostic biomarkers and therapeutic targets for cancer treatment. miRNAs may be one of the critical molecular therapeutic targets in future personalized medicine. This chapter summarizes the research progress of miRNA biogenesis, biological functions, mechanisms, and potential application and highlights the clinical challenges in this field. Also, this chapter summarizes the research progress of miRNAs in body fluids as breast cancer biomarkers and their potential application, highlighting the clinical challenges in this field.

Keywords: biomarker, breast cancer, gene, non-coding RNA, miRNA

1. Introduction

Cancer is a pathological condition that occurs through a genetic and developmental process, resulting in excessive proliferation of cells and loss of their apoptosis functions [1]. Breast cancer (BC) is the most common cause of female cancer-related deaths, causing approximately half a million deaths each year [2]. Despite the advances in methods used today for breast cancer treatment, such as surgery, chemotherapy, radiotherapy, and hormone replacement, the expected improvement in advanced-stage disease is not at the desired level [1]. Chemotherapy is a frequently used method in the fight against cancer, but disadvantages such as ineffectiveness, severe toxicity, and multidrug resistance reduce the success rate [3]. Therefore, new strategies are needed to overcome resistance to anticancer drugs [4].

MicroRNAs (miRNAs), which are in the small RNA class, are non-coding RNA molecules. miRNAs play a role in various functions, such as cell proliferation, apoptosis, development, and metabolism. Many studies have been conducted on the role of miRNAs in cancer and various diseases [5, 6]. These studies have shown that miRNAs have provided essential clues in elucidating the molecular pathology of many types of cancer. Loss of function of miRNAs or their impact on the onset and progression of cancer, correction of these miRNAs, and the genes they regulate change the behavior of cancer cells [7]. Therefore, miRNAs are good targets for developing new therapeutic approaches and offer significant hope for treatment.

This book chapter discusses the biogenesis and functions of miRNAs and emphasizes their functions in breast cancer. Additionally, potential miRNA approaches and their clinical use in diagnosing and treating breast cancer are presented.

2. miRNAs

The genomes of eukaryotes are widely duplicated. Many non-coding RNAs (ncRNAs) influence intricate molecular and cellular processes in addition to protein-coding RNAs. Although much research has been carried out on messenger RNAs (mRNAs) as templates for protein synthesis, ncRNAs have been viewed as the byproducts of enormous transcription with less biological importance. As critical players in gene regulatory networks, ncRNAs work with other biomolecules, including DNAs, and proteins [8]. Generally speaking, ncRNAs can be categorized based on their length into small (less than 200 nucleotides) and large (more than 200 nucleotides) RNAs, or based on the roles they play as regulatory and housekeeping RNAs. miRNAs are a small subclass of ncRNAs [9]. Since their discovery, miRNAs have garnered much interest in scientific research since it has been determined that they function as transcriptional or post-transcriptional moderators to control gene expression. By enhancing the stimulation of oncogenic pathways and reducing the expression of tumor suppressors, miRNAs can regulate critical genes involved in the genesis of cancer, thereby impacting tumor growth, spread, and metastasis. Moreover, miRNAs become crucial mediators in the pathways underlying drug sensitivity and resistance [9, 10].

In 1993, the Ambros and Ruvkun groups found the first miRNA, lin-4, in *Caenorhabditis elegans*. miRNAs are short RNA transcripts consisting of 18–24 nucleotides and regulate gene expression at the translational level [11]. These are some of the ncRNAs that have been studied the most and are the best described. According to the conventional perspective, miRNAs are regarded as negative regulators of the expression of genes. When they attach to the 3′-untranslated sequence of the targeted mRNA, they might cause a translation block or transcript destruction. It suggests that miRNAs shuttle between different intracellular compartments to control the translation and even the rate of transcription [12].

2.1 miRNA biogenesis

MicroRNA biogenesis begins with posttranscriptional or co-processing of RNA polymerase II/III transcripts [13]. About half of the miRNAs that have been discovered to date are intragenic, meaning that they are mainly processed from introns and a small number of exons of genes that code for proteins; the other half are intergenic, meaning that they are transcribed without the assistance of their host gene and are controlled by their regulators [13, 14]. miRNAs can occasionally be transcribed in lengthy transcripts known as clusters, regarded as a family and may share seed regions [12, 14]. The miRNA biogenesis is classified into canonical and non-canonical pathways, as shown in **Figure 1.**

The main mechanism by which miRNAs are translated is the canonical biogenesis pathway. The RNA-binding protein DiGeorge Syndrome Critical Region 8

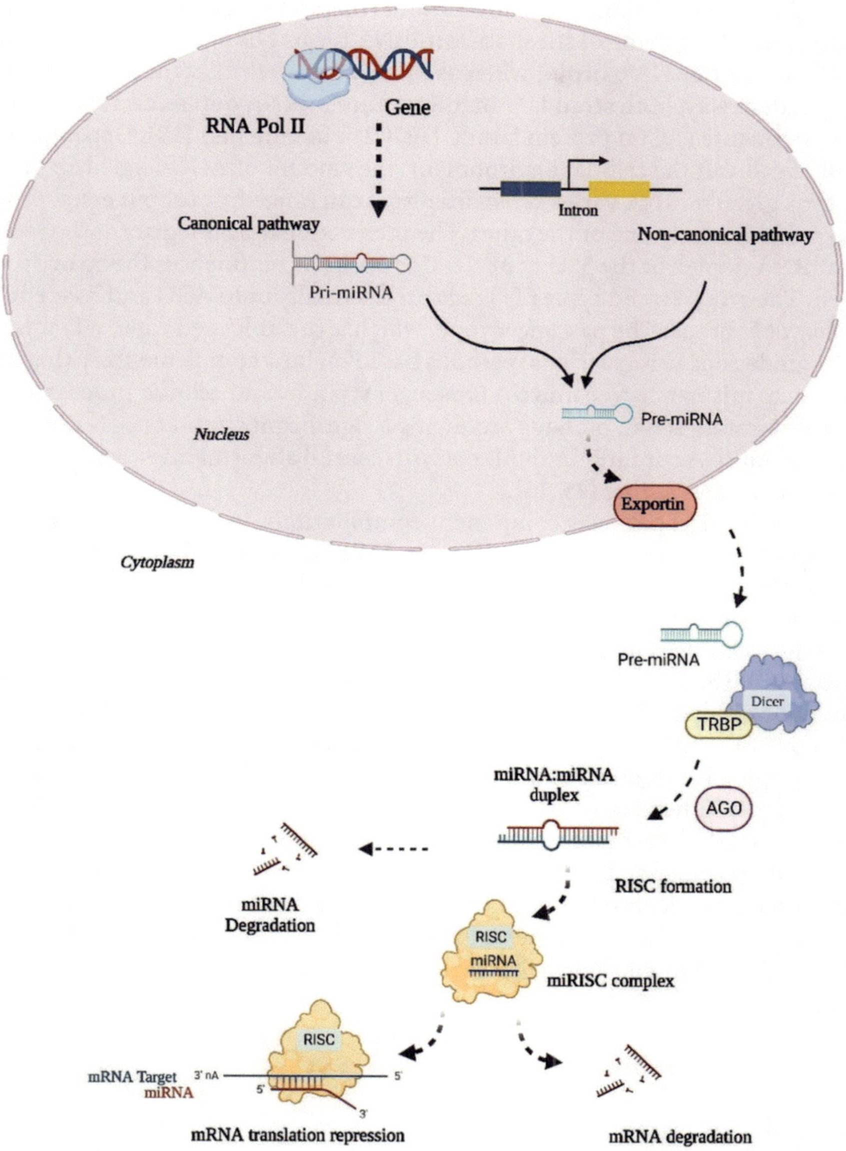

Figure 1.
Canonical/non-canonical miRNA biogenesis and miRNA-mediated gene silencing. pri-miRNA: primary miRNA, pre-miRNA: precursor microRNA, AGO: argonaute, TRBP: transactivation response element RNA-binding protein, RISC: RNA-induced silencing complex, miRISC; miRNA-induced silencing complex. This figure was created using BioRender.

(DGCR8) and the ribonuclease III enzyme Drosha form the microprocessor complex in this pathway, which converts pri-miRNAs that are transcribed from their genes into pre-miRNAs [15]. Drosha separates the pri-miRNA duplex at the base of its distinctive hairpin structure, whereas DGCR8 identifies additional motifs and an N6-methyladenylated GGAC within pri-miRNA. Consequently, the pre-miRNA develops a 2 nt 3′overhang [16]. An exportin 5 (XPO5)/RanGTP complex transports the newly formed pre-miRNAs into the cytoplasm, where the RNase III endonuclease Dicer breaks them down. This procedure causes the production of a mature miRNA duplex and involves the removal of the terminal loop. The directionality of the miRNA chain determines the name of the mature miRNA form. The 5p strand starts at the 5′ end of the pre-miRNA hairpin, whereas the 3p strand starts at the 3′ end. In an ATP-dependent way, both strands from the mature miRNA duplex can be transported into the Argonaute (AGO) protein family (AGO1-4 in humans) [15]. Depending on the kind of cell and the cellular environment, the amount of AGO-loaded 5p or 3p strand for a given miRNA varies substantially; it can range from about equal proportions to predominately one or the other. The thermodynamic integrity at the 5′ ends of the miRNA duplex or the 5′ U at nucleotide position 1 influences the 5p or 3p strand selection. The guide strand typically loads preferentially onto AGO and has reduced 5′ stability or 5′ uracil. The passenger rope, which is the unloaded rope, will unwind from the guide rope using various methods based on how complementary they are. AGO2 cleaves mismatch-free miRNA passenger strands, and cellular processes then break these strands down, perhaps producing a significant strand bias. If not loaded with AGO2, miRNAs or miRNA duplexes with central abnormalities are destroyed through passive unwinding [15, 16].

Various canonical pathway component combinations, including Drosha, Dicer, Exportin 5, and AGO2, are used in several non-canonical miRNA synthesis pathways. Non-canonical miRNA biogenesis may be broadly classified into routes that are Dicer-independent and those that are Drosha/DGCR8-independent. Pre-miRNAs derived from the Drosha/DGCR8-independent pathway bear similarities to substrates of the Dicer pathway. Mirtrons, created during splicing from mRNA introns, are one type of pre-miRNA [15, 17]. The pre-miRNA 7-methylguanosine (m7G) is one of them. Without undergoing Drosha cleavage, exportin 1 transports these developing RNAs straight to the cytoplasm. Strong 3p thread bias is probably caused by the m7G header, which prevents 5p threads from entering into AGO [16]. Conversely, Drosha processes endogenous short hairpin RNA (shRNA) transcripts to produce dicer-independent miRNAs [17]. Because these pre-miRNAs are short enough to become Dicer-substrates, they need AGO2 to finish maturing in the cytoplasm [15]. This facilitates the full loading of pre-miRNA onto AGO2 and the 3p chain's AGO2-dependent slicing. The 5p strand's maturation is finished by cutting its 3′–5′ segment [17].

2.1.1 Biological function and regulation of miRNAs

The biogenesis and function of miRNAs are associated with the molecular mechanisms of various clinical diseases. miRNAs are widely expressed and regulate many biological functions. They accomplish their purpose by adjusting translational and transcriptional processes. Specifically, they can control all facets of cellular activity, particularly the genesis and creation of tumors, differentiation and growth, metabolism, cell division, apoptosis, viral infection, and cellular activity [18]. miRNAs serve as tumor suppressors or oncogenes in cancer by acting as regulatory molecules. Previous studies have shown that miRNAs could play a role in the initiation and progression of specific cancer types by inhibiting the synthesis of oncogenes or anti-oncogenes [19]. miRNAs can function as oncogenes or tumor suppressors in specific situations. Dysregulated miRNAs have been shown to influence hallmarks of cancer, including sustaining proliferative signaling, evading growth suppressors, resisting cell death, activating invasion and metastasis, and inducing angiogenesis [18, 19].

3. Breast cancer and miRNAs

The condition known as BC is complicated and is marked by a variety of genetic changes. When skin cancers are excluded, BC accounts for about one in three cancer diagnoses among women in the United States, making it a particularly prevalent illness among women, according to the American Cancer Society. Over the past 10 years, technological advancements have improved researchers' understanding of this complicated illness. There are six main subtypes of BC based on phenotypic and gene expression profiles: basal-like, normal-like, claudin-low subtype, human epidermal growth factor receptor 2 (Her2)-enriched tumor, and luminal A, B, and C [20–22]. Luminal A is the most frequently absent subtype among them. Her2, B-cell lymphoma 2 (Bcl-2) expression, progesterone receptor (PR), and estrogen receptor (ER) are absent in it. About 50–60% of all BC cases are made up of it [21]. Research is still being conducted to link patterns of miRNA expression to a particular subtype. For instance, in ER, PR, and Her2 kinds of BC, miR-21, miR210, and miR-221 are highly overexpressed, whereas miR-10b, miR-145, miR-205, and miR-122a are significantly underexpressed. Furthermore, miR-21, miR-210, and miR-221 are crucial in triple-negative primary breast tumors (TNBC) because they are linked to the worse patients free of illness and overall survival (OS) [23, 24]. miRNAs may help determine BC subtype and prognosis, specifically using cancer samples to determine the status of ER, PR, and Her2. Crucially, this miRNA signature identifies targets for therapy and prognostic markers in addition to assisting in determining the BC phenotype [25].

3.1 Key miRNAs in breast cancer

Many miRNAs play a role in BC's initiation, progression and metastasis. In particular, three groups of miRNAs that can function as oncogenes or tumor suppressors or play a role in BC treatment resistance have a crucial role in BC. **Figure 2** summarizes the functional role of miRNAs in BC [24].

Regarding apoptosis, cell proliferation, migration and invasion, and metastasis, tumor suppressor gene(s) expression is often suppressed by oncogenic miRNAs, which are often overexpressed in cancer. Many noteworthy miRNAs are present as an oncomiR in cancer [26]. miR-10a and miR-10b consist of the miR-10 family, which is still in the Homeobox (Hox) cluster of evolutionary regulators. Since this group of miRNAs controls the transcripts encoding Hox, they probably have significant effects on development. Through miR-10a and miR-10b, respectively, the miR-10 family is reported to have a role in development and metastasis in the BC. The Homeobox D10 (HoxD10) gene has been reported to be significantly expressed and cause cell invasion and migration in a mouse xenograft model of BC. miR-10b may target e-cadherin, and there is a positive correlation between miR-10b expression and miR-10b. miR-10b's suppression of E-cadherin may influence BC metastasis. As a result, miR-10b might be one of the markers for BC's later stages and metastases [27].

One of the crucial miRNAs linked to BC cell invasion and migration is miR-21, which promotes tumor growth and metastasis. It was reported that microarray and northern blot investigations had revealed the abnormal expression of miR-21 and other miRNAs, such as miR-125b, miR-145, and miR-155, in human BC. Compared to corresponding normal breast tissues, miR-21 is significantly expressed in BC [28]. Maspin, a breast serine protease inhibitor, is well documented for its ability to prevent invasion and metastasis in BC by inducing apoptosis and suppressing invasion ability and angiogenesis.

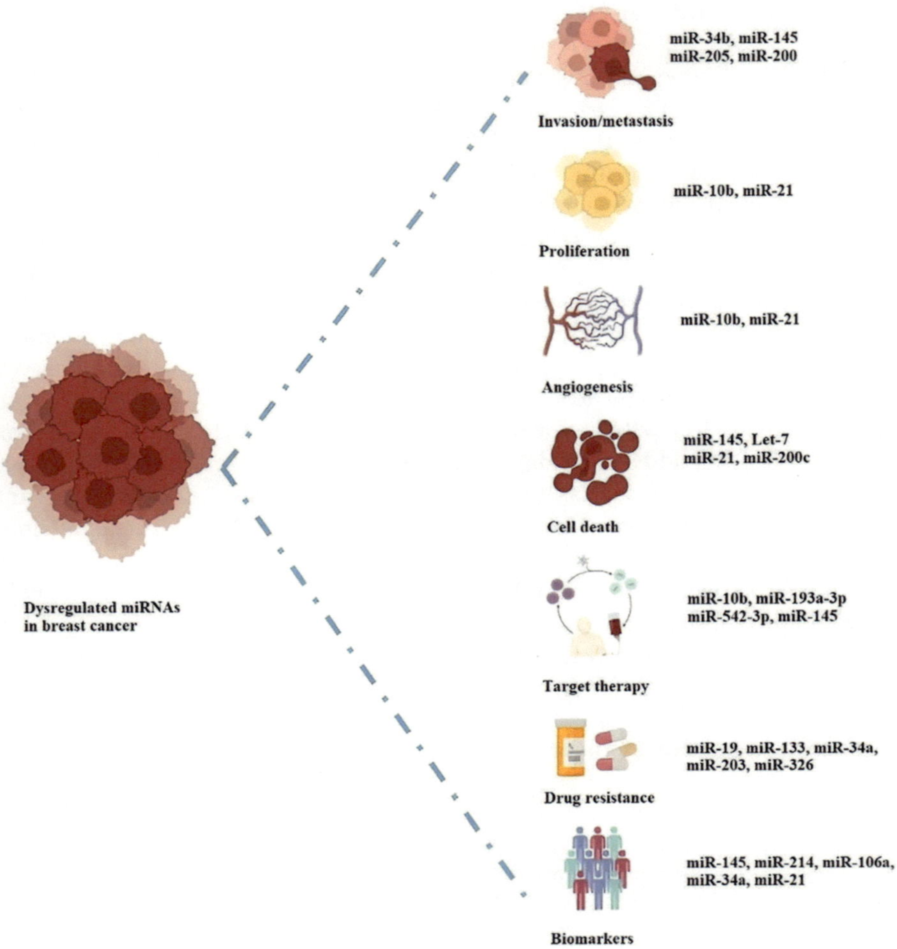

Figure 2.
miRNAs have many functional roles in BC, such as cell proliferation, tumor invasion, migration, angiogenesis, immune evasion, and chemotherapy resistance. This figure was created using BioRender.

Phosphatase and tensin homolog (PTEN) and miR-21 expression are inversely correlated in the breast cancer. Additionally, poor survival and advanced-stage metastases are linked to it. Transforming growth factor-β (TGF-β) is increased in BC [29, 30].

One polycistron in a DNA region that is elevated from human B-cell lymphomas is the miR-17–92 cluster. Six mature miRNAs are present, comprising miR-18b, miR-19b, miR-20a, and miR-92 in the miR-17–92 cluster. In lymphomas, this miRNA group is increased. Furthermore, the miRNA cluster might function as a suppressor of metastasis. However, unlike non-invasive MCF-7, invasive MDA-MB-231 BC cells have high levels of miR-17-5p expression. It has been demonstrated that breast cancer cells do not contain it. The HBP1/β-catenin pathway may be the target of ectopic production of such miRNA in MCF-7 cells, which could result in more invasive and migratory behaviors. Similarly, MDA-MB-231 cell migration and invasion are inhibited *in vitro* by downregulating miR-17-5p [31, 32].

The let-7 family consists of 10 members identified in humans, including let-7a, let-7b, let-7c, and let-7d. Normal physiological functions of Let-7 include muscle formation, cell adhesion, and gene expression and development regulation. It has been demonstrated that Lin28 functions as a post-transcriptional regulator to control let-7 biogenesis [33, 34]. Let-7 in breast cancer stem cells stimulates breast tumor-initiating cells and breast tumor-initiating cells (BT-IC) from primary BC for self-renewal, differentiation, and tumorigenesis. It was discovered that Let-7 family miRNAs were considerably lower in BT-IC and increased with differentiation. When overexpressed, let-7 decreases proliferation, BT-IC mammosphere development *in vitro*, carcinogenesis, and metastasis in NOD/SCID animals. This implies that let-7 modulates the stem cell-like characteristics of BT-IC by inhibiting several targets [33].

The miR-200 family consists of five members, including miR-200a, miR-200b, miR-200c, miR-141, and miR-429. The miR-200 family is a suppressor of epithelial-to-mesenchymal transition (EMT), partly mediated by regulating the E-cadherin transcriptional repressors ZEB1 and ZEB2 (also known as SIP1). The expression of E-cadherin is markedly increased by abnormal production of the miR-200 family, which also causes the cell shape to change into an epithelial phenotype. In this instance, the regulation of BC cell motility, stress fiber production, invasion, extension, and metastasis is attributed to miR-200c. The miR-200 family regulates many tumor suppressor genes. Conversely, this class of miRNAs controls the transcription factor ZEB (zinc finger) [35].

miR-145 is significantly downregulated in the BC sample compared to normal breast tissue. Similar to miR-205, there is a notable decrease in the expression of miR-145 in BC compared to normal breast tissue. The early appearance of elevated miR-145 expression in BC suggests that this miRNA may be an innovative biomarker for early-stage cancer identification with clinical diagnostic relevance. Through direct contact, miR-145 can directly target the production of the estrogen receptor-α (ER-α) protein and induce apoptosis in BC cells that express tumor protein 53 (TP53) in both the wild-type and ER-α positive forms [36].

3.2 miRNAs involved in breast cancer treatment resistance

Chemoresistance is one of the main drawbacks and challenges associated with treating BC. The majority of this resistance's causes are genetic and epigenetic changes. Multidrug resistance 1 (MDR1), which codes for P-glycoprotein, multidrug resistance-associated protein (MRPs), BC resistance protein (BCRP), and glutathione S-transferase π (GSTπ) are essential genes linked to drug resistance in BC [25]. The MDR1 gene is directly regulated in doxorubicin-resistant and sensitive MCF-7 and MDA-MB-231 cells by miR-451 and miR-298. These miRNAs can downregulate P-glycoprotein when overexpressed, which increases the cytotoxicity and nuclear localization of doxorubicin in resistant BC cells [37, 38]. The participation of breast cancer stem cells (BCSCs) is one of the challenges facing chemotherapy for BC. Cancer stem cells are also thought to play a role in the initiation, spread, and chemoresistance of BC. The ATP-binding cassette transporter proteins shield cells against chemotherapy through efflux pumping processes [39]. Thus, despite making up a minor portion of the BC population, BCSCs may have a significant role in chemoresistance. Here, miRNAs play a critical role in regulating the course of cancer growth and directly influencing resistance genes and cell expression [39, 40].

Since BC has been the most well-studied malignancy with regard to pathobiology, subtypes, and treatment, the function of miRNAs in BC is well-established. Most importantly, miRNAs elicit tissue- or cell-type-specific phenotypes through a complex mechanism that may depend on the cellular environment in which they exert their silencing roles. A better understanding of the miRNA network will open new approaches for diagnosing and treating BC. Under these circumstances, miRNAs could be useful biomarkers for forecasting prognosis and systemic therapeutic response in clinical settings. One promising strategy for treating drug resistance in BC is to target particular miRNAs within the drug resistance network. Specifically, combining various anticancer drugs with miRNA reagents, such as anti-miR-21, could lead to more successful treatment strategies. Thus, the development of miRNA-based targeted treatments and the effective identification of miRNA as cancer markers may be necessary for the clinical use of miRNA investigations [24, 40].

4. Therapeutic use of miRNAs

Understanding the role of miRNAs in BC's progression has enabled the development of targeted miRNA-based therapeutic strategies [41]. Therapeutic methods for miRNAs can be divided into two categories. The first is to inhibit oncogenes and oncogenic signaling pathways, and the second is to restore the expression of tumor suppressor genes [41, 42]. In order to recover miRNAs that are lost or down-regulated in cancer cells, miRNA mimics are employed in miRNA replacement therapy. Furthermore, carcinogenic miRNAs are inhibited or have their function lost by miRNA antagonists [42].

4.1 miRNA replacement therapy

MicroRNA mimics are used as miRNA-based therapies to increase anticancer activity. miRNA mimics, which are double-stranded structures, are small, synthetic sequences that can precisely match endogenous miRNAs. The objective is to restore or enhance suppressor miRNA expression that has been lost or decreased in diseases [43]. Studies conducted *in vivo* and *in vitro* have demonstrated promising results demonstrating the effectiveness of this treatment [41]. Strong tumor suppressor miR-542-3p targets the apoptotic suppressor survivin as well as p53. It has been observed that intracellular miR-542-3p substitute therapy increases apoptosis in TNBC cells through p53 activation and decreases survivin expression [44]. Another tumor suppressor molecule, miR-145, has therapeutic applications in treating BC, among other cancers. The miR-145 mimic investigation revealed that MCF-7 cell proliferation was inhibited [45]. It has been established that in TNBC patients, miR-4306 expression is linked to metastases of lymph nodes and poor patient survival. It has been observed that TNBC cell proliferation, angiogenesis, spread, and migration are considerably inhibited by increased expression of miR-4306 [46].

4.2 miRNA inhibitors

Oncogenic miRNAs are inhibited by anti-miRNA oligonucleotides (AMOs, antagomiRs) antagomiRs, miRNA sponges, and masks. The most common way to block miRNA function is to synthesize antisense oligonucleotides whose sequences match those of endogenous miRNAs. Antisense oligonucleotides that bind directly to miRNA and inhibit its function are collectively referred to as AMOs [47]. AMOs modify the amount of expression of genes and cellular activities that miRNA regulates by efficiently blocking its action. These highly stable compounds and particular oligonucleotides have undergone chemical modification [41]. Steric antisense oligonucleotides (ASOs) can inhibit the effect of miRNAs on target mRNAs because they have a high degree of specificity and affinity for particular miRNAs [48]. ASOs are chemically modified single-stranded molecules that imitate DNA. Their target is to mimic a particular mRNA and obstruct its translation; the length of these molecules ranges from 17 to 22 nt [47]. According to recent findings, antagomiRs' nucleotide backbone has undergone chemical modifications that improve their binding affinity, stability, and target regulation effects [43]. The 2′-O-methyl group (OMe) is one of the most frequently occurring chemical modifications to oligonucleotides. Because of their low toxicity, economical cost of synthesis, and strong affinity for targeting miRNAs, 2′-O-Me-modified AMOs are the most often employed compounds [49]. Compared to OMe analogs, other 2′-O-Methoxyethyl (MOE)-modified oligonucleotides exhibit greater binding affinity and selectivity to RNA. Modified oligonucleotides are becoming increasingly favored in clinical research [50]. Locked nucleic acids (LNA) are molecules that establish a duplex configuration with RNA molecules to give dynamic thermostability. As backbone oligonucleotides, miRNAs must be detected [51], and they could represent a novel class of therapeutics [47].

Analyzing the literature reveals that antisense miR-429 suppresses tumor growth in the HER2+ mouse model [52], while miR-10b antagonists have been demonstrated to reduce tumor formation in BC mouse models [53]. It has been shown that 2-O-methyl AMOs target miR-21 and are used as antagonists in BC [28]. According to a different study, antisense miR-21 oligonucleotide could help BC patients become trastuzumab-sensitive again [54].

Single-stranded miRNAs without a translational initiation codon are known as miRNA sponges. These synthetic miRNAs prevent the miRNA from binding to its intended target by having many binding regions for endogenous miRNAs. As a result, they have indirect influence over gene expression [41, 55]. Sponge inhibitors are used in long-term miRNA loss of function studies and *in vivo* analyses [47]. Adriamycin-based chemotherapy can more effectively target tumor cells when miR-3609 is implanted into MCF-7/ADR cells [56]. According to Lin et al., chemotherapeutic sensitivity was markedly enhanced by enhancing miR-133 production in cisplatin-resistant TNBC cells [57]. Consequently, focusing on oncomiRs presents a viable therapeutic strategy to raise BC cell susceptibility to chemotherapy [41]. By controlling the E-cadherin gene, Ma et al. demonstrated that miRNA sponges significantly prevented metastasis formation by suppressing miR-9 levels in BC cells [58]. The importance of miRNA sponges in cancer therapy is to mimic the downregulation of specific released miRNAs [47].

Target mRNA is degraded when miRNA masks attach to it with great affinity, creating a duplex in the process [59]. The effect of miRNAs in masking target mRNA is gene-specific [60]. The high efficiency of miRNA masking is based on target gene selection [47]. Recent advancements in miRNA treatment technology have shown the existence of miRNA masking oligonucleotide medicines (ONDs) that bind to mRNA [60]. Because many miRNAs operate as oncogenes or tumor suppressors, these molecules are regarded as effective therapeutic agents even if the medical application of miRNA remains in the preclinical and beginning clinical stages. Studies on miRNA's potential as a treatment is day by day [47].

5. miRNA-based delivery strategies

Despite recent advancements in miRNA treatments, many obstacles remain to be overcome before these molecules can be successfully used in clinical settings [41].

The main obstacle to the clinical application of miRNA therapeutics is the lack of an optimal miRNA delivery mechanism. High loading capacity, strong stability, extended half-life in circulation, gradual breakdown of miRNA payload, and minimal toxicity are desirable characteristics of miRNA transport mechanisms [59]. It is crucial to improve the long-term viability of miRNA mimics or antimiR and develop safe and effective delivery methods in order to introduce miRNA therapies into the clinic [42]. Currently, miRNA is transported effectively using viral and non-viral vectors [59]. The different systems available for miRNA delivery are shown in **Figure 3**.

Although these systems have various limitations, such as immune response, off-target effects, and poor endosomal escape, overcoming them holds great promise for personalized cancer therapy in the near future. However, comprehensive studies are needed to optimize and validate these strategies before drawing definitive conclusions and recommending miRNA-based cancer therapies for clinical practice [42, 59].

5.1 Viral-based miRNA delivery system

One of the most essential delivery methods for treating diseases is the employment of viral vectors, which are particularly good at delivering miRNA genes to particular target cells or tissues [61]. Gene therapy has long been used modified genetically viral vectors, retroviruses, lentiviruses, adenoviruses (ADVs), and adeno-associated viruses (AAVs). Transgenes encoding miRNA mimics or antagonists are intended to be delivered *via* them [62]. ADVs are viruses from the adenoviridae family with linear double-stranded DNA (dsDNA) [63]. They may set off immune responses that obstruct efficient gene transfer and ADV vector recycling [61]. According to Kim et al., *in vitro* and *in vivo*, transfected miR-145 imitating double-stranded

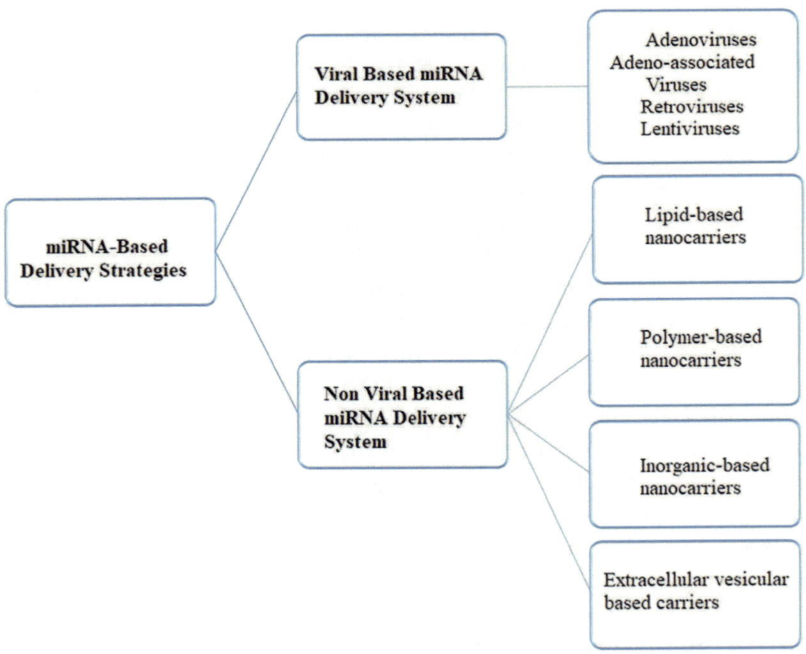

Figure 3.
Frequently used delivery techniques for RNA-based therapeutics. The many available miRNA delivery techniques can be divided into two categories: viral and non-viral vectors.

oligonucleotides decreased cell growth and infiltration upon transfection into BC cells [37]. Single-stranded linear DNA (ssDNA) is present in AAVs. Because these viruses can transduce proliferating and non-dividing cells, they are used as vectors in gene therapy. It is also essential that AAVs cannot be pathogenic and are not responsible for human cancer another crucial feature [61, 64]. It has been demonstrated that AAV systems provide a secure and practical approach to cancer treatment. Trepel et al. demonstrated that using a dual-target AAV vector to treat BC effectively inhibits tumor formation and manages adverse effects linked to collateral tropism [65, 66].

A family of enclosed viruses with single-stranded RNA (ssRNA) is known as retroviruses and lentiviruses, which are a subclass of retroviruses. These viruses use the reverse transcriptase enzyme to transcribe their genome into DNA. The integrase enzyme integrates the produced DNA into the host cell's genome. The steady production of target genes benefits significantly from this activity of retroviruses [61, 67]. Unlike retroviruses, lentiviruses can permanently transduce proliferating and non-dividing cells into the host genome [68]. Because they encourage fusion at active transcription locations, these vectors exhibit improved immunogenicity [64]. In a mouse model of BC, it has been demonstrated that intravenously administered lentivirus encoding miR-494 antagonists dramatically reduces tumor-infiltrating myeloid-derived suppressor cells (MDSCs), inhibiting tumor development and metastasis [69]. Despite their excellent transfection efficiency, the viral vectors have several issues, including immunogenicity, cytotoxicity, and production complexity [42]. These difficulties have made it possible to create and employ synthetic non-viral vectors that are safer and more efficient for the *in vivo* administration of RNA-based therapies [70].

5.2 Non-viral-based miRNA delivery system

Although effective, viral-based miRNA delivery systems have been replaced with less harmful and biocompatible non-viral delivery systems based on lipids, polymers, liposomes, and inorganic vectors [54].

5.2.1 Lipid-based nanocarriers

Lipid-based nanoparticles (LNPs) with biodegradability and low toxicity are one of the most preferred non-viral delivery systems for drug delivery, including miRNA delivery. To date, a variety of LNPs have been described, such as liposomes, micelles, solid lipid nanoparticles (SLNs), and stable nucleic acid-lipid particles (SNALPs) [70]. The core component of all LNPs is a liposome, which is chemically modified with hyaluronic acid (HA) and polyethylene glycol (PEG) to improve tumor-targeting properties and stability [47]. Phospholipid compositions, shapes, sizes, and surface charge properties can vary among liposomes. Depending on their size, liposomes are multilayered vesicles (MLVs) type liposomes with onion structure have a size range of 500 nm to 5 um, small monolayer vesicles (SUVs) have a size range of 20–200 nm, while large monolayer vesicles (LUVs) have a size range of 200 nm to 1 μm [70]. Owing to their strong affinity for the cell membrane, cationic, anionic, and neutral liposomes are utilized extensively [47]. miR-1296 was reportedly delivered to the MDA-MB-231 cells by Albakr et al. *via* a positively charged nano-liposome containing cholesterol and 1,2-dioleoyl-3 trimethylammonium-propane (DOTAP). miR-1296 enhanced BC cells' susceptibility to cisplatin by targeting Cyclin D1 (CCND1) [71]. According to Yang et al., antisense miR-191 has demonstrated a substantial potential for therapeutic benefit. Antisense miR-191 was reported to have boosted apoptotic cell death and decreased invasion in MCF-7 and ZR-75-1 cells, and its administration was accomplished by utilizing a stearylamine (SA)-based cationic liposome carrier system [72]. Another study found systemic liposomal miR-603 nanoparticle treatment for TNBC xenograft animal models decreased tumor formation and inhibited invasion [73]. Colloidal particles known as SLNs have a solid lipid core encircled by surfactants. Because cationic lipids are present, they have a strong affinity for nucleic acids [74]. SNALPs are FDA-approved instruments for siRNA drug delivery. Using PEG and siRNA that are 120 nm in size, SNALPs are lipid-based systems [75, 76]. For the *in vitro* and *in vivo* administration of siRNA and miRNA [77] for many tumor types, such as breast [78], prostate [79], cervical [80], and glioblastoma [70, 77], micelles represent a potential class of therapeutic lipid-based systems for administration.

Although miRNA delivery systems have proven to be a reliable platform for miRNA-based therapies, they can trigger hypersensitivity responses due to preferential accumulation in the reticuloendothelial system [61].

5.2.2 Polymer-based nanocarriers

Polymeric vectors are effective delivery systems for miRNA therapeutics due to their properties, such as high stability, low toxicity, biocompatibility, and biodegradability [47, 66]. Synthetic polymers such as polyethyleneimines (PEIs), poly lactic-co-glycolic acid (PLGA), dendrimers, and polyamidoamine (PAMAM) have shown effective in delivering miRNA-based cancer therapy [47]. PEIs are one of the most frequently used cationic polymers for miRNA delivery. Due to its high positive charge, PEI easily binds to negatively charged nucleic acids, protecting miRNAs from degradation and facilitating cell uptake. Due to their high charge density, they allow miRNAs to reach the cytoplasm by allowing endosomal escape [66]. miR-21 has an oncogenic effect on breast cancer. Gao et al. showed that it is possible to deliver anti-miR-21 with PLL. The G1 cell cycle arrest and enhanced production of caspase-3 mediated by the modified PEI complex (PEI-PLL) resulted in BC cell death [81]. It was reported that targeted transcription of miR-145 in metastatic breast cancer cells, mediated by cell-penetrating peptide (DS4-3) coupled branching PE (DS-bPEI), significantly inhibited cell proliferation and invasion [82].

As an FDA-approved transport vector that effectively facilitates miRNA transfer in cancer treatment, PLGAs have an established composition, are biodegradable and biocompatible, and permit regulated drug release into organs [47, 61]. Active targeting in cells or long-term circulation is made possible by LGA polymers modified with PEG, peptides, or antibodies. Antisense miR-21 and miR-10b were found to be efficiently transported by PLGA-PEG in triple-negative BC; as a result, the use of antisense miR-21 and miR-10b considerably reduced *in vitro* cell migration and invasiveness [83]. When delivered by PLGA nanoparticles in PLL, miR-34a was demonstrated to cause cell death in TNBC by targeting CCND1 and other receptors [84]. Another study found that antisense miR-21 coupled with orlistat-loaded PLGA nanoparticles increased the mortality of cancer and apoptotic cells [85]. Branched polymers having symmetrical structures or branches that start at the center and go outward toward the tip are known as dendrimers. The dendritic effect is a distinctive characteristic of dendrimers, since it is contingent upon the dimensions, composition, and level of collaboration among the outer functional categories of dendrimers [86]. The few polymers suitable for effective dispersion are polypropyleneimine (PPI), carbosilane, phosphorus-derived dendrimers, PAMAM, and PLL [87]. The most used delivery method for miRNA is PAMAM dendrimers [88]. One use of dendrimers as non-viral vectors for miRNA distribution is PAMAM, employed in BC treatment to deliver miR-205 mimics and antagomiR-221 [61, 84, 89]. It has been demonstrated that PAMAMs expressing miR-205 and 5-fluorouracil prevent BC from proliferating *in vivo* and *in vitro* [90]. Mei and colleagues employed PAMAM dendrimers to deliver miR-21 and taxol to BC cells. There was a notable enhancement in the cytotoxicity of taxol and a notable rise in MCF-7 cell apoptosis. Furthermore, it resulted in a significant reduction in the invasiveness of tumor cells [91].

5.2.3 Inorganic-based nanocarriers

Nanoparticles are one of the carrier systems that can help effectively deliver miRNA to target tissues or cells and achieve the necessary therapeutic effects [88]. Diabetes, neurological illnesses, metabolic problems, cardiovascular illnesses, and cancer can all be treated with these compounds [92]. miRNA is also transported by inorganic-based nanoparticles, including phosphate (CaP) [93], iron oxide [94], calcium gold [95], silica [96], carbon nanotubes [97], and carbon nanoparticles [94]. These structures offer a more significant concentration of miRNA to target cells or tissues, are more resistant to degradation, and are more accessible and faster in cellular delivery-specific qualities that vary depending on the material utilized [98, 99]. Numerous researches on using gold nanoparticles (AuNPs) for miRNA distribution in the treatment of BC have been conducted recently. According to Ekin et al., miR-145-loaded AuNPs elevated the expression miR-145 in prostate and BC cells [100]. In another investigation, replacement treatment resulting from the production of miR-708 mimics suppressed TNBC metastasis. PLL, miR-708 mimics, and gold nanoparticles were utilized [101]. Jing et al. developed AuNP-conjugated GNP-2′-2’-O-methyl DNA probes (AuNP-2’-OMe-DNA probes) to realize miR-21 detection and inhibition. Anti-miR-21 was shown to be effectively delivered to cells and inhibited its function by degrading miR-21, thus inhibiting proliferation and apoptotic cell death. A chemically modified miR-21 inhibitor based on gold nanoparticles could be a clinically promising diagnostic and therapeutic platform for BC [102].

5.2.4 Extracellular vesicular based carriers

Gene therapy also employs extracellular vesicles (EVs) as a delivery mechanism. EVs are divided into three groups: apoptotic bodies, microparticles, and exosomes [103]. The vesicle containing miRNAs is transported by exosomes, which are produced by the cell and act as a unique carrier system [104]. According to Ohno et al., delivering let-7a, a tumor suppressor, *via* exosomes stopped the growth and development of BC tumors [61]. Doxorubicin and miR-159-loaded exosomes have been shown in another study to improve anticancer activity and restrict invasion in TNBC cells [105].

6. miRNAs as biomarkers of breast cancer

One of the most effective ways to improve the performance of BC treatment and prevent death from this disease is to have an early/accurate diagnosis and sensitive/specific biomarkers that can predict effective treatments or measure the response to treatment [41, 106]. Early diagnosis of the disease, assessment of disease risk, and characterization of the prognosis for patients diagnosed with cancer are essential [106]. Therefore, new and more accurate biomarkers must be discovered to achieve the desired properties of personalized medicine [107]. miRNAs have become attractive prognostic diagnostic biomarkers because of their excellent stability and simplicity of detection in whole-blood, plasma, and serum samples specific to particular tissues or cell types [107, 108]. Many studies have shown that circulating miRNAs are valuable, non-invasive biomarkers for BC (**Table 1**). Currently, some clinical investigations look at circulating miRNAs as potential biomarkers for human BC liquid biopsies. These investigations are expected to demonstrate the potential of circulating miRNAs as a BC biomarker for prognosis and diagnosis [41].

miRNA	Source	Type of study	Potentials	AUC	Ref.
miR-214	Serum	Clinical study	Diagnostic	0.924	[109]
miR-106a	Serum	Prospective-non-randomize	Diagnostic	0.947	[110]
miR-10b	Serum	Clinical study	Diagnostic	0.98	[111]
miR-373	Serum	Clinical study	Diagnostic	0.98	[112]
miR-9 miR-34a	Tissues	Case-control	Diagnostic	0.71 and 0.72	[113]
miR-126-5p miR-144-5p miR-144 3p miR-301a-3p miR-126-3p miR-101-3p miR-664b-5p	Blood	Clinical trial	Diagnostic	0.814	[114]
miR-21 miR-27a	Blood	Case-control	Diagnostic	0.737 and 0.771	[115]
miR-1246 miR-1307 3p miR-4634 miR-6861-5p miR-6875-5p	Serum	Cohort study	Diagnostic	0.971	[116]
miR-1246 miR-206 miR-24 miR-373	Plasma	Cohort study	Diagnostic	0.992	[117]
miR-185-5p miR-362-5p	Plasma	Clinical trial	Diagnostic	0.957	[117]
miR21	Serum and tissues	Clinical trial	Prognostic	NR	[120]
miR-181a	Tissues	*In vitro* *In vivo*	Prognostic	NR	[121]
miR-21	Tissues	Retrospective cohort study	Prognostic	NR	[123]
miR-493	Tissues	Retrospective cohort study	Prognostic	NR	[124]
miR-210	Tissues	Experimental study	Prognostic	NR	[125]
miR-195	Tissue and blood	Cohort study	Prognostic	NR	[126]
miR-145	Blood	Cohort study	Prognostic	NR	[127]

AUC, area under the ROC curve; NR, information not reported.

Table 1.
miRNAs as diagnostic and prognostic biomarkers in BC.

When the literature is analyzed, numerous studies have demonstrated the usefulness of circulating miRNAs in diagnosing BC. Newly discovered miRNAs associated with BC include miR-214 [109], miR-106a [110], miR-10b [111], and miR-373 [112]. According to Orangi and Motovali-Bashi, BC Tissues exhibit downregulated levels of miR-9 and miR-34a. They claimed that in BC tumor samples, both miRNAs might be connected to tumor identification and stage [113]. Seven miRNA molecules (miR-126-5p, miR-144-5p, miR-144 3p, miR-301a-3p, miR-126-3p, miR-101-3p, and miR-664b-5p) were investigated for their diagnostic potential in a different study. According to TNBC [114], the miRNA molecules had the following values: specificity (74.2%), sensitivity (83.8%), accuracy (79%), and AUC (0.814). Li et al. also looked into the potential for miR-21 and miR-27a to be breast cancer detection tools. Both miRNAs were found to have high expressions in plasma; ROC curve analysis revealed that the AUC values for each miRNA were 0.737 and 0.771, respectively [115]. As an early diagnostic sign for breast cancer, a miRNA panel including the genes miR-1246, miR-1307 3p, miR-4634, miR-6861-5p, and miR-6875-5p has been discovered. The study examined the expression of miRNA in serum samples taken from patients suffering from benign breast illnesses, patients with breast cancer, and healthy controls. The high specificity and sensitivity of the miRNA panel have been demonstrated [116]. In their study by Jang et al., the combination of four miRNAs (miR-1246, miR-206, miR-24, and miR-373) showed an AUC of 0.992 [117]. According to Zhang et al.'s miRNA microarray studies in the blood of BC patients and healthy controls, miR-185-5p and miR-362-5p have marker potential [118]. As our knowledge of tumor biology develops, increasing miRNAs seem to function as prognostic indicators in BC [108]. Prognostic indicators include essential parameters such as OS, recurrence-free survival (RFS), response to specific treatment regimens, and metastasis [119].

This proactive approach can significantly improve patient outcomes and reduce the burden of recurrent BC [41]. For BC, miR-21 [120], miR-181a [121], and the miR-221/miR-222 cluster [122] are the most potentially prognostic miRNAs. Given that their overexpression is associated with advanced tumor stage, lymph node metastases, and poor patient survival, high expression of miR-21 in the tumor stroma was linked to a significantly worse clinical outcome in TNBC, and high expression of miR-21 in the tumor epithelium in ER+ and PR + HER2 patients was linked to a poor clinical outcome in another study [123]. Yao et al. demonstrated that the production level of miR-493 remained a critical predictive factor in BC even after adjusting for common clinicopathological variables [124]. Investigations were conducted on the gene expressions of miR-21 and miR-210 in BC tissue and their associations with clinicopathological characteristics and prognosis. According to reports, there is a substantial correlation between these molecules and differentiation, clinical stage, and lymph node metastases [125]. miR-195 was found to have prognostic qualities for the disease and considerably higher tumor expression in stage IV BC malignancies compared to stages I and II [126]. McGuire et al. stated that increased miR-21 and miR-145 expression was associated with non-response to neoadjuvant chemotherapy in luminal BC. These data highlight the exciting potential of miRNAs to help determine which patients will benefit from neoadjuvant chemotherapy and to help avoid unnecessary side effects in patients unlikely to respond [127].

Future research should examine sizable, thoroughly described, and stratified patient cohorts to assess the clinical value of miRNAs in BC fully. This method will provide a more precise and trustworthy assessment of miRNAs' prognostic and predictive potential in treating BC. Furthermore, these investigations should try to find new miRNAs that may function as useful biomarkers. In addition to deepening our knowledge of miRNAs' role in BC, the hunt for unidentified miRNAs may help future researchers create ground-breaking methods for diagnosis and treatment. Furthermore, it is critical to quantify miRNAs in extensive prospective multicenter studies comprising a range of patient groups spanning different tumor stages to completely ascertain the clinical value of miRNAs as diagnostic, prognostic, and predictive biomarkers. To guarantee the validity and dependability of the results, these investigations must be carried out independently.

7. Clinical use of miRNA

Surgery, radiation therapy, endocrine therapy, and chemotherapy are used to treat BC; nevertheless, problems such as drug resistance and adverse effects from long-term use of chemotherapeutic drugs remain, making the treatment of BC more difficult than expected. A successful therapeutic strategy must be created because of the significant morbidity and mortality rates associated with BC [128]. miRNAs are being studied for potential benefits in the treatment of BC since they are involved in the pathophysiology and progression of the disease [129]. The clinical application of miRNAs is still in its infancy, even though it has been established that miRNA-based treatments may represent the next wave of pharmaceuticals for treating numerous illnesses, including BC [130]. Although there are incredibly few clinical studies using miRNAs to treat BC, the fact that more research is being done in clinical trials is encouraging [129]. TransCode Therapeutics Inc. developed the anti-miR-10b nanoparticle formulation (TTX-MC138) for BC treatment and is a miR-10b inhibitor conjugated with dextran-coated iron oxide nanoparticles (https://www.transcodetherapeutics.com). TTX-MC138 is currently being tested in the preclinical stage for the treatment of metastatic breast cancer [131–134]. A synthetically modified miR-193a-3p mimic is called 1B3. INT-1B3, a different medication, is made with LNP and a miR-193a-3p mimic [135]. A phase 1 clinical trial is now being conducted on INT-1B3 (ClinicalTrials.gov identifier: NCT04675996). Many cancer cells, including TNBC, non-small-cell lung cancer, melanoma, colon cancer, and hepatocellular carcinoma were evaluated with the novel synthetic miR-193a-3p mimic 1B3. Reports state that 1B3 treatment inhibits the expression of many oncogenic pathways while promoting the PTEN tumor suppressor pathway. The difficulties in creating miRNA medications for cancer treatment are also evident in the clinical trials [134, 136]. Some of the difficulties include distributing miRNAs to target cells, guaranteeing their stability in blood circulation, and requiring efficient delivery mechanisms [137]. Many novel medications based on miRNA-based therapies will soon be available when these obstacles are removed. In particular, therapeutic miRNA regulation seems to be a great new option for systems that will be used in the future [130]. However, more research is required to validate recent discoveries and develop new miRNAs that can be used in therapeutic settings. This could result in better patient outcomes and offer insightful information on BC biology.

8. Conclusion

Breast cancer is a heterogeneous disease and is the most common cause of cancer death in women. Despite recent advances, cancer treatment requires extensive research and new strategies, given the limitations and side effects facing traditional treatments. The development of diagnostic, prognostic, and predictive techniques is crucial for the accurate diagnosis and management of breast cancer. The discovery of miRNAs as new therapeutic agents in breast cancer patient management, profiling these molecules in the disease, and understanding their mechanisms are significant. Studies have revealed that miRNAs regulate BC onset, progression, and treatment response by controlling many biological processes such as cell differentiation, cell cycle, apoptosis, angiogenesis, and metastasis. Therefore, it is inevitable that miRNAs will be used in BC diagnosis, prognosis, and prediction of recurrence and treatment response. In recent years, with the discovery of RNAi-based gene silencing strategy, there has been an increase in therapeutic applications for a wide range of diseases, including cancer. It is possible to increase many tumor suppressor miRNAs or inhibit oncogenic miRNAs using various techniques to target and suppress cancer-related genes. However, miRNA modulators need to be delivered to the target tissue precisely, efficiently, and securely to tumor locations for miRNAs to exhibit practical therapeutic effects. Various novel nanocarrier delivery systems have been developed for miRNA therapeutics.

Conflict of interest

The authors declare no conflict of interest.

Author details

Sema Misir[1*], Serap Ozer Yaman[2], Osman Akidan[3], Ceylan Hepokur[1] and Yuksel Aliyazicioglu[2]

1 Faculty of Pharmacy, Department of Biochemistry, Sivas Cumhuriyet University, Sivas, Turkey

2 Faculty of Medicine, Department of Medical Biochemistry, Karadeniz Technical University, Trabzon, Turkey

3 Department of Hematology, Mengücek Gazi Education and Research Hospital, Erzincan, Turkey

*Address all correspondence to: smisir@cumhuriyet.edu.tr

References

[1] Misir S, Aliyazicioglu Y, Demir S, Turan I, Hepokur C. Effect of Turkish propolis on miRNA expression, cell cycle, and apoptosis in human breast cancer (MCF-7) cells. Nutrition and Cancer. 2020;**72**(1):133-145. DOI: 10.1080/01635581.2019.1616100

[2] Power EJ, Chin ML, Haq MM. Breast cancer incidence and risk reduction in the Hispanic population. Cureus. 2018;**10**(2):e2235. DOI: 10.7759/cureus.2235

[3] Duo J, Ying GG, Wang GW, Zhang L. Quercetin inhibits human breast cancer cell proliferation and induces apoptosis via Bcl-2 and Bax regulation. Molecular Medicine Reports. 2012;**5**(6):1453-1456. DOI: 10.3892/mmr.2012.845

[4] McGuire A, Brown JAL, Kerin MJ. Metastatic breast cancer: The potential of miRNA for diagnosis and treatment monitoring. Cancer Metastasis Reviews. 2015;**34**(1):145-155. DOI: 10.1007/s10555-015-9551-7

[5] Su Z, Yang Z, Xu Y, Chen Y, Yu Q. MicroRNAs in apoptosis, autophagy and necroptosis. Oncotarget. 2015;**6**(11):8474-8490. DOI: 10.18632/ONCOTARGET.3523

[6] Li C, Hashimi SM, Good DA, Cao S, Duan W, Plummer PN, et al. Apoptosis and microRNA aberrations in cancer. Clinical and Experimental Pharmacology & Physiology. 2012;**39**(8):739-746. DOI: 10.1111/J.1440-1681.2012.05700.X

[7] Acunzo M, Romano G, Wernicke D, Croce CM. MicroRNA and cancer - A brief overview. Advances in Biological Regulation. 2015;**57**:1-9. DOI: 10.1016/J.JBIOR.2014.09.013

[8] Zhang P, Wu W, Chen Q, Chen M. Non-coding RNAs and their integrated networks. Journal of Integrative Bioinformatics. 2019;**16**(3):1-12. DOI: 10.1515/jib-2019-0027

[9] Ratti M, Lampis A, Ghidini M, Salati M, Mirchev MB, Valeri N, et al. MicroRNAs (miRNAs) and long non-coding RNAs (lncRNAs) as new tools for cancer therapy: First steps from bench to bedside. Targeted Oncology. 2020;**15**(3):261-278. DOI: 10.1007/s11523-020-00717-x

[10] He L, Hannon GJ. MicroRNAs: Small RNAs with a big role in gene regulation. Nature Reviews. Genetics. 2004;**5**(7):522-531. DOI: 10.1038/nrg1379

[11] Bartel DP. MicroRNAs: Genomics, biogenesis, mechanism, and function. Cell. 2004;**116**(2):281-297. DOI: 10.1016/s0092-8674(04)00045-5

[12] Brien JO, Hayder H, Zayed Y, Peng C. Overview of microRNA biogenesis, mechanisms of actions, and circulation. Frontiers in Endocrinology. 2018;**9**:1-12. DOI: 10.3389/fendo.2018.00402

[13] Ha M, Kim VN. Regulation of microRNA biogenesis. Nature Reviews. Molecular Cell Biology. 2014;**15**(8):509-524. DOI: 10.1038/nrm3838

[14] Kim YK, Kim VN. Processing of intronic microRNAs. The EMBO Journal. 2007;**26**(3):775-783. DOI: 10.1038/sj.emboj.7601512

[15] Ruby JG, Jan CH, Bartel DP. Intronic microRNA precursors that bypass Drosha processing. Nature. 2007;**448**(7149):83-86. DOI: 10.1038/nature05983

[16] Yang S, Maurin T, Robine N, Rasmussen KD, Jeffrey KL, Chandwani R,

et al. Conserved vertebrate mir-451 provides a platform for dicer-independent, Ago2-mediated microRNA biogenesis. Proceedings of the National Academy of Sciences of the United States of America. 2010;**107**(34):15163-15168. DOI: 10.1073/pnas.1006432107

[17] Cheloufi S, Dos SCO, Chong MMW, Hannon1 GJ. A dicer-independent miRNA biogenesis pathway that requires ago catalysis. Nature. 2010;**465**(7298):584-589. DOI: 10.1038/nature09092

[18] Huang Y, Shen XJ, Zou Q, Wang SP, Tang SM, Zhang GZ. Biological functions of microRNAs: A review. Journal of Physiology and Biochemistry. 2011;**67**(1):129-139. DOI: DOI

[19] Shenouda SK, Alahari SK. MicroRNA function in cancer: Oncogene or a tumor suppressor? Cancer Metastasis Reviews. 2009;**28**(3-4):369-378. DOI: 10.1007/s10555-009-9188-5

[20] Sørlie T, Tibshirani R, Parker J, Hastie T, Marron JS, Nobel A, et al. Repeated observation of breast tumor subtypes in independent gene expression data sets. Proceedings of the National Academy of Sciences of the United States of America. 2003;**100**(14):8418-8423. DOI: 10.1073/pnas.0932692100

[21] Sørliea T, Peroua CM, Tibshiranie R, Aasf T, Geislerg S, Johnsenb H, et al. Gene expression patterns of breast carcinomas distinguish tumor subclasses with clinical implications. The Journal of the Pakistan Medical Association. 2001;**98**(19):10869-10874. DOI: 10.1073/pnas.191367098

[22] Eroles P, Bosch A, Alejandro Pérez-Fidalgo J, Lluch A. Molecular biology in breast cancer: Intrinsic subtypes and signaling pathways. Cancer Treatment Reviews. 2012;**38**(6):698-707. DOI: 10.1016/j.ctrv.2011.11.005

[23] Radojicic J, Zaravinos A, Vrekoussis T, Kafousi M, Spandidos DA, Stathopoulos EN. MicroRNA expression analysis in triple-negative (ER, PR and Her2/neu) breast cancer. Cell Cycle. 2011;**10**(3):507-517. DOI: 10.4161/cc.10.3.14754

[24] Singh R, Mo Y-Y. Role of microRNAs in breast cancer. Cancer Biology & Therapy. 2013;**14**(3):201-212. DOI: 10.4161/cbt.23296

[25] Lowery AJ, Miller N, Devaney A, McNeill RE, Davoren PA, Lemetre C, et al. MicroRNA signatures predict oestrogen receptor, progesterone receptor and HER2/neu receptor status in breast cancer. Breast Cancer Research. 2009;**11**(3):1-18. DOI: 10.1186/bcr2257

[26] Zhang B, Pan X, Cobb GP, Anderson TA. microRNAs as oncogenes and tumor suppressors. Developmental Biology. 2007;**302**(1):1-12. DOI: 10.1016/j.ydbio.2006.08.028

[27] Lund AH. miR-10 in development and cancer. Cell Death and Differentiation. 2010;**17**(2):209-214. DOI: 10.1038/cdd.2009.58

[28] Si ML, Zhu S, Wu H, Lu Z, Wu F, Mo YY. miR-21-mediated tumor growth. Oncogene. 2007;**26**(19):2799-2803. DOI: 10.1038/sj.onc.1210083

[29] Bailey CM, Khalkhali-Ellis Z, Seftor EA, Hendrix MJC. Biological functions of maspin. Journal of Cellular Physiology. 2006;**209**:617-624. DOI: 10.1002/jcp.20782

[30] Guan-LI H, Zhang X-H, Guo G-L, Huang K-T, Kai-Yan Y, Shen X, et al. Clinical significance of miR-21 expression in breast cancer: SYBR-Green I-based real-time RT-PCR study of invasive ductal carcinoma. Oncology Reports. 2009;**21**(3):673-679. DOI: 10.3892/or_00000270

[31] Fassina A, Marino F, Siri M, Zambello R, Ventura L, Fassan M, et al. The miR-17-92 microRNA cluster: A novel diagnostic tool in large B-cell malignancies. Laboratory Investigation. 2012;**92**(11):1574-1582. DOI: 10.1038/labinvest.2012.129

[32] Hayashita Y, Osada H, Tatematsu Y, Yamada H, Yanagisawa K, Tomida S, et al. A polycistronic microRNA cluster, miR-17-92, is overexpressed in human lung cancers and enhances cell proliferation. Cancer Research. 2005;**65**(21):9628-9632. DOI: 10.1158/0008-5472.CAN-05-2352

[33] Yu F, Yao H, Zhu P, Zhang X, Pan Q, Gong C, et al. Let-7 regulates self renewal and tumorigenicity of breast cancer cells. Cell. 2007;**131**(6):1109-1123. DOI: 10.1016/j.cell.2007.10.054

[34] Wang X, Cao L, Wang Y, Wang X, Liu N, You Y. Regulation of let-7 and its target oncogenes (review). Oncology Letters. 2012;**3**(5):955-960. DOI: 10.3892/ol.2012.609

[35] Gregory PA, Bert AG, Paterson EL, Barry SC, Tsykin A, Farshid G, et al. The miR-200 family and miR-205 regulate epithelial to mesenchymal transition by targeting ZEB1 and SIP1. Nature Cell Biology. 2008;**10**(5):593-601. DOI: 10.1038/ncb1722

[36] Spizzo R, Nicoloso MS, Lupini L, Lu Y, Fogarty J, Rossi S, et al. miR-145 participates with TP53 in a death-promoting regulatory loop and targets estrogen receptor-α in human breast cancer cells. Cell Death and Differentiation. 2010;**17**(2):246-254. DOI: 10.1038/cdd.2009.117

[37] Kim SJ, Oh JS, Shin JY, Lee KD, Sung KW, Nam SJ, et al. Development of microRNA-145 for therapeutic application in breast cancer. Journal of Controlled Release. 2011;**155**(3):427-434. DOI: 10.1016/j.jconrel.2011.06.026

[38] Bao L, Hazari S, Mehra S, Kaushal D, Moroz K, Dash S. Increased expression of P-glycoprotein and doxorubicin chemoresistance of metastatic breast cancer is regulated by miR-298. The American Journal of Pathology. 2012;**180**(6):2490-2503. DOI: 10.1016/j.ajpath.2012.02.024

[39] Hirschmann-Jax C, Foster AE, Wulf GG, Nuchtern JG, Jax TW, Gobel U, et al. A distinct "side population" of cells with high drug efflux capacity in human tumor cells. Proceedings of the National Academy of Sciences of the United States of America. 2004;**101**(39):14228-14233. DOI: 10.1073/pnas.0400067101

[40] Ghafouri-Fard S, Khanbabapour Sasi A, Abak A, Shoorei H, Khoshkar A, Taheri M. Contribution of miRNAs in the pathogenesis of breast cancer. Frontiers in Oncology. 2021;**11**:1-20. DOI: 10.3389/fonc.2021.768949

[41] Muñoz JP, Pérez-Moreno P, Pérez Y, Calaf GM. The role of microRNAs in breast cancer and the challenges of their clinical application. Diagnostics. 2023;**13**(19):3072. DOI: 10.3390/diagnostics13193072

[42] El SSR, Cristante J, Guyon L, Denis J, Chabre O, Cherradi N. MicroRNA therapeutics in cancer: Current advances and challenges. Cancers (Basel). 2021;**13**(11):1-28. DOI: 10.3390/cancers13112680

[43] Rupaimoole R, Slack FJ. MicroRNA therapeutics: Towards a new era for the management of cancer and other diseases. Nature Reviews. Drug Discovery. 2017;**16**(3):203-221. DOI: 10.1038/nrd.2016.246

[44] Wang S, Zhang J, Wang Y, Chen M. Hyaluronic acid-coated PEI-PLGA nanoparticles mediated co-delivery of doxorubicin and miR-542-3p for

triple negative breast cancer therapy. Nanomedicine. 2016;**12**(2):411-420. DOI: 10.1016/j.nano.2015.09.014

[45] Tekie FSM, Atyabi F, Soleimani M, Arefian E, Atashi A, Kiani M, et al. Chitosan polyplex nanoparticle vector for miR-145 expression in MCF-7: Optimization by design of experiment. International Journal of Biological Macromolecules. 2015;**81**:828-837. DOI: 10.1016/j.ijbiomac.2015.09.014

[46] Zhao Z, Li L, Du P, Ma L, Zhang W, Zheng L, et al. Transcriptional downregulation of miR-4306 serves as a new therapeutic target for triple negative breast cancer. Theranostics. 2019;**9**(5):1401-1416. DOI: 10.7150/thno.30701

[47] Pagoni M, Cava C, Sideris DC, Avgeris M, Zoumpourlis V, Michalopoulos I, et al. miRNA-based technologies in cancer therapy. Journal of Personalized Medicine. 2023;**13**(11):1586. DOI: 10.3390/jpm13111586

[48] Lennox KA, Behlke MA. Chemical modification and design of anti-miRNA oligonucleotides. Gene Therapy. 2011;**18**(12):1111-1120. DOI: 10.1038/gt.2011.100

[49] Lennox KA, Owczarzy R, Thomas DM, Walder JA, Behlke MA. Improved performance of anti-miRNA oligonucleotides using a novel non-nucleotide modifier. Molecular Therapy Nucleic Acids. 2013;**2**:e117. DOI: 10.1038/mtna.2013.46

[50] Gleave ME, Monia BP. Antisense therapy for cancer. Nature Reviews. Cancer. 2005;**5**(6):468-479. DOI: 10.1038/nrc1631

[51] Válóczi A, Hornyik C, Varga N, Burgyán J, Kauppinen S, Havelda Z. Sensitive and specific detection of microRNAs by northern blot analysis using LNA-modified oligonucleotide probes. Nucleic Acids Research. 2004;**32**(22):e175. DOI: 10.1093/nar/gnh171

[52] Cava C, Novello C, Martelli C, Lodico A, Ottobrini L, Piccotti F, et al. Theranostic application of miR-429 in HER2+ breast cancer. Theranostics. 2020;**10**(1):50-61. DOI: 10.7150/thno.36274

[53] Zhang Q, Ran R, Zhang L, Liu Y, Mei L, Zhang Z, et al. Simultaneous delivery of therapeutic antagomirs with paclitaxel for the management of metastatic tumors by a pH-responsive anti-microbial peptide-mediated liposomal delivery system. Journal of Controlled Release. 2015;**197**:208-218. DOI: 10.1016/j.jconrel.2014.11.010

[54] Si H, Sun X, Chen Y, Cao Y, Chen S, Wang H, et al. Circulating microRNA-92a and microRNA-21 as novel minimally invasive biomarkers for primary breast cancer. Journal of Cancer Research and Clinical Oncology. 2013;**139**(2):223-229. DOI: 10.1007/s00432-012-1315-y

[55] Ebert MS, Sharp PA. MicroRNA sponges: Progress and possibilities. RNA. 2010;**16**(11):2043-2050. DOI: 10.1261/rna.2414110

[56] Li D, Wang X, Yang M, Kan Q, Duan Z. miR3609 sensitizes breast cancer cells to adriamycin by blocking the programmed death-ligand 1 immune checkpoint. Experimental Cell Research. 2019;**380**(1):20-28. DOI: 10.1016/j.yexcr.2019.03.025

[57] Lin Y, Lin F, Anuchapreeda S, Chaiwongsa R, Duangmano S, Ran B, et al. Effect of miR-133b on progression and cisplatin resistance of triple-negative breast cancer through FGFR1-Wnt-β-catenin axis. American Journal of Translational Research. 2021;**13**(6):5969-5984. eCollection 2021

[58] Ma L, Young J, Prabhala H, Pan E, Mestdagh P, Muth D, et al. miR-9, a MYC/MYCN-activated microRNA, regulates E-cadherin and cancer metastasis. Nature Cell Biology. 2010;**12**(3):247-256. DOI: 10.1038/ncb2024

[59] Menon A, Abd-Aziz N, Khalid K, Poh CL, Naidu R. miRNA: A promising therapeutic target in cancer. International Journal of Molecular Sciences. 2022;**23**(19):11502. DOI: 10.3390/ijms231911502

[60] Murakami K, Miyagishi M. Tiny masking locked nucleic acids effectively bind to mRNA and inhibit binding of microRNAs in relation to thermodynamic stability. Biomedical Reports. 2014;**2**(4):509-512. DOI: 10.3892/br.2014.260

[61] Yang M, Zhang Y, Li M, Liu X, Darvishi M. The various role of microRNAs in breast cancer angiogenesis, with a special focus on novel miRNA-based delivery strategies. Cancer Cell International. 2023;**23**(1):1-22. DOI: 10.1186/s12935-022-02837-y

[62] Fu Y, Chen J, Huang Z. Recent progress in microRNA-based delivery systems for the treatment of human disease. ExRNA. 2019;**1**:1-14. DOI: 10.1186/s41544-019-0024-y

[63] Douglas JT. Adenoviral vectors for gene therapy. Molecular Biotechnology. 2007;**36**(1):71-80. DOI: 10.1007/s12033-007-0021-5

[64] Pouya FD, Rasmi Y, Gazouli M, Zografos E, Nemati M. MicroRNAs as therapeutic targets in breast cancer metastasis. Drug Delivery and Translational Research. 2022;**12**(5):1029-1046. DOI: 10.1007/s13346-021-00999-2

[65] Trepel M, Körbelin J, Spies E, Heckmann MB, Hunger A, Fehse B, et al. Erratum: Treatment of multifocal breast cancer by systemic delivery of dual-targeted adeno-associated viral vectors. Gene Therapy. 2015;**22**(10):848. DOI: 10.1038/gt.2015.52

[66] Ahmadi SM, Amirkhanloo S, Yazdian-Robati R, Ebrahimi H, Pirhayati FH, Almalki WH, et al. Recent advances in novel miRNA mediated approaches for targeting breast cancer. Journal of Drug Targeting. 2023;**31**(8):777-793. DOI: 10.1080/1061186X.2023.2240979

[67] Pagès JC, Bru T. Toolbox for retrovectorologists. The Journal of Gene Medicine. 2004;**6**(1):67-82. DOI: 10.1002/jgm.498

[68] Greber UF, Fassati A. Nuclear import of viral DNA genomes. Traffic. 2003;**4**(3):136-143. DOI: 10.1034/j.1600-0854.2003.00114.x

[69] Liu Y, Lai L, Chen Q, Song Y, Xu S, Ma F, et al. MicroRNA-494 is required for the accumulation and functions of tumor-expanded myeloid-derived suppressor cells via targeting of PTEN. Journal of Immunology. 2012;**188**(11):5500-5510. DOI: 10.4049/jimmunol.1103505

[70] Kara G, Calin GA, Ozpolat B. RNAi-based therapeutics and tumor targeted delivery in cancer. Advanced Drug Delivery Reviews. 2022;**182**:114113. DOI: 10.1016/j.addr.2022.114113

[71] Albakr L, Alqahtani FY, Aleanizy FS, Alomrani A, Badran M, Alhindas H, et al. Improved delivery of miR-1296 loaded cationic nanoliposomes for effective suppression of triple negative breast cancer. Saudi Pharmaceutical Journal. 2021;**29**(5):446-455. DOI: 10.1016/j.jsps.2021.04.007

[72] Sharma S, Rajendran V, Kulshreshtha R, Ghosh PC. Enhanced

efficacy of anti-miR-191 delivery through stearylamine liposome formulation for the treatment of breast cancer cells. International Journal of Pharmaceutics. 2017;**530**(1-2):387-400. DOI: 10.1016/j.ijpharm.2017.07.079

[73] Bayraktar R, Pichler M, Kanlikilicer P, Ivan C, Bayraktar E, Kahraman N, et al. MicroRNA 603 acts as a tumor suppressor and inhibits triplenegative breast cancer tumorigenesis by targeting elongation factor 2 kinase. Oncotarget. 2017;**8**(7):11641-11658. DOI: 10.18632/oncotarget.14264

[74] Scheideler M, Vidakovic I, Prassl R. Lipid nanocarriers for microRNA delivery. Chemistry and Physics of Lipids. 2020;**226**:104837. DOI: 10.1016/j.chemphyslip.2019.104837

[75] Sarisozen C, Salzano GP, Torchilin V. Lipid-based siRNA delivery systems: Challenges, promises and solutions along the long journey. Current Pharmaceutical Biotechnology. 2016;**17**(8):728-740. DOI: 10.2174/1389201017666160401145319

[76] Singh A, Trivedi P, Jain NK. Advances in siRNA delivery in cancer therapy. Artificial Cells, Nanomedicine, and Biotechnology. 2018;**46**(2):274-283. DOI: 10.1080/21691401.2017.1307210

[77] Costa DF, Torchilin VP. Micelle-like nanoparticles as siRNA and miRNA carriers for cancer therapy. Biomedical Microdevices. 2018;**20**(3):59. DOI: 10.1007/s10544-018-0298-0

[78] Essex S, Navarro G, Sabhachandani P, Chordia A, Trivedi M, Movassaghian S, et al. Phospholipid-modified PEI-based nanocarriers for in vivo siRNA therapeutics against multidrug-resistant tumors. Gene Therapy. 2015;**22**(3):257-266. DOI: 10.1038/gt.2014.97

[79] Liu X, Liu C, Zhou J, Chen C, Qu F, Rossi JJ, et al. Promoting siRNA delivery via enhanced cellular uptake using an arginine-decorated amphiphilic dendrimer. Nanoscale. 2015;**7**(9):3867-3875. DOI: 10.1039/c4nr04759a

[80] Cunningham AJ, Gibson VP, Banquy X, Zhu XX, Jeanne LC. Cholic acid-based mixed micelles as siRNA delivery agents for gene therapy. International Journal of Pharmaceutics. 2020;**578**:119078. DOI: 10.1016/j.ijpharm.2020.119078

[81] Gao S, Tian H, Guo Y, Li Y, Guo Z, Zhu X, et al. MiRNA oligonucleotide and sponge for miRNA-21 inhibition mediated by PEI-PLL in breast cancer therapy. Acta Biomaterialia. 2015;**25**:184-193. DOI: 10.1016/j.actbio.2015.07.020

[82] Lee HJ, Namgung R, Kim WJ, Il KJ, Park IK. Targeted delivery of microRNA-145 to metastatic breast cancer by peptide conjugated branched PEI gene carrier. Macromolecular Research. 2013;**21**(11):1201-1209. DOI: 10.1007/s13233-013-1161-z

[83] Devulapally R, Sekar NM, Sekar TV, Foygel K, Massoud TF, Willmann JK, et al. Polymer nanoparticles mediated codelivery of AntimiR-10b and AntimiR-21 for achieving triple negative breast cancer therapy. ACS Nano. 2015;**9**(3):2290-2302. DOI: 10.1021/nn507465d

[84] Dzmitruk V, Apartsin E, Ihnatsyeu-Kachan A, Abashkin V, Shcharbin D, Bryszewska M. Dendrimers show promise for siRNA and microRNA therapeutics. Pharmaceutics. 2018;**10**(3):126. DOI: 10.3390/pharmaceutics10030126

[85] Song C, Xiao Y, Ouyang Z, Shen M, Shi X. Efficient co-delivery of microRNA 21 inhibitor and doxorubicin to cancer

cells using core-shell tecto dendrimers formed via supramolecular host-guest assembly. Journal of Materials Chemistry B. 2020;**8**(14):2768-2774. DOI: 10.1039/d0tb00346h

[86] Goyal R, Tripathi SK, Tyagi S, Sharma A, Ram KR, Chowdhuri DK, et al. Linear PEI nanoparticles: Efficient pDNA/siRNA carriers in vitro and in vivo. Nanomedicine. 2012;**8**(2):167-175. DOI: 10.1016/j.nano.2011.06.001

[87] Xing J, Jia J, Cong X, Liu Z, Li Q. N-isopropylacrylamide-modified polyethylenimine-mediated miR-29a delivery to inhibit the proliferation and migration of lung cancer cells. Colloids Surfaces B Biointerfaces. 2021;**198**:111463. DOI: 10.1016/j.colsurfb.2020.111463

[88] Shinde SS, Ahmed S, Malik JA, Hani U, Khanam A, Ashraf Bhat F, et al. Therapeutic delivery of tumor suppressor miRNAs for breast cancer treatment. Biology (Basel). 2023;**12**(3):467. DOI: 10.3390/biology12030467

[89] Conde J, Oliva N, Atilano M, Song HS, Artzi N. Self-assembled RNA-triple-helix hydrogel scaffold for microRNA modulation in the tumour microenvironment. Nature Materials. 2016;**15**(3):353-363. DOI: 10.1038/nmat4497

[90] Tang Q, Liu D, Chen H, He D, Pan W, Li Q, et al. Functionalized PAMAM-based system for targeted delivery of miR-205 and 5-fluorouracil in breast cancer. Journal of Drug Delivery Science and Technology. 2022;**67**:102959. DOI: 10.1016/j.jddst.2021.102959

[91] Mei M, Ren Y, Zhou X, Yuan XB, Han L, Wang GX, et al. Downregulation of miR-21 enhances chemotherapeutic effect of taxol in breast carcinoma cells. Technology in Cancer Research & Treatment. 2010;**9**(1):77-86. DOI: 10.1177/153303461000900109

[92] Puricelli C, Gigliotti CL, Stoppa I, Sacchetti S, Pantham D, Scomparin A, et al. Use of poly lactic-co-glycolic acid nano and micro particles in the delivery of drugs modulating different phases of ınflammation. Pharmaceutics. 2023;**15**(6):1772. DOI: 10.3390/pharmaceutics15061772

[93] Qiu C, Wei W, Sun J, Zhang HT, Ding JS, Wang JC, et al. Systemic delivery of siRNA by hyaluronan-functionalized calcium phosphate nanoparticles for tumor-targeted therapy. Nanoscale. 2016;**8**(26):13033-13044. DOI: 10.1039/c6nr04034a

[94] Luo X, Peng X, Hou J, Wu S, Shen J, Wang L. Folic acid-functionalized polyethylenimine superparamagnetic iron oxide nanoparticles as theranostic agents for magnetic resonance imaging and PD-L1 siRNA delivery for gastric cancer. International Journal of Nanomedicine. 2017;**12**:5331-5343. DOI: 10.2147/IJN.S137245

[95] Ding Y, Jiang Z, Saha K, Kim CS, Kim ST, Landis RF, et al. Gold nanoparticles for nucleic acid delivery. Molecular Therapy. 2014;**22**(6):1075-1083. DOI: 10.1038/mt.2014.30

[96] Wang Y, Xie Y, Kilchrist KV, Li J, Duvall CL, Oupický D. Endosomolytic and tumor-penetrating mesoporous silica nanoparticles for siRNA/miRNA combination cancer therapy. ACS Applied Materials & Interfaces. 2020;**12**(4):4308-4322. DOI: 10.1021/acsami.9b21214

[97] Mohammadi M, Salmasi Z, Hashemi M, Mosaffa F, Abnous K, Ramezani M. Single-walled carbon nanotubes functionalized with aptamer

and piperazine-polyethylenimine derivative for targeted siRNA delivery into breast cancer cells. International Journal of Pharmaceutics. 2015;**485**(1-2):50-60. DOI: 10.1016/j.ijpharm.2015.02.031

[98] Conde J, Ambrosone A, Hernandez Y, Tian F, McCully M, Berry CC, et al. 15 years on siRNA delivery: Beyond the state-of-the-art on inorganic nanoparticles for RNAi therapeutics. NanoToday. 2015;**10**(4):421-450. DOI: 10.1016/j.nantod.2015.06.008

[99] Jiang Y, Huo S, Hardie J, Liang§ X-J, Rotello VM. Progress and perspective of inorganic nanoparticles based siRNA delivery system. Expert Opinion on Drug Delivery. 2016;**13**(4):547-559. DOI: 10.1517/17425247.2016.1134486

[100] Ekin A, Karatas OF, Culha M, Ozen M. Designing a gold nanoparticle-based nanocarrier for microRNA transfection into the prostate and breast cancer cells. The Journal of Gene Medicine. 2014;**16**:331-335. DOI: 10.1002/jgm.2810

[101] Ramchandani D, Lee SK, Yomtoubian S, Han MS, Tung C-H, Mittal V. Nanoparticle delivery of miR-708 mimetic impairs breast cancer metastasis. Molecular Cancer Therapeutics. 2019;**18**(3):579-591. DOI: 10.1158/1535-7163.MCT-18-0702

[102] Li J, Huang J, Yang X, Yang Y, Quan K, Xie N, et al. Gold nanoparticle-based 2′-O-methyl modified DNA probes for breast cancerous theranostics. Talanta. 2018;**183**:11-17. DOI: 10.1016/j.talanta.2018.02.036

[103] Kosaka N, Iguchi H, Yoshioka Y, Takeshita F, Matsuki Y, Ochiya T. Secretory mechanisms and intercellular transfer of microRNAs in living cells. The Journal of Biological Chemistry. 2010;**285**(23):17442-17452. DOI: 10.1074/jbc.M110.107821

[104] Ohno SI, Takanashi M, Sudo K, Ueda S, Ishikawa A, Matsuyama N, et al. Systemically injected exosomes targeted to EGFR deliver antitumor microrna to breast cancer cells. Molecular Therapy. 2013;**21**(1):185-191. DOI: 10.1038/mt.2012.180

[105] Gong C, Tian J, Wang Z, Gao Y, Wu X, Ding X, et al. Functional exosome-mediated co-delivery of doxorubicin and hydrophobically modified microRNA 159 for triple-negative breast cancer therapy. Journal of Nanobiotechnology. 2019;**17**(1):1-18. DOI: 10.1186/s12951-019-0526-7

[106] Tarighati E, Keivan H, Mahani H. A review of prognostic and predictive biomarkers in breast cancer. Clinical and Experimental Medicine. 2023;**23**(1):1-16. DOI: 10.1007/s10238-021-00781-1

[107] Condrat CE, Thompson DC, Barbu MG, Bugnar OL, Boboc A, Cretoiu D, et al. miRNAs as biomarkers in disease: Latest findings regarding their role in diagnosis and prognosis. Cell. 2020;**9**(2):276. DOI: 10.3390/cells9020276

[108] Anilkumar KV, Rema LP, John MC, Vanesa John T, George A. miRNAs in the prognosis of triple-negative breast cancer: A review. Life Sciences. 2023;**333**:122183. DOI: 10.1016/j.lfs.2023.122183

[109] Schwarzenbach H, Milde-Langosch K, Steinbach B, Müller V, Pantel K. Diagnostic potential of PTEN-targeting miR-214 in the blood of breast cancer patients. Breast Cancer Research and Treatment. 2012;**134**(3):933-941. DOI: 10.1007/s10549-012-1988-6

[110] Mohmmed EA, Shousha WG, El-Saiid AS, Ramadan SS. A clinical evaluation of circulating miR-106a and Raf-1 as breast cancer diagnostic and prognostic markers. Asian Pacific. Journal of Cancer Prevention. 2021;**22**(11):3513-3520. DOI: 10.31557/APJCP.2021.22.11.3513

[111] Dwedar FI, Shams-Eldin RS, Nayer Mohamed S, Mohammed AF, Gomaa SH. Potential value of circulatory microRNA10b gene expression and its target E-cadherin as a prognostic and metastatic prediction marker for breast cancer. Journal of Clinical Laboratory Analysis. 2021;**35**(8):e23887. DOI: 10.1002/jcla.23887

[112] Bakr NM, Mahmoud MS, Nabil R, Boushnak H, Swellam M. Impact of circulating miRNA-373 on breast cancer diagnosis through targeting VEGF and cyclin D1 genes. Journal, Genetic Engineering & Biotechnology. 2021;**19**(1):84. DOI: 10.1186/s43141-021-00174-7

[113] Orangi E, Motovali-Bashi M. Evaluation of miRNA-9 and miRNA-34a as potential biomarkers for diagnosis of breast cancer in Iranian women. Gene. 2019;**687**:272-279. DOI: 10.1016/j.gene.2018.11.036

[114] Kahraman M, Röske A, Laufer T, Fehlmann T, Backes C, Kern F, et al. MicroRNA in diagnosis and therapy monitoring of early-stage triple-negative breast cancer. Scientific Reports. 2018;**8**(1):11584. DOI: 0.1038/s41598-018-29917-2

[115] Li M, Li Q, Yin Q, Wang Y, Shang JM, Wang LH. Evaluation of color doppler ultrasound combined with plasma miR-21 and miR-27a in the diagnosis of breast cancer. Clinical & Translational Oncology. 2021;**23**(4):709-717. DOI: 10.1007/s12094-020-02501-9

[116] Shimomura A, Shiino S, Kawauchi J, Takizawa S, Sakamoto H, Matsuzaki J, et al. Novel combination of serum microRNA for detecting breast cancer in the early stage. Cancer Science. 2016;**107**(3):326-334. DOI: 10.1111/cas.12880

[117] Jang JY, Kim YS, Kang KN, Kim KH, Park YJ, Kim CW. Multiple microRNAs as biomarkers for early breast cancer diagnosis. Molecular and Clinical Oncology. 2021;**14**(2):31. DOI: 10.3892/mco.2020.2193

[118] Zhang K, Wang YY, Xu Y, Zhang L, Zhu J, Si PC, et al. A two-miRNA signature of upregulated miR-185-5p and miR-362-5p as a blood biomarker for breast cancer. Pathology, Research and Practice. 2021;**222**:153458. DOI: 10.1016/j.prp.2021.153458

[119] Tariq M, Richard V, Kerin MJ. MicroRNAs as molecular biomarkers for the characterization of basal-like breast tumor subtype. Biomedicine. 2023;**11**(11):3007. DOI: 10.3390/biomedicines11113007

[120] Li J, Zhang Y, Zhang W, Jia S, Tian R, Kang Y, et al. Genetic heterogeneity of breast cancer metastasis may be related to miR-21 regulation of TIMP-3 in translation. International Journal of Surgical Oncology. 2013;**2013**:875078. DOI: 10.1155/2013/875078

[121] Taylor MA, Sossey-Alaoui K, Thompson CL, Danielpour D, Schiemann WP. TGF-β upregulates miR-181a expression to promote breast cancer metastasis. The Journal of Clinical Investigation. 2013;**123**(1):150-163. DOI: 10.1172/JCI64946

[122] Chen WX, Hu Q, Qiu MT, Zhong SL, Xu JJ, Tang JH, et al. MiR-221/222: Promising biomarkers for breast cancer. Tumor Biology.

2013;**34**(3):1361-1370. DOI: 10.1007/s13277-013-0750-y

[123] Mackenzie TA, Schwartz GN, Calderone HM, Graveel CR, Winn ME, Hostetter G, et al. Stromal expression of miR-21 identifies high-risk group in triple-negative breast cancer. The American Journal of Pathology. 2014;**184**(12):3217-3225. DOI: 10.1016/j.ajpath.2014.08.020

[124] Yao L, Liu Y, Cao Z, Li J, Huang Y, Hu X, et al. MicroRNA-493 is a prognostic factor in triple-negative breast cancer. Cancer Science. 2018;**109**(7):2294-2301. DOI: 10.1111/cas.13644

[125] Wu X. Expressions of MiR-21 and MiR-210 in breast cancer and their predictive values for prognosis. Iranian Journal of Public Health. 2020;**49**(1):21-29

[126] Heneghan HM, Miller N, Lowery AJ, Sweeney KJ, Newell J, Kerin MJ. Circulating micrornas as novel minimally invasive biomarkers for breast cancer. Annals of Surgery. 2010;**251**(3):499-505. DOI: 10.1097/SLA.0b013e3181cc939f

[127] McGuire A, Casey MC, Waldron RM, Heneghan H, Kalinina O, Holian E, et al. Prospective assessment of systemic microRNAs as markers of response to neoadjuvant chemotherapy in breast cancer. Cancers (Basel). 2020;**12**(7):1820. DOI: 10.3390/cancers12071820

[128] Zhang K, Zhang Y, Liu C, Xiong Y, Zhang J. MicroRNAs in the diagnosis and prognosis of breast cancer and their therapeutic potential (review). International Journal of Oncology. 2014;**45**(3):950-958. DOI: 10.3892/ijo.2014.2487

[129] Tomar D, Yadav AS, Kumar D, Bhadauriya G, Kundu GC. Non-coding RNAs as potential therapeutic targets in breast cancer. Biochimica et Biophysica Acta-Gene Regulatory Mechanisms. 2020;**1863**(4):194378. DOI: 10.1016/j.bbagrm.2019.04.005

[130] Chakraborty C, Sharma AR, Sharma G, Lee SS. Therapeutic advances of miRNAs: A preclinical and clinical update. Journal of Advanced Research. 2021;**28**:127-138. DOI: 10.1016/j.jare.2020.08.012

[131] Yoo B, Ghosh SK, Kumar M, Moore A, Yigit MV, Medarova Z. Design of nanodrugs for miRNA targeting in tumor cells. Journal of Biomedical Nanotechnology. 2014;**10**(6):1114-1122. DOI: 10.1166/jbn.2014.1795

[132] Farzin A, Etesami SA, Quint J, Memic A, Tamayol A. Magnetic nanoparticles in cancer therapy and diagnosis. Advanced Healthcare Materials. 2020;**9**(9):e1901058. DOI: 10.1002/adhm.201901058

[133] Weissleder R, Lee AS, Fischman AJ, Reimer P, Shen T, Wilkinson R, et al. Polyclonal human immunoglobulin G labeled with polymeric iron oxide: Antibody MR imaging. Radiology. 1991;**181**(1):245-249. DOI: 10.1148/radiology.181.1.1887040

[134] Kim T, Croce CM. MicroRNA: Trends in clinical trials of cancer diagnosis and therapy strategies. Experimental & Molecular Medicine. 2023;**55**(7):1314-1321. DOI: 10.1038/s12276-023-01050-9

[135] Telford BJ, Yahyanejad S, de Gunst T, den Boer HC, Vos RM, Stegink M, et al. Multi-modal effects of 1B3, a novel synthetic miR-193a-3p mimic, support strong potential for therapeutic intervention in oncology. Oncotarget. 2021;**12**(5):422-439. DOI: 10.18632/oncotarget.27894

[136] van den Bosch MTJ, Yahyanejad S, Alemdehy MF, Telford BJ, de Gunst T, den Boer HC, et al. Transcriptome-wide analysis reveals insight into tumor suppressor functions of 1B3, a novel synthetic miR-193a-3p mimic. Molecular Therapy Nucleic Acids. 2021;**23**:1161-1171. DOI: 10.1016/j.omtn.2021.01.020

[137] Raue R, Frank A-C, Syed SN, Brüne B. Therapeutic targeting of microRNAs in the tumor microenvironment. International Journal of Molecular Sciences. 2021;**22**(4):2210. DOI: 10.3390/ijms22042210

Chapter 13

Natural Polysaccharides in Breast Cancer: Fucoidan's Role in Enhancing Cisplatin Cytotoxicity and Reducing Chemotherapy Resistance

Reza Taghipour, Hadi Hassannia, Hesamoddin Arabnozari, Seyed Ehsan Enderami and Emran Habibi

Abstract

Cancer is one of the leading causes of death worldwide. Recent advancements in chemotherapy, particularly using natural drug-based strategies, have shown promise. This study evaluated the antitumor and anti-inflammatory effects of a combination of the brown alga *Sargassum ilicifolium* with cisplatin *in vitro*. After collecting and identifying the algae, fucoidan and alginate were extracted. The antioxidant activity was assessed using DPPH and Ferric Reducing Ability of Plasma (FRAP) assays. The cytotoxic effects on the MDA-MB-231 breast cancer cell line were evaluated in both 2D and 3D cultures using the XTT assay. Fucoidan and alginate yielded 7203 and 441 mg per 100 grams of dried algae, respectively. Total polysaccharide content in the fraction was estimated to be 89.39 mg/g dried algae weight. Fucoidan-rich extract exhibited higher antioxidant properties compared to alginate-rich extract. Also, the combination treatment significantly enhanced cytotoxicity, with the IC_{50} of fucoidan-rich extract reduced from 177.9 ± 8.7 to 79.3 ± 4.6 μg/ml in 2D culture when combined with cisplatin. In 3D culture, the IC_{50} decreased from over 800 ± 78.5 to 364.5 ± 41.7 μg/ml. Additionally, the fucoidan-rich extract significantly decreased IL-1β and IL-6 cytokine secretion in macrophages. These findings suggest combining cisplatin with fucoidan-rich extract enhances antitumor efficacy and may reduce chemotherapy side effects.

Keywords: alginate, breast cancer, cisplatin, fucoidan, MDA-MB-231

1. Introduction

Cancer remains one of the most critical global health challenges, with over 10 million new cases diagnosed annually. Cancer development is primarily driven by mutations in oncogenes that lead to a dominant gain of function, along with the dysfunction of tumor suppressor genes [1, 2]. Among women, breast cancer is the most common malignancy worldwide and is the leading cause of death from cancer. The incidence of breast cancer continues to increase globally, with more than one million new cases each year, accounting for approximately 25% of all cancers in women [3, 4].

Triple-negative breast cancer (TNBC) includes various diseases that differ in histologic, genomic, and immunologic profiles but share a lack of estrogen, progesterone, and HER2 receptors. TNBCs generally have a 5-year survival rate of 8–16% lower than hormone receptor-positive cancers and exhibit aggressive clinical behavior. They are more common in younger women and those of African or Hispanic descent, and they are the most frequent invasive breast cancer type in patients with BRCA1 germline mutations [5, 6]. MDA-MB-231 cells serve as a critical model for the mesenchymal subtype of triple-negative breast cancer (MES-TNBC). Due to its representative features, this cell line is widely used to study the characteristics and behaviors typical of MES-TNBC [7].

Chemotherapy often targets DNA, causing mutations or genome instability, a hallmark of cancer and aging. Various chemotherapeutic drugs are genotoxic, disrupting DNA metabolism through different mechanisms, each with unique biodistribution and kinetics [8]. Chemotherapeutic drugs are administered either before surgery (neoadjuvant therapy) or after surgery (adjuvant treatment) to selectively inhibit cancer cell proliferation and induce apoptosis. However, patients often experience moderate to severe side effects and may develop acquired drug resistance due to prolonged treatment [9]. Cisplatin, a platinum-based drug, works by binding to DNA and forming platinum-DNA adducts, which cause DNA damage, lead to G1/S phase arrest, and trigger apoptosis. Despite its side effects, cisplatin remains a crucial component of first-line treatments and is also used for patients with recurrent or metastatic cancer. While cisplatin is initially effective at destroying cancer cells, resistance to the drug eventually develops [10]. Cells resist cisplatin through various mechanisms, such as altering drug accumulation by reducing its uptake or increasing efflux. Additionally, they can neutralize the drug via redox-based detoxification, repair the cisplatin-induced DNA damage using excision repair pathways, or downregulate the apoptotic processes that the drug typically triggers [11]. Today, cancer treatment options include chemotherapy and radiotherapy, but plant-based phytotherapy also significantly contributes to cancer management. Phytotherapy can enhance the effectiveness of conventional treatments and may help mitigate side effects [12].

Sargassum ilicifolium (Turner) C. Agardh, a member of the *Sargassaceae* family, is a brown seaweed notable for its diverse biochemical constituents. This alga contains essential photosynthetic pigments, including chlorophyll and carotene. It also possesses a range of other compounds, such as steroids, terpenoids, mannitol, polysaccharides, and alginic acid. Additionally, its cell walls are rich in algin, and the cells feature plastids with thylakoidal lamellae, which are crucial for photosynthesis [12]. Fucoidan, a sulfated polysaccharide rich in fucose from brown algae like Sargassum, exhibits diverse biological activities, including antitumor, antioxidant, anti-inflammatory, anticoagulant, antiviral, and immune-regulating properties. Similarly, sodium alginate, derived from alginic acid and found in the cell walls, is valued in the food and pharmaceutical industries for its gelation and hydrophilic properties [13].

In vitro and *in vivo* studies on the ethyl acetate fraction (ETF) of brown algae *S. ilicifolium* demonstrated significant immunostimulatory effects on human neutrophils. Testing across concentrations from 10 to 100 µg/ml, the ETF notably enhanced chemotaxis, phagocytosis, and intracellular killing activities, particularly at 100 µg/ml. These findings highlight *S. ilicifolium*'s potential as a potent immunomodulator [14]. Fucoidans extracted from *Sargassum ilicifolium* show significant potential in inhibiting oxidative stress and gastric cancer pathogenesis in rats. The protective effects observed, including the improvement in mitochondrial structure, suggest that these benefits may be due to the high sulfate content in the fucoidans [15]. Phlorotannins, marine polyphenols abundant in brown seaweeds, enhance chemotherapy by promoting cancer cell apoptosis while protecting normal cells. When combined, phlorotannin (dieckol)-rich extracts from *Ecklonia cava* and cisplatin amplify apoptosis through increased reactive oxygen species (ROS) and inhibition of the Akt/NF-κB pathway. Additionally, these extracts help prevent cisplatin-induced kidney cell damage [16].

This study aims to evaluate and compare the anti-proliferative and anti-inflammatory effects of purified fucoidan and alginate extracted from *Sargassum ilicifolium* with the effects of the chemotherapeutic drug cisplatin on the MDA-MB-231 breast cancer cell line, a model for TNBC.

2. Materials and methods

2.1 Materials

The MDA-MB 231 human breast cancer cell line was supplied by the National Cell Bank of Iran (Pasteur Institute of Iran, Tehran, Iran). 2,2-Diphenyl-1-picrylhydrazyl (DPPH) polycaprolactone (PCL) (80,000 Mn), 2,4,6-Tri (2-pyridyl)-s-triazine (TPTZ), ammonium persulfate ($(NH_4)_2 S_2O_8$), *In vitro* Toxicology Assay Kit (XTT based), penicillin-streptomycin and butylated hydroxyanisole (BHA) were purchased from Sigma Aldrich™ (USA). Roswell Park Memorial Institute (RPMI) and fetal bovine serum (FBS) were purchased from GIBCO™ (USA). Acrylamide was purchased from Pharmacia™ (USA). The Total RNA Isolation kit (Hybrid RTM) was purchased from GeneAll™ (South Korea). SYBR® Premix Ex Taq (Tli RNase H Plus) was purchased from Takara Bio™ (Japan). High Capacity cDNA Reverse Transcription Kit was purchased from Applied Biosystems™ (USA). Pierce bicinchoninic acid (BCA) Protein Assay Kit was purchased from Thermo scientific™ (USA). Agarose gel, ethanol 96%, acetic acid (CH_3COOH), trypsin-ethylene diamine tetra acetic Acid (EDTA), and tetramethylethylenediamine (TEMED), Triton X-100, and Tris were purchased from Merck™ (Germany). All other chemicals and solvents were of the highest grade commercially available.

2.2 Sample preparation

S. ilicifolium was collected from the Persian Gulf Beach in Hormozgan province, Iran. The Taxonomy Laboratory at the Faculty of Pharmacy, Mazandaran University of Medical Science, Iran, identified and confirmed the sample to ensure accurate taxonomic classification. The brown algae were meticulously cleaned to remove epiphytes, waste, and necrotic tissue. After rinsing with fresh water, the algae were sun-dried and placed in an oven at 40°C for 2 days to ensure thorough dehydration. Then, a freeze dryer (Christ™, Germany) was employed at −20°C for 3 days. The dried algae were then finely cut and ground into a fine powder using a mixer grinder

(Yazicilar™, Turkey). The resulting powder was stored in a dry, clean, and sealed container to maintain its integrity.

2.3 Extraction and purification of sodium alginates

Alginate extraction from *S. ilicifolium* was conducted following a high-temperature alkaline extraction method, according to Bouissil et al. Initially, 85 grams of depigmented and dried algae were subjected to two rounds of treatment with 500 ml of 0.1 M HCl at 60°C, maintaining a pH of 2.0 with continuous stirring (Drawell™, China) at 250 rpm for 2 hours. The mixture was centrifuged (Kaida™, China) at 5000 rpm for 15 minutes at 4°C. The resulting residue, or pellet, was rinsed with distilled water and subsequently treated with a 3% w/v solution of sodium carbonate (Na_2CO_3) at pH 11.0 for 2 hours at 60°C, again under constant stirring. The supernatants from this process were collected and precipitated using three volumes of ice-cold 96% ethanol. The precipitate was further centrifuged and resuspended in distilled water before being acidified with 6 M HCl to a pH below 3.0, precipitating alginic acid. This acid was then redissolved in distilled water and neutralized to pH 7.5. The final purification of alginates involved three successive precipitations using ice-cold 96% ethanol. The resulting precipitate was resuspended in distilled water and lyophilized to produce powdered sodium alginates from *S. ilicifolium* algae [17].

2.4 Extraction and purification of fucoidan

Since fucoidans are polar, hydrophilic, and water-soluble macromolecules, water is an excellent solvent for their extraction. Fucoidan was extracted from 180 g of *S. ilicifolium* powder using 40 ml of water heated to 70°C. The extract was then purified through ethanol precipitation. To further remove alginate, 1.5 ml of 3 M $CaCl_2$ was added. Lipids and pigments were effectively eliminated using a solvent mixture of acetone and diethyl ether. Finally, the sediment was dried at 40°C for 24 hours, yielding a concentrated fucoidan extract [18, 19].

2.5 Preparation of polysaccharides from the algae

About 10 g of dried and finely *S. ilicifolium* algae was subjected to extraction using distilled water heated to 90°C in a water bath for 3 hours. Following this initial extraction, the mixture was filtered, and the remaining solid residue underwent a second extraction using distilled water under the same conditions for another 3 hours. The combined extracts were then centrifuged to eliminate any impurities. The clear supernatant obtained from this process was concentrated using rotary evaporation to refine the extract further [20].

2.6 Total carbohydrate determination

The phenol-sulfuric acid method was used to quantify the total carbohydrate content in polysaccharides. In this procedure, 2.5 ml of 96% sulfuric acid was added to 10 μL of the sample at a concentration of 1 mg/ml and to a series of standard glucose solutions ranging from 5 to 200 μg/ml. Then, 500 μL of a 4% phenol solution was quickly added into each tube. The resulting mixture was then incubated in a water bath at 90°C for 5 minutes. A standard curve was created using various concentrations of D-glucose to ensure accurate quantification [21].

2.7 Structural analysis of fucoidan and alginate

The UV–Vis absorbance spectrum of alginate extracted from *S. ilicifolium* was measured using a Double Beam T80 series spectrophotometer (PG Instruments™, China) across the 200–800 nm wavelength range. To analyze the composition and block structure of the extracted alginate, ^{1}H NMR spectroscopy was employed, with the alginate sample prepared at a concentration of 6 mg/ml in deuterium oxide (D_2O). For infrared (IR) analysis, the dried alginate sample was finely ground and mixed with anhydrous potassium bromide (KBr) to form pellets. The IR spectra were then recorded at room temperature, covering a frequency range of 650–4000 cm^{-1} using a Fourier-transform infrared (FTIR) spectrometer [22].

2.8 Determination of antioxidant capacity

2.8.1 DPPH assay

The DPPH assay is a widely used technique to assess the radical-scavenging potential of various compounds. DPPH exhibits a deep purple color in its stable form, which diminishes when it interacts with antioxidants that donate electrons to neutralize the free radicals. In this assay, 8 mg of a DPPH solution is mixed with 100 ml of methanol, and 2 ml of the test extract is added at various concentrations alongside ascorbic acid as a reference antioxidant. The mixtures are then incubated in the dark at room temperature for 30 minutes to allow the reaction to occur. After incubation, the absorbance of the solutions is measured at 517 nm. The inhibition percentage of the DPPH radical is determined using the following formula:

$$\text{Scavenging rate} = \left(\left(A_0 - A_S \right) / A_0 \right) \times 100 \tag{1}$$

A_0 represents the absorbance of the DPPH solution without the sample, and A_S is the absorbance with the sample present. The IC_{50} value, indicating the concentration required to neutralize 50% of the DPPH radicals, is then calculated from the standard curve [23].

2.8.2 Measurement of FRAP

Total antioxidant activity was assessed using the FRAP (ferric reducing ability of plasma) method, which measures the reduction of ferric ions (Fe^{3+}) to ferrous ions (Fe^{2+}) by antioxidants present in biological samples. In this procedure, 50 μL of serum was combined with 1.5 ml of FRAP reagent, prepared from 25 ml of 300 mM acetate buffer (pH 3.6), 2.5 ml of 10 mM TPTZ solution in 40 mM HCl, and 2.5 ml of 20 mM $FeCl_3$. The mixture was vortexed to ensure thorough mixing and then incubated at 37°C in a water bath for 5 minutes. The reaction's progress was monitored by measuring the absorbance at 593 nm, which corresponds to the formation of the Fe^2-TPTZ complex. A standard curve was generated using stock solutions of $FeSO_4{\cdot}7H_2O$ to quantify antioxidant activity at concentrations of 125, 250, 500, 750, and 1000 μM. The results were expressed as mM of Fe^{2+} per gram of dried mass [24].

2.9 Cell culture

MDA-MB 231 cells were cultured in RPMI-1640 medium enriched with 10% heat-inactivated fetal bovine serum (FBS), 100 IU/ml penicillin, and 100 μg/ml streptomycin. The cultures were maintained in a controlled environment at 37°C with 5%

CO_2 to ensure optimal growth conditions. The cells were subcultured twice weekly, starting at approximately 5 × 10^5 cells/ml density. Cell viability was assessed using the trypan blue exclusion method, which selectively stains non-viable cells, allowing for accurate viability measurements [25].

2.9.1 Cryopreservation of MDA-MB-231 cells

Cryopreservation is a critical method used to preserve the viability and functionality of cell lines for extended durations. The procedure begins by harvesting cells during their logarithmic growth phase. This is achieved by detaching the cells from the culture flask using 0.25% trypsin and EDTA. The detached cells are then washed with RPMI-1640 medium to remove residual trypsin and other impurities. The cells are counted using a hemocytometer to assess cell viability and concentration. Subsequently, 3 million cells are transferred into conical tubes and subjected to centrifugation at 1500 rpm for 5 minutes. After centrifugation, the supernatant is carefully discarded, leaving behind the cell pellet thoroughly resuspended in a suitable buffer. For each 3 million cells, 1 milliliter of freezing medium is added to cryovials. The vials are then cooled at a controlled rate, typically 1°C per minute, using a specialized freezer container (Mr. Frosty™, USA) down to −20°C for 1 hour. Subsequently, the vials are transferred to a −70°C freezer for 24 hours. Finally, the cryovials are stored in liquid nitrogen tanks for long-term preservation. Each cryovial is meticulously labeled with key information, including the cell type, date of freezing, and passage number [26].

2.9.2 Thawing procedure for cryopreserved cells

The thawing protocol is critical for the successful recovery of cryopreserved cells, ensuring they are viable for future experiments and applications in cell culture studies. Unlike the slow freezing process, thawing must be done quickly to avoid cellular damage from dimethyl sulfoxide (DMSO). The process begins with preparing the necessary equipment and culture medium under sterile conditions. Cryovials containing frozen cells are swiftly removed from liquid nitrogen storage and immersed in a 37°C water bath. This rapid thawing process is carefully monitored, with attention to the melting of DMSO, which has a higher freezing point. Once the ice crystals have fully dissolved, the cells are quickly transferred to a sterile conical tube containing RPMI medium supplemented with 10% FBS. The tube is then centrifuged at 1500 rpm for 5 minutes at room temperature to separate the cells from the residual DMSO. The supernatant, now containing the DMSO, is gently discarded to preserve the integrity of the cell pellet. Cell counting and viability assessments are then performed, typically using trypan blue exclusion or automated cell counting methods. The viable cells are seeded at the appropriate density into a T25 flask (SPL™, South Korea) containing a medium with 10% FBS. After a 24-hour incubation period, the culture medium is replaced to remove any remaining DMSO, and the cell's morphology is assessed using an inverted microscope.

2.10 Cytotoxicity evaluation of fucoidan, sodium alginates, and cisplatin on MDA-MB-231 cancer cells

To assess their response, MDA-MB-231 cell lines were exposed to a range of fucoidan (0–800 μg/ml), sodium alginates (0–350 μg/ml), and cisplatin (0–20 μg/ml) concentrations. IC50 was determined using the 2, 3-bis-(2-methoxy-4-nitro-5-sulfophenyl)-2H-tetrazolium-5-carboxanilide (XTT) colorimetric assay, which measures cell viability based on metabolic activity. In the experiment, 2×10^4 MDA-MB-231 cells were seeded into each well of a 96-well plate, followed by adding 0.1 ml of medium containing different concentrations of fucoidan, sodium alginates, and cisplatin. After incubating the cells for 48 hours at 37°C in a 5% CO_2 atmosphere, the XTT reagent was introduced to each well. The absorbance was then measured at 450 and 620 nm using a multifunctional ELISA reader. To ensure the reliability of the results, all experiments were repeated three times to ensure accuracy [27].

2.11 Drug interaction analysis in MDA-MB-231 cells

The analysis of drug interactions was conducted using CompuSyn software, which utilizes the modified Chou-Talalay Combination Index (CI) method. This software helps calculate the required doses of drugs, individually and in combination, to achieve specific levels of cytotoxicity. The software calculates a Combination Index (CI) for each cytotoxicity level to evaluate the drug interaction. In the study, MDA-MB-231 cells were treated with 3.6 μg (IC_{20}) of cisplatin and various concentrations of fucoidan and sodium alginates-rich extract to assess the interactions. The CI values were used to determine the type of interaction: synergistic ($CI < 1$), additive ($CI = 1$), or antagonistic ($CI > 1$).

The outcomes of these interactions were visualized using several plots:

i. *Dose-effect curve*: This plot shows the dose-response relationship for both the drug and the extract, individually and in combination.

ii. *Fa-CI plot*: It differentiates between antagonism ($CI > 1$) and synergism ($CI < 1$) based on the Combination Index.

iii. *Median-effect plot*: This plot illustrates the relationship between the drug dose (Log D) and the effect (Log Fa/Fu). The IC_{50} value is identified where the curve intersects the X-axis.

iv. *Dose-normalized isobologram*: Points on this plot show the interaction between the drug and the extract, indicating synergism, antagonism, or an additive effect based on their position relative to the diagonal line [28].

2.12 Measurement of IL-1 and IL-6 from a THP-1 monocyte cell line stimulated with bacterial lipopolysaccharide (LPS) and treated with non-toxic concentrations of an alginate and fucoidan-rich extract

Human acute monocytic leukemia cells (THP-1) supplied by Pasteur Institute of Iran were cultured in RPMI 1640 medium with 10% fetal bovine serum and 100 μM penicillin-streptomycin under conditions of 95% air and 5% CO_2. In the experiment, 4×10^4 Differentiated THP-1 cells were seeded into each well of a 96-well plate and then exposed to 1 μg/ml of bacterial LPS for 24 hours along with concentrations of 5 and 50 μg/ml of fucoidan-rich extract and with concentrations of 25 and 250 μg/ml of alginate-rich extract given in duplicate for each cultured sample. After 48 hours, the cells were collected, and the supernatants were stored at −20°C for cytokine analysis. The cell pellets were washed with phosphate-buffered saline (PBS), centrifuged at

1000 rpm for 8 minutes, and then stored at −20°C. According to the manufacturer's instructions, IL-1 and IL-6 levels were evaluated using commercially available ELISA kits [29].

2.13 Cytotoxicity evaluation of alginate and fucoidan-rich extract in a 3D culture model

The fabrication and design of the nano-scaffold were performed using an electrospinning device (Fanavaran Nano Meghyas™, Iran). The setup involved an injection flow rate of 1 ml/h, a needle distance of 15 cm, and a total volume of 10 ml. The structural characteristics of the Electrospun Polycaprolactone (PCL) nano-scaffolds were analyzed using scanning electron microscopy (SEM), which provided detailed visualization of the fiber alignment and diameter. To improve the surface properties of the PCL nanofibers, they were treated with O_2 plasma to increase hydrophilicity. This modification was performed for 5 minutes at a pressure of 0.4 millibars and a power of 30 W in a microwave plasma chamber. The plasma treatment was critical for enhancing cell adhesion and proliferation by making the nanofiber surface more wettable. For sterilization, the PCL nanofibers were treated with 70% ethanol, eliminating microbial contaminants. Post-sterilization, the nanofibers were rinsed three times with phosphate-buffered saline (PBS) to remove any ethanol residues. The nanofibers were then freeze-dried, preserving the scaffold's structural integrity while maintaining its mechanical properties. Combining SEM analysis, plasma surface modification, ethanol sterilization, and freeze-drying produced high-quality PCL nano-scaffolds ideal for applications in 3D cell culture [30].

2.14 Cytotoxicity evaluation of fucoidan-rich extract and cisplatin on MDA-MB-231 cells in a PCL polymeric nano-scaffold

After determining the IC_{50} values for both the fucoidan-rich extract and cisplatin in prior experiments, the cells were treated with varying concentrations—ranging from 0 to 1000 μg/ml of the fucoidan-rich extract and 2.1 μM of cisplatin—under conditions that closely resemble the physiological environment. 3×10^4 cells were seeded into each well of a 96-well plate and allowed to adhere to a polymeric scaffold for 24 hours. Subsequently, different concentrations of the extract and paclitaxel were added in triplicate to each well. An equivalent volume of PBS was added in triplicate for the negative control. The cells were incubated for 48 hours at 37°C with 5% CO_2. Following incubation, cell viability was assessed using the XTT assay, with absorbance readings taken at 450 and 620 nm using an ELISA reader. The entire experiment was conducted three times to ensure reproducibility and accuracy [31].

2.15 Data analysis and statistics

Results are expressed as the mean ± standard deviation (SD). Statistical analyses were conducted utilizing GraphPad Prism version 6 and SPSS version 16. The Kolmogorov-Smirnov test was applied to assess the normality of data distribution. For analyzing the data, paired t-tests were used for normally distributed variables, while the Wilcoxon signed-rank test was employed for non-parametric data. A P-value <0.05 was considered statistically significant in all analyses.

3. Results

3.1 Total sodium alginates and fucoidan determination

The extraction yields of fucoidan and alginate from the dried algae extract were determined to be 7203 and 441 mg per 100 grams of dried extract, respectively. This indicates that 7.2% of the algae extract's dried weight consisted of fucoidan, while 0.44% was alginate.

3.2 Total carbohydrate determination

The polysaccharide fraction from *S. ilicifolium* was obtained through a series of processes, including hot water extraction, ethanol precipitation, and dialysis. Using a calibration curve ($y = 0.0621x + 0.0084$, $r^2 = 0.999$) in absorbance of 490 nm created with standard glucose solutions, the total polysaccharide content in the fraction was estimated to be 89.39 mg/g dried algae weight.

3.3 Antioxidant properties of fucoidan and alginate

3.3.1 FRAP assay

In the reducing power assay, antioxidants present in the samples facilitate the conversion of ferric ions (Fe^{3+}) to ferrous ions (Fe^{2+}) through electron donation. Based on the standard curve equation ($y = 0.6685x + 0.0005$, $r^2 = 0.99$), the quantities of iron reduced by alginate and fucoidan-rich extract of *S. ilicifolium* are detailed in **Table 1**, suggesting higher antioxidant properties in fucoidan-rich extract compare to alginate-rich extract.

3.3.2 DPPH assay

The IC_{50} value for DPPH was assessed for different concentrations of algae's fucoidan-rich and alginate-rich extracts. The calculations were based on the standard curve equation ($y = 14.497x + 28.764$, $r^2 = 0.9962$) for ascorbic acid as a reference antioxidant.

For fucoidan, the standard curve equation was ($y = 21.35x + 0.1283$, $r^2 = 0.9955$), which exhibited a 33.9% inhibition at a concentration of 100 μg/ml as the highest percentage of inhibition with IC_{50} of 180.6 ± 26.3 μg/ml.

For alginate, the standard curve equation was ($y = 1.3217x + 0.076$, $r^2 = 0.9976$), which demonstrated a 16.7% inhibition at a concentration of 200 μg/ml as the highest percentage of inhibition, with IC_{50} of 640 ± 37.4 μg/ml.

Extract	FRAP at Concentration 0.1 mg/ml	FRAP at Concentration 1 mg/ml
Fucoidan-rich	153.6 ± 8.4 (μg/ ml)	865.5 ± 23.2 (μg/ ml)
Alginate-rich	43.8 ± 3.7 (μg/ ml)	105.3 ± 9.4 (μg/ ml)

Table 1.
The ferric-reducing ability of plasma of different concentrations of fucoidan and alginate-rich extract of S. ilicifolium.

3.4 FTIR spectrum of sodium alginate

The FTIR spectrum of sodium alginate (**Figure 1**) identified various chemical functional groups. A prominent broad absorption band at 3465 cm^{-1} indicates the hydroxyl group's (–OH) stretching vibrations. Additionally, peaks within the 2845 to 2930 cm^{-1} range correspond to the stretching vibrations of the methylidyne group (–CH). Significant peaks observed within 1599 ± 4 and 1410 ± 4 cm^{-1} are associated with asymmetric and symmetric stretching of carboxylate anions (COO–), respectively. The spectrum also displays a shoulder band at 1083.444 cm^{-1}, reflecting C–C and C–O stretching vibrations, which suggest cross-linking within the alginate structure. Moreover, the peak at 1022.493 cm^{-1} is attributed to C–C stretching vibrations, further characterizing the molecular framework.

3.5 FTIR spectrum of fucoidan

The FTIR spectrum of fucoidan revealed several key chemical functional groups (**Figure 2**). A broad and intense absorption band within the 3000 to 3600 cm^{-1} range signifies the stretching vibrations of hydroxyl groups (–OH), indicative of hydrogen bonding, commonly associated with polysaccharides. Additionally, absorption peaks between 2845 and 2930 cm^{-1} correspond to the stretching vibrations of the methylidyne (–CH) group. Further analysis shows spectral peaks between 1610 and 1651 cm^{-1}, attributed to carbonyl (C=O) and carbon-carbon double bond (C=C) stretching vibrations. These are linked to the presence of uronic acids, suggesting alginic acid as part of the alginate polymers in the sample. Peaks between 1420 and 1445 cm^{-1} are possibly related to C–H deformation or –OH rocking vibrations in monosaccharides. The FTIR spectrum also indicates the presence of C-O-C and C-O-S bonds, with observed peaks ranging from 387 to 1030 cm^{-1}. Specifically, a peak

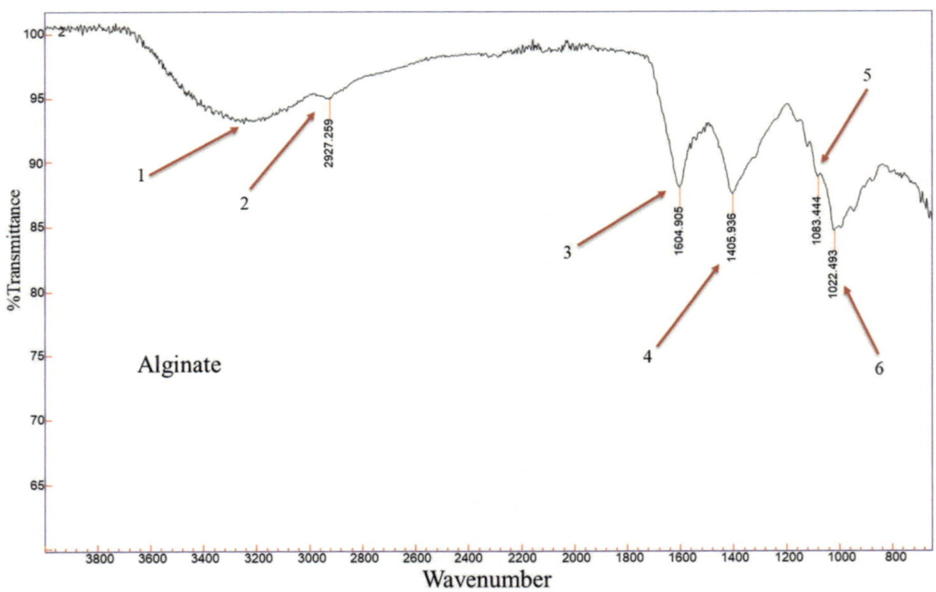

Figure 1.
FTIR analysis of sodium alginate.

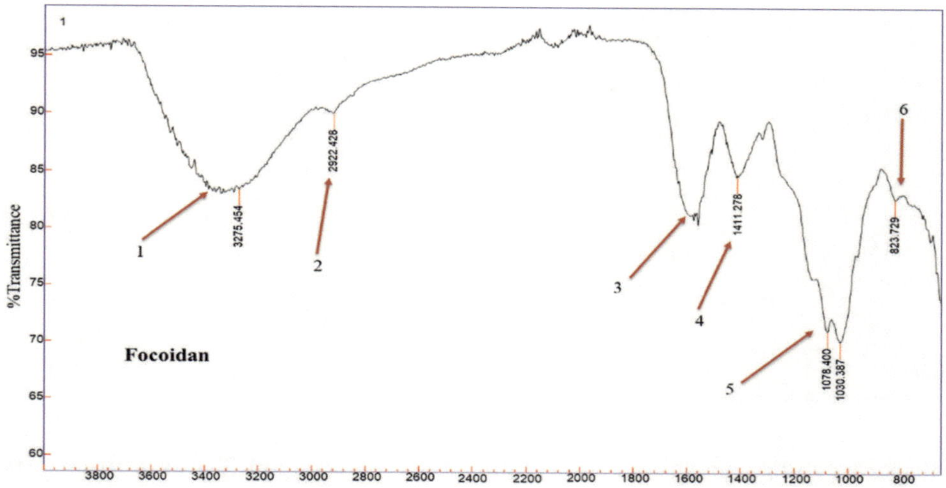

Figure 2.
FTIR analysis of fucoidan.

near 1078.4 cm^{-1} signifies C–O, C–C, and C–O–H stretching vibrations in hydrocarbon structures. Lastly, the sharp absorption bands between 729 and 823 cm^{-1} are attributed to C–O–S bending vibrations, pointing to sulfate substitution.

3.6 UV-visible analysis

The UV-visible spectrogram of the alginate extract (**Figure 3**) displayed absorption peaks within the 200–400 nm range, which are indicative of carboxylate groups and protein-related components. Peaks observed at 280, 370, and 405 nm suggest the presence of phenolic compounds, flavonoids, and their derivatives. The data further highlighted absorption bands between 280 and 410 nm, characteristic of aromatic and polycyclic aromatic compounds, including proteins and amino acids, supporting complex organic structures in the extract.

The spectrogram of the fucoidan extract (**Figure 4**) in the 300 to 400 nm range appears abnormal, possibly due to impurities, sample preparation issues, or instrumental problems. Polysaccharides in their pure form are generally optically

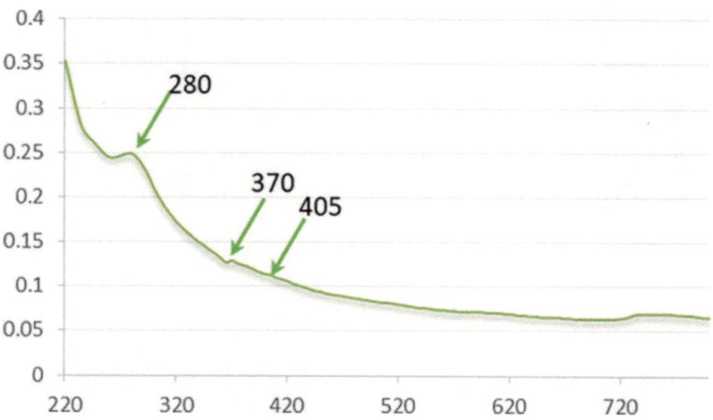

Figure 3.
UV spectrogram of alginate extract.

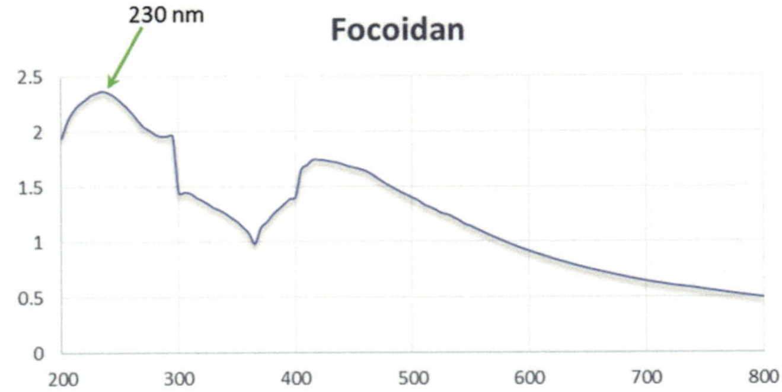

Figure 4.
UV spectrogram of fucoidan extract.

transparent and do not exhibit absorption in the UV-Vis region. The absorption peak around 230 nm may indicate the presence of polyphenols in the sample.

3.7 Cytotoxicity evaluation of cisplatin on MDA-MB-231 cancer cell line

The XTT assay was employed to assess the cytotoxic effects of cisplatin on MDA-MB-231 breast cancer cells. According to the results depicted in **Figure 5**, different concentrations of cisplatin, ranging from 0 to 20 μg/ml, were administered to the cells over 48 hours. Cisplatin demonstrated an evident dose-dependent cytotoxicity, with the IC_{20} and IC_{50} values calculated at 3.6 ± 0.4 and 15.33 ± 0.9 μg/ml, respectively.

3.8 Cytotoxicity evaluation of fucoidan-rich extract and its drug interaction analysis with cisplatin on MDA-MB-231 cancer cell line

The XTT assay was initially conducted to evaluate the impact of a fucoidan-rich extract on the viability of MDA-MB-231 breast cancer cells. As illustrated in **Figure 6** (green line), various extract concentrations, ranging from 0 to 800 μg/ml, were tested over 48 hours. The results revealed that the fucoidan-rich extract induced a dose-dependent cytotoxic effect on the cells, with an IC_{20} value (the

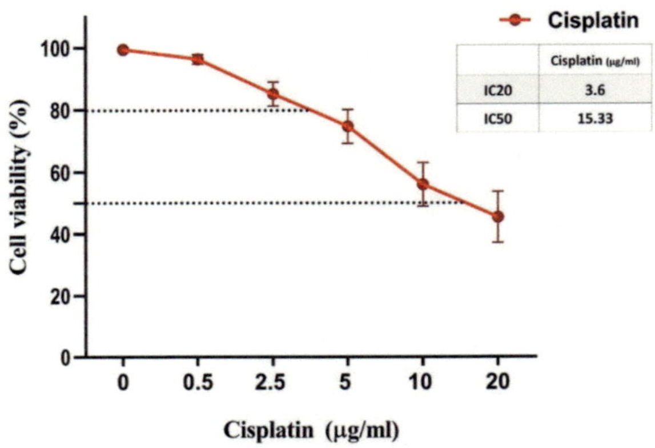

Figure 5.
Cytotoxicity evaluation of different concentrations of cisplatin on MDA-MB-231 cancer cells.

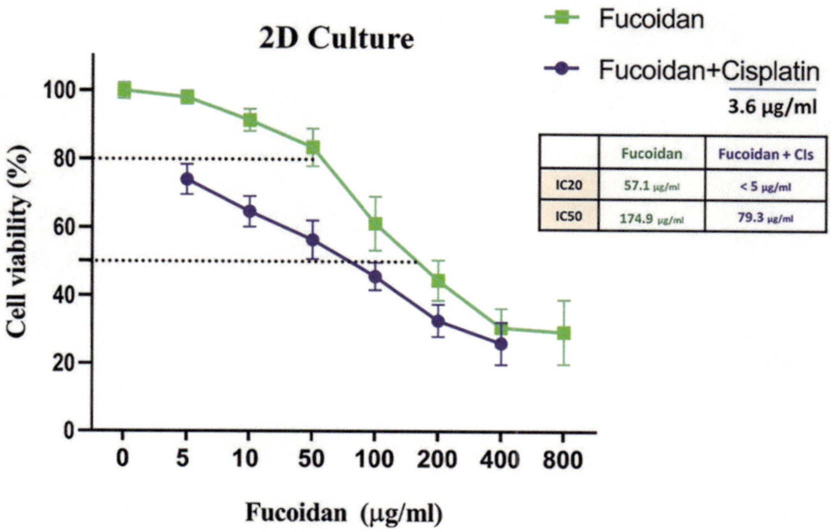

Figure 6.
Cytotoxicity evaluation of fucoidan-rich extract and in combination with cisplatin on MDA-MB-231 cancer cells.

concentration at which 80% of cells remain viable) of 57.1 ± 2.9 µg/ml and an IC_{50} value of 174.9 ± 8.7 µg/ml.

Subsequently, the effects of combining different concentrations of the fucoidan-rich extract (ranging from 5 to 400 µg/ml) with 3.6 ± 0.4 µg/ml (IC_{20}) of cisplatin were analyzed. As shown in **Figure 6** (blue line), after 48 hours of treatment, the combination significantly enhanced cytotoxicity, reducing the IC_{50} from 174.9 ± 8.7 to 79.3 ± 4.6 µg/ml and lowering the IC_{20} from 57.1 ± 2.9 µg/ml to below 5.0 ± 0.8 µg/ml. This indicates a synergistic effect between the fucoidan-rich extract and cisplatin.

The synergistic interaction between the fucoidan-rich extract and cisplatin was validated through CompuSyn software analysis. This software calculated the Combination Index (CI) values for all tested concentrations, with values less than one consistently indicating a synergistic effect (as shown in **Table 2**). Among the tested concentrations, 200 µg/ml demonstrated the highest synergy, with a CI value of 0.28518.

A detailed analysis using CompuSyn software generated several insightful plots (**Figure 7**).

1. *Dose-effect curve* (**Figure 7A**): The combination treatment demonstrated a more substantial dose-dependent effect than the extract alone. The green points, representing the combined treatment of cisplatin and extract, were positioned lower on the graph than the blue line, corresponding to the extract alone. This positioning indicates enhanced cytotoxicity when the treatments are combined.

2. *Combination index plot* (**Figure 7B**): All Fa-CI points fell below the line at 1, signifying synergistic effects at all concentrations tested. This confirms that combining treatments is more effective than either treatment alone.

3. *Median-effect plot* (**Figure 7C**): The log-transformed data revealed positive slope lines, indicating that higher doses correlate with increased cellular response. The point where the lines intersect the X-axis represents the combined IC_{50} value, calculated at 79.3 ± 4.6 µg/ml.

Fucoidan concentration (µg/ml)	CI	Effect
5	0.69302	Synergism
10	0.41359	Synergism
50	0.47320	Synergism
100	0.38466	Synergism
200	0.28518	Synergism
400	0.32998	Synergism

Table 2.
Combination index of different concentrations of fucoidan-rich extract in combination with IC_{20} concentration (3.6 ± 0.4 µg/ml) of cisplatin.

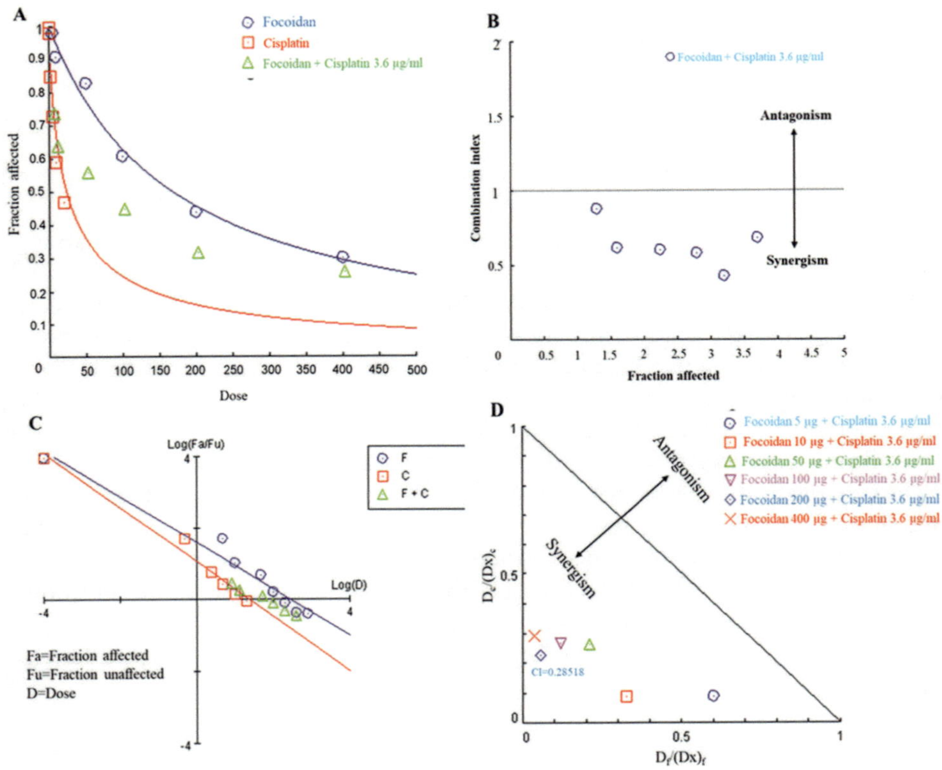

Figure 7.
Plot analysis of fucoidan-rich extract and cisplatin on MDA-MB-231 cells using CompuSyn software. (A) Dose-effect curve (B) Combination index plot (C) Median-effect plot (D) Dose-normalized isobologram.

4. *Dose-normalized isobologram* (**Figure 7D**): This plot demonstrated that all combined doses, represented by colored points within the triangle, displayed synergistic effects, with CI values consistently below one, reinforcing the enhanced effectiveness of the combination therapy. The colored points represent the concentration of the combined drug. The closer a point is to the left and bottom, the lower its CI number and the more potent its synergistic effect. Since all five concentrations combined with cisplatin fall within the triangle, each concentration demonstrates a synergistic effect with a CI of less than one.

3.9 Cytotoxicity evaluation of alginate-rich extract and its drug interaction analysis with cisplatin on MDA-MB-231 cancer cell line

As mentioned for fucoidan-rich extract, the XTT assay was used to assess the effects of an alginate-rich extract on the viability of MDA-MB-231 breast cancer cells. **Figure 8** (blue line) shows that varying extract concentrations, ranging from 0 to 350 μg/ml, were tested over 48 hours. The findings indicated that the alginate-rich extract exhibited minimal toxicity toward the MDA-MB-231 cell line, with significant cytotoxicity observed only at concentrations exceeding 280 μg/ml, surpassing the IC_{20} threshold.

The combined effects of the various concentrations of alginate-rich extract (ranging from 0 to 350 μg/ml) with 3.6 μg/ml of cisplatin (IC_{20}) were evaluated. As shown in **Figure 8** (green line), after 48 hours of treatment, the combination did not result in any notable increase in cytotoxicity, suggesting that the alginate-rich extract did not enhance the cytotoxic effects of cisplatin in this cell line.

The interaction between the alginate-rich extract and cisplatin was further analyzed using CompuSyn software. The Combination Index (CI) values, calculated across all tested concentrations, revealed that the alginate-rich extract displayed both weak synergistic and antagonistic effects when combined with the IC_{20} concentration of cisplatin (**Table 2**). Notably, the 50 μg/ml concentration exhibited the strongest synergy, with a CI value of 0.83198 (**Table 3**).

A detailed analysis using CompuSyn software generated several detailed plots (**Figure 9**).

1. *Dose-effect curve* (**Figure 9A**): The combination of alginate and cisplatin did not increase toxic effects as the alginate concentration was raised. This is evident from the horizontal trend of the green triangles in the dose-effect plot, representing the combination of the alginate extract and cisplatin, which indicates that alginate has an insignificant impact on enhancing cisplatin's toxicity. Moreover, the red line, which denotes the cytotoxic effect of various concentrations of cisplatin alone, demonstrates the potent toxicity of the drug.

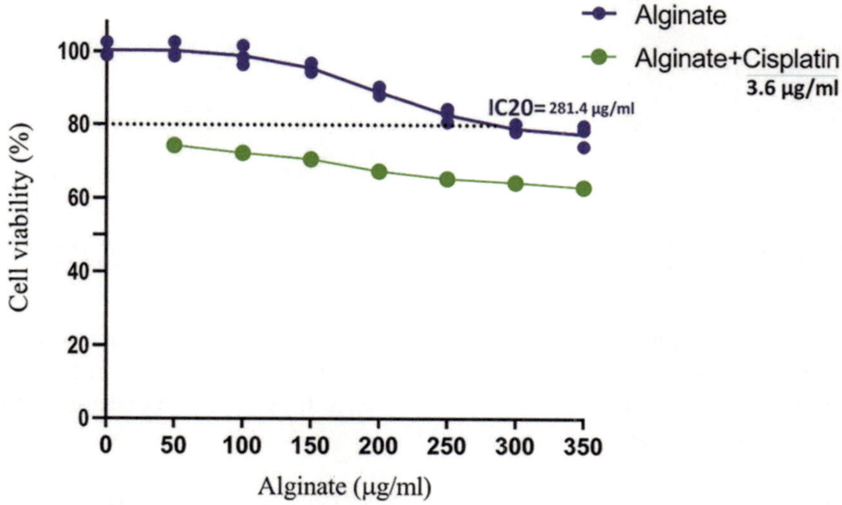

Figure 8.
Cytotoxicity evaluation of alginate-rich extract and in combination with cisplatin on MDA-MB-231 cancer cells.

Alginate concentration (μg/ml)	CI	Effect
50	0.83198	Synergism
100	0.94180	Synergism
150	1.05919	Antagonism
200	1.12509	Antagonism
250	1.22702	Antagonism

Table 3.
CI of different concentrations of fucoidan-rich extract in combination with IC20 concentration (3.6 ± 0.4 μg/ml).

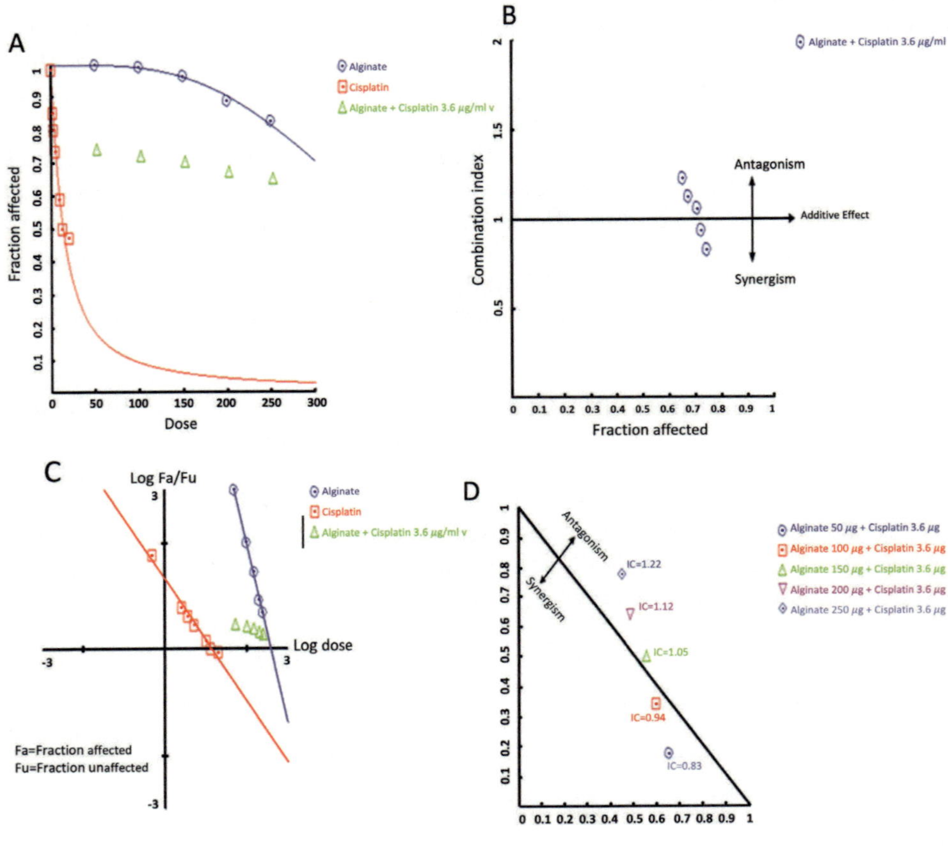

Figure 9.
Plot analysis of alginate-rich extract and cisplatin on MDA-MB-231 cells using CompuSyn software. (A) Dose-effect curve (B) Combination index plot (C) Median-effect plot (D) Dose-normalized isobologram.

2. *Combination index plot* (**Figure 9B**): In the Fa-CI diagram, two data points fell below the line, indicating a synergistic interaction at these two concentrations. However, an antagonistic interaction occurs at three other concentrations of Fa-CI points positioned above the line at 1.

3. *Median-effect plot* (**Figure 9C**): The log-transformed data revealed that increasing the dose does not lead to a significant rise in cytotoxic response due to the shallow slope of the combination curve for the drug and the extract. This indicates that the

tested alginate concentrations did not reach the IC_{50} threshold. Furthermore, the combination of alginate with cisplatin also failed to achieve an IC_{50}, reflecting the limited enhancement in cytotoxicity when these two agents are used together.

4. *Dose-normalized isobologram* (**Figure 9D**): Doses represented within the triangle display a synergistic effect when combined with cisplatin, while the doses plotted outside the triangle exhibit antagonistic effects. The colored points represent the concentration of the combined drug. The closer a point is to the left and bottom, the lower its CI number and the more potent its synergistic effect. Two concentrations, which lie inside the triangle and close to the diagonal line, show only a weak synergistic effect. In contrast, three concentrations situated outside the triangle demonstrate antagonistic interactions.

3.10 IL-1β and IL-6 cytokine secretion from THP-1 monocyte cell line stimulated with *S. ilicifolium* fucoidan-rich extract

The impact of non-toxic doses (5 and 50 μg/ml) of *S. ilicifolium* fucoidan-rich extract on cytokine secretion was evaluated using the THP-1 monocyte cell line. Lipopolysaccharide (LPS, 1 μg/ml) was used as a positive control to stimulate cytokine secretion. The results revealed that, compared to the untreated control group, both the 5 and 50 μg/ml doses of the extract significantly reduced IL-1β cytokine secretion by 14% (p-values = 0.0411) and 37% (p-values = 0.0022), respectively (**Figure 10**).

Similarly, for IL-6 cytokine, the 5 and 50 μg/ml doses of the extract led to significant reductions of 16% (p-values = 0.0411) and 42% (p-values = 0.0022), respectively, as shown in **Figure 11**.

3.11 IL-1β and IL-6 cytokine secretion from THP-1 monocyte cell line stimulated with *S. ilicifolium* alginate-rich extract

The effect of non-toxic doses (50 and 250 μg/ml) of *S. ilicifolium* alginate-rich extract on cytokine secretion was assessed using the THP-1 monocyte cell line, with

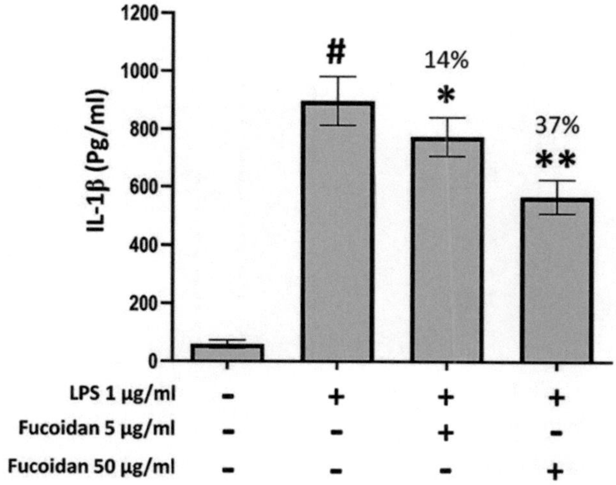

Figure 10.
The effect of non-toxic doses of S. ilicifolium *fucoidan-rich extract on the secretion of IL-1β cytokine from THP-1 monocyte cell line, # control group, * and ** P value<0.05 compared to the control group.*

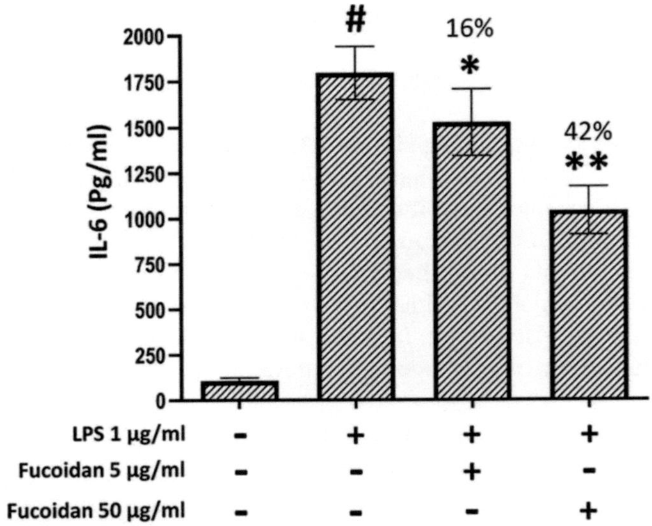

Figure 11.
The effect of non-toxic doses of S. ilicifolium *fucoidan-rich extract on the secretion of IL-6 cytokine from THP-1 monocyte cell line, # control group, * and ** P value<0.05 compared to the control group.*

lipopolysaccharide (LPS, 1 μg/ml) serving as a positive control to induce cytokine production. The findings indicated that, compared to the untreated control group, both the 50 and 250 μg/ml concentrations of the extract significantly decreased IL-1β cytokine secretion by 8 and 15%, with p-values of 0.0411 and 0.0022, respectively (**Figure 12**).

Similarly, the extract significantly reduced IL-6 cytokine levels by 5 and 13% at doses of 50 and 250 μg/ml, with corresponding p-values of 0.0411 and 0.0022, as depicted in **Figure 13**.

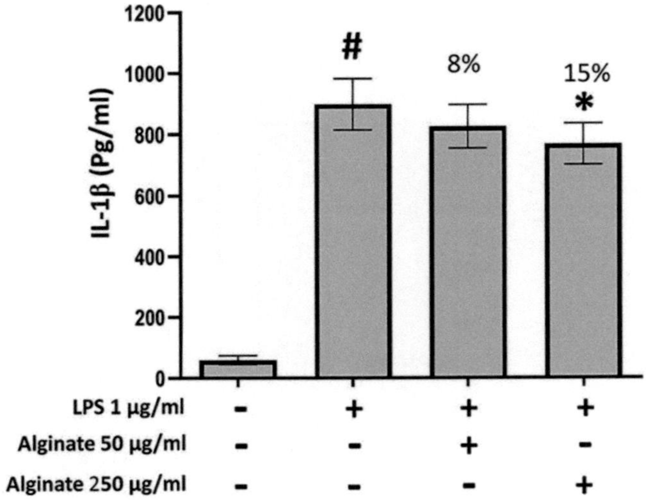

Figure 12.
The effect of non-toxic doses of S. ilicifolium *alginate-rich extract on the secretion of IL-1β cytokine from THP-1 monocyte cell line, # control group, * and ** P value<0.05 compared to the control group.*

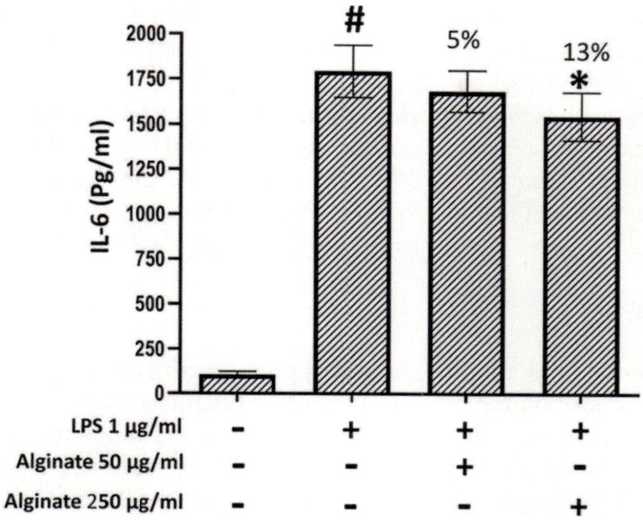

Figure 13.
The effect of non-toxic doses of S. ilicifolium *alginate-rich extract on the secretion of IL-6 cytokine from THP-1 monocyte cell line, # control group, * and ** P value<0.05 compared to the control group.*

3.12 Cytotoxicity evaluation of fucoidan-rich extract on cancer cells and its drug interaction analysis with paclitaxel on MDA-MB-231 cell line in a PCL polymeric nano-scaffold

Cell viability was measured using the XTT assay across a range of extract concentrations to assess the cytotoxic potential of a fucoidan-rich extract on MDA-MB-231 breast cancer cells. As depicted in **Figure 14** (green line), after 48 hours of treatment with concentrations between 0 and 800 µg/ml, the extract exhibited evident

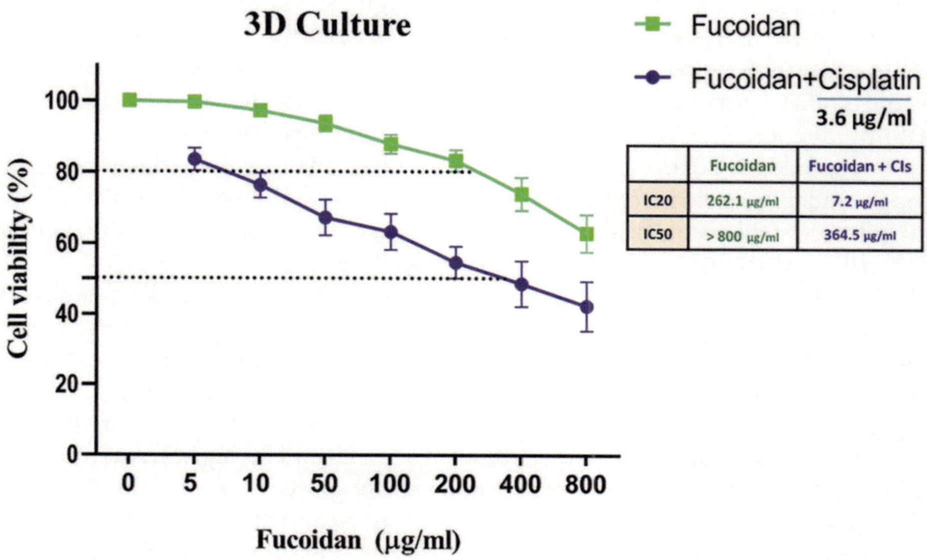

Figure 14.
Cytotoxicity evaluation of fucoidan-rich extract in combination with cisplatin on MDA-MB-231 cells in a 3D culture model.

dose-dependent cytotoxicity against MDA-MB-231 cells. The IC_{20}, or the concentration required to inhibit 20% of cell growth, was calculated at 262.1 ± 19.7 µg/ml, while the IC_{50} exceeded 800 ± 78.5 µg/ml.

Furthermore, as shown in **Figure 14** (blue line), the cytotoxic effect was notably enhanced when the extract was combined with 3.6 µg/ml cisplatin for 48 hours. The IC_{20} dropped sharply from 262.1 ± 19.3 to 7.2 ± 1.4 µg/ml, and the IC_{50} decreased significantly from over 800 ± 78.5 to 364.5 ± 41.7 µg/ml.

4. Discussion

Breast cancer remains a significant global public health challenge and stands as the most prevalent cancer among women. Predictions estimate that by 2040, the global incidence of breast cancer will exceed 3 million new cases annually, accompanied by nearly 1 million deaths each year. Among the various subtypes, triple-negative breast cancer (TNBC) is particularly aggressive, known for its high mortality rates and a pronounced tendency to metastasize beyond the breast to distant organs. This makes TNBC one of the most challenging forms of breast cancer to treat and underscores the urgent need for improved therapeutic strategies [32, 33]. The application of immunostimulants, particularly as adjuvants to chemotherapy, offers significant potential for controlling and preventing cancers. There is growing interest in exploring bioactive compounds from marine-derived drugs as immunomodulatory agents in alternative medicine [14]. This study evaluated the fucoidan and alginate-rich extract of *S. ilicifolium* for their potential impact on immune function along with cisplatin as a chemotherapeutic agent, highlighting their promise in enhancing immune response and supporting therapeutic interventions.

The antioxidant, cytotoxic, and apoptotic properties of fucoidan and alginate from the brown algae *Colpomenia sinuosa* have shown promising anticancer effects across various cancer cell lines. Notably, highly sulfated fucoidans exhibited more potent antioxidant and cytotoxic activities than alginate. Human colon cancer cells were susceptible to these treatments, with fucoidan demonstrating a lower IC_{50} value (618.9 µg/ml) than alginate (690 µg/ml). The treatment of HCT-116 cells with fucoidan and alginate from *C. sinuosa* led to a significant increase in reactive oxygen species (ROS) production. This elevated ROS production indicates that these compounds may induce oxidative damage within the cells, which can ultimately trigger cell death through oxidative stress mechanisms. Moreover, when combined with vitamin C, the algal polysaccharides significantly enhanced nuclear degeneration and increased the $subG_1$ cell population, indicating induced cell death [34].

S. ilicifolium, a seaweed native to the coastal regions of the Persian Gulf, is rich in polysaccharides like fucoidan, which exhibit potential anticancer properties, explored through various assays, including MTT, cell culture, viability, and apoptosis tests. The findings demonstrated that within 24 hours, cell viability decreased by 2% at 1 mg/mL of the fucoidan-rich extract, while concentrations of 60 mg/mL reduced cell viability by less than 30%, with an IC_{50} between 20 and 30 mg/ml. Additionally, ELISA results confirmed that the extract induced apoptosis in cancer cells [35].

Fucoidan, a sulfated polysaccharide from brown algae, exhibits various biological activities, including antitumor effects. *In vitro* investigation of fucoidan's crude impact on mouse breast cancer significantly reduced the viability of 4 T1 cells, induced apoptosis, and downregulated VEGF expression. It also decreased Bcl-2 expression, lowering the Bcl-2/Bax ratio, and reduced levels of Survivin and phosphorylated ERKs. Additionally, fucoidan triggered cytochrome C release from mitochondria and increased cleaved Caspase-3 levels. *In vivo*, intraperitoneal fucoidan injections in breast cancer models reduced tumor volume and weight, enhancing antitumor effects by decreasing angiogenesis and increasing apoptosis [36].

The difference in antioxidant performance between fucoidan and sodium alginate can be attributed to their distinct chemical structures. Both fucoidan and sodium alginate exhibit strong binding affinities to lead, which enables them to restore antioxidant enzyme activity and mitigate oxidative damage by absorbing lead *in vivo*. While sodium alginate is known to have a superior lead adsorption capacity compared to fucoidan, the latter demonstrates greater antioxidant properties. This is likely due to the presence of sulfhydryl groups in fucoidan, which have a strong ability to neutralize excessive free radicals generated by lead-induced toxicity. This unique structural feature of fucoidan may explain its enhanced antioxidant performance in this study, despite both compounds showing similar efficacy in repairing lead-induced oxidative damage in rats [37].

The anticancer effects of fucoidan on human breast cancer MCF-7 cells include inhibition of proliferation and induction of apoptosis in adult Sprague–Dawley rats treated with fucoidan (200 or 400 mg/kg daily) for 3 days show significantly suppressed MCF-7 cell proliferation, enhanced apoptosis, and reduced cell migration and invasion in serum from these fucoidan-treated rats. These effects were linked to the upregulation of E-cadherin and downregulation of MMP-9, suggesting that fucoidan may inhibit the epithelial-mesenchymal transition (EMT) process, thereby reducing cancer cell invasiveness [38]. These results align with our findings and underscore the potential of fucoidan as a potent anticancer agent.

The sodium alginate-curcumin bioconjugate (AA-CUR) shows great potential as an anticancer drug system due to its simple synthesis, high colloidal stability, and effective curcumin release profile. It demonstrates significant cytotoxicity against cancer cells while maintaining low toxicity in normal cells, making it a promising candidate for therapeutic applications [39]. Alginate/lignin is a promising antioxidant material with potential applications in pharmaceuticals, functional foods, and diabetes management. The acute toxicity test of alginate/lignin in mice presented an LD_0 of (3.91 g/kg) and LD_{100} of (9.77 g/kg). It demonstrates strong total antioxidant activity and effective α-glucosidase inhibition, crucial for controlling blood sugar levels. Although it shows minimal effects on cancer cells, its thermal stability, spherical structure, and unique composition of metals and non-metals enhance its suitability for therapeutic uses, particularly in treating aging-related conditions, diabetes, and digestive system disorders. Additionally, its low toxicity profile further supports its potential for safe use in medical applications [40]. These results are consistent with the beneficial attributes observed in the present study of alginate.

The results regarding alginate's lack of significant enhancement in cisplatin's cytotoxicity, while less impactful compared to fucoidan, raise important points for further exploration. Alginate's primary role is often as a drug delivery matrix or protective agent rather than a direct enhancer of cytotoxicity. Studies have shown that alginate can reduce drug efficacy due to its ability to encapsulate and slow drug release, limiting immediate cytotoxic action [41]. In contrast, fucoidan's sulfated structure allows for better interaction with cellular components and may enhance chemotherapy effects by promoting apoptosis and oxidative stress [42].

Fucoidan exhibits notable anti-inflammatory activity, demonstrated through its ability to inhibit various inflammatory pathways. It reduces the production of key pro-inflammatory cytokines, such as TNF-α, IL-1β, and IL-6, *in vitro* and *in vivo* models [43]. For instance, fucoidan from different algae species has shown efficacy in decreasing cytokine levels in stimulated human cells and macrophages. Specifically, low molecular weight fucoidan subfractions are particularly effective, as seen in the anti-inflammatory effects of LJSF4 from Saccharina japonica [44] and EMSF6 from Ecklonia maxima [45]. These fucoidans work by modulating signaling pathways like MAPK and NF-κB, highlighting their potential for therapeutic applications against inflammation. These results are consistent with the beneficial anti-inflammatory effects observed in the present study of fucoidan.

Alginate exhibits significant anti-inflammatory activity across various models. Alginate oligosaccharides reduce nitric oxide and pro-inflammatory cytokines such as TNF-α, IL-1β, and IL-6 in LPS-induced RAW 264.7 cells, showing peak anti-inflammatory effects after 36 hours of incubation. They also reduce NF-κB p65, iNOS, and COX-2 expression, decreasing ear edema and mast cell numbers [46]. Additionally, alginate microspheres enhance phagocytosis and modulate M1 macrophage responses, leading to a moderate reduction in bacterial viability and increased secretion of pro-inflammatory cytokines [47]. Sodium alginate, administered orally, significantly reduces inflammation and cytokine levels in a rat model of ulcerative colitis, demonstrating its therapeutic potential in managing chronic inflammatory conditions [48]. These findings highlight alginate's potential as an anti-inflammatory agent, which aligns with the findings of this study.

Seaweed bioactive compounds, such as fucoidan, exhibit diverse anticancer activities when tested alone or in combination with drugs like cisplatin. In 3D cultures, where cells often display greater resistance to treatments due to factors like hypoxia and altered drug diffusion, the effects of these compounds can differ significantly from those observed in 2D cultures. For instance, while fucoidan alone may have varying impacts on cytotoxicity, its combination with cisplatin can enhance or diminish drug effectiveness depending on the specific cell line and experimental conditions. This variability underscores the importance of 3D models for more accurate evaluations of drug interactions and therapeutic potentials [49]. 3D cell culture systems are becoming more precise drug testing models than traditional two-dimensional (2D) cultures. Studies have shown that 3D cultures, particularly those forming dense multicellular spheroids (MCSs), exhibit greater resistance to chemotherapeutic drugs like paclitaxel and doxorubicin due to factors such as hypoxia and altered apoptosis pathways. For example, breast cancer cell lines with dense MCSs in 3D cultures demonstrated reduced drug-induced apoptosis and changes in drug sensitivity compared to their 2D counterparts. This resistance is linked to higher proportions of dormant cells (G_0 phase) and lower levels of apoptotic markers [50]. Analysis of colon cancer spheroids showed lower activity in key signaling pathways like AKT, mTOR, and S6K in 3D models. Spatial variations in signaling were observed, with reduced phosphorylation of RPS6 at the spheroid core, mirroring *in vivo* tumor conditions. 3D cultures displayed enhanced antitumor responses to pathway inhibitors, such as increased ERK phosphorylation when AKT-mTOR-S6K was inhibited, contrary to 2D cultures. Additionally, MEK1 inhibition decreased AKT-mTOR-S6K signaling in 3D but not in 2D [51]. These findings highlight the distinct signaling rewiring in 3D models and their potential to mimic tumor behavior and improve anticancer drug evaluation.

This study has several limitations that warrant acknowledgment. First, the use of only one cell line (MDA-MB-231) limits the generalizability of the findings across different cancer subtypes. Second, the abnormal spectrogram data observed in the FTIR analysis of fucoidan points to potential impurities or instrumental limitations. While this analysis was conducted to confirm the presence of fucoidan, the spectroscopic anomalies suggest that further refinement of the extraction process or improved purification methods may be needed.

5. Conclusion

This study highlights the potential of fucoidan extract of *S. ilicifolium* in overcoming cisplatin resistance, reducing drug dosage, and enhancing its effectiveness. The results demonstrate that fucoidan-rich extract exhibits dose-dependent antiproliferative effects and significantly improves the antitumor efficacy of cisplatin in both 2D and 3D models. Additionally, this extract shows notable anti-inflammatory and antioxidant properties, considerably reducing the secretion of cytokines IL-6 and IL-1β. Consequently, this study underscores the potential of fucoidan in addressing drug resistance, a significant challenge in cancer treatment, and may lead to more effective therapeutic strategies, thereby improving prognosis and quality of life for patients with drug-resistant breast cancer. The evidence suggests that combining fucoidan with cisplatin could enhance survival rates and reduce the social and economic burden of triple-negative breast cancer (TNBC), offering hope for more effective alternative treatments. Further investigation into these mechanistic differences between alginate and fucoidan and also can investigate the impact of these compounds on additional cancer cell lines.

Acknowledgements

The authors would like to express their gratitude to the research team members who contributed their time and expertise.

Conflict of interest

The authors declare no conflict of interest.

Author details

Reza Taghipour[1], Hadi Hassannia[2], Hesamoddin Arabnozari[3], Seyed Ehsan Enderami[4] and Emran Habibi[5]*

1 Faculty of Pharmacy, Mazandaran University of Medical Sciences, Sari, Iran

2 Immunogenetic Research Center, Faculty of Medicine and Amol Faculty of Paramedical Sciences, University of Medical Sciences, Sari, Iran

3 School of Medicine, Babol University of Medical Sciences, Babol, Iran

4 Immunogenetics Research Center, Department of Medical Biotechnology, School of Advanced Technologies in Medicine, Mazandaran University of Medical Sciences, Sari, Iran

5 Medicinal Plants Research Center, Mazandaran University of Medical Sciences, Sari, Iran

*Address all correspondence to: emrapharm@yahoo.com

References

[1] Shokrzadeh M, Rajabali F, Habibi E, Modanloo M. Survey cytotoxicity and genotoxicity of hydroalcoholic extract of Stevia rebaudiana in breast cancer cell line (MCF7) and human fetallung fibroblasts (MRC-5). Journal of Cancer Research Metastasis. 2018;**1**(2):12-17

[2] Sanjeewa KA, Lee J-S, Kim W-S, Jeon Y-J. The potential of brown-algae polysaccharides for the development of anticancer agents: An update on anticancer effects reported for fucoidan and laminaran. Carbohydrate Polymers. 2017;**177**:451-459

[3] Smolarz B, Nowak AZ, Romanowicz H. Breast cancer—Epidemiology, classification, pathogenesis and treatment (review of literature). Cancers. 2022;**14**(10):2569

[4] Makki J. Diversity of breast carcinoma: Histological subtypes and clinical relevance. Clinical Medicine Insights: Pathology. 2015;**8**:23-31

[5] Derakhshan F, Reis-Filho JS. Pathogenesis of triple-negative breast cancer. Annual Review of Pathology: Mechanisms of Disease. 2022;**17**(1):181-204

[6] Howard FM, Olopade OI. Epidemiology of triple-negative breast cancer: A review. The Cancer Journal. 2021;**27**(1):8-16

[7] Liu S, Dong Y, Wang Y, Hu P, Wang J, Wang RY. Pristimerin exerts antitumor activity against MDA-MB-231 triple-negative breast cancer cells by reversing of epithelial-mesenchymal transition via downregulation of integrin β3. Biomedical Journal. 2021;**44**(6):S84-S92

[8] Van den Boogaard W, Komninos D, Vermeij W. Chemotherapy side-effects: Not all DNA damage is equal. Cancers. 2022;**14**(3):627

[9] Varghese E, Samuel SM, Líšková A, Samec M, Kubatka P, Büsselberg D. Targeting glucose metabolism to overcome resistance to anticancer chemotherapy in breast cancer. Cancers. 2020;**12**(8):2252

[10] Romani AM. Cisplatin in cancer treatment. Biochemical Pharmacology. 2022;**206**:115323

[11] Hill DP, Harper A, Malcolm J, McAndrews MS, Mockus SM, Patterson SE, et al. Cisplatin-resistant triple-negative breast cancer subtypes: Multiple mechanisms of resistance. BMC Cancer. 2019;**19**:1-13

[12] Sumithra M, Chitra V, Ramasamy R. Spectral analysis of Sargassum ilicifolium (turner) C. Agardh and *in vitro* anti-proliferative study of its ethanolic extract and chloroform fraction against colon cancer (HT-29) and lung cancer (A549) cell lines. Marmara. The Pharmaceutical Journal. 2017;**21**(2):269-277

[13] Tsou M-H, Lee C-C, Wu Z-Y, Lee Z-H, Lin H-M. Bioactivity of crude fucoidan extracted from *Sargassum ilicifolium* (turner) C. Agardh. Scientific Reports. 2022;**12**(1):15916

[14] Chandraraj S, Prakash B, Navanath K. Immunomodulatory activities of ethyl acetate extracts of two marine sponges *Gelliodes fibrosa* and *Tedania anhelans* and brown algae *Sargassum ilicifolium* with reference to phagocytosis. Research Journal of Pharmaceutical, Biological and Chemical Sciences. 2010;**1**:302-307

[15] Al-Muqbali MHS, Al-Alawi A, Waly MI, Rahman MS. Anticancer

properties of fucoidans extracted from brown seaweed (*Sargassum ilicifolium*) in a rat model of gastric cancer. Canadian Journal of Clinical Nutrition. 2019;**7**(2):43-61

[16] Simón L, Arazo-Rusindo M, Quest AF, Mariotti-Celis MS. Phlorotannins: Novel orally administrated bioactive compounds that induce mitochondrial dysfunction and oxidative stress in cancer. Antioxidants. 2023;**12**(9):1734

[17] Bouissil S, El Alaoui-Talibi Z, Pierre G, Michaud P, El Modafar C, Delattre C. Use of alginate extracted from Moroccan brown algae to stimulate natural defense in date palm roots. Molecules. 2020;**25**(3):720

[18] Li B, Wei X-J, Sun J-L, Xu S-Y. Structural investigation of a fucoidan containing a fucose-free core from the brown seaweed, Hizikia fusiforme. Carbohydrate Research. 2006;**341**(9):1135-1146

[19] Flórez-Fernández N, Balboa EM, Domínguez H. Extraction and purification of fucoidan from marine sources. Encyclopedia of Marine Biotechnology. 2020;**2**:1093-1125

[20] Xi X, Wei X, Wang Y, Chu Q, Xiao J. Determination of tea polysaccharides in *Camellia sinensis* by a modified phenol-sulfuric acid method. Archives of Biological Sciences. 2010;**62**(3):669-676

[21] Jouybari HB, Valadan R, Mirzaee F, Karizno FB, Habibi E. Immunomodulatory activity of polysaccharide from *Trametes gibbosa* (Pers.) Fr (Basidiomycota, fungi) mediated by TLR4 signaling pathway. Advanced Biomedical Research. 2023;**12**(1):127

[22] Dalal SR, Hussein MH, El-Naggar NE-A, Mostafa SI, Shaaban-Dessuuki SA. Characterization of alginate extracted from *Sargassum latifolium* and its use in *Chlorella vulgaris* growth promotion and riboflavin drug delivery. Scientific Reports. 2021;**11**(1):16741

[23] Amerifar M, Arabnozari H, Shokrzadeh M, Habibi E. Evaluation of antioxidant properties and cytotoxicity of brown algae (nizamuddinia zanardinii) in uterine (hela) and pancreatic cancer cell lines (paca-2). Human & Experimental Toxicology. 2024;**43**:09603271241227228

[24] Arabnozari H, Shaki F, Najjari A, Sharifianjazi F, Sarker SD, Habibi E, et al. The effect of *Polygonum hyrcanicum* Rech. f. Hydroalcoholic extract on oxidative stress and nephropathy in alloxan-induced diabetic mice. Scientific Reports. 2024;**14**(1):18117

[25] Habibi E, Hemmati P, Arabnozari H, Khalili HA, Sharifianjazi F, Enderami SE, et al. Phytochemical analysis and immune-modulatory potential of *Trichaptum biforme* polysaccharides: Implications for cancer. International Journal of Biological Macromolecules. 2024;**280**:135691

[26] Geraghty R, Capes-Davis A, Davis J, Downward J, Freshney R, Knezevic I, et al. Guidelines for the use of cell lines in biomedical research. British Journal of Cancer. 2014;**111**(6):1021-1046

[27] Park DC, Yeo SG, Shin EY, Mok SC, Kim DH. Clusterin confers paclitaxel resistance in cervical cancer. Gynecologic Oncology. 2006;**103**(3):996-1000

[28] El Hassouni B, Mantini G, Petri GL, Capula M, Boyd L, Weinstein HN, et al. To combine or not combine: Drug interactions and tools for their analysis. Reflections from the EORTC-PAMM course on preclinical and early-phase clinical pharmacology. Anticancer Research. 2019;**39**(7):3303-3309

[29] Cutone A, Frioni A, Berlutti F, Valenti P, Musci G, Bonaccorsi di Patti MC. Lactoferrin prevents LPS-induced decrease of the iron exporter ferroportin in human monocytes/macrophages. Biometals. 2014;**27**:807-813

[30] Siddiqui N, Asawa S, Birru B, Baadhe R, Rao S. PCL-based composite scaffold matrices for tissue engineering applications. Molecular Biotechnology. 2018;**60**:506-532

[31] Ata FK, Yalcin S. The cisplatin, 5-fluorouracil, irinotecan, and gemcitabine treatment in resistant 2D and 3D model triple negative breast cancer cell line: ABCG2 expression data. Anti-Cancer Agents in Medicinal Chemistry (Formerly Current Medicinal Chemistry-Anti-Cancer Agents). 2022;**22**(2):371-377

[32] Arnold M, Morgan E, Rumgay H, Mafra A, Singh D, Laversanne M, et al. Current and future burden of breast cancer: Global statistics for 2020 and 2040. The Breast. 2022;**66**:15-23

[33] He L, Wick N, Germans SK, Peng Y. The role of breast cancer stem cells in chemoresistance and metastasis in triple-negative breast cancer. Cancers. 2021;**13**(24):6209

[34] Al Monla R, Dassouki Z, Sari-Chmayssem N, Mawlawi H, Gali-Muhtasib H. Fucoidan and alginate from the brown algae *Colpomenia sinuosa* and their combination with vitamin C trigger apoptosis in colon cancer. Molecules. 2022;**27**(2):358

[35] Niknejad F, Kordjazi M, Asadi Farsani O, Sinehsepehr K. Cytotoxic effects of the fucoidan extracted from Persian gulf brown algae *Sargassum ilicifolium* inducing apoptosis in breast cancer cell line. Journal of Fisheries. 2022;**75**(1):63-73

[36] Xue M, Ge Y, Zhang J, Wang Q, Hou L, Liu Y, et al. Anticancer properties and mechanisms of fucoidan on mouse breast cancer *in vitro* and *in vivo*. PLoS One. 2012;**7**(8):e43483

[37] Gao W, Guo Y, Wang L, Jiang Y, Liu Z, Lin H. Ameliorative and protective effects of fucoidan and sodium alginate against lead-induced oxidative stress in Sprague Dawley rats. International Journal of Biological Macromolecules. 2020;**158**:662-669

[38] He X, Xue M, Jiang S, Li W, Yu J, Xiang S. Fucoidan promotes apoptosis and inhibits EMT of breast cancer cells. Biological and Pharmaceutical Bulletin. 2019;**42**(3):442-447

[39] Lachowicz D, Karabasz A, Bzowska M, Szuwarzyński M, Karewicz A, Nowakowska M. Blood-compatible, stable micelles of sodium alginate–curcumin bioconjugate for anti-cancer applications. European Polymer Journal. 2019;**113**:208-219

[40] Hoan NX, Anh LTH, Ha HT, Cuong DX. Antioxidant activities, anticancer activity, physico-chemistry characteristics, and acute toxicity of alginate/lignin polymer. Molecules. 2023;**28**(13):5181

[41] Sun J, Tan H. Alginate-based biomaterials for regenerative medicine applications. Materials. 2013;**6**(4):1285-1309

[42] Ale MT, Maruyama H, Tamauchi H, Mikkelsen JD, Meyer AS. Fucoidan from *Sargassum* sp. and Fucus vesiculosus reduces cell viability of lung carcinoma and melanoma cells *in vitro* and activates natural killer cells in mice *in vivo*. International Journal of Biological Macromolecules. 2011;**49**(3):331-336

[43] Ahmad T, Eapen MS, Ishaq M, Park AY, Karpiniec SS, Stringer DN,

et al. Anti-inflammatory activity of fucoidan extracts *in vitro*. Marine Drugs. 2021;**19**(12):702

[44] Ni L, Wang L, Fu X, Duan D, Jeon Y-J, Xu J, et al. *In vitro* and *in vivo* anti-inflammatory activities of a fucose-rich fucoidan isolated from *Saccharina japonica*. International Journal of Biological Macromolecules. 2020;**156**:717-729

[45] Lee H-G, Nagahawatta D, Liyanage N, Jayawardhana H, Yang F, Je J-G, et al. Structural characterization and anti-inflammatory activity of fucoidan isolated from *Ecklonia maxima* stipe. Algae. 2022;**37**(3):239-247

[46] Kim M-J, Bae N-Y, Bark S-W, Kim K-B-W-R, Park J-H, Park S-H, et al. Anti-inflammatory effect of alginate oligosaccharides produced by an alginate-degrading enzyme from *Shewanella oneidensis* PKA1008 on LPS-induced RAW 264.7 cells. Korean Journal of Fisheries and Aquatic Sciences. 2015;**48**(6):888-897

[47] Vaghasiya K, Eram A, Sharma A, Ray E, Adlakha S, Verma RK. Alginate microspheres elicit innate M1-inflammatory response in macrophages leading to bacillary killing. AAPS PharmSciTech. 2019;**20**:1-10

[48] Razavi A, Khodadadi A, Eslami MB, Eshraghi S, Mirshafiei A. Therapeutic effect of sodium alginate in experimental chronic ulcerative colitis. Iranian Journal of Allergy, Asthma, and Immunology. 2008;7(1):13-18

[49] Malhão F, Ramos AA, Macedo AC, Rocha E. Cytotoxicity of seaweed compounds, alone or combined to reference drugs, against breast cell lines cultured in 2D and 3D. Toxics. 2021;**9**(2):24

[50] Imamura Y, Mukohara T, Shimono Y, Funakoshi Y, Chayahara N, Toyoda M, et al. Comparison of 2D-and 3D-culture models as drug-testing platforms in breast cancer. Oncology Reports. 2015;**33**(4):1837-1843

[51] Riedl A, Schlederer M, Pudelko K, Stadler M, Walter S, Unterleuthner D, et al. Comparison of cancer cells in 2D vs 3D culture reveals differences in AKT–mTOR–S6K signaling and drug responses. Journal of Cell Science. 2017;**130**(1):203-218

Section 4

Clinical Advances and Therapeutic Innovation

Chapter 14

Key Landmark Clinical Trials Transforming the Therapeutic Landscape of Metastatic Breast Cancer: From Precision Medicine to Immunotherapy

Uzma Saddia Asghar, Yashna Nadkarni, Ryan Panchal and Navita Somaiah

Abstract

Metastatic breast cancer remains a leading cause of mortality among women, drawing substantial attention in drug development research. Landmark clinical trials are notable for their role in securing drug approvals, improving clinical practice and reflect the culmination of decades of scientific effort. This chapter focuses on pivotal, phase 3 interventional trials that have improved the standard of care in metastatic breast cancer. First line use of CDK4/6 inhibitors was a "game changing" breakthrough for metastatic hormone breast cancer because they helped overcome endocrine resistance and provide an effective alternative to chemotherapy. Licensing of PI3 kinase inhibitors is a success story for biomarker driven treatment strategies using *PIK3CA* mutations to select patients, and, combining immunotherapy with chemotherapy in triple negative breast cancer has improved clinical outcomes for women with aggressive disease. Consequently, women with metastatic breast cancer have more treatment options, are living longer but still anticipate a cure.

Keywords: metastatic breast cancer, landmark clinical trials, chemotherapy, CDK4/6 inhibitors, endocrine treatment, antibody drug conjugates, immunotherapy, patient outcomes (progression free survival = PFS overall survival = OS)

1. Introduction

In the western world approximately 5–10% of people present with de novo metastatic breast cancer and 90–95% of people relapse following a previous breast cancer diagnosis despite being treated with curative intent. Conventionally, breast cancer is classified into three main subtypes using immunohistochemistry scoring system for estrogen receptor (ER), progesterone receptor (PR), and the human epidermal growth factor receptor-2 (HER2). The three breast cancer subtypes, in order of prevalence are:

i. Hormone receptor-positive (ER+ve +/− PR+ve),

ii. HER2 amplified breast cancer (HER2+ve with/without ER+ve +/− PR+ve receptors), and

iii. Triple negative breast cancer (TNBC) which is negative for all three receptors (ER−ve, PR−ve and HER2−ve).

The overall survival (OS) for individuals with metastatic disease (stage IV) has improved due to the availability of more effective treatments. However, there remains a prognostic disparity across the breast cancer subtypes. The current median overall survival (mOS) is 4–5 years for the hormone positive (HR+ve) subgroup, 4–5 years for the HER2-positive disease and only 10–13 months for metastatic TNBC. Therapeutics which have significantly improved clinical outcomes for patients include antibody drug conjugates, immunotherapy combination with chemotherapy, and, targeted small molecules which are chemotherapy sparing and preferably used with hormone treatment prior to chemotherapy. The drive for precision medicine has pushed the development of new predictive molecular biomarkers which are embedded within companion diagnostic assays such as *PIK3CA* mutations, PD-L1 staining and pathogenic germline *BRCA* mutations. In this chapter we highlight the key landmark clinical trials which have led to drug approval, changed clinical practice and significantly reshaped the rapidly evolving therapeutic landscape for metastatic breast cancer over the last decade [1].

2. Hormone (HR+ve, HER2−ve) positive breast cancer

Hormone positive (HR+ve) breast cancer, also referred to as luminal A and B subtypes represents 70–80% of all breast cancers and can affect both women (~95%) and men (5%). HR+ve breast cancers are commoner in older, postmenopausal women, and although the prevalence is slightly lower in premenopausal women, it still represents the most common subtype across all age groups. An internationally accepted immunohistochemistry scoring system is used for estrogen receptor and progesterone receptor positivity, where 1–100% of the tumor cell percentage and staining is currently considered as positive. Breast tumors with 10% or more are considered clearly HR positive, and tumors with less than >1–<10% hormone receptor staining are considered to have a low estrogen/progesterone expression [2].

The current mOS for metastatic hormone positive breast cancers is approximately 4 years with 25% of individuals alive at 5 years despite the modern therapeutic landscape [3, 4]. Although endocrine therapy remains the gold standard treatment for HR+ metastatic breast cancer, there have been significant advances in drug development to help overcome endocrine resistance over the last 10 years which have improved patient prognosis. Clinical practice, where possible and not constrained by financial pressures has moved away from single agent hormone treatment, towards the routine use of drug combinations with endocrine treatment as the main therapeutic backbone, in combination with a targeted anti-cancer agent. Here, we outline the key practice changing landmark studies which have delivered effective drugs for routine administration like the CDK4/6 inhibitors and inhibitors of PI3 kinase—AKT—mTOR signaling pathway to mitigate endocrine resistance in the clinic (Summary in **Table 1** and **Figure 1**).

Trial	Author	Year	Line	Investigational Arm	Standard of care	1ery End-point	Median PFS months	PFS HR (95%CI)	P-VALUE	Median OS months	OS HR (95%CI)	P-value	Menopausal status
MONARCH-3	Goetz et al [5]	2017	1st	NSAI+ abemaciclib	NSAI+ placebo	PFS	NR vs. 14.7 m	0.54 (0.41–0.72)	<0.0001	Not mature	N/A	N/A	Post
	Johnston et al. [6]	2019					28.18 *vs.* 14.8 m	0.54 (0.418–0.698)	<0.0001	Not mature	N/A	N/A	
	Goetz et al. [7]	2024					29.0 *vs.* 14.8 m	0.535 (0.429–0.668)	<0.0001	66.8 *vs.* 53.7 m	0.804	0.0664	
MONALEESA-2	Hortobagyi et al. [8–10]	2016	1st	Letrozole + ribociclib	Letrozole + placebo	PFS	NR *vs.* 14.7 m	0.56 (0.43–0.72)	<0.0001	Not mature	N/A	N/A	Post
		2018					25.3 *vs.* 16 m	0.568 (0.457–0.704)	<0.0001	Not mature	N/A	N/A	
		2022					N/A	N/A	N/A	63.9 *vs.* 51.4 m	0.76 (0.63–0.93)	0.008	
MONALEESA-7	Tripathy et al. [11]	2018	1st	ET+ ribociclib	ET + placebo	PFS	23.8 *vs.* 13.0 m	0.55 (0.44–0.69)	<0.0001	N/A	N/A	N/A	Pre-
	Im S et al. [12]	2019					N/A	N/A	N/A	NR *vs.* 40.9 m	0.71 (0.54–0.95)	0.00973	
	Lu et al. [13]	2022					N/A	N/A	N/A	58.7 *vs.* 48 m	0.76 (0.61–0.96)	?	

Trial	Author	Year	Line	Investigational Arm	Standard of care	1ery End - point	Median PFS months	PFS HR (95%CI)	P-VALUE	Median OS months	OS HR (95%CI)	P-value	Menopausal status
PALOMA-2	Finn et al. [14]	2016	1st	Letrozole +palbociclib	Letrozole +placebo	PFS	24.8 *vs.* 14.5 m	0.58 (0.46–0.72)	<0.001	Not mature	N/A	N/A	Post
	Rugo et al. [15]	2019					27.6 *vs.* 14.5 m	0.563 (0.461 – 0.687)	<0.0001	Not mature	N/A	N/A	
	Slamon et al. [3]	2024					N/A	N/A	N/A	53.9 *vs.* 51.2 m	0.96 (0.78–1.18)	0.34	
PALOMA-3	Turner et al. [16, 17]	2015	2nd	Fulvestrant + palbociclib	Fulvestrant + palbociclib	PFS	9.2 *vs.* 3.8 m	0.42 (0.32–0.56)	< 0.001	Not mature	N/A	N/A	Pre-/post
		2018					11.2 *vs.* 4.6	0.50 (0.4–0.62)	<0.0001	34 *vs.* 28.0 m	0.81 (0.64–1.03)	0.09	
MONALEESA-3	Slamon et al. [18, 19]	2018	1st or 2nd	Fulvestrant + ribociclib	Fulvestrant + placebo	PFS	20.5 *vs.* 12.8 m	0.593 (0.48–0.732)	<0.001	Not mature	N/A	N/A	Post
		2020					20.6 *vs.* 12.8 m	0.59 (0.49–0.71)	N/A	NR *vs.* 40.0 m (placebo)	0.72 (0.57–0.92)	0.0045	
MONARCH-2	Sledge et al. [20, 21]	2017	2nd	Fulvestrant + Abemaciclib	Fulvestrant + placebo	PFS	16.4 *vs.* 9.3 m	0.553 (0.45–0.681)	<0.001	Not mature	N/A	N/A	Pre-/post
		2020					16.9 *vs.* 9.3 m	0.536 (0.45–0.645)	<0.001	46.7 *vs.* 37.3 m	0.757 (0.61–0.945)	0.0137	

Trial	Author	Year	Line	Investigational Arm	Standard of care	1ery End - point	Median PFS months	PFS HR (95%CI)	P-VALUE	Median OS months	OS HR (95%CI)	P-value	Menopausal status
BOLERO-2	Baselga et al. [22]	2012	2nd	Exemestane + everolimus	Exemestane + placebo	PFS	10.6 *vs.* 4.1 m Central assess	0.36 (0.27–0.47)	<0.001	Not mature	N/A	N/A	Post
	Piccart et al. [23]	2014					N/A	N/A	N/A	31.0 *vs.* 26.6 m	0.89 (0.73–1.10)	0.14	
SOLAR-1	Andre et al. [24, 25]	2019	2nd	Fulvestrant + alpelisib	Fulvestrant + placebo	PFS	*PIK3CA*-mut: 11 *vs.* 5.7 m	0.65 (0.50–0.85)	<0.001	Not mature	N/A	N/A	Post
							PIK3CA-wt: 7.4 *vs.* 5.6 m	0.85 (0.58–1.25)	N/A	Not mature	N/A	N/A	
		2021					N/A	N/A	N/A	*PIK3CA*-mut: 39.3 m *vs.* 31.4 m	0.86 (0.64–1.15)	0.15	

ET = endocrine treatment.

Table 1.
Selected key landmark studies in hormone positive (ER+ve, HER2−ve) metastatic breast cancer.

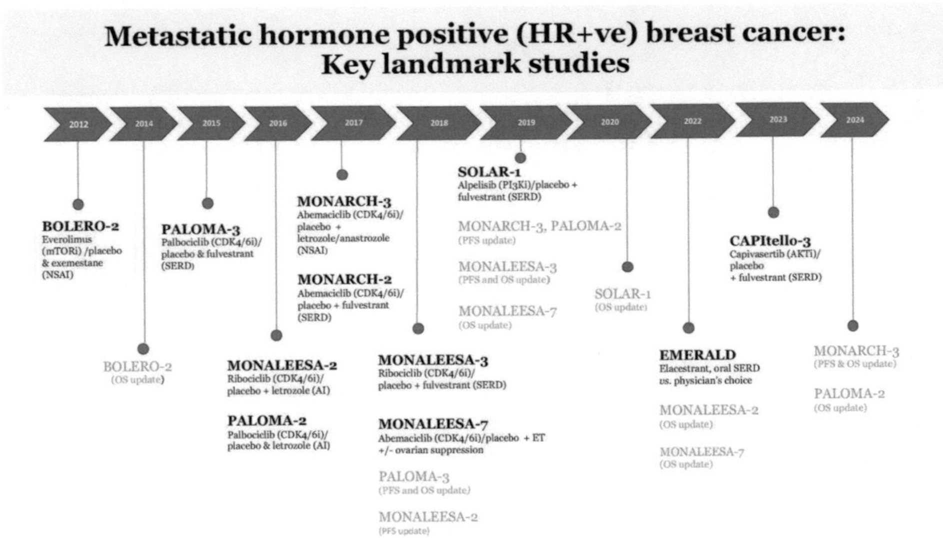

Figure 1.
Timeline for selected key landmark studies in metastatic hormone positive breast cancer. Abbreviations: AKTi = AKT inhibitor, AI = aromatase inhibitor, ET = endocrine treatment, mTORi = mammalian target of rapamycin inhibitor, NSAI = non-steroidal aromatase inhibitor, PFS = progression free survival, OS = overall survival, SERD = selective estrogen receptor degrader.

2.1 Cyclin dependent kinase 4/6 (CDK4/6) inhibitors

2.1.1 PALOMA-3 study

Targeted inhibition of both CDK4 and CDK6 arrests the cell cycle with reported drug synergy between CDK4/6 inhibitors and hormone inhibitors in pre-clinical cell models [26]. The PALOMA-3 study tested if the combination of palbociclib (Ibrance®, Pfizer)-with fulvestrant [Faslodex®, AstraZeneca]) could significantly overcome endocrine resistance.

PALOMA-3 was a randomized double blind, multi-center clinical trial which randomized (2:1) people to receive either palbociclib-fulvestrant or placebo-fulvestrant and included both pre- and postmenopausal women. The intended target population was hormone resistant because these individuals had progressed during or after endocrine treatment. The initial preplanned interim analysis (2015) reported a doubling of the median progression free survival (mPFS) by adding palbociclib to fulvestrant. With palbociclib, the mPFS improved to 9.2 months compared to 3.8 months for the control arm treated with placebo–fulvestrant (hazard ratio [HR] for disease progression or death, 0.42; 95% CI, 0.32–0.56; $P < 0.001$) [16].

Surprisingly, despite an absolute overall survival (OS) difference of +6.9 months between the two study arms, this [16, 17] difference was not statistically significant. The median OS was 34.9 months in the palbociclib-fulvestrant group and 28.0 months in the placebo-fulvestrant group (HR for death, 0.81; 95% CI, 0.64–1.03; $P = 0.09$) [17]. Many clinicians consider this difference in OS as clinically meaningful and continue to prescribe palbociclib with fulvestrant for their patients.

The key learnings from PALOMA-3, the first clinical study to formally report the benefits of combining CDK4/6 inhibition with endocrine blockade as an effective treatment strategy, was that adding a CDK4/6 inhibitor doubled the mPFS compared to the standard of care, single agent fulvestrant. This study revolutionized the treatment for metastatic HR+ve breast cancer by providing an effective solution to overcome hormone resistance, delay cancer progression and delay the use of chemotherapy. It was shortly followed by multiple positive studies reporting the benefits of CDK4/6 inhibitors in metastatic HR+ve breast cancer [16, 17].

2.1.2 PALOMA-2 study

PALOMA-2 was the game changing which altered first line treatment for HR+ve metastatic breast cancer from single agent aromatase inhibitor to a doublet combination of a CDK4/6 inhibitor with an aromatase inhibitor (2016).

PALOMA-2 (n = 666) was a double-blinded study which randomized (2:1) participants (post-menopausal women only or men) to either palbociclib-letrozole (n = 444) or, placebo-letrozole (n = 222). The palbociclib dose and regimen was the same as in PALOMA-3 which was 125 mg/day of palbociclib, taken orally over a 28-day treatment cycle, (21 days on treatment and 7 days off treatment) or a matching placebo. The dose for the aromatase inhibitor letrozole was 2.5 mg (Femara®, Novartis), taken orally, daily. The primary end point for the study was PFS, as assessed by the investigators.

The addition of palbociclib significantly improved the mPFS to 24.8 months in the palbociclib-letrozole group compared to 14.5 months in the placebo-letrozole group (HR, 0.58; 95%CI, 0.4–0.72; P < 0.001) [14]. Disappointingly this improvement in delaying breast cancer progression did not translate to a significant statistical improvement in survival (2024). The mOS was 53.9 months with palbociclib-letrozole *vs.* 51.2 months with placebo-letrozole (HR, 0.96, P = 0.34; refer to **Table 1** for more details) [3].

The key learnings from PALOMA-2 were that combining CDK4/6 inhibitors with hormone treatment significantly improved cancer control in the hormone sensitive population. Consequently, first line management of HR+ve breast cancer changed to this combination treatment. The lack of statistically significant OS difference impacted the choice of CDK4/6 inhibitor in the clinic. Palbociclib became less favorable as first choice and many, but not all switched to an alternative CDK4/6 inhibitor such as ribociclib with stronger survival data.

2.1.3 MONALEESA-2 study

The MONALEESA series of clinical studies tested the CDK4/6 inhibitor ribociclib (Kisqali®, Novartis) in breast cancer. The MONALEESA-2 study (n = 668) was conducted on a similar parallel timeline as PALOMA-2 and PALOMA-3. MONALEESA-2 evaluated ribociclib with letrozole, first line in postmenopausal women with hormone sensitive metastatic breast cancer. Women were randomly assigned to receive either oral ribociclib (600 mg/day 21 days on treatment and 7 days off; q28) plus letrozole (2.5 mg/day) or placebo-letrozole. The primary end point was investigator-assessed PFS.

Ribociclib improved PFS from 42.2% in the placebo group to 63.0% in the CDK4/6 inhibitor group (HR, 0.56; P < 0.001) [8]. After a median follow-up of 6.6 years (2022), the survival difference was reported to be statistically significant with an additional benefit of +1 year with ribociclib-letrozole. The mOS for individual treated with ribociclib-letrozole was 63.9 months (95% CI, 52.4–71.0) and 51.4 months in the control arm (95% CI, 47.2–59.7; HR, 0.76; two-sided P = 0.008) [9].

The key learnings from the MONALEESA-2 study were that the benefits of adding CDK4/6 inhibitors to endocrine treatment was a drug class effect and the use of ribociclib combination resulted in a significant survival benefit. The survival data from MONALEESA-2 shifted preference to prescribing ribociclib as the CDK4/6 inhibitor of choice, first line for metastatic hormone positive breast cancer.

2.1.4 MONALEESA-7 study

Historically pre-menopausal women were omitted from clinical studies testing novel drugs/combinations with aromatase inhibitors until the benefits of ovarian suppression were established. The MONALEESA-7 study is notable because this trial focused exclusively upon the pre-menopausal population. MONALEESA-7 was a phase 3, randomized, double-blind, placebo-controlled trial which recruited younger pre-menopausal women (n = 672) aged between 18 and 59 years. The study evaluated ribociclib-endocrine therapy (tamoxifen or a non-steroidal aromatase inhibitor) plus ovarian suppression with goserelin in HR+ve, HER2−ve, advanced breast cancer. Previous permissible treatments included endocrine therapy and chemotherapy in either the adjuvant or neoadjuvant setting, and one line of chemotherapy for advanced disease. The MONALEESA-7 study confirmed a similar beneficial improvement in both mPFS and mOS for the ribociclib treatment arm [11].

The key learnings from the MONALEESA-7 study were that ribociclib administered with an aromatase inhibitor and ovarian suppression had similar prognostic benefit in the pre-menopausal population. This enables clinicians to take a more patient-centric focus by confidently delaying chemotherapy use and the associated toxicities in younger women without compromising quality of life or cancer control (**Table 1**).

2.1.5 Drug toxicity profiles for CDK4/6 inhibitors

Most common drug associated adverse events for palbociclib, ribociclib and abemaciclib are shared across the three CDK4/6 inhibitors such as hematological toxicities and decreased immunosuppression. There are drug specific adverse events which may influence the choice of drug. For example, palbociclib is more likely to cause fatigue, alopecia and drop in blood counts. Ribociclib specific adverse events include QT prolongation and a derangement in the liver function tests (increase in alanine transaminase and aspartate aminotransferases). Abemaciclib has a higher incidence of gastrointestinal toxicities, such as diarrhea and mucosal toxicities. The advantage of having access to all three drugs are that the clinician can select the most tolerable CDK4/6 inhibitor for their patient and, switch CDK4/6 inhibitors if the initial choice is not tolerable [27].

2.2 PI3 kinase-AKT-mTOR signaling pathway

The crosstalk between the estrogen receptor and the PI3K-AKT-mTOR pathways has been a key strategic focus for circumventing or delaying endocrine resistance in metastatic HR+ve breast cancer. Inhibition of the **m**echanistic **T**arget **O**f **R**apamycin (mTOR) protein is a success story for using a targeted therapeutic approach illustrated in the BOLERO-2 study (2012). Decades of scientific research has delivered various types of PI3 kinase inhibitors and more recently AKT inhibitors. For the first time in history, there is now a licensed compound for each drug class: everolimus (mTOR inhibitor), alpelisib (PI3 kinase inhibitor) and capivasertib (AKT inhibitor), with several newer compounds in the pipeline.

2.2.1 BOLERO-2 study (breast cancer trials of oral everolimus-2)

Aberrant mTOR signaling through the PI3-mTOR pathway can drive endocrine resistance and in pre-clinical models, mTOR inhibition restores endocrine sensitivity. Everolimus (Afinitor®, Novartis) is the first and currently the only licensed mTOR inhibitor routinely used in combination with exemestane in metastatic HR+ve, HER2-ve breast cancer. Everolimus allosterically binds to mTORC1.

BOLERO-2 was the registration phase 3 clinical study (n = 724) which randomized (2:1) patients to everolimus-exemestane or placebo-exemestane. An essential eligibility requirement was recurrence or progression on a nonsteroidal aromatase inhibitor in the adjuvant or advanced disease setting, or both. Previous therapy included letrozole or anastrozole (100%), tamoxifen (48%), fulvestrant (16%), and chemotherapy (68%). In 2012, central assessment identified that everolimus-exemestane modestly improved mPFS from 4.1 to 10.6 months (HR, 0.36; 95% CI, 0.27–0.47; $P < 0.001$), meeting the primary study endpoint, and consequently entered routine clinical practice. After the drug was approved, later OS data showed no statistical improvement with the addition of everolimus (mOS 31 *vs.* 26.6 months, HR = 0.89; log-rank P = 0.14).

The key learnings from BOLERO-2, the earliest landmark study discussed in this chapter, conducted years prior to the current era of CDK4/6 inhibitors, were that targeting the PI3-kinase-mTOR signaling pathway could reverse hormone resistance when used in the second- or third-line setting. Currently, the body of evidence suggests that the everolimus-exemestane drug combination is active in the unselected patient population, including the *PIK3CA* wild-type population, not eligible for a *PIK3CA* inhibitor [22, 23].

2.2.2 SOLAR-1 (clinical studies of alpelisib in breast cancer 1) study

PIK3CA mutations are detectable in up to approximately 40% of patients with HR +ve, HER2-ve breast cancer. Breast cancer (HR+ve) patients with *PIK3CA* mutations have worse prognosis than individuals with *PIK3CA* wild-type cancers [28]. Alpelisib (Piqray®, Novartis) is an α-specific class I PI3K inhibitor available with fulvestrant in the clinic, specifically for the *PIK3CA* mutant, HR+ve population. SOLAR-1 was the phase 3 registration clinical study which led to the approval of alpelisib with fulvestrant (2019). In SOLAR-1 individuals who had previously received endocrine treatment were randomized to alpelisib (300 mg daily, oral) plus fulvestrant (500 mg every 28 days) or placebo-fulvestrant in both the *PIK3CA* mutant and *PIK3CA* wild-type populations.

Alpelisib-fulvestrant combination demonstrated superior clinical efficacy in the *PIK3CA* mutant population only. In the *PIK3CA* mutant cohort, the mPFS was 11.0 months (95% CI, 7.5–14.5) with alpelisib-fulvestrant group *vs.* 5.7 months (95% CI, 3.7–7.4) in the placebo-fulvestrant group (HR, 0.65, $P < 0.001$). There was a small benefit of only +1.8 months in the *PIK3CA* wild-type cohort. Surprisingly, the OS difference was not statistically significant despite a numerical improvement of +7.9 months (n = 341). The median OS was 39.3 months (95% CI, 34.1–44.9) for alpelisib-fulvestrant and 31.4 months (26.8–41.3) for placebo-fulvestrant (HR, 0.86, P = 0.15)] [24].

The key learnings from the SOLAR-1 study were that the PI3 kinase was finally druggable with alpelisib, the first PI3 kinase inhibitor to demonstrate clinical activity with fulvestrant in hormone resistant breast cancer, with *PIK3CA* mutations.

2.2.3 CAPItello-291 (AKT) study

AKT is a serine and threonine kinase considered an important signaling node in the PI3-AKT-mTOR pathway. Aberrant AKT signaling can drive hormone resistance following endocrine treatment in breast cancer. Genetic alterations in the tumor increase AKT signaling, most commonly activating *PIK3CA* or *AKT* mutations or inactivation of the tumor suppressor gene *PTEN*. Capivasertib (Truqap®, AstraZeneca) is the first in class oral AKT inhibitor which inhibits all three AKT isoforms.

Capivasertib was approved by the FDA (2023) for use in combination with fulvestrant following the positive phase 3 CAPItello-291 registration study and the phase 2 study FAKTION [29]. CAPItello-291 was a randomized (n = 708), double-blind trial which recruited individuals with HR+ve, HER2-negative advanced breast cancer who had relapsed or progressed during or after an aromatase inhibitor, with a CDK4/6 inhibitor (69.1%) or without (30.9%). Capivasertib/placebo dosing schedule was oral 400 mg, BD for 4 days on treatment followed by 3 days off treatment each week, over a 28-day treatment cycle. The primary end points were investigator-assessed PFS and OS in both the overall population and the subpopulation with AKT pathway-altered (*PIK3CA, AKT1* or *PTEN*) tumors (n = 289 patients, 40.8%) [30].

Capivasertib-fulvestrant delayed breast cancer progression by 40% and doubled the mPFS (+3.6 months) from 3.6 months in the placebo-fulvestrant group to 7.2 months in the capivasertib-fulvestrant group (HR, 0.60; $P < 0.001$). Capivasertib-fulvestrant demonstrated clinical activity in the broader population beyond the AKT pathway-altered (*PIK3CA*, *AKT1* or *PTEN*) cases.

The key learnings from the CAPItello-291 study were that AKT is a useful drug target in endocrine resistant disease with promising clinical activity. The impact of this novel combination upon OS is yet to be determined.

2.2.4 Drug toxicity for inhibitors of PI3-AKT-mTOR signaling pathway

Current clinical trial data suggests that alpelisib-fulvestrant combination is less tolerable with drug discontinuation rates up to 33% for alpelisib-fulvestrant [24], 25% for everolimus-exemestane [22] and 13% for capivasertib-fulvestrant [30]. Over a third of patients on alpelisib-fulvestrant developed hyperglycaemia (37%) needing anti-diabetic medication, 10% reported a rash and 7% experienced diarrhea. Hence, diabetic patients with breast cancer were preferentially excluded from administration of alpelisib. Although, the hyperglycemia rates were lower (16%) in individuals treated with capivasertib-fulvestrant, the rates of diarrhea (72%; Grade 1 46%) and rash were higher (38%). The everolimus combination appears to have the lowest rates of hyperglycaemia (4%) in the BOLERO-2 study, although currently there is no direct comparison of drug toxicity profiles for alpelisib *vs.* capivasertib *vs.* everolimus. Patients taking everolimus can experience severe mouth ulcers and stomatitis (8%) preventable through prophylactic steroid mouth washes and starting at a lower dose (5 mg) of everolimus. In summary, we have three drug combinations all competing in a similar clinical space, post CDK4/6 inhibition where the specific drug toxicity profiles and the patient's co-morbidities may be the deciding factor, especially if the OS data from the CAPItello-291 study is negative.

2.3 Oral selective estrogen receptor degraders (SERDS)

Acquisition of hormone resistance in breast cancer is underpinned by multiple different mechanisms including the development of mutations in the estrogen receptor gene-1, referred to as *ESR1* mutations. *ESR1* mutations occur in 20-40% of metastatic HR+ve breast cancer cases following exposure to aromatase inhibitors. *ESR1* mutations drive estrogen-independent, constitutive activation of estrogen receptor [31]. Selective estrogen receptor degraders (SERDs) bind to the estrogen receptor with or without *ESR1* mutations and induce receptor degradation reducing estrogen signaling. The second generation oral SERDS are estrogen receptor antagonists with better bioavailability than fulvestrant, a first-generation SERD administered intramuscularly [32]. Elacestrant (Orserdu®, Stemline Therapeutics, Inc.) is the first oral SERD (non-steroidal) to get FDA approval (2023) following the EMRALD registration study which is now available for use in the clinic with a ctDNA diagnostic assay, Guardant360®, used for detecting *ESR1* mutations from liquid biopsies.

2.3.1 EMRALD study

The EMRALD study was a randomized, open-label, phase 3 trial targeting the hormone resistant HR+ve, HER2-ve advanced population. The requirements were previous progression on a CDK4/6 inhibitor-endocrine treatment and had at least one (52.2%) or two (47.8%) lines of previous hormone therapy with no more than one line of chemotherapy. The treatment arms were either the oral SERD elacestrant 400 mg orally once daily (n = 239) or standard-of-care (SOC) endocrine monotherapy (n = 238). The primary end points were PFS by blinded independent central review in all patients and patients with detectable *ESR1* mutations (47.8%). Elacestrant demonstrated modest but greater drug activity in the *ESR1* mutant population (mPFS 3.8 *vs.* 1.9 months) compared to the *ESR1* wildtype population (mPFS 2.8 *vs.* 1.9 months) with an initial sharp drop in the Kaplan-Meier curves for both groups in the first 2 months suggesting intrinsic drug resistance to elacestrant in 40–60% of individuals. Elacestrant reduced risk of progression or death by 30% in the overall cohort (P = 0.002) and by 45% in patients with *ESR1* mutations (P = 0.0005) [33]. Similarly to the AKT inhibitor capivasertib, the release of the OS analyses is awaited.

The key learning from the EMRALD study was that elacestrant, the first approved oral SERD had better clinical efficacy than fulvestrant, the standard of care treatment choice in most cases. As a single agent, elacestrant demonstrated modest clinical activity in the hormone resistant *ESR1* mutant population and is under ongoing evaluation within different drug combinations in clinical studies.

3. HER2 positive (HER2+ve, HR+ve/−ve) breast cancer

Approximately 20% of breast cancers overexpress the transmembrane human epidermal growth factor receptor 2 (HER2+ve). Historically, HER2+ve breast cancers used to have the worst prognostic outcomes, however significant therapeutic advances over the past 20 years have dramatically improved the outlook for this breast cancer subtype. The mOS for HER2+ve breast cancer has significantly improved to 4–5 years with infrequent reports of durable complete responses in women with metastatic breast cancer. Unfortunately, despite the impressive success of monoclonal HER2 directed antibodies and the novel antibody drug conjugates outlined below (**Table 2** and **Figure 2**), most people with HER2-positive metastatic breast cancer

Trial	Author	Journal	Year	Line	Investigational arm	Standard of care	1ery end -point	Median PFS months	HR (95% CI)	P-value	Median OS months	OS HR (95% CI)	P-value
CLEOPATRA	Baselga et al. [34]	NEJM	2012	1st	Pertuzumab + trastuzumab + docetaxel	Placebo + trastuzumab + docetaxel	PFS	18.5 *vs.*12.4 m	0.62 (0.51–0.75)	<0.001	Not mature	N/A	N/A
	Swain et al. [35]	NEJM	2015				OS	18.7 *vs.*12.4 m	0.68 (0.58–0.80)	<0.001	56.5 *vs* 40.8 m	0.68 (0.56–0.84)	<0.001
EMILIA	Verma et al. [36]	NEJM	2012	2nd	Trastuzumab emtansine	Lapatinib + capecitabine	PFS	9.6 *vs.* 6.4 m	0.65 (0.55–0.77)	<0.001	30.9 *vs* 25.1 m	0.68 (0.55–0.85)	<0.001
	Dieras et al. [37]	Lancet Oncology	2017				OS	N/A	N/A	N/A	29.9 *vs* 25.9 m	0.75 (0.64–0.88)	N/A
DESTINY-Breast02	Andre et al. [38]	Lancet	2023	2nd	Trastuzumab deruxtecan	Physician's choice (capecitabine + trastuzumab, or capecitabine + lapatinib)	PFS	17.8 *vs.*6.9 m	0.36 (0.28–0.45)	<0.0001	39.2 *vs* 26.5 m	0.66 (0.50–0.86)	0.0021
DESTINY-Breast03	Cortes et al. [39]	NEJM	2022	2nd	Trastuzumab deruxtecan	Trastuzumab emtansine	PFS	NR *vs.* 6.8 m	0.28 (0.22–0.37)	<0.001	Not mature	N/A	N/A
	Hurvitz et al. [40]	Lancet	2023				OS	28.8 *vs.*6.8 m	0.33 (0.26–0.43)	<0.0001	NR (40.5 m-NE) *vs.* NR (34.0 m-NE)	0.64 (0.47–0.87)	0.0037
	Hamilton, et al. [41]	JCO	2024		OS		29.0 *vs.*7.2 m	N/A	N/A	52.6 *vs* 42.7 m	0.73 (0.56–0.94)	N/A	

DOI: http://dx.doi.org/10.5772/intechopen.1008863

Trial	Author	Journal	Year	Line	Investigational arm	Standard of care	1ery end -point	Median PFS months	HR (95% CI)	P-value	Median OS months	OS HR (95% CI)	P-value
DESTINY-Breast04	Modi et al. [42]	NEJM	2022	2nd	Trastuzumab deruxtecan	Physician's choice (capecitabine, eribulin, gemcitabine, paclitaxel or nab-paclitaxel)	PFS	9.9 *vs.* 5.1 m	0.50 (0.40–0.63)	<0.001	23.4 *vs* 16.8 m	0.64 (0.49–0.84)	0.001
	Modi et al. [43]	Annals of Oncology	2023					8.8 *vs.* 4.2 m	0.36 (0.29–0.45)	N/A	22.9 *vs.* 16.8 m	0.69 (0.55–0.86)	N/A
HER2CLIMB	Murthy et al. [44]	NEJM	2020	3rd	Tucatinib + trastuzumab + capecitabine	Placebo + trastuzumab + capecitabine	PFS	7.8 *vs.*5.6 m	0.54 (0.42–0.71)	<0.001	21.9 *vs* 17.4 m	0.66 (0.50–0.88)	0.005
TH3RESA	Krop et al. [45]	Lancet Oncology	2014	3rd	Trastuzumab emtansine	Physician's choice (chemotherapy, hormonal therapy, HER2-directed therapy, or combination)	PFS	6.2 *vs.*3.3 m	0.53 (0.42–0.66)	<0.0001	Not mature	N/A	N/A
	Krop et al. [46]	Lancet Oncology	2017				OS	N/A	N/A	N/A	22.7 *vs* 15.8 m	0.68 (0.54–0.85)	0.0007

N/A = not applicable, NR = not reached.

Table 2.
Selected key landmark studies in HER2+ve positive (HER2+ve) metastatic breast cancer.

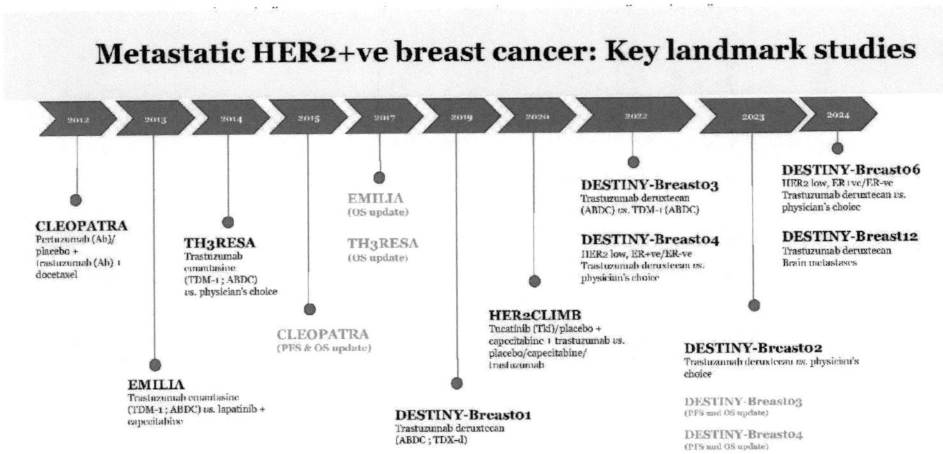

Figure 2.
Timeline for selected key landmark studies in metastatic HER2+ve breast cancer. Abbreviations: Ab = monoclonal antibody, ABDC = antibody drug conjugate, HER2 = Human epidermal growth receptor, HER2+ve = IHC HER2 3+ or -ISH+ve, HER2 low = IHC 1+ or 2+ but ISH−ve, TKi = tyrosine kinase inhibitor, PFS = progression free survival, OS = overall survival, SERD = selective estrogen receptor degrader.

continue to die from their cancer, re-enforcing the ongoing need for developing better drugs.

3.1 Monoclonal HER2 directed antibodies

3.1.1 CLEOPATRA study

The CLEOPATRA study (2015; n = 808) proved the combination of docetaxel chemotherapy plus dual HER2 inhibition with both pertuzumab (Perjeta®, Genentech) and trastuzumab (Herceptin®, Genentech) was more effective first line for metastatic HER2+ve breast cancer than trastuzumab alone with chemotherapy. The scientific rationale of combining pertuzumab with trastuzumab was the distinct HER2 binding sites of both antibodies. Pertuzumab binds to subdomain 2 of the extracellular portion of the HER2 receptor, and trastuzumab binds to the subdomain 4 of the HER2 receptor [47].

In CLEOPATRA, treatment naïve patients who had not received previous chemotherapy or anti-HER2 therapy for metastatic disease, were randomly assigned to docetaxel-trastuzumab-pertuzumab or docetaxel-trastuzumab-placebo. The primary end point was independently assessed PFS. Adding pertuzumab to docetaxel-trastuzumab improved PFS by +6.1 months from a mPFS of 12.4 (control group) to 18.5 months in the pertuzumab group (HR, 0.62; $P < 0.001$) [34]. There was a profound increase in OS by +15.7 months with a mOS of 56.5 months (95% CI, 49.3 to not reached) *vs.* 40.8 months (95% CI, 35.8–48.3) in the placebo group (HR, 0.68; $P < 0.001$).

The key learnings from the CLEOPATRA study were that dual inhibition of HER2 receptor was better without significant new drug toxicities, establishing taxane-trastuzumab-pertuzumab as the optimal treatment of choice for first line metastatic HER2+ve breast cancer. This regimen remained the standard of care over the last decade [35].

3.2 Antibody drug conjugates

3.2.1 EMILIA study

Trastuzumab emtansine (T-DM1; Kadcyla®, Genentech) was the first antibody-drug conjugate to get approval for HER2+ve breast cancer at least 10 years ago. Trastuzumab emtansine targets HER2 receptor on the cell surface. Trastuzumab emtansine consists of one molecule of trastuzumab conjugated by a non-cleavable linker to approximately 3.5 molecules of a cytotoxic payload emtansine, a derivative of maytansine with anti-microtubule properties [48].

The Phase 3 EMILIA study (n = 991) evaluated the efficacy of trastuzumab emtansine (2013) before the CLEOPATRA study had established docetaxel-trastuzumab-pertuzumab as the standard of care, first line. Patients with HER2-positive advanced breast cancer, who had progressed on taxane-trastuzumab were randomly assigned (1:1) second line treatment to either trastuzumab emtansine (3.6 mg/kg, IV) or the control arm with lapatinib (oral, 1250 mg daily) plus capecitabine (oral 1000 mg, BD 14 days on and 7 days off treatment, q21). The primary end points for the study were met with a positive increase in PFS, OS, and tolerable safety. The median PFS assessed by an independent review was 9.6 months with trastuzumab emtansine treatment *vs.* 6.4 months with lapatinib-capecitabine (HR, 0.65; $P < 0.001$). Median OS (second interim analysis) was 30.9 months with trastuzumab emtansine *vs.* 25.1 months with lapatinib-capecitabine (HR, 0.68; $P < 0.001$).

The key learnings from the EMILIA study were than the antibody drug conjugate trastuzumab emtansine was more effective than the existing standard of care despite developing resistance to previous antibody induced HER2 blockade. Trastuzumab emtansine displaced lapatinib-capecitabine to third line and onwards [36]. The EMILIA study secured the commitment needed for ongoing research and development of the next generation antibody-drug conjugates.

3.2.2 DESTINY Breast-03 study

Approximately 10 years following FDA approval of the antibody-drug conjugate trastuzumab emtansine, a third generation highly potent HER2 directed antibody-drug conjugate was approved in 2023 called trastuzumab deruxtecan (T-DXd, DS-8201, Enhurtu®, Daiichi Sankyo-AstraZeneca). Trastuzumab deruxtecan is composed of a trastuzumab antibody linked via a cleavable linker to deruxtecan (payload), a potent topoisomerase I inhibitor with a drug to antibody ratio of 8:1 [49].

Trastuzumab deruxtecan was recently evaluated in the landmark study DESTINY Breast-03 study against the current standard of care, trastuzumab emtansine. Trastuzumab deruxtecan demonstrated durable antitumor activity in heavily pretreated patients in DESTINY-Breast02 [38]. DESTINY-Breast03 was a phase 3, multicenter, open-label, randomized (1:1) trial (n = 524) which compared the efficacy and safety of trastuzumab deruxtecan (n = 261; 5.4 mg/kg, IV, q21) against trastuzumab emtansine (n = 263; 3.6 mg/kg, IV, q21), the standard of care, in patients with HER2+ve metastatic breast cancer previously treated with first line trastuzumab-taxane combination. Overall response rates were significantly higher for trastuzumab deruxtecan at 79.7% compared to 34.2% with trastuzumab emtansine. The median PFS by investigator assessment was 29.0 *vs.* 7.2 months (HR, 0.30; 95% CI, 0.24–0.38 [39, 40]. The median OS was 52.6 *vs.* 42.7 months (HR, 0.73; 95% CI, 0.56–0.94) for trastuzumab deruxtecan and trastuzumab emtansine, respectively. The evidence overwhelming supported the need to switch from trastuzumab emtansine to trastuzumab deruxtecan as the new standard of care, in the second line, due to the profound superior clinical efficacy.

There are multiple promising ongoing DESTINY trials testing trastuzumab deruxtecan in different clinical indications. Recently, positive clinical data was reported for *DESTINY-Breast04* in HER2 low populations previously treated with 1-2 lines of chemotherapy, and *DESTINY-Breast06* in the HER2 low and ultralow populations after one line of endocrine therapy before chemotherapy (**Table 2** and **Figure 2**) [**42, 50**]. *DESTINY-Breast012* a single arm phase 3b/4 confirmed CNS activity of trastuzumab deruxtecan in women with brain metastases [51].

3.3 Tyrosine kinase inhibitors

Small molecules such as tyrosine kinase inhibitors can also effectively target the HER2 receptor and disrupt HER2 signaling. Examples include tucatinib (Tukysa®; Seagen/Pfizer), neratinib (Neralynx®; Pierre Fabre) or lapatinib (Tykerb®; Novartis), each of which has demonstrated clinical efficacy when combined with capecitabine chemotherapy in the metastatic setting. The tucatinib-trastuzumab-capecitabine drug regimen is a popular alternative treatment option if oral administration is preferable, especially for individuals with brain metastases.

3.3.1 HER2CLIMB study

HER2CLIMB was a randomized (2:1), double-blinded study comparing tucatinib plus trastuzumab-capecitabine against placebo plus trastuzumab-capecitabine in the third line setting. The tucatinib dose was 300 mg twice daily (oral) in combination with trastuzumab-capecitabine (1000 mg/m^2 oral BD, 14 days on, 7 days off) in patients with HER2+ve metastatic breast cancer previously treated with taxane-trastuzumab-pertuzumab (1st line), and trastuzumab emtansine (2nd line). The primary end point was PFS [44].

In the heavily pre-treated population, the mPFS for tucatinib-trastuzumab-capecitabine regimen was 7.8 months (95% CI, 7.5–9.6) *vs.* 5.6 months (95% CI, 4.2–7.1) for placebo-trastuzumab-capecitabine. The mPFS was similar for patients with brain metastases, 7.6 and 5.4 months, respectively (HR, 0.48; $P < 0.001$). After 1 year of treatment, approximately a quarter of the patients with brain metastases (24.9%) were estimated to continue to benefit from tucatinib combination whereas all the patients in the placebo arm had progressed. There was a survival benefit for women treated with tucatinib combination by +4.5 months because the mOS improved from 17.4 months [95% CI, 13.6–19.9] to 21.9 months [95% CI, 18.3–31.0] [44].

The key learnings from the HER2CLIMB study were that tucatinib provided additional prognostic value when added to trastuzumab-capecitabine in the third line setting and has been adopted as a new standard of care. For patients with brain metastases, the tucatinib combination can be considered earlier, as an alternative drug treatment choice to trastuzumab deruxtecan, in the second line [52].

3.4 Drug toxicities for anti-HER2 therapies

In the CLEOPATRA study, the addition of pertuzumab, a monoclonal antibody to trastuzumab-docetaxel did not significantly increase the incidence of symptomatic cardiac dysfunction (~2%; asymptomatic 13%). The toxicity profile was largely driven by docetaxel chemotherapy with mucosal inflammation (27%), diarrhea (69%), rash (39%) and alopecia (61%), with an increase in severity of some of the adverse reactions [35]. The safety profile for the antibody drug conjugate trastuzumab emtansine tested in the EMILIA study suggested a better tolerability profile than the first line regimen with docetaxel-pertuzumab-trastuzumab with less neutropenia (5.9 *vs.* 53%), less anemia (8 *vs.* 25%) less diarrhea (23 *vs.* 69%) and vomiting (19 *vs.* 27%). The incidence of cardiac toxicity and fatigue were similar across both regimens [36]. The antibody drug conjugate trastuzumab deruxtecan which displaced trastuzumab emtansine in DESTINY-Breast03 study, is currently considered one of the most potent single agent anti-cancer therapies with an overall response rate of 80%, however relative to trastuzumab emtansine, is also associated with a higher incidence of nausea (72.8 *vs.* 27.6%), vomiting (44 *vs.* 5.7%) and drug induced interstitial lung disease (10.5–15 *vs.*5%) which clinicians are getting better at identifying and managing. The incidence of death from interstitial lung disease in the DESTINY-Breast studies is approximately 2–3% [40, 41].

4. Triple Negative breast cancer

Triple Negative breast cancer (TNBC) represents approximately 10–15% of all breast cancers. Triple Negative refers to the lack or reduced expression of the three receptors routinely tested for in breast cancer, the estrogen receptor (ER−ve), progesterone (PR−ve) and HER2 overexpression (HER2−ve). Recognition that TNBC is a distinct subtype became widespread in the early 2000, when key papers characterizing breast cancer reported aggressive subtypes lacking ER, PR and HER2 expression. Generally, women diagnosed with either early or metastatic TNBC have poorer outcomes compared to women with HR+ve breast cancer, with lower 5-year survival rates by 8–16% for matched cases [53]. Despite modern treatments, the current mOS for TNBC is only 10.2 months. At 5 years from diagnosis only 11% of people are alive with metastatic TNBC and only 65% of women diagnosed with local disease are alive [54]. Higher mortality rates re-enforce the need for ongoing research and drug development for TNBC.

Over the last 10 years, the therapeutic landscape for metastatic TNBC has significantly evolved and now includes combination therapies with immunotherapy plus chemotherapy and antibody drug conjugates in the clinic. Due to the delicate balance between drug efficacy and drug toxicities, there is a strong drive to understand how best to stratify treatments using biomarkers such as PD-L1 (IHC testing) for immunotherapy and *BRCA* status (germline testing) for PARP inhibition (**Table 3** and **Figure 3**).

4.1 Antibody drug conjugates

4.1.1 ASCENT study

Sacituzumab govitecan is a novel antibody drug conjugate designed to target Trop2 a surface glycoprotein expressed on cancer cells. Once internalized, the SN-38 payload which is an irinotecan metabolite, is released. ASCENT was a prospectively conducted, phase 3 randomized (1:1) study which led to full FDA approval of sacituzumab govitecan (February 2023; Trodelvy®, Gilead Sciences, Inc.) for metastatic TNBC. ASCENT evaluated sacituzumab govitecan against single agent

Trial	Author	Journal	Year	Line	Investigational arm	Standard of care	1ery endpoint	Median PFS /ORR months	PFS HR (95% CI)	P-value	Median OS months	OS HR (95% CI)	P-value
Impassion-130	Schmid et al. [55]	NEJM	2018	1st	nab-paclitaxel+atezolizumab	nab-paclitaxel+placebo	PFS	Unselected 7.2 *vs.* 5.5 m	0.8 (0.69–0.92)	0.002	21.3 *vs.*17.6 m	0.84 (0.69–1.02)	0.08
								PD-L1 + ve: 7.5 *vs.* 5.0 m	0.62 (0.49–0.78)	<0.001	25 m *vs.* 15.5 m	0.62 (0.45–0.86)	NR
Impassion-131	Miles et al. [56]	Annals of Oncology	2021	1st	paclitaxel+ atezolizumab	paclitaxel+placebo	PFS in PD-L1	PD-L1 + ve: 6.0 *vs.*5.7 m	0.82 (0.60–1.12)	0.2	22.1 *vs.* 28.3 m	1.11 (0.76–1.64)	NR
KEYNOTE-355	Cortes et al. [57, 58]	Lancet [57]	2020	1st	chemo (nab-paclitaxel or paclitaxel or gemcitabine +carboplatin) + pembrolizumab	chemo (nab-paclitaxel or paclitaxel or gemcitabine +carboplatin) + placebo	PFS CPS ≥ 10	9·7 *vs.* 5·6 m	0·65 (0·49–0·86)	0.0012	NR	NR	NR
							PFS CPS ≥ 1	7·6 *vs.* 5·6 m	0·74 (0·61–0·90)	0.0014			
							ITT	7·5 *vs.* 5·6 m	0·82 (0·69–0·97)	NR			
		NEJM [58]	2022				OS CPS ≥ 10	NR	NR	NR	23.0 *vs.* 16.1 m	0.73, (0.55–0.95)	0.019
							OS CPS ≥ 1				17.6 *vs.* 16.0 m	0.86, (0.72–1.04)	0.1125
							OS ITT				17.2 *vs.* 15.5 m	0.89, (0.76–1.05)	NR

DOI: http://dx.doi.org/10.5772/intechopen.1008863

Trial	Author	Journal	Year	Line	Investigational arm	Standard of care	1ery endpoint	Median PFS /ORR months	PFS HR (95% CI)	P-value	Median OS months	OS HR (95% CI)	P-value
TNT study	Tutt et al. [59]	Nature Medicine	2018	1st	carboplatin	docetaxel	ORR - unselected	31.4 *vs.* 34%	NA	0.66	NR	NR	NR
							ORR *gBRCA*-BC	68 *vs.* 33%	NA	0.01	NR	NR	NR
ASCENT	Bardia et al. [60, 61]	NEJM [60]	2021	2nd/ 3rd	sacituzumab govitecan	Physician's choice (eribulin vinorelbine capecitabine gemcitabine)	PFS	5.6 *vs.* 1.7 m	0.41, (0.32–0.52)	<0.001	NR	NR	NR
		JCO [61]	2024				PFS and OS	4.8 *vs.*1.7 m	0.41 (0.33–0.52)	NR	11.8 *vs.* 6.9 m	0.51 (0.42–0.63)	NR
EMBRACE	Cortes et al. [62]	Lancet	2011	3rd	eribulin mesilate	chemotherapy	PFS and OS	3·7 *vs.* 2·2 m	0·87, (0·71–1·05)	0.137	13.1 *vs.* 10.6 m	0·81 (0·66–0·99)	0.041
	Kaufm et al. [63]	JCO	2015	3rd	eribulin mesilate	capecitabine		4.1 *vs.* 4.2 m ORR 11 *vs.* 11.5%	1.08, (0.93–1.25)	0.3	15.9 *vs.* 14.5 m	0.88, (0.77–1.00)	0.56

CPS = combine positive score for PD-L1; ORR = overall response rates.

Table 3.
Selected key landmark studies in metastatic triple negative breast cancer.

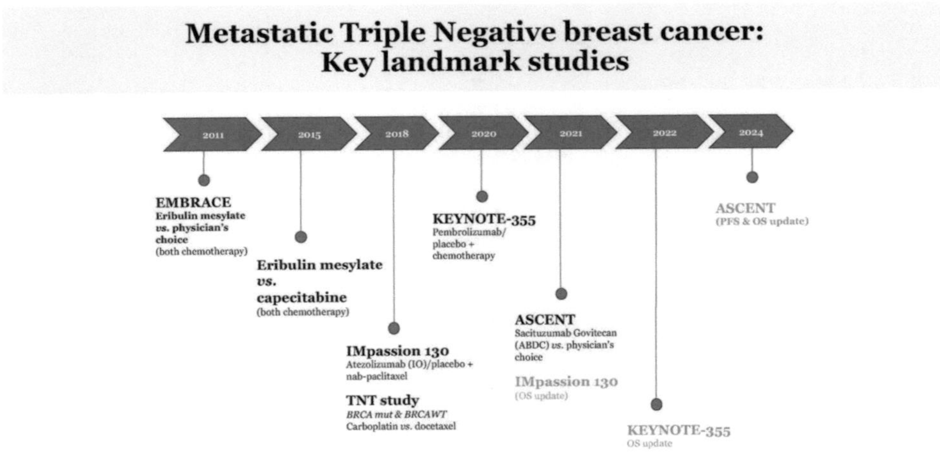

Figure 3.
Timeline for selected key landmark studies in metastatic TNBC breast cancer. Abbreviations: ABDC = antibody drug conjugate, IO = immunotherapy, PFS = progression free survival, OS = overall survival, SERD = selective estrogen receptor degrader.

chemotherapy which clinicians considered standard of care (capecitabine, eribulin, vinorelbine or gemcitabine) [60].

ASCENT recruited women with metastatic TNBC (n = 529) refractory to two or more previous lines of chemotherapy (no upper limit) including a taxane. Dosing schedule for sacituzumab govitecan was 10 mg/kg, IV, on days 1 and 8 of each 21-day cycle. The study stratified for the number of previous chemotherapy regimens for advanced disease (2 or 3 *vs.* >3), the presence of known brain metastases at baseline (yes n = 61 *vs.* no; 15% recruitment cap), and geographic region (North America *vs.* rest of the world). No crossover to the sacituzumab govitecan arm was allowed on progression with chemotherapy.

The first set of analyses reported upon women without known baseline brain metastases (2021) with a median follow up time of 17.7 months. There was a +3.9-months benefit in mPFS with sacituzumab govitecan from 1.7 months for control arm to 5.6 months (95% CI, 4.3–6.3) with sacituzumab govitecan (HR, 0.41; $P < 0.001$). Sacituzumab govitecan treatment also improved the mOS by +5.4 months from 6.7 months to 12.1 months (95% CI, 10.7–14.0) compared the standard of care (HR, 0.48; $P < 0.001$).

The key findings of the ASCENT study were that using the antibody drug conjugate sacituzumab govitecan in metastatic TNBC was superior to existing chemotherapy options, was tolerable and needed to become the new standard of care in the 2nd or 3rd line setting [60].

4.2 Immunotherapy with chemotherapy (combination)

4.2.1 IMpassion130 study

The monoclonal antibody (IgG) atezolizumab (Tecentriq®, Genentech) selectively targets the programmed death ligand-1 (PD-L1). Inhibition of PD-L1 prevents its interaction with the PD-1 receptor and B7-1, a costimulatory cell-surface receptor. This reverses T-cell suppression. IMpassion130 was the phase 3 landmark study

(2018) which demonstrated that combining immunotherapy with first line chemotherapy in PD-L1+ve metastatic TNBC improved clinical outcomes. Nanoparticle albumin-bound (nab)-paclitaxel was selected as the chemotherapy backbone to avoid steroid premedication. There was concern that concomitant use of steroids could negatively affect immunotherapy efficacy.

IMpassion130 was a phase 3 randomized double blinded study which recruited treatment naïve women with metastatic TNBC. Participants were randomly assigned (1: 1; both arms n = 451) to nab-paclitaxel (100 mg/m^2, IV, D1, D8 and D15, q28) with atezolizumab (840 mg, IV, D1 and D15), or nab-paclitaxel + placebo. The PD-L1 population was selected using the companion diagnostic VENTANA PD-L1 assay. The atezolizumab-nab-paclitaxel combination significantly improved mPFS in the PD-L1 positive cohort compared to the placebo-nab-paclitaxel by +2.5 months (7.0 *vs.* 5.0 months; HR, 0.62; P = <0.001). Surprisingly OS did not reach statistical significance in the intention-to-treat population, despite a meaningful improvement in mOS by +9.5 months in the PD-L1-positive subgroup treated with atezolizumab-nab-paclitaxel (25.0 *vs.* 15.5 months). The safety profile was consistent with known effects of each drug, with higher rates of immune-related adverse events in the atezolizumab group [55].

They key findings of IMpassion130 were that a biomarker stratification using tumor PD-L1 status to identify individuals with higher probabilities of response to immunotherapy was a promising approach and there was clinical benefit of combining atezolizumab with nab-paclitaxel first line treatment for metastatic TNBC.

IMpassion131 is an important negative study because atezolizumab was tested with paclitaxel, a more widely available chemotherapy than nab-paclitaxel. In a similar PD-L1+ve population, the addition of atezolizumab demonstrated no significant benefit in mPFS or mOS compared to the placebo arm (HR, 0.82, 95% CI; P = 0.20) [56]. The outcomes of IMpassion131 contrasted to those reported for the IMpassion130 study. The conflicted study outcomes could be due to different immunogenic responses induced by paclitaxel *vs.* nab-paclitaxel. Also, immune suppression due to prophylactic use of corticosteroids with paclitaxel may have affected drug efficacy in IMpassion131, whereas nab-paclitaxel was specifically selected because it was steroid sparing [64]. An important impact of the negative IMpassion131 results were that the FDA withdrew accelerated approval, and Roche withdrew atezolizumab for TNBC in the USA, but it remains available in parts of Europe and is accessible via off label use.

4.2.2 KEYNOTE-355 study

Pembrolizumab is a humanized antibody which inhibits the programmed cell death protein-1 (PD-1), a receptor found on the cell surface of immune cells. PD-1 is an immune checkpoint inhibitor which downregulates the immune system. The Combined Positive Score (CPS) score quantifies PD-L1+ve cells within a tissue section, specifically tumor cells, lymphocytes and macrophages relative to all viable tumor cells.

The phase 3 KEYNOTE-355 study led to the approval of pembrolizumab (Keytruda®, Merck) combination with chemotherapy for first-line treatment of advanced PD-L1+ve TNBC with a CPS ≥10. KEYNOTE-355 was a placebo-controlled, double-blinded study which randomized women (2:1) to pembrolizumab (200 mg, IV, every 3 weeks) plus chemotherapy (nab-paclitaxel, paclitaxel, or gemcitabine-carboplatin; n = 566) or placebo plus chemotherapy (n = 281). Stratification factors were chemotherapy type, PD-L1 expression (CPS ≥1 or < 1), and previous neo/adjuvant setting treatment within the same class of chemotherapy [57].

Initial analyses reported women with higher CPS scores had better clinical outcomes than women with lower CPS scores with immunotherapy. In the CPS ≥10 population, the mPFS was 9.7 months (pembrolizumab-chemotherapy) *vs.* 5.6 months (placebo-chemotherapy; HR of 0.65, P = 0.0012) [57]. Overall survival analyses reported better prognosis for women treated with pembrolizumab-chemotherapy by +6.9 months in the CPS ≥10 subgroup (23.0 *vs.* 16.1 months with placebo-chemotherapy; HR, 0.73; P = 0.019). There was no survival benefit for immunotherapy in the CPS ≥1 subgroup (HR, 0.86, P = 0.11).

The key findings of the KEYNOTE-355 study were that pembrolizumab, a PD-1 inhibitor combined with chemotherapy improved clinical outcomes for women with TNBC and was more effective than administrating first line chemotherapy alone. The mOS difference in the CPS ≥10 subpopulation was statistically significant. KEYNOTE-355 confirmed that quantification of PD-L1 using a CPS ≥10 was a useful biomarker to help identify women with highest probability of response.

4.3 Chemotherapy

Until the recent successes of targeted approaches described above, traditional cytotoxic treatment has remained the cornerstone of metastatic TNBC treatment. Single agent chemotherapy is preferred when patient quality of life is important. Chemotherapy drugs frequently administered are either taxanes (paclitaxel, docetaxel), anthracyclines (epirubicin, doxorubicin) if they have not recently been used in the neo/adjuvant setting, anti-metabolites (capecitabine, gemcitabine) or platinum treatment (carboplatin, cisplatin). Here, we outline two important studies supporting the use of carboplatin, and eribulin in metastatic TNBC.

4.3.1 TNT (triple negative trial) study

The TNT was an academic study which demonstrated how genetic profiling, specifically *BRCA* testing in breast cancer identified women more likely to benefit from carboplatin chemotherapy. It was a randomized phase 3 trial comparing single agent carboplatin against docetaxel (taxane), the standard of care for first line metastatic TNBC population. A pre-specified biomarker analyses for germline *BRCA1/2* mutations and 'BRCAness' subgroups (tumor *BRCA*1 methylation; *BRCA1* mRNA-low; Homologous recombination deficiency mutational signatures and basal phenotypes) were planned as part of the study design [59].

The study enrolled 376 patients who were randomized to receive either first line carboplatin (n = 188) or docetaxel (n = 188). In the unselected population, carboplatin was not more active than docetaxel regarding drug response (ORR: 31.4 *vs.* 34.0; P = 0.66) with similar median PFS and OS outcomes. The mPFS with carboplatin was 3·1 months [95% CI: 2.4–4.2] and 4·4 months [95%CI: 4.1–5.1] with docetaxel. In the unselected population, the mOS for carboplatin was 12·8 months [95% CI: 10.6, 15.3] and 12.0 months with docetaxel [95% CI: 10.2, 13.0], indicating that either drug can be used first line for metastatic TNBC in the *BRCA* wild type population.

In the biomarker selected population for germline *BRCA1/BRCA2* deleterious mutations, the overall response rate doubled for carboplatin (n = 43) to 68% but not for docetaxel (33.3%, P = 0.03). The mPFS for carboplatin was 6.8 months, this was a +2.2-month improvement compared to docetaxel (p = 0.002) but with no clear survival benefit. Interestingly, neither the *BRCA1* methylation status nor *the* low mRNA levels significantly influenced response to carboplatin or docetaxel.

The key learning from the TNT study was that germline *BRCA* mutations were predictive biomarkers for carboplatin response, providing a strong rationale for routine germline testing in TNBC. Carboplatin should be considered preferentially first line choice of chemotherapy in the *BRCA* mutant population [59].

4.3.2 EMBRACE study (Eisai Metastatic Breast Cancer Study Assessing Physician's Choice Versus Eribulin)

EMBRACE was the phase 3 (n = 762), registration study which led to the approval and routine use of eribulin, a non-taxane anti-microtubule agent in heavily pretreated (≥2 chemotherapy lines; median = 4 lines) metastatic breast cancer including metastatic TNBC (2011). This study mandated previous treatments with an anthracycline and a taxane. Women were randomly allocated (2:1) to eribulin mesylate (n = 762; 1·4 mg/m^2, IV 2–5 min, D1 and D8 q21) or treatment of physician's choice (TPC n = 254). TPC choice included single agent vinorelbine (n = 61, 25%), gemcitabine (n = 46, 19%), capecitabine (n = 44, 18%), taxanes (n = 38, 15%), anthracyclines (n = 24, 10%) and other chemotherapies (n = 24, 10%). Randomization was stratified by geographical region, previous capecitabine treatment, and HER2 status. The EMBRACE study met its primary end point because there was an improvement in mOS by +2.5 months in women assigned to eribulin (mOS = 13.1 months, 95% CI 11.8–14.3) compared with TPC (mOS =10.6 months, 9.3–12.5; HR, 0.81, p = 0.041) [62].

A subsequent phase 3 (n = 1, 102; 2011) compared eribulin (n = 554, dosing schedule as above) with capecitabine (n = 548, 1250 mg/m^2, oral BD, on D1 to 14, q21) as first-, second-, or third-line therapy for advanced breast cancer. There were no significant differences in objective response rates (11.0% for eribulin and 11.5% for capecitabine), no difference in mPFS (HR, 1.08; P = 0.30) or mOS for eribulin (15.9 months) and capecitabine respectively (14.5 months, HR, 0.88; P = 0.056) [63]. Eribulin had similar activity to capecitabine.

The key findings of these studies were that eribulin was an active chemotherapy drug in the third line setting for metastatic TNBC. At this timepoint, eribulin was a new treatment and provided an additional choice when effective anti-cancer therapeutics were scarce for TNBC.

4.4 Drug toxicity profiles observed in TNBC

The routine use of immunotherapy with chemotherapy in breast cancer has lagged several years behind other cancer types. The addition of atezolizumab to nab-paclitaxel introduced immune-related adverse events (irAEs) such as hypothyroidism, colitis, hepatitis, pneumonitis, adrenal insufficiency, in addition to higher frequency of adverse events typically associated with nab-paclitaxel chemotherapy such as nausea, neutropenia and peripheral neuropathy [55]. A similar profile of irAEs were observed in KEYNOTE-355 study with higher incidences of hypothyroidism (15.8 *vs.* 3.2%), hyperthyroidism (4.3 *vs.* 4.3%) and pneumonitis (2.5 *vs.* 0%) [58]. IrAEs are challenging to manage because they can be permanent, affect multiple organs, occur after treatment discontinuation and the chronic use of steroids to manage the specific irAEs is associated with significant morbidity.

5. Conclusion and discussion

Despite the significant number of drugs approved for use in metastatic breast cancer over the last 10 years (>10), breast cancer remains the most common cause of death for women globally [1]. The majority of the pivotal phase 3 studies conducted in the metastatic breast cancer population reflect the incidence of breast cancer subtypes with the most number of new drugs approved for luminal breast cancer (HR+ve), the most common subtype (palbociclib, ribociclib, abemaciclib, everolimus, alpelisib, capivasertib, fulvestrant, elacestrant) followed by HER2+ve breast cancer (pertuzumab, trastuzumab emtansine, trastuzumab deruxtecan, tucatinib, phesgo) and lastly metastatic TNBC (eribulin, sacituzumab govitecan and pembrolizumab combination with chemotherapy). Over time the treatment strategies for the three breast cancer subtypes have diverged, reflecting the differences in the underlying tumor biology. For example, there is a strong emphasis to combine targeted therapy with hormone treatment for HR+ve breast cancer and target the HER2 receptor by antibodies and/or tyrosine kinases in combination with chemotherapy. Unfortunately, the management of metastatic TNBC remains a challenge and chemotherapy remain the gold standard. The two major therapeutic breakthroughs for TNBC are: immunotherapy with chemotherapy combination [65] and secondly, single agent sacituzumab govitecan, the first successful antibody drug conjugated to demonstrate clinical efficacy in metastatic TNBC (**Figure 3** and **Table 3**).

In HR+ve breast cancer, CDK4/6 inhibition with endocrine treatment has been "game changing". Numerous pivotal phase 3 studies (PALOMA-2 [14], PALOMA-3 [16], MONALEESA-2 [9], MONALEESA-7 [12], MONARCH-2 [20] and MONARCH-3 [6]) have evaluated the three CDK4/6 inhibitors palbociclib, ribociclib or abemaciclib in combination with endocrine treatment. Consequently, treatment with CDK4/6 inhibitor with a non-steroidal aromatase inhibitor such as letrozole or anastrozole has become standard practice, first line for hormone sensitive population. The current mPFS for people treated with a CDK4/6 inhibitor first line is approximately 2 years compared to 12–14 months with hormone treatment alone. Despite similar clinical data for all three CDK4/6 inhibitors, clinical trials with ribociclib consistently report statistically significant improvement in mOS, despite numerically similar outcomes for palbociclib and abemaciclib. Several reasons have been proposed for why ribociclib has the strongest survival data, including subtle differences in drug activity and mechanism of action for the CDK4/6 inhibitors [26], differences in statistical approaches used to analyze the data and, missing data which may affect survival analyses especially in the PALOMA-2 study.

In metastatic breast cancer, the sequencing order of treatment has become topical, and precision medicine focused approaches to help match treatments to patients (**Figure 4**). For example, in the metastatic HR+ve population following progression on a CDK4/6 inhibitor, whether the tumor harbors *PIK3CA* or *BRCA-1/-2* mutations becomes important when making treatment decisions about the next appropriate therapy (**Figures 5–7**). For the *PIK3CA* mutant population (~40%), the data from the registration study SOLAR-1 supports the administration of the selective p110α alpha PI3 inhibitor alpelisib with fulvestrant (mPFS 11 months *vs.* 5.7 months placebo-fulvestrant). Due to the timing of the SOLAR-1 study, only 5.3–6.4% of the patients were previously exposed to a CDK4/6 inhibitor [24]. Therefore, the BYLieve study was conducted to test and confirm the efficacy of alpelisib-fulvestrant combination in a *PIK3CA*-mutated population which had progressed on a CDK4/6 inhibitor plus an aromatase inhibitor [68].

There are multiple drug regimen options post CDK4/6 inhibition in the *PIK3CA wild-type* population including the "older" everolimus-exemestane regimen (BOLERO-2 study [23]), the novel AKT inhibitor capivasertib with fulvestrant (CAPitello [30]) or an oral SERD such as elacestrant if an *ESR1* mutation is detectable (EMRALD [33]). Multiple factors influence clinical decisions about treatment choices such as drug toxicities, patient co-morbidities, drug interactions, patient preferences, genetic profiles and which drug is associated with the best clinical outcome. Currently neither everolimus-exemestane (+4.4 months) and nor alpelisib-fulvestrant (+7.9 months) drug combinations have statistically positive OS data, hence the need for ongoing development of future next generation compounds. The OS data for capivasertib and elacestrant is currently immature. In summary, the current prescribing trend for HR+ve breast cancer is delaying the administration of chemotherapy and increasing the number of "non-chemotherapy" lines with targeted drug regimens and hormone treatment, upstream to preserve quality of life.

The treatment landscape for metastatic HER2+ve breast cancer is dominated by drugs targeting the HER2 receptor. These include the monoclonal antibodies pertuzumab with trastuzumab (CLEOPATRA [35]), antibody drug conjugates such as trastuzumab emtansine (EMELIA [36]) and trastuzumab deruxtecan (DESTINY-Breast-03 [40]) and small molecules like tucatinib with trastuzumab-capecitabine (HER2CLIMB [44]). Trastuzumab deruxtecan is currently the most impressive drug available for treating metastatic HER2+ve breast cancer with a +22-month (4×) improvement in mPFS against trastuzumab emtansine the previous standard of care in DESTINY-Breast03 [40]. Emerging data suggests that trastuzumab deruxtecan will continue to reshape the treatment landscape with promising signal in the HER2 low and the ER low populations.

Currently biomarkers with the most robust supportive data for metastatic breast cancer are somatic mutations in *PIK3CA* (**Figures 5** and **6**), *ESR1* (**Figure 8**), germline mutations in *BRCA1&-2* (**Figure 7**) [66], and immunohistochemical staining of the PD-L1 protein. There is now a justification for germline *BRCA* testing of metastatic

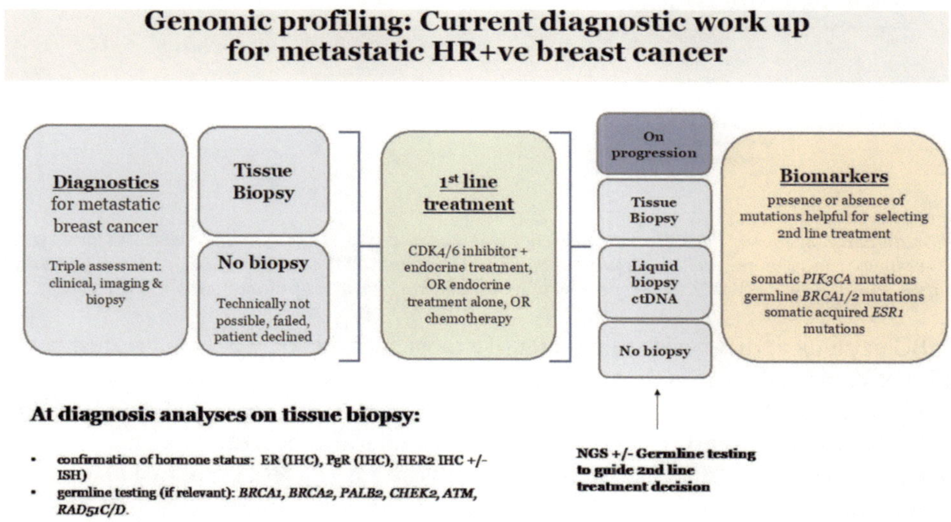

Figure 4.
The current diagnostic work up for metastatic hormone positive (HR+ve) breast cancer (2024).

Mutation	Hereditary risk	Prognostic in metastatic breast cancer	Predictive of drug response
PIK3CA (somatic)	No	Poorer prognosis	Level 1 evidence: predictive of drug response to PI3 kinase inhibitors
BRCA-1 & -2 (germline)	Yes, carriers have an increased risk of developing breast cancer	Not prognostic	Level 1 evidence: predictive of drug response to PARP inhibitors
ESR1 (somatic)	No	Poorer prognosis	Level 1 evidence: predictive of drug response to oral SERD inhibitors

Figure 5.
Summary of the three current actionable mutations in HR+ve metastatic breast cancer in 2024 with a matching drug/drug combination. PIK3CA *(somatic),* BRCA-1/BRCA-2 *(germline),* ESR1 *(somatic). References: ESCAT scale [66], OncoKB™ [67].*

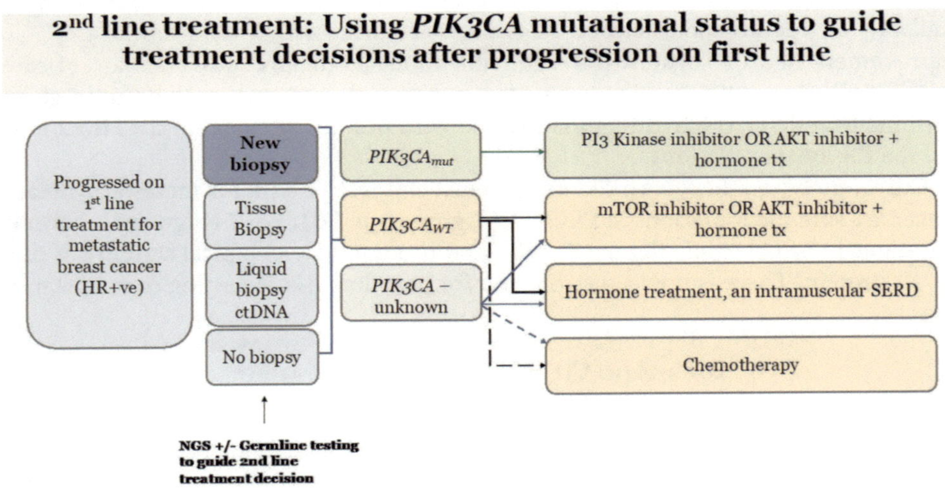

Figure 6.
Schematic outlining the possible different treatment options according to PIK3CA *mutational status for metastatic HR+ve breast cancer patients who have progress on first line systemic treatment.* PIK3CA$_{mut}$ = PIK3CA *mutation positive,* PIK3CA$_{WT}$ = PIK3CA *wild-type,* PIK3CA- *unknown = genetic test failed or unable to test patient.*

TNBC patients at diagnosis to help identify those individuals with the greatest probability of response to carboplatin (**Figure 4**). We can now also justify tumor profiling of HR+ve metastatic breast cancer patients after they have progressed on a first line CDK4/6 inhibitor to test for *PIK3CA* and *ESR1* mutations because this impacts whether these patients can access alpelisib-fulvestrant (*PIK3CA* mutant) *vs.* everolimus-exemestane (*PIK3CA* wildtype) or capivasertib/fulvestrant (*PIK3CA* mutant or wildtype) or an oral SERD. Overall, in this chapter, selected fundamental landmark studies have been highlighted because these studies clinically validated novel drugs which became the new standard of care and improved clinical outcomes for metastatic breast cancer. Drug development in breast cancer is a rapidly evolving

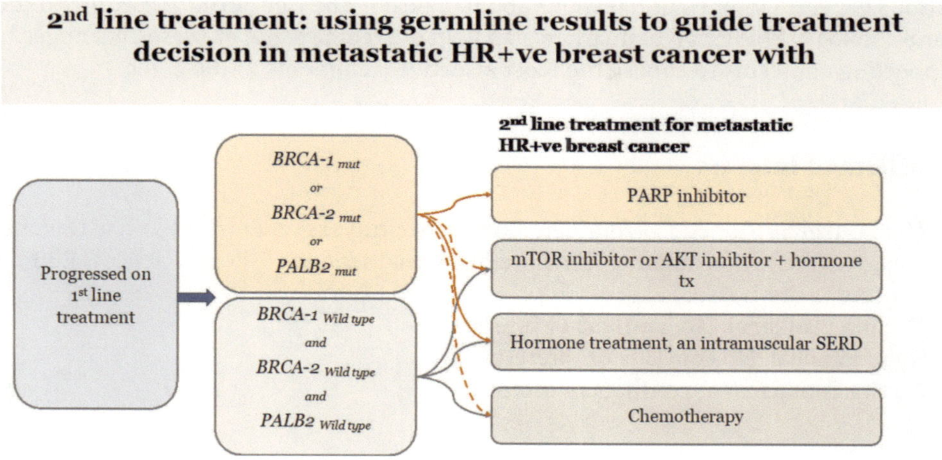

Figure 7.
Schematic outlining the possible different treatment options according to germline BRCA-1, BRCA-2 *and* PALB2 *mutational status for metastatic HR+ve breast cancer patients who progress on first line systemic treatment.* $_{\text{mut}}$ *= mutation positive,* $_{\text{Wild type}}$ *= mutation negative.*

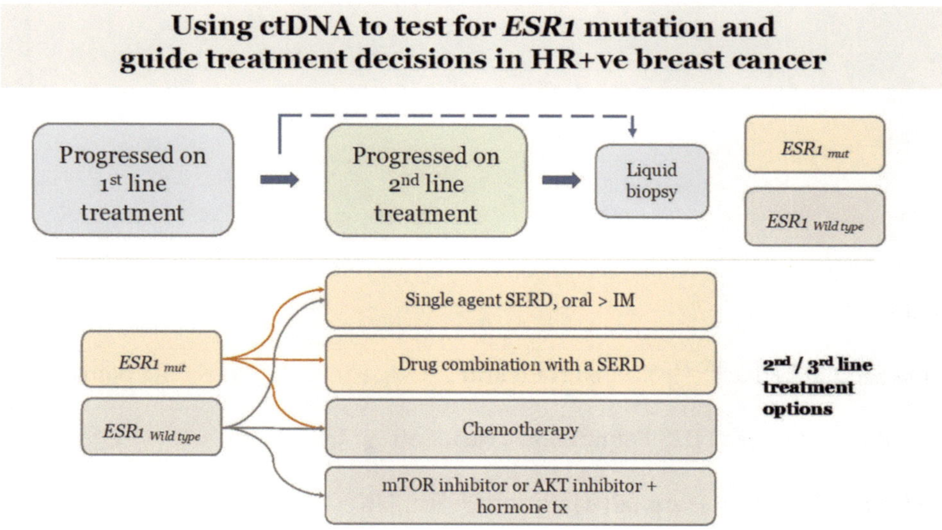

Figure 8.
Schematic outlining the possible different treatment options according to acquisition of an ESR1 *mutation on hormone treatments for metastatic HR+ve breast cancer patients who have progressed on first line or second line systemic treatment.* $_{\text{mut}}$ *= mutation positive,* $_{\text{Wild type}}$ *= mutation is not present.*

field benefiting patients due to the fierce competition. Hopefully, with ongoing progress, metastatic breast cancer can be considered a chronic medical condition whilst cancer researchers continue to search for a "cure".

In conclusion, people with metastatic breast cancer have more treatment options with better prognoses. Health care professionals are now facing new complexities associated with precision medicine such how to integrate tumor profiling (**Figures 4–8**) and access to drugs with overlapping clinical indications. Numerous options generate important questions about choosing the right drug according to the tumor biology. Predictive biomarkers can help overcome some of these challenges by supporting clinicians to choose the most effective treatments in the clinic.

Conflicts of interest

Uzma Asghar: Concr: Co-founder, Conference travel grants from Concr, Daiichi Sankyo, Novartis. Consultancy fees for educational sessions: Gilead Sciences, Eli Lilly, Seagen. Advisory board: Seagen.

Yashna Nadkarni: No conflicts of interest.

Ryan Panchal: No conflicts of interest.

Navita Somaiah: No conflicts of interest.

Author details

Uzma Saddia Asghar[1,2,3*], Yashna Nadkarni[1], Ryan Panchal[1] and Navita Somaiah[1,4]

1 The Royal Marsden NHS Foundation Trust, Sutton, UK

2 Croydon University Hospital, Thornton Heath, UK

3 Concr LTD, Esher, UK

4 The Institute of Cancer Research, Sutton, UK

*Address all correspondence to: uzma.asghar@rmh.nhs.uk

References

[1] Duranti S, Fabi A, Filetti M, Falcone R, Lombardi P, Daniele G, et al. Breast cancer drug approvals issued by EMA: A review of clinical trials. Cancers (Basel). 16 Oct 2021;**13**(20):5198. DOI: 10.3390/cancers13205198. PMID: 34680350; PMCID: PMC8533780

[2] Allison KH, Hammond MEH, Dowsett M, McKernin SE, Carey LA, Fitzgibbons PL, et al. Estrogen and progesterone receptor testing in breast cancer: ASCO/CAP guideline update. Journal of Clinical Oncology. 2020;**38**(12):1346-1366

[3] Slamon DJ, Diéras V, Rugo HS, Harbeck N, Im SA, Gelmon KA, et al. Overall survival with palbociclib plus letrozole in advanced breast cancer. Journal of Clinical Oncology. 2024;**42**(9):994-1000

[4] CRUK. Cancer Research UK Website. Breast-Cancer/Survival; 2024. Available from: https://www.cancerresearchuk.org/about-cancer/breast-cancer/survival

[5] Goetz MP, Toi M, Campone M, Trédan O, Bourayou N, Sohn J, et al. MONARCH 3: Abemaciclib as initial therapy for advanced breast cancer. Journal of Clinical Oncology. 2017;**35**(32):3638-3646

[6] Johnston S, Martin M, Di Leo A, Im SA, Awada A, Forrester T, et al. MONARCH 3 final PFS: A randomized study of abemaciclib as initial therapy for advanced breast cancer. NPJ Breast Cancer. 17 Jan 2019;**5**:5. DOI: 10.1038/s41523-018-0097-z

[7] Goetz MP, Toi M, Huober J, Sohn J, Trédan O, Park IH, et al. Abemaciclib plus a nonsteroidal aromatase inhibitor as initial therapy for HR+, HER2- advanced breast cancer: Final overall survival results of MONARCH 3. Annals of Oncology. 2024;**35**(8):718-727. DOI: 10.1016/j.annonc.2024.04.013

[8] Hortobagyi GN, Stemmer SM, Burris HA, Yap YS, Sonke GS, Paluch-Shimon S, et al. Ribociclib as first-line therapy for HR-positive, advanced breast cancer. New England Journal of Medicine. 2016;**375**(18):1738-1748

[9] Hortobagyi GN, Stemmer SM, Burris HA, Yap YS, Sonke GS, Hart L, et al. Overall survival with ribociclib plus letrozole in advanced breast cancer. New England Journal of Medicine. 2022;**386**(10):942-950

[10] Hortobagyi GN, Stemmer SM, Burris HA, Yap YS, Sonke GS, Paluch-Shimon S, et al. Updated results from MONALEESA-2, a phase III trial of first-line ribociclib plus letrozole versus placebo plus letrozole in hormone receptor-positive, HER2-negative advanced breast cancer. Annals of Oncology. 2018;**29**(7):1541-1547

[11] Tripathy D, Im SA, Colleoni M, Franke F, Bardia A, Harbeck N, et al. Ribociclib plus endocrine therapy for premenopausal women with hormone-receptor-positive, advanced breast cancer (MONALEESA-7): A randomised phase 3 trial. The Lancet Oncology. 2018;**19**(7):904-915

[12] Im SA, Lu YS, Bardia A, Harbeck N, Colleoni M, Franke F, et al. Overall survival with ribociclib plus endocrine therapy in breast cancer. New England Journal of Medicine. 2019;**381**(4):307-316

[13] Lu YS, Im SA, Colleoni M, Franke F, Bardia A, Cardoso F, et al. Updated overall survival of Ribociclib plus endocrine therapy versus endocrine

therapy alone in pre- and perimenopausal patients with HR+/HER2- advanced breast cancer in MONALEESA-7: A phase III randomized clinical trial. Clinical Cancer Research. 2022;**28**(5):851-859

[14] Finn RS, Martin M, Rugo HS, Jones S, Im SA, Gelmon K, et al. Palbociclib and letrozole in advanced breast cancer. New England Journal of Medicine. 2016; **375**(20):1925-1936

[15] Rugo HS, Finn RS, Diéras V, Ettl J, Lipatov O, Joy AA, et al. Palbociclib plus letrozole as first-line therapy in estrogen receptor-positive/human epidermal growth factor receptor 2-negative advanced breast cancer with extended follow-up. Breast Cancer Research and Treatment. 2019;**174**(3):719-729

[16] Turner NC, Ro J, André F, Loi S, Verma S, Iwata H, et al. Palbociclib in hormone-receptor–positive advanced breast cancer. New England Journal of Medicine. 2015;**373**(3):209-219

[17] Turner NC, Slamon DJ, Ro J, Bondarenko I, Im SA, Masuda N, et al. Overall survival with palbociclib and fulvestrant in advanced breast cancer. New England Journal of Medicine. 2018; **379**(20):1926-1936

[18] Slamon DJ, Neven P, Chia S, Fasching PA, De Laurentiis M, Im SA, et al. Phase III randomized study of ribociclib and fulvestrant in hormone receptor-positive, human epidermal growth factor receptor 2-negative advanced breast cancer: MONALEESA-3. Journal of Clinical Oncology. 2018;**36** (24):2465-2472

[19] Slamon DJ, Neven P, Chia S, Fasching PA, De Laurentiis M, Im SA, et al. Overall survival with ribociclib plus fulvestrant in advanced breast cancer. New England Journal of Medicine. 2020; **382**(6):514-524

[20] Sledge GW, Toi M, Neven P, Sohn J, Inoue K, Pivot X, et al. MONARCH 2: Abemaciclib in combination with fulvestrant in women with HR+/HER2- advanced breast cancer who had progressed while receiving endocrine therapy. Journal of Clinical Oncology. 2017;**35**(25):2875-2884

[21] Sledge GW, Toi M, Neven P, Sohn J, Inoue K, Pivot X, et al. The effect of abemaciclib plus fulvestrant on overall survival in hormone receptor-positive, ERBB2-negative breast cancer that progressed on endocrine therapy - MONARCH 2: A randomized clinical trial. JAMA Oncologia. 2020;**6**(1):116-124

[22] Baselga J, Campone M, Piccart M, Burris HA, Rugo HS, Sahmoud T, et al. Everolimus in postmenopausal hormone-receptor–positive advanced breast cancer. New England Journal of Medicine. 2012;**366**(6):520-529. DOI: 10.1056/NEJMoa1109653

[23] Piccart M, Hortobagyi GN, Campone M, Pritchard KI, Lebrun F, Ito Y, et al. Everolimus plus exemestane for hormonereceptor- positive, human epidermal growth factor receptor-2-negative advanced breast cancer: Overall survival results from BOLERO-2. Annals of Oncology. 2014;**25**(12):2357-2362

[24] André F, Ciruelos EM, Juric D, Loibl S, Campone M, Mayer IA, et al. Alpelisib plus fulvestrant for PIK3CA-mutated, hormone receptor-positive, human epidermal growth factor receptor-2–negative advanced breast cancer: Final overall survival results from SOLAR-1. Annals of Oncology. 2021;**32**(2):208-217

[25] André F, Ciruelos E, Rubovszky G, Campone M, Loibl S, Rugo HS, et al. Alpelisib for PIK3CA -mutated, hormone

receptor–positive advanced breast cancer. New England Journal of Medicine. 2019;**380**(20):1929-1940

[26] Asghar U, Witkiewicz AK, Turner NC, Knudsen ES. The history and future of targeting cyclin-dependent kinases in cancer therapy. Nature Reviews Drug Discovery. 2015;**14**:130-146

[27] Lin W, Zeng Y, Weng L, Yang J, Zhuang W. Comparative analysis of adverse events associated with CDK4/6 inhibitors based on FDA's adverse event reporting system: A case control pharmacovigilance study. BMC Pharmacology & Toxicology. 2024;**25**(1):47

[28] Fuentes-Antrás J, Martínez-Rodríguez A, Guevara-Hoyer K, López-Cade I, Lorca V, Pascual A, et al. Real-world use of highly sensitive liquid biopsy monitoring in metastatic breast cancer patients treated with endocrine agents after exposure to aromatase inhibitors. International Journal of Molecular Sciences. 2023;**24**(14):11419

[29] Howell SJ, Casbard A, Carucci M, Ingarfield K, Butler R, Morgan S, et al. Fulvestrant plus capivasertib versus placebo after relapse or progression on an aromatase inhibitor in metastatic, oestrogen receptor-positive, HER2-negative breast cancer (FAKTION): Overall survival, updated progression-free survival, and expanded biomarker analysis from a randomised, phase 2 trial. The Lancet Oncology. 2022;**23**(7):851-864

[30] Turner NC, Oliveira M, Howell SJ, Dalenc F, Cortes J, Gomez Moreno HL, et al. Capivasertib in hormone receptor–Positive advanced breast cancer. New England Journal of Medicine. 2023;**388**(22):2058-2070

[31] Gheysen M, Kevin P, Wildiers H, Patrick N. Oral SERDs changing the scenery in hormone receptor positive breast cancer, a comprehensive review. Cancer Treatment Reviews. 2024;**130**: 102825. Available from: https://www.cancertreatmentreviews.com/article/S0305-7372(24)00153-1/fulltext

[32] Neupane N, Bawek S, Gurusinghe S, Ghaffary EM, Mirmosayyeb O, Thapa S, et al. Oral SERD, a novel endocrine therapy for estrogen receptor-positive breast cancer. Cancers. 2024;**16**(3):619

[33] Bidard FC, Kaklamani VG, Neven P, Streich G, Montero AJ, Forget F, et al. Elacestrant (oral selective estrogen receptor degrader) versus standard endocrine therapy for Estrogen receptor-positive, human epidermal growth factor receptor 2-negative advanced breast cancer: Results from the randomized phase III EMERALD trial. Journal of Clinical Oncology. 1 Oct 2022;**40**(28): 3246-3256

[34] Baselga J, Cortés J, Kim SB, Im SA, Hegg R, Im YH, et al. Pertuzumab plus trastuzumab plus docetaxel for metastatic breast cancer. New England Journal of Medicine. 2012;**366**(2): 109-119

[35] Swain SM, Miles D, Kim SB, Im YH, Im SA, Semiglazov V, et al. Pertuzumab, trastuzumab, and docetaxel for HER2-positive metastatic breast cancer (CLEOPATRA): End-of-study results from a double-blind, randomised, placebo-controlled, phase 3 study. The Lancet Oncology. 2020;**21**(4):519-530

[36] Verma S, Miles D, Gianni L, Krop IE, Welslau M, Baselga J, et al. Trastuzumab emtansine for HER2-positive advanced breast cancer. New England Journal of Medicine. 2012;**367**(19):1783-1791

[37] Diéras V, Miles D, Verma S, Pegram M, Welslau M, Baselga J, et al. Trastuzumab emtansine versus

capecitabine plus lapatinib in patients with previously treated HER2-positive advanced breast cancer (EMILIA): A descriptive analysis of final overall survival results from a randomised, open-label, phase 3 trial. The Lancet Oncology. 2017;**18**(6):732-742

[38] André F, Hee Park Y, Kim SB, Takano T, Im SA, Borges G, et al. Trastuzumab deruxtecan versus treatment of physician's choice in patients with HER2-positive metastatic breast cancer (DESTINY-Breast02): A randomised, open-label, multicentre, phase 3 trial. The Lancet. 2023;**401** (10390):1773-1785

[39] Cortés J, Kim SB, Chung WP, Im SA, Park YH, Hegg R, et al. Trastuzumab deruxtecan versus trastuzumab emtansine for breast cancer. New England Journal of Medicine. 2022;**386** (12):1143-1154

[40] Hurvitz SA, Hegg R, Chung WP, Im SA, Jacot W, Ganju V, et al. Trastuzumab deruxtecan versus trastuzumab emtansine in patients with HER2-positive metastatic breast cancer: Updated results from DESTINY-Breast03, a randomised, open-label, phase 3 trial. The Lancet. 2023;**401** (10371):105-117

[41] Hamilton EP, Hurvitz SA, Im SA, Iwata H, Curigliano G, SBK K, et al. Trastuzumab deruxtecan (T-DXd) vs trastuzumab emtansine (T-DM1) in patients (pts) with HER2+ metastatic breast cancer (mBC): Updated survival results of DESTINY-Breast03. Journal of Clinical Oncology. 2024;**42**(Number 16_ Suppl). Available from: https://ascopubs.org/doi/10.1200/JCO.2024.42.16_suppl.1025

[42] Modi S, Jacot W, Yamashita T, Sohn J, Vidal M, Tokunaga E, et al. Trastuzumab deruxtecan in previously treated HER2-low advanced breast cancer. New England Journal of Medicine. 2022;**387**(1):9-20

[43] Modi S, Jacot W, Iwata H, Park YH, Losada MJV, Li W, et al. 376O Trastuzumab deruxtecan (T-DXd) versus treatment of physician's choice (TPC) in patients (pts) with HER2-low unresectable and/or metastatic breast cancer (mBC): Updated survival results of the randomized, phase III DESTINY-Breast04 study. Annals of Oncology. Oct 2023;**34**(Supplement 2):S334-S335. DOI: 10.1016/j.annonc.2023.09.553

[44] Murthy RK, Loi S, Okines A, Paplomata E, Hamilton E, Hurvitz SA, et al. Tucatinib, trastuzumab, and capecitabine for HER2-positive metastatic breast cancer. New England Journal of Medicine. 2020;**382**(7):597-609

[45] Krop IE, Kim SB, González-Martín A, LoRusso PM, Ferrero JM, Smitt M, et al. Trastuzumab emtansine versus treatment of physician's choice for pretreated HER2-positive advanced breast cancer (TH3RESA): A randomised, open-label, phase 3 trial. The Lancet Oncology. 2014; **15**(7):689-699

[46] Krop IE, Kim SB, Martin AG, LoRusso PM, Ferrero JM, Badovinac-Crnjevic T, et al. Trastuzumab emtansine versus treatment of physician's choice in patients with previously treated HER2-positive metastatic breast cancer (TH3RESA): Final overall survival results from a randomised open-label phase 3 trial. The Lancet Oncology. 2017;**18**(6):743-754

[47] Franklin MC, Carey KD, Vajdos FF, Leahy DJ, De Vos AM, Sliwkowski MX. Insights into ErbB signaling from the structure of the ErbB2-pertuzumab complex. Cancer Cell. 2004;**5**(4): 317-328

[48] Barok M, Joensuu H, Isola J. Trastuzumab emtansine: Mechanisms of action and drug resistance. Breast Cancer Research. 2014;**16**(2):209

[49] Guidi L, Pellizzari G, Tarantino P, Valenza C, Curigliano G. Resistance to antibody-drug conjugates targeting HER2 in breast cancer: Molecular landscape and future challenges. Cancers. 2023;**15**(4):1130

[50] Curigliano G, Hu X, Dent RA, Yonemori K, Barrios S, O'Shaughnessy J, et al. Trastuzumab deruxtecan (T-DXd) vs physician's choice of chemotherapy (TPC) in patients (pts) with hormone receptor-positive (HR+), human epidermal growth factor receptor 2 (HER2)-low or HER2-ultralow metastatic breast cancer (mBC) with prior endocrine therapy (ET): Primary results from DESTINY-Breast06 (DB-06). Journal of Clinical Oncology. 2024;**42**(Number 17_Suppl). DOI: 10.1200/JCO.2024.42.17_suppl. LBA1000

[51] Harbeck N, Ciruelos E, Jerusalem G, Müller V, Niikura N, Viale G, et al. Trastuzumab deruxtecan in HER2-positive advanced breast cancer with or without brain metastases: A phase 3b/4 trial. Nature Medicine. Dec 2024;**30**(12): 3717-3727

[52] Gennari A, André F, Barrios CH, Cortés J, de Azambuja E. DeMichele A, et al. ESMO Clinical Practice Guideline for the diagnosis, staging and treatment of patients with metastatic breast cancer 2024. Available from: https://www.annalsofoncology.org/article/S0923-7534(21)04498-7/fulltext

[53] Won KA, Spruck C. Triple-negative breast cancer therapy: Current and future perspectives. International Journal of Oncology. 2020;**57**(6):1245-1261

[54] Janeva S, Zhang C, Kovács A, Parris TZ, Crozier JA, Pezzi CM, et al. Adjuvant chemotherapy and survival in women aged 70 years and older with triple-negative breast cancer: A Swedish population-based propensity score-matched analysis. Lancet Healthy Longevity. 2020;**1**(3):e117-e124

[55] Schmid P, Adams S, Rugo HS, Schneeweiss A, Barrios CH, Iwata H, et al. Atezolizumab and nab-paclitaxel in advanced triple-negative breast cancer. New England Journal of Medicine. 2018; **379**(22):2108-2121

[56] Miles D, Gligorov J, André F, Cameron D, Schneeweiss A, Barrios C, et al. Primary results from IMpassion131, a double-blind, placebo-controlled, randomised phase III trial of first-line paclitaxel with or without atezolizumab for unresectable locally advanced/metastatic triple-negative breast cancer. Annals of Oncology. 2021;**32**(8):994-1004

[57] Cortes J, Cescon DW, Rugo HS, Nowecki Z, Im SA, Yusof MM, et al. Pembrolizumab plus chemotherapy versus placebo plus chemotherapy for previously untreated locally recurrent inoperable or metastatic triple-negative breast cancer (KEYNOTE-355): A randomised, placebo-controlled, double-blind, phase 3 clinical trial. The Lancet. 2020;**396**(10265):1817-1828

[58] Cortes J, Rugo HS, Cescon DW, Im SA, Yusof MM, Gallardo C, et al. Pembrolizumab plus chemotherapy in advanced triple-negative breast cancer. New England Journal of Medicine. 2022; **387**(3):217-226

[59] Tutt A, Tovey H, Cheang MCU, Kernaghan S, Kilburn L, Gazinska P, et al. Carboplatin in BRCA1/2-mutated and triple-negative breast cancer BRCAness

subgroups: The TNT trial. Nature Medicine. 2018;**24**(5):628-637

[60] Bardia A, Hurvitz SA, Tolaney SM, Loirat D, Punie K, Oliveira M, et al. Sacituzumab govitecan in metastatic triple-negative breast cancer. New England Journal of Medicine. 2021;**384**(16):1529-1541

[61] Bardia A, Rugo HS, Tolaney SM, Loirat D, Punie K, Oliveira M, et al. Final results from the randomized phase III ASCENT clinical trial in metastatic triple-negative breast cancer and association of outcomes by human epidermal growth factor receptor 2 and trophoblast cell surface antigen 2 expression. Journal of Clinical Oncology. 2024;**42**(15):1738-1744

[62] Cortes J, O'Shaughnessy J, Loesch D, Blum JL, Vahdat LT, Petrakova K, et al. Eribulin monotherapy versus treatment of physician's choice in patients with metastatic breast cancer (EMBRACE): A phase 3 open-label randomised study. The Lancet. 2011;**377**(9769):914-923

[63] Kaufman PA, Awada A, Twelves C, Yelle L, Perez EA, Velikova G, et al. Phase III open-label randomized study of eribulin mesylate versus capecitabine in patients with locally advanced or metastatic breast cancer previously treated with an anthracycline and a taxane. Journal of Clinical Oncology. 2015;**33**(6):594-601

[64] Voorwerk L, Kok M. "IMpassionate conflicts" in immunotherapy trials for metastatic triple-negative breast cancer. Annals of Oncology. 2021;**32**(8):947-949

[65] Romero D. KEYNOTE-355 — OS benefit now reported. Nature Reviews Clinical Oncology. 2022;**19**(10):616

[66] Condorelli R, Mosele F, Verret B, Bachelot T, Bedard PL, Cortes J, et al. Genomic alterations in breast cancer: Level of evidence for actionability according to ESMO scale for clinical actionability of molecular targets (ESCAT). Annals of Oncology. 2019;**30**(3):365-373

[67] Chakravarty D, Gao J, Phillips S, Kundra R, Zhang H, Wang J, et al. OncoKB: A precision oncology knowledge Base. JCO Precision Oncology. Jul 2017;**2017**:PO.17.00011

[68] Rugo HS, Lerebours F, Ciruelos E, Drullinsky P, Ruiz-Borrego M, Neven P, et al. Alpelisib plus fulvestrant in PIK3CA-mutated, hormone receptor-positive advanced breast cancer after a CDK4/6 inhibitor (BYLieve): One cohort of a phase 2, multicentre, open-label, non-comparative study. The Lancet Oncology. 2021;**22**(4):489-498

Chapter 15

Innovations in Drug Delivery Strategies for Breast Cancer

Mani Sharma, Rama Satya Sri Kotipalli, Nemala Siva Kumar, Abhiram Kumar, Mohini Rawat, Chhavi Dhiman and Madhaw Kumar

Abstract

This chapter provides a detailed overview of innovative drug delivery strategies in breast cancer therapeutics, emphasizing emerging and futuristic approaches. Current modalities, including conventional chemotherapy, targeted therapies, and hormone treatments, are critically assessed regarding their mechanisms and clinical efficacy. The chapter highlights advancements in drug delivery systems, such as nanotechnology-based formulations, liposomal carriers, and implantable devices, which enhance therapeutic effectiveness and minimize systemic toxicity. Futuristic strategies, particularly precision medicine, are explored for their potential to tailor treatments based on genomic and molecular profiling, thereby optimizing therapeutic responses and reducing adverse effects. The role of nanotechnology in achieving targeted delivery of therapeutics to cancer cells while sparing healthy tissues is examined. Additionally, gene editing technologies, such as CRISPR, are discussed for their ability to selectively modulate cancer-related genes, promising precise and lasting therapeutic effects. The chapter also covers immunotherapeutic innovations, including CAR T-cell therapy and cancer vaccines, which leverage the immune system's capacity to target and eliminate cancer cells. In summary, this chapter elucidates the transformative potential of novel drug delivery strategies in breast cancer, highlighting the integration of advanced technologies to foster effective, personalized treatment paradigms.

Keywords: drug delivery, breast cancer, precision medicine, nanotechnology, biomarkers, immunotherapy

1. Introduction

Breast cancer (BC) accounts for around 25% of all cancer cases worldwide, making it the most common cancer among women. Approximately 2.3 million new cases and 685,000 deaths were reported in 2020 [1, 2]. Because it is resistant to HER2-targeted therapy, triple-negative breast cancer (TNBC), which lacks progesterone (PR), estrogen (ER), and HER2 receptors, is particularly aggressive and challenging

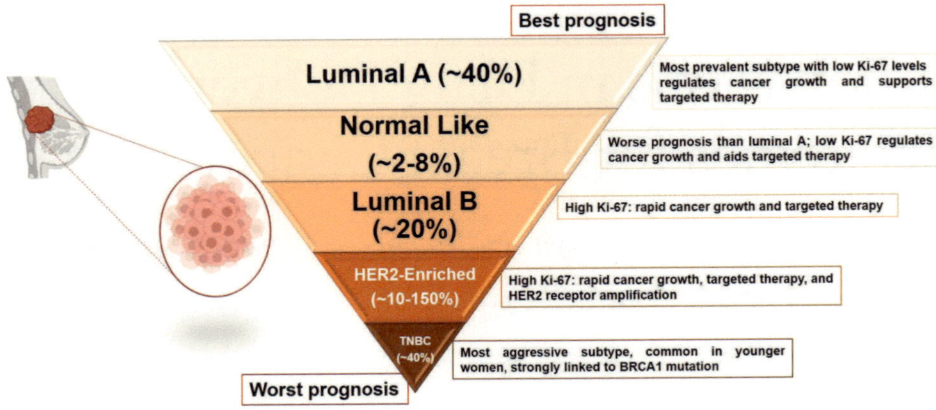

Figure 1.
Illustration of prognosis across breast cancer molecular subtypes.

to treat [3, 4]. In **Figure 1,** the chart illustrates how different molecular subtypes, including Luminal A, Luminal B, HER2-positive, and Triple-negative, impact patient outcomes and survival rates. Treatment approaches for BC differ depending on the receptor status, including hormone receptor-positive and HER2-positive subtypes [5]. BC is a diverse disease. Surgery, radiation, chemotherapy, hormone therapy, and targeted medicines, depending on the particular subtype, are frequently used in combination for the treatment of BC [6].

Traditional therapies for cancer often encounter significant challenges, primarily due to their lack of specificity and resulting systemic toxicity. Chemotherapy, for instance, can lead to severe adverse effects such as nausea, alopecia, and myelosuppression, while hormone therapies are commonly associated with hot flashes and bone loss. Additionally, targeted therapies, despite their precision, can still cause cardiotoxicity and other complications [7]. These drawbacks highlight the critical need for advanced drug delivery systems that not only enhance the efficacy of treatments but also mitigate the collateral damage to healthy tissues. Developing more refined delivery methods is essential to improving patient outcomes by reducing side effects and increasing the overall safety of cancer therapies [8].

Emerging drug delivery technologies, such as nanoparticles, liposomes, and micelles, are designed to address the limitations of traditional therapies by enhancing targeted drug delivery and minimizing systemic toxicity. Nanoparticles, for instance, can be precisely engineered to recognize and bind to specific cancer biomarkers, which facilitate more efficient accumulation of therapeutic agents at tumor sites while reducing exposure to healthy tissues. This targeted approach not only improves the therapeutic efficacy of the drugs but also helps in mitigating adverse systemic effects. Similarly, liposomes and micelles offer advantages such as enhanced stability and controlled drug release, further contributing to the precision of treatment and minimizing collateral damage. Collectively, these advanced delivery systems represent a significant advancement in overcoming the shortcomings of conventional therapies, aiming for more effective and safer cancer treatment options [9]. Liposomal formulations, which encapsulate drugs, allow for prolonged release and enhanced bioavailability. Antibody-drug conjugates (ADCs) combine monoclonal antibodies and genes like MAPK with cytotoxic drugs to deliver therapies directly to cancer cells, sparing

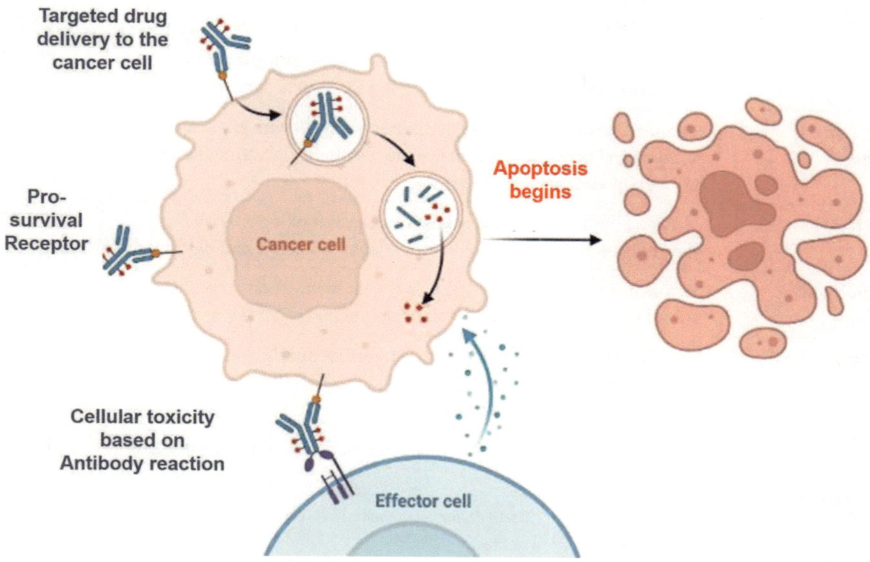

Figure 2.
Figure illustrates how targeted antibody-drug conjugates trigger programmed cell death in cancer cells. Source: [12].

healthy tissues [10]. Additionally, precise control of therapeutic release is possible with intelligent drug delivery devices that react to environmental cues like temperature changes or pH shifts [11].

Technological advancements in drug delivery systems, such as nanotechnology and precision medicine, are transforming breast cancer treatment by enabling more targeted and effective therapies in real words. These innovations allow for precise drug delivery to tumor sites, by increasing the apoptosis mechanism as shown in **Figure 2** with reduced side effects and toxicity to the healthy cells. As a result, patients benefit from more personalized and efficient care, leading to better management of the disease and enhanced quality of life. Advancements in personalized medicine further refine these approaches, tailoring drug delivery systems to individual genetic and molecular profiles. This personalization enhances targeting precision and reduces off-target effects, optimizing treatment outcomes. Recent advancements in breast cancer treatment have been promising. For example, as of late 2023, the five-year survival rate for breast cancer has reached approximately 90%, reflecting significant progress in early detection and targeted therapies. Newer treatments, such as targeted therapies and immunotherapies, have shown increased effectiveness, particularly for HER2-positive and triple-negative breast cancers. Additionally, advancements in genetic research and personalized medicine have led to more tailored treatment plans, improving outcomes and reducing side effects. Overall, these innovations are contributing to more effective and personalized care for patients [13].

Collectively, these advancements in drug delivery technology have the potential to revolutionize the way that breast cancer is treated by increasing therapeutic specificity, decreasing side effects, and eventually improving patient outcomes [14]. Sustained investigation and advancement are essential for tackling present therapeutic constraints and enhancing patients' quality of life (**Table 1**) [33].

Aspect	Description	References
Genetic Factors	Genetic mutations (e.g., BRCA1, BRCA2) significantly increase breast cancer risk. Inherited mutations account for 5–10% of cases.	[15, 16]
Hormonal Factors	A higher risk of breast cancer has been associated with exposure to estrogen and progesterone, such as via hormone replacement therapy, late menopause, or early menarche.	[17, 18]
Lifestyle Factors	Obesity, physical inactivity, alcohol use, and smoking are risk factors. Elevated risk is also correlated with sedentary lifestyle and high-fat diet.	[19, 20]
Reproductive History	Factors like nulliparity, late age at first childbirth, and short duration of breastfeeding are associated with increased risk of breast cancer.	[21, 22]
Environmental Factors	Exposure to environmental pollutants and chemicals, such as pesticides and endocrine disruptors, has been suggested to influence breast cancer risk, though evidence is still emerging.	[23, 24]
Age	Age is a major risk factor, with incidence increasing significantly after age 50.	[25]
Family History	A family history of breast cancer increases risk, particularly if first-degree relatives are affected.	[26, 27]
Geographic Variation	Geographically speaking, incidence rates differ; North America and Western Europe have greater rates than Asia and Africa.	[28, 29]
Prevalence	Globally, breast cancer is the most common cancer among women; 2.3 million new cases are expected to be reported in 2020.	[2, 30]
Mortality	Breast cancer is a leading cause of cancer-related deaths among women worldwide, with approximately 685,000 fatalities recorded globally in 2020.	[31, 32]

Table 1.
Etiology and epidemiology of breast cancer.

2. Conventional drug delivery modalities

Chemotherapy remains foundational in breast cancer treatment, utilizing cytotoxic agents like doxorubicin, paclitaxel, and cyclophosphamide to target rapidly proliferating cancer cells [34]. These drugs disrupt critical cellular processes—doxorubicin intercalates DNA, paclitaxel stabilizes microtubules, and cyclophosphamide cross-links DNA—thereby inhibiting tumor growth. However, their non-specific action leads to substantial off-target toxicity, including myelosuppression, nausea, and alopecia. The emergence of drug resistance through genetic mutations or enhanced drug efflux mechanisms further complicates treatment, necessitating advanced delivery systems to enhance specificity and reduce adverse effects [35].

Targeted Therapies aim to selectively disrupt oncogenic pathways. For instance, trastuzumab (Herceptin) targets HER2-positive breast cancer cells by binding to HER2 receptors, inhibiting tumor growth and promoting immune-mediated cell death [36]. Additionally, small molecule inhibitors like lapatinib and palbociclib block key signaling pathways and cell cycle regulators. Despite their precision, issues such as drug resistance and variable efficacy highlight the need for ongoing innovation in targeted delivery mechanisms [37].

Hormone therapy is employed for hormone receptor-positive breast cancer, where tumor growth is driven by estrogen and progesterone. Agents like tamoxifen act as estrogen receptor modulators, while aromatase inhibitors such as letrozole block estrogen synthesis. Long-term hormone therapy, while effective in reducing recurrence and improving survival rates, often comes with significant side effects such as hot flashes, bone loss, and increased cardiovascular risks. These adverse effects underscore the urgent need for more advanced drug delivery strategies that enhance the therapeutic benefits of hormone therapy while minimizing systemic toxicity. Innovations in drug delivery could include targeted therapies that localize treatment effects, controlled-release formulations, or novel carriers designed to reduce side effects. By improving the precision and safety of hormone therapy, these strategies aim to optimize patient outcomes and reduce the negative impact on overall health [38].

Recent innovations in drug delivery strategies have significantly enhanced the efficacy of breast cancer treatments, surpassing traditional modalities. One notable advancement is the development of antibody-drug conjugates (ADCs), such as Enhertu (trastuzumab deruxtecan), which combines the HER2-targeted monoclonal antibody trastuzumab with a cytotoxic drug, enabling targeted delivery of chemotherapy directly to HER2-positive tumor cells. This approach has demonstrated impressive clinical outcomes, including substantial improvements in progression-free survival compared to conventional therapies. Another promising innovation is the use of nanoparticle-based delivery systems, exemplified by the Nanoparticle Albumin-Bound Paclitaxel (nab-paclitaxel), which enhances the bioavailability and tumor penetration of paclitaxel while reducing systemic toxicity. Furthermore, novel liposomal formulations, such as Doxil, have improved the delivery of doxorubicin to tumor sites, minimizing cardiotoxicity and extending treatment options for patients with advanced breast cancer. These advancements in drug delivery are redefining treatment paradigms, offering more precise and effective therapeutic options [39].

3. Nanotechnology-based formulations

Nanotechnology operates at the nanoscale (1–100 nanometers), enabling precise manipulation of materials to create novel carriers for drug delivery [40]. Nanoscale carriers, such as nanoparticles and nanorods, are meticulously engineered to address the challenges associated with drug delivery by significantly enhancing the solubility, stability, and bioavailability of therapeutic agents. These advanced carriers are designed to facilitate controlled and sustained release of drugs specifically at tumor sites, allowing for a more targeted approach to treatment. By localizing the delivery of therapeutic agents, nanoscale carriers not only improve the efficacy of the treatment but also substantially reduce the systemic toxicity that can result from conventional drug delivery methods. This targeted delivery system ensures that higher concentrations of the drug are available precisely where needed, thereby maximizing therapeutic outcomes while minimizing adverse effects on healthy tissues. Some of the advanced nanotechnology-based drug delivery formulations are represented in **Figure 3**.

One notable example is the use of liposomal formulations, such as Doxil, which has been instrumental in reducing the cardiotoxicity associated with doxorubicin. Liposomes encapsulate the drug, which not only enhances its accumulation in tumor tissues but also mitigates adverse effects on the heart. A 2023 study in Clinical Cancer Research illustrated that liposomal doxorubicin provided better therapeutic outcomes and reduced cardiotoxicity in patients with advanced breast cancer compared to free doxorubicin [41].

Liposomes are lipid-based vesicles designed to encapsulate hydrophilic drugs, thereby enhancing their stability and extending their circulation time. Dendrimers,

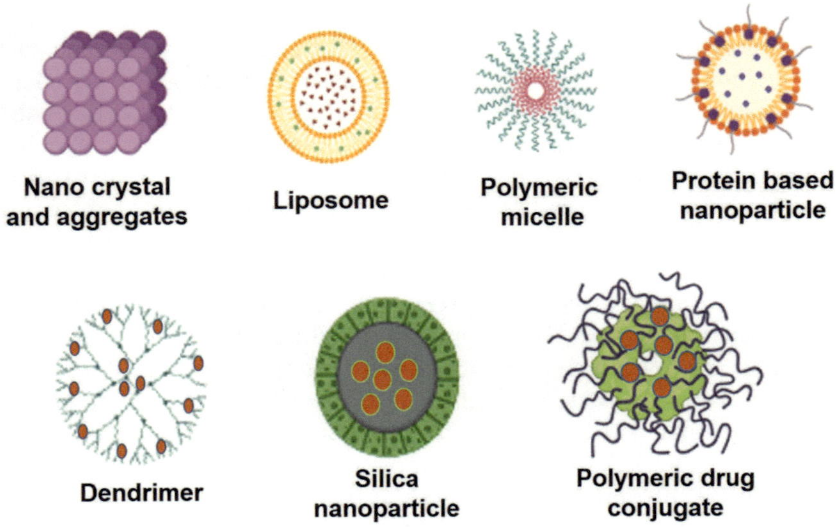

Figure 3.
Figure depicts various nanotechnology-based formulations.

with their branched polymeric structure, allow for precise drug loading and release control [42]. Gold nanoparticles can be functionalized with targeting ligands to achieve selective binding to cancer cells, facilitating targeted therapy. Each nanoparticle type provides unique benefits, such as improved targeting, reduced off-target effects, and enhanced ability to traverse biological barriers [43]. Nanotechnology-based formulations, such as liposomal doxorubicin *(Doxil)*, have demonstrated enhanced efficacy and reduced cardiotoxicity compared to traditional formulations. Engineered nanoparticles can target drugs more precisely, lowering off-target toxicity and improving therapeutic outcomes. Ongoing clinical trials are evaluating these advanced formulations, with preliminary data suggesting significant improvements in both efficacy and patient tolerability (**Table 2**) [60].

4. Liposomal drug delivery systems

Liposomes are spherical vesicles composed of lipid bilayers that can encapsulate a diverse range of therapeutic agents, including both hydrophilic and hydrophobic drugs. This versatile structure closely resembles cellular membranes, which allows liposomes to facilitate controlled drug release and enhance cellular uptake. The bilayer encapsulation provides a protective environment for the drugs, ensuring stability and preventing premature degradation. This controlled release mechanism not only improves the bioavailability of the drugs but also ensures that they are delivered more effectively to target cells [61]. Surface modifications of liposomes can further enhance their performance by improving their stability, increasing their drug-loading capacity, and optimizing their targeting abilities. Techniques such as PEGylation, where polyethylene glycol chains are attached to the liposome surface, can extend circulation time and reduce immune recognition, while ligand conjugation can direct liposomes to specific tumor sites. These modifications allow for more precise delivery of therapeutic agents, minimizing systemic exposure and reducing associated side effects. This targeted approach ensures that higher concentrations of

Nanotechnology-based system	Mechanism of action	Advantages	References
Liposomes	Lipid bilayers encapsulate drugs, allowing controlled release and improved cellular uptake.	Enhanced drug solubility, extended circulation time, reduced toxicity.	[44, 45]
Polymeric Nanoparticles	Drug-loaded polymeric matrices release drugs through diffusion or degradation.	High drug loading capacity, controlled release, and prolonged circulation.	[46, 47]
Dendrimers	Branched polymer structures that release drugs through their functional groups.	Precise drug delivery, high drug loading, and versatile surface modifications.	[48, 49]
Gold Nanoparticles	Drug attachment to gold nanoparticles, targeting specific cancer cell receptors.	Surface functionalization, enhanced cellular uptake, and imaging capabilities.	[50, 51]
Carbon Nanotubes	Drug loading within nanotubes with release via surface interactions or degradation.	High surface area for drug loading, targeted delivery, and cellular penetration.	[52, 53]
Silica Nanoparticles	Drug encapsulation in mesoporous silica with controlled release through pore channels.	High stability, tunable pore size for controlled release, and easy functionalization.	[54, 55]
Micelles	Self-assembled amphiphilic molecules forming core-shell structures that encapsulate drugs.	Improved solubility of hydrophobic drugs, targeted delivery, and reduced toxicity.	[56, 57]
Stimuli-Responsive Nanoparticles	Release drugs in response to specific environmental triggers (e.g., pH, temperature).	Enhanced targeting to tumor microenvironment, reduced side effects.	[58, 59]

Table 2.
Different nanoformulations with mechanism of action and their advantages.

the drug are available at the tumor site, enhancing therapeutic efficacy and improving patient outcomes [62].

Liposomal formulations provide significant benefits over traditional drug delivery methods. They enhance the solubility of poorly soluble drugs and extend circulation time in the bloodstream, thus improving bioavailability and therapeutic efficacy. Engineered liposomes can be functionalized with targeting ligands, facilitating selective drug delivery to cancer cells while minimizing off-target effects. This targeted delivery reduces systemic toxicity and optimizes patient outcomes [63].

Several liposomal formulations have been successfully implemented in clinical settings. *Doxil*, a liposomal formulation of doxorubicin, is utilized for treating breast cancer and other malignancies, offering reduced cardiotoxicity compared to free doxorubicin and efficacy in refractory cases. Another example is *Myocet* (non-pegylated liposomal doxorubicin), which has been evaluated in several clinical trials for its efficacy in treating breast cancer. Other liposomal drugs, such as those containing paclitaxel and daunorubicin, are also under development or in clinical use, with ongoing evaluations to enhance efficacy and minimize adverse effects in breast cancer therapy [64].

5. Implantable drug delivery devices

Implantable drug delivery devices are engineered to release therapeutic agents over extended periods within the body. Key examples include intratumoral implants and programmable infusion pumps. Intratumoral implants, such as those containing chemotherapeutic agents or radioisotopes, are inserted directly into or adjacent to tumors, enabling localized treatment. Programmable infusion pumps deliver precise, controlled doses of drugs over time, facilitating sustained and adjustable therapy [65].

Implantable devices utilize various drug-release mechanisms, including diffusion, erosion, and mechanical pumping. Polymer-based implants often release drugs through diffusion from a polymer matrix or gradual polymer degradation. Infusion pumps, which can be mechanically or electronically controlled, regulate medication flow to provide continuous delivery. This approach is particularly beneficial for managing chronic conditions and reducing the frequency of drug administration [66].

Clinical evidence indicates that implantable drug delivery devices enhance patient compliance and therapeutic efficacy. For instance, hormone-releasing implants effectively manage hormone-sensitive breast cancer by providing continuous hormone suppression. Programmable infusion pumps deliver targeted therapies, such as analgesics or chemotherapeutics, with greater precision and fewer side effects compared to conventional methods. Advances in technology and materials are anticipated to further expand the applications of these devices. Recent technological innovations in breast cancer treatment include the use of *Trastuzumab Deruxtecan* (Enhertu), an antibody-drug conjugate that has significantly improved outcomes for HER2-positive breast cancer, showing higher progression-free survival rates in recent trials. Additionally, *Oncotype DX genomic assays* have enabled more personalized treatment plans by assessing recurrence risk and guiding adjuvant therapy decisions with greater precision [67].

6. Futuristic approaches in drug delivery

Precision medicine: Precision medicine in breast cancer leverages next-generation sequencing (NGS) to identify specific genetic mutations, guiding personalized treatments. Recent breakthroughs include targeted therapies for HER2-positive breast cancer, such as trastuzumab, which directly targets HER2-overexpressing cells. Ongoing research into liquid biopsies enables real-time monitoring of tumor DNA, allowing for adaptable treatment adjustments. Additionally, integrating multi-omics data—combining genetic, proteomic, and metabolic profiles—further refines personalized therapies, enhancing treatment efficacy and patient outcomes [68].

Nanotechnology advancements: Recent advances in nanotechnology have led to the development of sophisticated nanocarriers and delivery systems. Stimuli-responsive nanoparticles release drugs in response to specific tumor triggers like pH changes or temperature variations. Advanced surface modifications, including stealth coatings and targeting ligands, improve the precision and penetration of nanocarriers into tumor tissues, enhancing the efficacy of breast cancer treatments [69].

Gene editing technologies: Gene editing technologies, notably CRISPR-Cas9, offer the potential to directly alter genes associated with cancer. CRISPR-Cas9 allows precise DNA editing of oncogenes and tumor suppressor genes, potentially transforming breast cancer treatment by correcting mutations and disrupting cancer pathways. For example, it can correct mutations in genes like BRCA1 and disrupt pathways driving tumor growth, potentially revolutionizing breast cancer treatment by directly targeting and modifying genetic abnormalities [70].

Immunotherapy and cell-based therapies: Immunotherapy leverages the immune system's capability to identify and eliminate cancer cells. Immunotherapy harnesses the immune system to target and destroy cancer cells. For example, CAR T-cell therapy, which involves engineering patient T-cells to express receptors targeting cancer cells, has shown promise in hematological cancers and is being explored for breast cancer. Additionally, cancer vaccines aim to induce immune responses against tumor-specific antigens. These therapies represent a significant shift toward utilizing the body's own immune defenses to combat cancer, offering new therapeutic possibilities (**Table 3**) [85].

Approach	Description	Integration with conventional therapy	References
Precision Medicine	Tailoring treatments based on genetic, genomic, and molecular profiles of the patient's tumor.	Enhances efficacy of conventional therapies by selecting the most appropriate treatment based on genetic alterations.	[71, 72]
Nanotechnology	Utilizes nanoscale carriers like nanoparticles and liposomes for targeted drug delivery and controlled release.	Combined with chemotherapy to increase drug accumulation in tumors and reduce systemic toxicity.	[73, 74]
Stimuli-Responsive Nanoparticles	Nanoparticles engineered to release drugs in response to specific stimuli such as pH or temperature changes in the tumor microenvironment.	Integrates with conventional therapies to enhance drug release at the tumor site while reducing side effects.	[75, 76]
Gene Editing Technologies	Uses tools like CRISPR-Cas9 to modify genes associated with cancer, potentially correcting mutations or disrupting oncogenes.	Can be used alongside conventional therapies to target specific genetic mutations and improve treatment efficacy.	[77, 78]
Immunotherapy	Enhances the immune system's ability to target and destroy cancer cells, including CAR T-cell therapy and cancer vaccines.	Combines with conventional therapies to boost immune response against cancer cells and improve overall treatment outcomes.	[79, 80]
Antibody-Drug Conjugates (ADCs)	Combines monoclonal antibodies with cytotoxic drugs to target and kill cancer cells specifically.	Integrated with traditional therapies to deliver targeted cytotoxic agents directly to cancer cells, enhancing treatment efficacy.	[81, 82]
Smart Drug Delivery Systems	Employs systems responsive to environmental stimuli (e.g., pH changes) for controlled drug release.	Can be used in conjunction with chemotherapy and other conventional therapies to optimize drug release at the tumor site.	[83, 84]

Table 3.
Futuristic approaches in integration with conventional therapy.

7. Integration with conventional therapies

Combination therapies use multiple modalities to enhance efficacy and overcome resistance. For instance, integrating advanced drug delivery systems with conventional treatments, like nanoparticles with chemotherapy, can significantly improve targeting and reduce toxicity. This multi-modal strategy addresses various facets of cancer biology, aiming to improve therapeutic outcomes and minimize resistance development [86].

Synergistic effects are observed when combining different treatments results in outcomes that surpass those achieved with individual therapies alone. For instance, the integration of targeted therapies with immunotherapy exemplifies this synergy, as the combination enhances the immune system's capacity to identify and eradicate cancer cells while concurrently disrupting critical molecular pathways that drive tumor growth. This dual approach not only amplifies the immune response but also addresses the underlying mechanisms of cancer proliferation. Similarly, the amalgamation of various drug delivery systems, such as nanoparticles and liposomes, exemplifies another form of synergy. By utilizing these advanced carriers in conjunction, it is possible to optimize drug delivery, ensuring more precise targeting and sustained release of therapeutic agents. This combined strategy enhances overall therapeutic efficacy, leading to more effective treatment outcomes and improved patient responses compared to using a single drug delivery method [87].

Clinical case studies demonstrate the effectiveness of combination therapies. The synergy of trastuzumab (HER2-targeted therapy) with chemotherapy has led to improved outcomes in HER2-positive breast cancer patients. Additionally, combining nanoparticle-based delivery systems with established treatments has shown promising results in preclinical studies and early-phase clinical trials. These examples underscore the potential of combination approaches to enhance treatment efficacy and address challenges in breast cancer therapy [88].

8. Challenges and future directions

Despite progress, several technical challenges persist in drug delivery for breast cancer. Key challenges include drug resistance, variability in tumor response, and targeting precision. Ongoing research into advanced drug delivery technologies and innovative combinations is crucial for overcoming these issues [89].

Developing and approving new drug delivery systems require rigorous regulatory and ethical scrutiny. Comprehensive clinical trials ensure safety and efficacy, while ethical concerns, especially in gene editing, must be carefully assessed to ensure responsible use of new technologies [90].

Emerging trends in drug delivery are driven by advancements in artificial intelligence (AI) and machine learning, which enhance treatment planning and patient response prediction. Innovations in bioengineering and materials science are also advancing the development of novel drug delivery systems with improved capabilities. These trends promise to significantly advance breast cancer treatment and enhance patient outcomes.

9. Conclusion

This chapter examined the progression of drug delivery systems in breast cancer treatment, highlighting a shift from traditional methods to advanced approaches like nanotechnology and precision medicine. Traditional drug delivery often struggles with limitations in efficacy and side effects. However, recent innovations, such as nanoparticles, have significantly improved drug solubility, stability, and targeted delivery. These nanoscale carriers enable precise, controlled release of therapeutics directly at tumor sites, enhancing effectiveness and minimizing overall toxicity. Such advancements are creating a major shift toward more targeted and personalized therapies.

As research continues, new technologies are expected to further refine breast cancer treatment. Emerging trends such as precision medicine, which customizes treatment based on individual genetic and molecular profiles, gene editing to correct cancer-related mutations, and immunotherapy to harness the immune system's power, are poised to revolutionize the field. These innovations promise to deliver more effective and personalized treatment options, significantly improving patient outcomes and quality of life. The ongoing evolution in drug delivery systems marks a significant advancement in breast cancer care, promising a future with more tailored, effective, and patient-centered treatments.

Acknowledgements

The author acknowledges the use of AI tools Perplexity and Liner for language polishing of the manuscript.

Author details

Mani Sharma[1*], Rama Satya Sri Kotipalli[1], Nemala Siva Kumar[2], Abhiram Kumar[3], Mohini Rawat[4], Chhavi Dhiman[3] and Madhaw Kumar[5]

1 CSIR-Indian Institute of Chemical Technology, Hyderabad, Secunderabad, Telangana, India

2 Sri Vasavi Institute of Pharmaceutical Sciences, Tadepalligudem, Andhra Pradesh, India

3 Birla Institute of Technology and Science, Pilani—Hyderabad Campus, Secunderabad, Telangana, India

4 Himalayan Institute of Pharmacy and Research, Atak Farm, Dehradun, Uttarakhand, India

5 Goel Instiute of Pharmacy and Sciences, Lucknow, Uttar Pradesh, India

*Address all correspondence to: mninup2015@gmail.com

References

[1] Arnold M, Singh D, Laversanne M, Vignat J, Vaccarella S, Meheus F, et al. Global burden of cutaneous melanoma in 2020 and projections to 2040. JAMA Dermatology. 2022;**158**(5):495-503

[2] DeSantis CE, Ma J, Gaudet MM, Newman LA, Miller KD, Goding Sauer A, et al. Breast cancer statistics, 2019. CA: A Cancer Journal for Clinicians. 2019;**69**(6):438-451

[3] Nisticò G. Consistent theories of free Dirac particle without singular predictions. Particles. 2022;**6**(1):1-16

[4] Thacker I. Climate change by the numbers: Leveraging mathematical skills for science learning online. Learning and Instruction. 2023;**86**:101782

[5] Thanopoulou E, Khader L, Caira M, Wardley A, Ettl J, Miglietta F, et al. Therapeutic strategies for the management of hormone receptor-positive, human epidermal growth factor receptor 2-positive (HR+/HER2+) breast cancer: A review of the current literature. Cancers. 2020;**12**(11):3317

[6] Waks AG, Winer EP. Breast cancer treatment: A review. JAMA. 2019;**321**(3):288-300

[7] Mustapha A, Ismail A, Abdullahi SU, Hassan ON, Ugwunnaji PI, Berinyuy EB. Cancer chemotherapy: A review update of the mechanisms of actions, prospects and associated problems. Journal of Biomedical. 2022;**1**(01):001-016

[8] Mao X, Wu S, Huang D, Li C. Complications and comorbidities associated with antineoplastic chemotherapy: Rethinking drug design and delivery for anticancer therapy. Acta Pharmaceutica Sinica B. 2024;**14**:2901-2926

[9] Ashfaq UA, Riaz M, Yasmeen E, Yousaf MZ. Recent advances in nanoparticle-based targeted drug-delivery systems against cancer and role of tumor microenvironment. Critical Reviews™ in Therapeutic Drug Carrier Systems. 2017;**34**(4):317-353

[10] Kotipalli RSS, Tirunavalli SK, Pote AB, Sahu BD, Kuncha M, Jerald MK, et al. Sinigrin attenuates the dextran sulfate sodium-induced colitis in mice by modulating the MAPK pathway. Inflammation. 2023;**46**(3):787-807

[11] Sharma M, Chouhan NK, Vaidya S. Hepatocellular carcinoma: A pharmacological aspect. In: Liver Pathology. London, UK: IntechOpen; 2020

[12] Datta A, Deng S, Gopal V, Yap KCH, Halim CE, Lye ML, et al. Cytoskeletal dynamics in epithelial-mesenchymal transition: Insights into therapeutic targets for cancer metastasis. Cancers (Basel). 2021;**13**(8):1882. DOI: 10.3390/cancers13081882

[13] Puccetti M, Pariano M, Schoubben A, Giovagnoli S, Ricci M. Biologics, theranostics, and personalized medicine in drug delivery systems. Pharmacological Research. 2024;**201**:107086

[14] Sharma M, Chouhan NK, Vaidya S, Talati MN. Lipids, peptides, and polymers as targeted drug delivery vectors in cancer therapy. In: Handbook of Research on Advancements in Cancer Therapeutics. Hershey, Pennsylvania: IGI Global; 2021. pp. 255-275

[15] Козлитин АМ. Www://risk-2005. Narod. ru/kammov@ gmail. Com. Безопасностьтруда в промышленности. 2004;**10**:35-42

[16] Miki Y, Swensen J, Shattuck-Eidens D, Futreal PA, Harshman K, Tavtigian S, et al. A strong candidate for the breast and ovarian cancer susceptibility gene BRCA1. Science. 1994;**266**(5182):66-71

[17] Cramer W, Kicklighter DW, Bondeau A, Iii BM, Churkina G, Nemry B, et al. Comparing global models of terrestrial net primary productivity (NPP): Overview and key results. Global Change Biology. 1999;**5**(S1):1-15

[18] Lee S, Colditz GA, Berkman LF, Kawachi I. Caregiving and risk of coronary heart disease in US women: A prospective study. American Journal of Preventive Medicine. 2003;**24**(2): 113-119

[19] Willett WC, Howe GR, Kushi LH. Adjustment for total energy intake in epidemiologic studies. The American Journal of Clinical Nutrition. 1997;**65**(4):1220S-1228S

[20] Yang Y, Sharma R, Sharma A, Awasthi S, Awasthi Y. Lipid peroxidation and cell cycle signaling: 4-hydroxynonenal, a key molecule in stress mediated signaling. Acta Biochimica Polonica. 2003;**50**(2):319-336

[21] Rohan M, Parow A, Stoll AL, Demopulos C, Friedman S, Dager S, et al. Low-field magnetic stimulation in bipolar depression using an MRI-based stimulator. American Journal of Psychiatry. 2004;**161**(1):93-98

[22] Key TJ, Appleby PN, Rosell MS. Health effects of vegetarian and vegan diets. Proceedings of the Nutrition Society. 2006;**65**(1):35-41

[23] Rudel RA, Camann DE, Spengler JD, Korn LR, Brody JG. Phthalates, alkylphenols, pesticides, polybrominated diphenyl ethers, and other endocrine-disrupting compounds in indoor air and dust. Environmental Science and Technology. 2003;**37**(20):4543-4553

[24] Cohn AC, MacNeil JR, Harrison LH, Hatcher C, Theodore J, Schmidt M, et al. Changes in Neisseria meningitidis disease epidemiology in the United States, 1998-2007: Implications for prevention of meningococcal disease. Clinical Infectious Diseases. 2010;**50**(2):184-191

[25] Siegel RL, Miller KD, Goding Sauer A, Fedewa SA, Butterly LF, Anderson JC, et al. Colorectal cancer statistics, 2020. CA: A Cancer Journal for Clinicians. 2020;**70**(3):145-164

[26] Hartmann WK, Neukum G. Cratering chronology and the evolution of Mars. In: Chronology and Evolution of Mars: Proceedings of an ISSI Workshop, 10-14 April 2000, Bern, Switzerland. Netherlands: Springer; 2001. pp. 165-194

[27] Goldgar DE, Easton DF, Byrnes GB, Spurdle AB, Iversen ES, Greenblatt MS, et al. Genetic evidence and integration of various data sources for classifying uncertain variants into a single model. Human Mutation. 2008;**29**(11):1265-1272

[28] Parkin DM, Bray F, Ferlay J, Pisani P. Global cancer statistics, 2002. CA: A Cancer Journal for Clinicians. 2005;**55**(2):74-108

[29] Deo SVS, Sharma J, Kumar S. GLOBOCAN 2020 report on global cancer burden: Challenges and opportunities for surgical oncologists. Annals of Surgical Oncology. 2022;**29**(11):6497-6500

[30] Arnold BJ, Huang IT, Hanage WP. Horizontal gene transfer and adaptive

evolution in bacteria. Nature Reviews Microbiology. 2022;**20**(4):206-218

[31] Ferlay J, Colombet M, Soerjomataram I, Mathers C, Parkin DM, Piñeros M, et al. Estimating the global cancer incidence and mortality in 2018: GLOBOCAN sources and methods. International Journal of Cancer. 2019;**144**(8):1941-1953

[32] Feigin VL, Stark BA, Johnson CO, Roth GA, Bisignano C, Abady GG, et al. Global, regional, and national burden of stroke and its risk factors, 1990-2019: A systematic analysis for the Global Burden of Disease Study 2019. The Lancet Neurology. 2021;**20**(10):795-820

[33] Laudet AB. The case for considering quality of life in addiction research and clinical practice. Addiction Science and Clinical Practice. 2011;**6**(1):44

[34] Meher JG, Dixit S, Pathan DK, Singh Y, Chandasana H, Pawar VK, et al. Paclitaxel-loaded TPGS enriched self-emulsifying carrier causes apoptosis by modulating survivin expression and inhibits tumour growth in syngeneic mammary tumours. Artificial Cells, Nanomedicine, and Biotechnology. 2018;**46**(Suppl_3):344-358

[35] Swain SM, Shastry M, Hamilton E. Targeting HER2-positive breast cancer: Advances and future directions. Nature Reviews Drug Discovery. 2023;**22**(2):101-126

[36] Gámez-Chiachio M, Sarrió D, Moreno-Bueno G. Novel therapies and strategies to overcome resistance to anti-HER2-targeted drugs. Cancers. 2022;**14**(18):4543

[37] Sharma M, Kansal S. A comprehensive study of multi-drug resistance in tuberculosis: Help desk for researchers, doctors, and patients. In: Contemporary Issues in Global Medicine and Moving toward International Healthcare Equity. Hershey, Pennsylvania: IGI Global; 2022. pp. 317-347

[38] Md S, Kotta S. Advanced drug delivery technologies for postmenopausal effects. Journal of Controlled Release. 2024;**373**:426-446

[39] Lee J, Choi MK, Song IS. Recent advances in doxorubicin formulation to enhance pharmacokinetics and tumor targeting. Pharmaceuticals. 2023;**16**(6):802

[40] Hossen S, Hossain MK, Basher MK, Mia MNH, Rahman MT, Uddin MJ. Smart nanocarrier-based drug delivery systems for cancer therapy and toxicity studies: A review. Journal of Advanced Research. 2019;**15**:1-18

[41] Gabizon AA. Pegylated liposomal doxorubicin: Metamorphosis of an old drug into a new form of chemotherapy. Cancer Investigation. 2001;**19**(4):424-436

[42] Sharma M, Ambadipudi SS, Chouhan NK, Nayak VL, Pabbaraja S, Andugulapati SB, et al. Design, synthesis and biological evaluation of novel cationic liposomes loaded with melphalan for the treatment of cancer. Bioorganic and Medicinal Chemistry Letters. 2024;**97**:129549

[43] Gowda R, Jones NR, Banerjee S, Robertson GP. Use of nanotechnology to develop multi-drug inhibitors for cancer therapy. Journal of Nanomedicine and Nanotechnology. 2013;**4**(6):2-16

[44] Gabizon A, Horowitz AT, Goren D, Tzemach D, Shmeeda H, Zalipsky S. In vivo fate of folate-targeted polyethylene-glycol liposomes in tumor-bearing mice. Clinical Cancer Research. 2003;**9**(17):6551-6559

[45] Vauthier C, Bouchemal K. Methods for the preparation and manufacture of polymeric nanoparticles. Pharmaceutical Research. 2009;**26**:1025-1058

[46] Fantin E, Niemeyer K, Dufresne-Deslières C. Nostalgies et remédiations du passé enpolitique, ou le danger des abus de la mémoire. Questions de communication. 2023;**44**:263-282

[47] Tomalia DA. In quest of a systematic framework for unifying and defining nanoscience. Journal of Nanoparticle Research. 2009;**11**:1251-1310

[48] Hu Y, Mignani S, Majoral JP, Shen M, Shi X. Construction of iron oxide nanoparticle-based hybrid platforms for tumor imaging and therapy. Chemical Society Reviews. 2018;**47**(5):1874-1900

[49] Hergt R, Dutz S, Müller R, Zeisberger M. Magnetic particle hyperthermia: Nanoparticle magnetism and materials development for cancer therapy. Journal of Physics: Condensed Matter. 2006;**18**(38):S2919

[50] Huang J, Li Q, Sun D, Lu Y, Su Y, Yang X, et al. Biosynthesis of silver and gold nanoparticles by novel sundried Cinnamomumcamphora leaf. Nanotechnology. 2007;**18**(10):105104

[51] Iijima S. Helical microtubules of graphitic carbon. Nature. 1991;**354**(6348):56-58

[52] Chen IC, Hill JK, Ohlemüller R, Roy DB, Thomas CD. Rapid range shifts of species associated with high levels of climate warming. Science. 2011;**333**(6045):1024-1026

[53] Vallet-Regí M, Balas F, Arcos D. Mesoporous materials for drug delivery. Angewandte Chemie International Edition. 2007;**46**(40):7548-7558

[54] Xie J, Sreenivasan S, Korniss G, Zhang W, Lim C, Szymanski BK. Social consensus through the influence of committed minorities. Physical Review E—Statistical, Nonlinear, and Soft Matter Physics. 2011;**84**(1):011130

[55] Maeda S, Chang L, Li ZW, Luo JL, Leffert H, Karin M. IKKβ is required for prevention of apoptosis mediated by cell-bound but not by circulating TNFα. Immunity. 2003;**19**(5):725-737

[56] Torchilin VP. Multifunctional nanocarriers. Advanced Drug Delivery Reviews. 2006;**58**(14):1532-1555

[57] Tran C, Ouk S, Clegg NJ, Chen Y, Watson PA, Arora V, et al. Development of a second-generation antiandrogen for treatment of advanced prostate cancer. Science. 2009;**324**(5928):787-790

[58] Davis AP, King BL, Mockus S, Murphy CG, Saraceni-Richards C, Rosenstein M, et al. The comparative toxicogenomics database: Update 2011. Nucleic Acids Research. 2010;**39**(Suppl_1):D1067-D1072

[59] Farooque F, Wasi M, Mughees MM. Liposomes as drug delivery system: An updated review. Journal of Drug Delivery and Therapeutics. 2021;**11**(5-S):149-158

[60] Allen TM, Cullis PR. Liposomal drug delivery systems: From concept to clinical applications. Advanced Drug Delivery Reviews. 2013;**65**(1):36-48

[61] Milling L, Zhang Y, Irvine DJ. Delivering safer immunotherapies for cancer. Advanced Drug Delivery Reviews. 2017;**114**:79-101

[62] Ghosh S, Lalani R, Patel V, Bhowmick S, Misra A. Surface engineered liposomal delivery of

therapeutics across the blood brain barrier: Recent advances, challenges and opportunities. Expert Opinion on Drug Delivery. 2019;**16**(12):1287-1311

[63] Rivera E. Liposomal anthracyclines in metastatic breast cancer: Clinical update. The Oncologist. 2003;**8**(S2):3-9

[64] Sharma M, Joshi J, Chouhan NK, Talati MN, Vaidya S, Kumar A. Liposome-a comprehensive approach for researchers. In: Molecular Pharmacology. London, UK: IntechOpen; 2020

[65] Pons-Faudoa FP, Ballerini A, Sakamoto J, Grattoni A. Advanced implantable drug delivery technologies: Transforming the clinical landscape of therapeutics for chronic diseases. Biomedical Microdevices. 2019;**21**:1-22

[66] Sharma R, Singh D, Gaur P, Joshi D. Intelligent automated drug administration and therapy: Future of healthcare. Drug Delivery and Translational Research. 2021;**11**:1-25

[67] Hussen BM, Abdullah ST, Salihi A, Sabir DK, Sidiq KR, Rasul MF, et al. The emerging roles of NGS in clinical oncology and personalized medicine. Pathology-Research and Practice. 2022;**230**:153760

[68] Mi P. Stimuli-responsive nanocarriers for drug delivery, tumor imaging, therapy and theranostics. Theranostics. 2020;**10**(10):4557

[69] Chan CW, Law BM, So WK, Chow KM, Waye MM. Novel strategies on personalized medicine for breast cancer treatment: An update. International Journal of Molecular Sciences. 2017;**18**(11):2423

[70] Mohanty R, Chowdhury CR, Arega S, Sen P, Ganguly P, Ganguly N. CAR T cell therapy: A new era for cancer treatment. Oncology Reports. 2019;**42**(6):2183-2195

[71] Garber J, Clarke GN, Weersing VR, Beardslee WR, Brent DA, Gladstone TR, et al. Prevention of depression in at-risk adolescents: A randomized controlled trial. JAMA. 2009;**301**(21):2215-2224

[72] Peer D, Zhu P, Carman CV, Lieberman J, Shimaoka M. Selective gene silencing in activated leukocytes by targeting siRNAs to the integrin lymphocyte function-associated antigen-1. Proceedings of the National Academy of Sciences. 2007;**104**(10):4095-4100

[73] Reddy LH, Arias JL, Nicolas J, Couvreur P. Magnetic nanoparticles: Design and characterization, toxicity and biocompatibility, pharmaceutical and biomedical applications. Chemical Reviews. 2012;**112**(11):5818-5878

[74] Zhang Y, Wallace B. A sensitivity analysis of (and practitioners' guide to) convolutional neural networks for sentence classification. arXiv preprint arXiv:1510.03820. 2015;**14**

[75] Lammers T, Aime S, Hennink WE, Storm G, Kiessling F. Theranosticnanomedicine. Accounts of Chemical Research. 2011;**44**(10):1029-1038

[76] Doudna JA, Charpentier E. The new frontier of genome engineering with CRISPR-Cas9. Science. 2014;**346**(6213):1258096

[77] Sander JD, Joung JK. CRISPR-Cas systems for editing, regulating and targeting genomes. Nature Biotechnology. 2014;**32**(4):347-355

[78] June CH, O'Connor RS, Kawalekar OU, Ghassemi S, Milone MC. CAR T cell immunotherapy for human cancer. Science. 2018;**359**(6382):1361-1365

[79] Rosenberg SA, Yang JC, Sherry RM, Kammula US, Hughes MS, Phan GQ, et al. Durable complete responses in heavily pretreated patients with metastatic melanoma using T-cell transfer immunotherapy. Clinical Cancer Research. 2011;**17**(13):4550-4557

[80] Ponomarev AV. Electron-beam radiolysis of gaseous alkanes under circulation conditions: Gas-to-liquid transformation. Radiation Physics and Chemistry. 2009;**78**(1):48-56

[81] Jain SL. Malignant: How Cancer Becomes Us. London, England: University of California Press; 2013

[82] Kwon AT, Hoos HH, Ng R. Inference of transcriptional regulation relationships from gene expression data. In: Proceedings of the 2003 ACM Symposium on Applied Computing. Melbourne, Australia: Association for Computing Machinery (ACM) Digital Library; 2003. pp. 135-140

[83] Wang X, Shen Y, Wang S, Li S, Zhang W, Liu X, et al. PharmMapper 2017 update: A web server for potential drug target identification with a comprehensive target pharmacophore database. Nucleic Acids Research. 2017;**45**(W1):W356-W360

[84] Hu Q, Sun W, Wang C, Gu Z. Recent advances of cocktail chemotherapy by combination drug delivery systems. Advanced Drug Delivery Reviews. 2016;**98**:19-34

[85] Collins FS, Varmus H. A new initiative on precision medicine. New England Journal of Medicine. 2015;**372**(9):793-795

[86] Patnaik SS, Kotipalli R, Jerald MK, Muralidharan K. Combination treatment of recombinant growth differentiation factor-9 and Cetrorelix improves gestational origin of the polycystic ovarian syndrome in female rats. Life Sciences. 2023;**321**:121638

[87] Block KI, Gyllenhaal C, Lowe L, Amedei A, Amin AR, Amin A, et al. Designing a broad-spectrum integrative approach for cancer prevention and treatment. In: Seminars in Cancer Biology. Vol. 35. New York, USA: Academic Press; 2015. pp. S276-S304

[88] Salemme V, Centonze G, Avalle L, Natalini D, Piccolantonio A, Arina P, et al. The role of tumor microenvironment in drug resistance: Emerging technologies to unravel breast cancer heterogeneity. Frontiers in Oncology. 2023;**13**:1170264

[89] Brokowski C, Adli M. CRISPR ethics: Moral considerations for applications of a powerful tool. Journal of Molecular Biology. 2019;**431**(1):88-101

[90] Han HJ, Ekweremadu C, Patel N. Advanced drug delivery system with nanomaterials for personalised medicine to treat breast cancer. Journal of Drug Delivery Science and Technology. 2019;**52**:1051-1060

Section 5

Translational Immunology and Specialized Topics

Chapter 16

Understanding the Relationship between Bone-Remodeling T Cells and Microbiota in Breast Cancer Bone Metastases

Maria Eduarda Globa Masset, Fábio B. Canto and Ana Carolina Monteiro

Abstract

Breast cancer remains a major threat to women's health, with bone metastases affecting ~70% of patients with advanced disease. These metastases lead to skeletal-related events (SREs) that severely impact quality of life and survival. Although anti-resorptive therapies—such as bisphosphonates and the anti-RANKL antibody denosumab—reduce skeletal morbidity, they are not curative. A limited understanding of the molecular and risk factors driving breast cancer bone metastases impairs both prevention and treatment strategies. Patients with estrogen receptor-positive (ER^+) tumors typically receive adjuvant endocrine therapy—tamoxifen or aromatase inhibitors—to block estrogen-driven tumor growth. While effective in controlling disease, these therapies can accelerate bone loss in premenopausal women, promoting early-onset osteoporosis and increasing fracture risk. This raises the possibility that treatment-induced osteoporosis may create a favorable niche for tumor cell colonization and bone metastasis. Interestingly, ER^+ breast cancer is associated with a higher long-term incidence of bone metastases compared to triple-negative subtypes, possibly due to the combined effects of endocrine therapy and changes in bone microenvironment. Recent studies reveal that osteoporosis linked to sex steroid deficiency is microbiota dependent. Expansion of intestinal Th17 and TNF-α^+ $CD4^+$ T cells under estrogen deprivation migrates to bone marrow, disrupting bone remodeling. This chapter explores the hypothesis that estrogen deprivation may act as a risk factor for bone metastases, modulated by individual microbiota profiles. We also discuss how microbiota-dependent T cells may contribute to pre-metastatic niche formation in bone, linking cancer therapies, immune responses, and bone homeostasis.

Keywords: breast cancer, bone metastasis, microbiota, immunophenotypes, premetastatic niche

1. Introduction

Breast cancer stands as the most common malignancy among women, with rising incidence and notable mortality rates [1]. However, recent advancements in early tumor screening/diagnosis and adjuvant treatments have contributed to a decline in mortality due to metastatic disease [1]. The identification of molecular tumor subtypes, distinguished by the expression of estrogen receptor (ER), progesterone receptor (PR), and human epidermal growth factor receptor 2 (HER2), holds critical importance for prognosis and rationalizing therapy approaches [2]. Furthermore, the PAM50 classification delineates four additional molecular subtypes (luminal A, luminal B, HER2-enriched, and basal type) based on a 50-gene signature, with the majority categorized as basal type—frequently triple-negative breast tumors (TNBC)—characterized by aggressive metastatic phenotypes and high recurrence rates [3]. Despite significant strides in comprehending disease subtypes, the challenge persists in aligning patients' clinical attributes with molecular histological patterns and available therapeutic options, along with predicting metastatic outcomes [1].

Bone metastases affect around 70% of breast cancer patients with advanced disease and are linked to various skeletal complications, such as pain, pathological fractures, hypercalcemia, and spinal cord compression [4–7]. These complications often demand surgical interventions, radiotherapy for bone-related issues, and adjustments to antineoplastic therapy to manage bone pain [4–7]. Collectively, these adverse features are referred to as skeletal-related events (SREs) and negatively impact patients' quality of life and overall survival [5, 6, 8]. Despite significant progress in tumor detection and treatment, patients diagnosed with breast cancer-derived bone metastases now have a median survival time of 40 months [4]. Patients with PR^+ breast tumors were shown to have a relatively lower risk of developing bone metastases (45.9%), as compared to those with $HER2^+$ mammary neoplasia (>77.6%) [9]. Additionally, the risk of bone metastases escalates with positive node metastases (99.7%) and advancing disease stages, with patients in stage II (1.99 times), stage III (4.74 times), or stage IV (14.57 times) exhibiting higher risks compared to those in stage I [9]. Notably, patients with estrogen receptor-positive (ER+) tumors in advanced stages have a significantly higher incidence of bone metastases (>87%) compared to those with ER-negative (ER-) breast cancer (<56%) [10].

Despite the remarkable advances previously described, breast cancer-derived bone metastasis remains an incurable condition [4]. Currently, there is limited understanding of the molecular signatures and risk factors associated with the establishment of bone metastases, both of which are crucial for disease prevention and treatment effectiveness. Some known risk factors include molecular and histopathological tumor features, patient age, serum markers of bone resorption, lymph node status (greater than 4), large tumor size (>2 cm), and menopausal status [4]. Recent retrospective studies have further explored the correlation between various clinical-pathological parameters in breast cancer patients and the risk factors for bone metastases. Studies reveal that the combination of axillary lymph node metastases, elevated levels of cancer antigen 153 (CA153) exceeding 25.42 u/mL, alkaline phosphatase (ALP) greater than 100.5 u/mL, and reduced hemoglobin concentrations (<49 g/L) provide the highest accuracy in predicting the risk of bone metastases in breast cancer [11].

Bone metastases in breast cancer predominantly manifest as osteolytic lesions, characterized by extensive bone destruction. However, 15–20% of cases may exhibit an osteoblastic pattern, leading to dysregulated bone formation [4, 6, 12]. Common anatomical sites for bone metastases include the spine, ribs, pelvis, and sternum [11, 13].

In osteolytic lesions, which tend to be more aggressive and have been associated with a higher incidence of pathologic fractures, tumor colonization of the bone is a consequence of an imbalanced tissue remodeling [8, 14]. Under physiological condition, this process is regulated by mechanical forces of gravity, sex-steroid, parathyroid and thyroid hormones, calcitonin, calcitriol, insulin-like growth factor, cortisol and, mainly, by the RANK/RANKL/OPG molecular axis.

The RANK/RANKL/OPG circuitry is coordinated by a complex cellular network comprising (i) bone-resorbing osteoclasts (OCs), (ii) bone-forming osteoblasts (OBs), (iii) OB-derived mature osteocytes embedded in mineralized bone matrix and (iv) chondrocytes (**Figure 1**) [15]. Since chondrocytes have been essentially implicated in skeletal growth [REF], their role in bone homeostasis will not be further detailed in the current review. It has been well characterized that, from embryonic period to post-birth lifetime, OBs and osteocytes serve as the main sources of both OPG (the RANKL decoy receptor) and RANKL itself, which initiates bone remodeling [16–18]. The binding of RANKL to $RANK^+$ hematopoietic-derived OC precursors causes their differentiation into mature OCs that resorb bone [19]. At the end of this stage, OPG, the main counter-regulator of RANKL-driven osteoclastogenesis, inhibits bone resorption [20]. The mesenchymal-derived OBs then initiate the complex process of bone deposition—consisting of both production of inorganic matrix and cellular specialization—dependent on Wnt signaling, critical for their own function and survival [21]. In addition, osteocytes secrete sclerostin, which suppresses Wnt signaling and terminates this phase of the process (**Figure 1**) [22]. Estrogens also play crucial roles in the maintenance of bone homeostasis, by causing OB activation and differentiation, keeping a higher OPG to RANKL ratio and inhibiting OC activity [19].

Of note, it has recently been shown that bone remodeling is also regulated by other cellular and molecular components residing at, or migrating to, bone marrow (BM), such as lymphocytes, macrophages, and hematopoietic cells [23]. Notably, molecules that regulate breast tumor cell migration to the bone and primary mammary tumor overlap [24]. When bone remodeling becomes imbalanced under non-homeostatic conditions, metastatic tumor cells initiate excessive osteoclastogenesis and bone resorption. This process releases growth factors stored in the bone matrix, which subsequently promotes tumor growth. Consequently, a self-perpetuating cycle is established between the disrupted bone remodeling system and the malignant cells, fostering an environment conducive to tumor progression (**Figure 2**) [14].

The colonization of breast tumor cells is thought to be preceded by alterations in the target tissue, which establishes a favorable microenvironment for the formation of metastatic foci, commonly referred to as the pre-metastatic niche [25–27]. Currently, only a few studies have proposed how pre-metastatic niches arise in bone tissue [25]. For example, our group demonstrated that the development of spontaneous bone metastases from the 4 T1 triple-negative breast cancer (TNBC) in mice depends on the production of RANKL by tumor-primed $CD3^+$ T cells [28], as the adoptive transfer of these lymphocytes to nude recipients induced an osteolytic pre-metastatic disease even in the absence of tumor [28]. The suppression of RANKL expression in tumor-primed T cells successfully safeguarded mice against osteolytic disease and completely inhibited the onset of bone metastases [28]. These findings suggest that the tissue degradation facilitated by pre-metastatic T cells establishes a microenvironment conducive to the subsequent colonization of the bone cavity by metastatic clones (**Figure 3**) [28]. Recently, our studies explored the role of dendritic cells (DCs) in sustaining tumor-specific T cell activity, which drives the formation of pre-metastatic

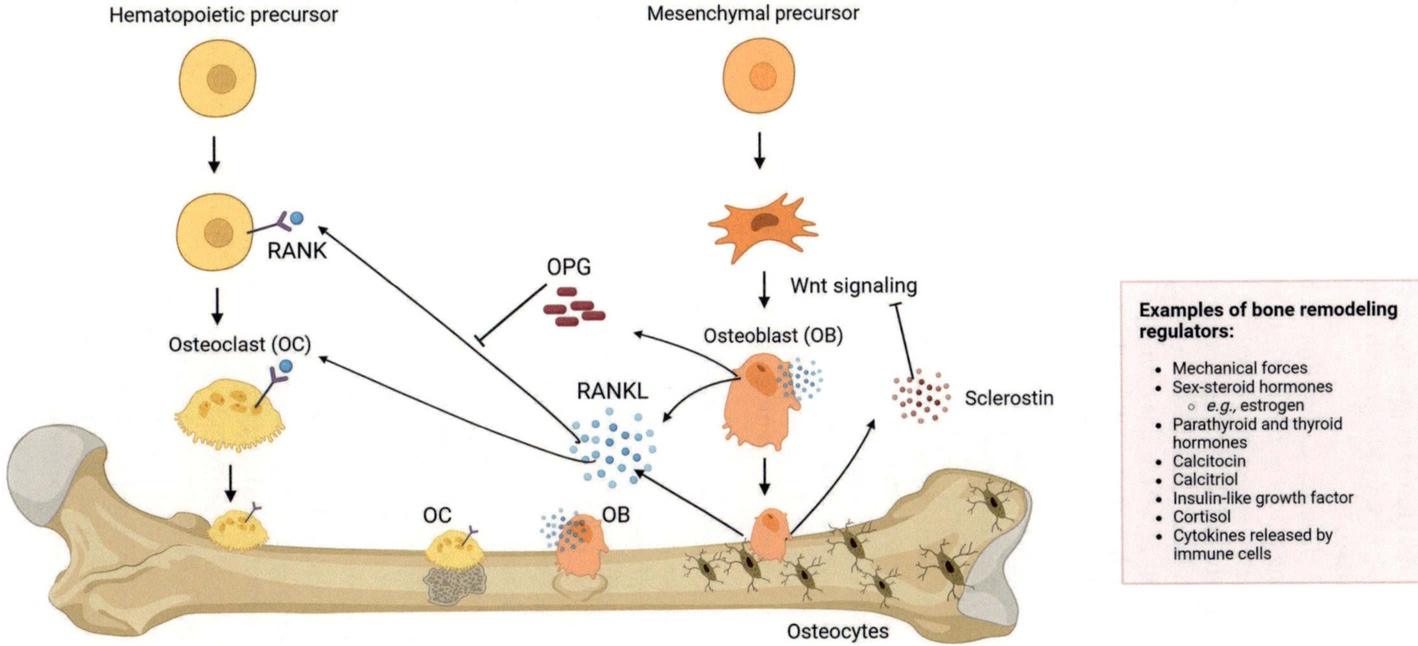

Figure 1.
RANK/RANKL/OPG molecular system. The RANK/RANKL/OPG molecular system is the major regulator of bone metabolism. Osteoclasts (OCs) derived from hematopoietic precursors act as bone-resorbing cells. Osteoblasts (OBs) are bone-forming cells derived from mesenchymal precursors. Osteocytes are mature OBs embedded in mineralized bone matrix. The interaction between RANK and RANKL stimulates osteoclastogenesis and osteoclastic activity. At this point, OPG, produced by both OBs and osteocytes, acts as a counter-regulator of osteoclastogenesis and bone resorption. Therewith, OBs initiate bone formation via *Wnt signaling that is critical for OB function and survival. Osteocytes, on the other hand, secrete sclerostin that suppresses Wnt signaling, terminating the process of bone remodeling.*

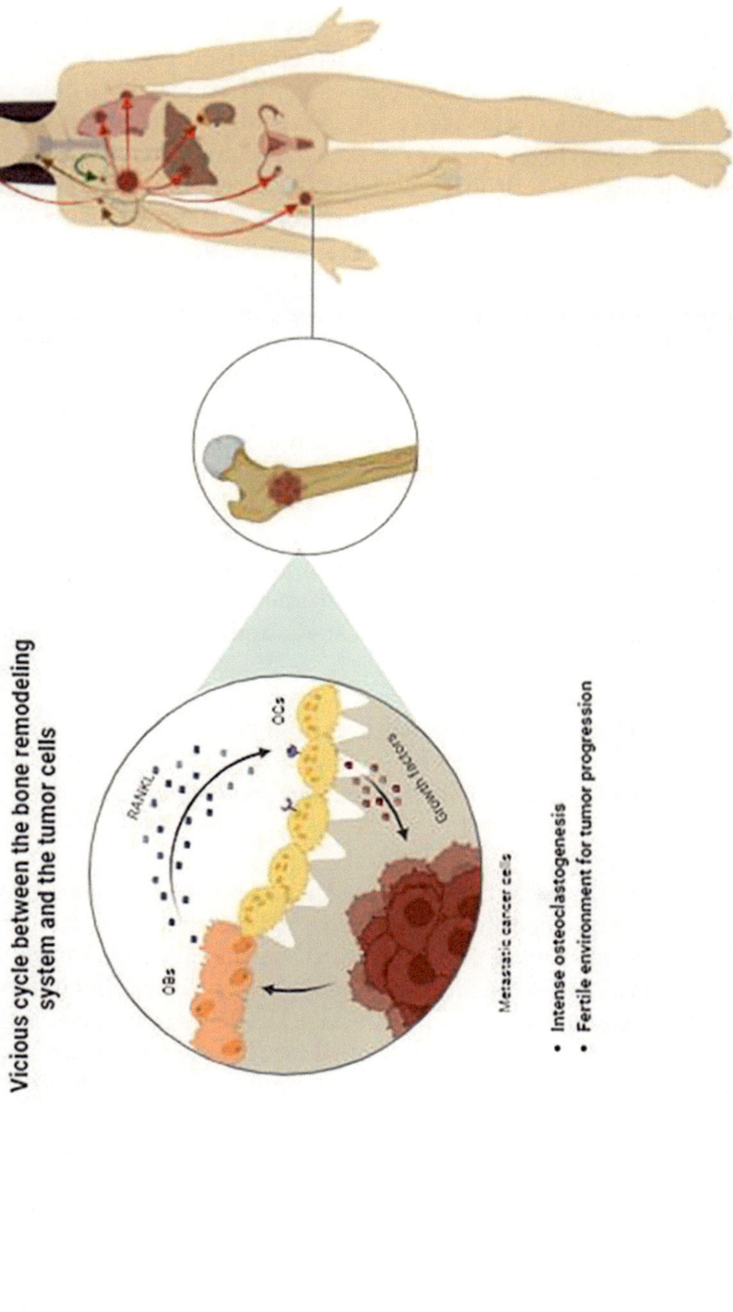

Figure 2.
Vicious cycle of bone metastasis. Upon disruption of the bone remodeling process under non-homeostatic conditions, metastatic cells stimulate intense osteoclastogenesis and bone consumption, resulting in the release of growth factors from bone matrix, which in turn feed the tumor and establishes a vicious cycle between the bone remodeling system and the tumor cells themselves, providing a fertile environment for cancer progression.

niches in the bone marrow (BM). Our findings revealed that DCs not only act as antigen-presenting cells (APCs) for 4 T1 tumor-specific T cells but also differentiate into osteoclast-like cells (DC-OC), thereby intensifying osteolytic processes prior to the colonization of the bone by tumor cells (**Figure 3**) [29]. Additionally, we discovered that 4 T1 tumor-reactive B cells are another source of RANKL and collaborate with T cells to establish the pre-metastatic niche environment in the bone [30]. Furthermore, our group recently found that *in situ* breast carcinoma can modify distant sites in a T-cell-driven manner, promoting physiological alterations in the bone [31]: IFN-γ- and IL-10-producing $CD8^+$ T lymphocytes previously primed by the non-metastatic 67NR tumor cell line (a sibling of 4 T1 tumor cells) effectively regulate the crosstalk between osteoclasts (OCs) and osteoblasts (OBs), contributing to both bone homeostasis, favoring bone deposition and, as a result, antagonizing pre-metastatic bone niche formation [31]. Taken together, our research highlights critical cellular and molecular immunological interactions underlying the development of these niches in breast cancer pre-metastatic bone niche formation [32]. However, many questions remain regarding the factors determining cell chemotaxis, the required antigens or ligands for T cells, and the modulating elements of the distal site.

Herein, we provide an overview of the knowledge concerning the direct and indirect effects of tissue-remodeling T cell immunophenotypes related to pre-metastatic niche formation in the bone [28–30, 32, 33], as well as those associated with osteoporosis (OP) [34–38] prior to breast cancer diagnosis and/or induced by treatment (**Figure 4**). Particularly, we hypothesize that interactions between gut and/or breast microbiomes and the immune system, which have been largely neglected in the context of tumor progression over the past years, may significantly impact the establishment of bone metastases. Understanding the roles of microbiota in modulating functions, expanding numbers and driving migration of tumor-specific bone-damaging or bone-protective T cells could be instrumental in predicting individuals at higher risk for the development of bone metastases and/or devising strategies for their prevention.

1.1 The state of the art on ER^+ breast cancer treatments

1.1.1 Bone loss induced by hormonal-ablative treatments or adjuvant endocrine therapy

The prognosis for women with breast cancer has significantly advanced in the recent decades, as a consequence of early detection and enhanced treatment options [1, 7]. Nonetheless, the persistence of breast cancer's recurrence and mortality are attributed to factors such as disease severity, tumor characteristics, and individual response [1, 7]. While patients diagnosed with stage I node-negative disease generally have a favorable outlook, those with stages II or III face heightened risks of recurrence. Treatment strategies encompass targeted therapies tailored to ER^+ or $HER2^+$ tumors, as well as broad-spectrum adjuvant chemotherapy for TNBC [1].

Women diagnosed with the ER^+ histological subtype may benefit from the adjuvant endocrine therapy (AET), comprising either tamoxifen—a selective antagonist that blocks estrogen binding to the ER+ breast tissue, usually indicated for pre-menopausal patients—or aromatase inhibitors (AIs), which are recommended when cancer is diagnosed after menopause due to their role in inactivating the rate-limiting enzyme responsible for converting androgens to estrogens in many tissues, including adipose tissue, ovary, breast, bone and brain [39]. In a series of randomized trials,

DOI: http://dx.doi.org/10.5772/intechopen.1010215

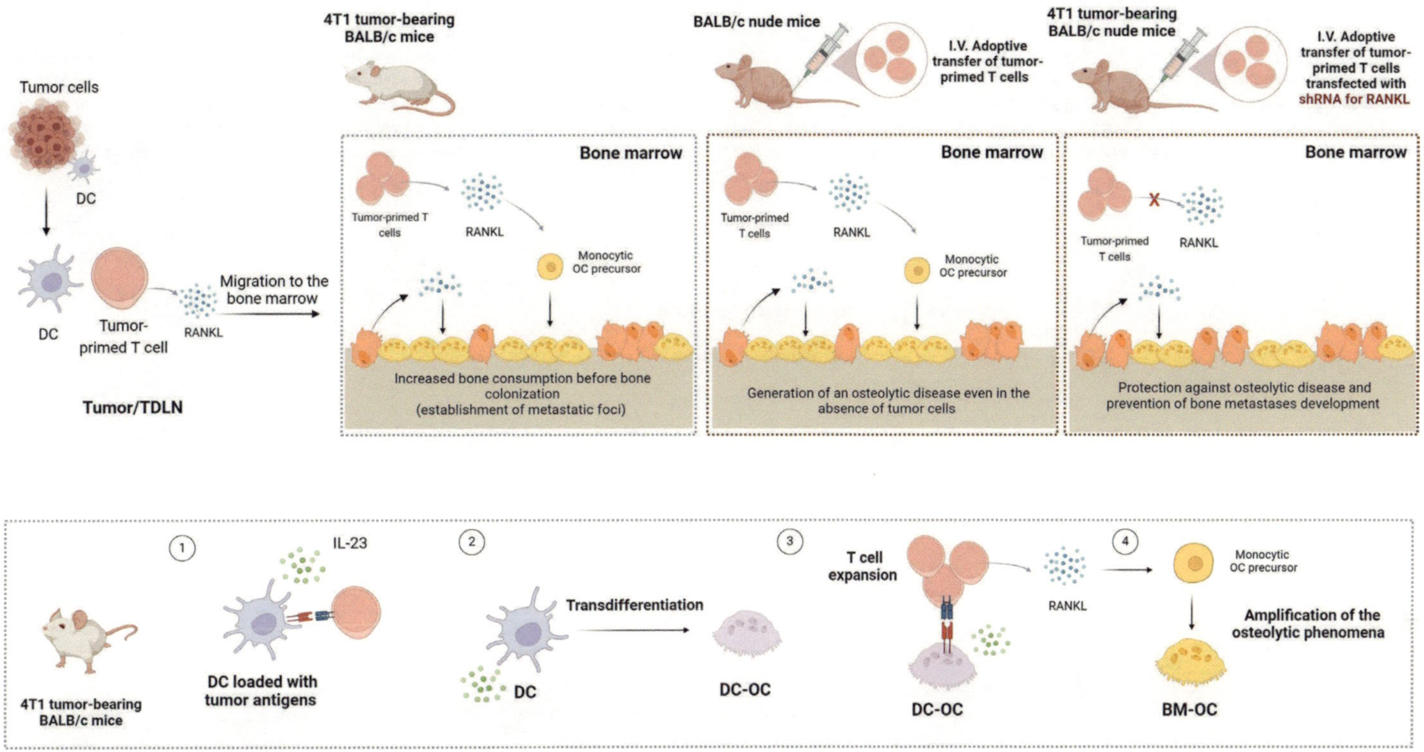

Figure 3.
T cells induce a pre-metastatic osteolytic disease that precedes and favors bone metastasis in the 4 T1 mice model of breast cancer. A. The development of bone metastases in 4 T1 triple negative breast cancer (TNBC) tumor model depends on RANKL production by tumor-primed $CD3^+$ T cells. When BALB/c nude mice are reconstituted with tumor-primed $CD3^+$ T cells, they develop an osteolytic disease, even in the absence of the primary tumor. BALB/c nude mice reconstituted with tumor-primed $CD3^+$ T cells develop an osteolytic disease even in the absence of the primary tumor, osteolytic disease is prevented, and the development of bone metastasis is abolished. B. (1) DCs loaded with tumor antigen derived from 4 T1 tumor-bearing mice produce IL-23 that maintains $RANKL^+$ T cells; (2) these DCs undergo trans-differentiation into DC-OCs; (3) DC-OCs contribute to the expansion of $RANKL^+$ T cells; (4) $RANKL^+$ T cells induce osteoclastogenesis, contributing to the amplification of the osteolytic phenomenon.

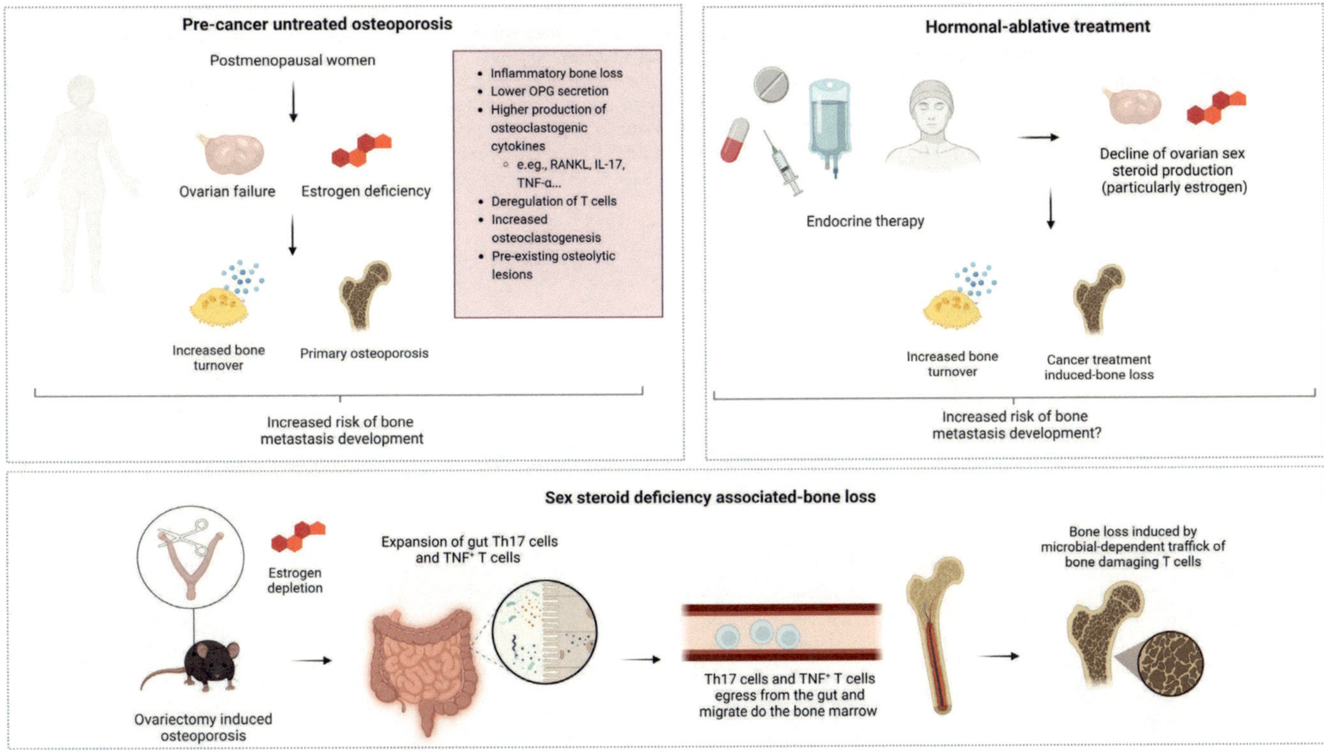

Figure 4.
Cancer therapy-induced bone loss in hormonal-ablative treatments. (A) Untreated pre-cancer osteoporosis: A decrease in bone mass density may enhance the risk for developing bone metastases. In the absence of a bone-protective intervention, a high bone turnover state increases the development of bone metastases. (B) Osteoporosis-induced cancer treatment: Endocrine therapies, based on the administration of aromatase inhibitors and tamoxifen, induce bone turnover and accelerate bone loss in premenopausal women. Therefore, endocrine therapy is associated with osteoporosis and muscle weakness, and, in some scenarios, likely to accelerate the progression of bone metastases. (C) Microbial-dependent bone loss in hormonal-ablative model of osteoporosis: Ovariectomy-induced osteoporosis generates the expansion of intestinal Th17 and T TNF-α^+ *$CD4^+$* T cells that migrate to the bone marrow in a microbial-dependent manner and promote inflammatory bone loss.*

both AIs and tamoxifen have shown significant enhancements in disease-free and overall survival rates [40, 41]. However, breast cancer survivors after under AET are at an increased risk for developing low bone mass density and OP [40–47], and can occur either as a direct consequence of the dysregulation in osteoblast (OB) and/or osteoclast (OC) differentiation and activity or indirectly, through conditions such as chronic renal disorders, onset of hypogonadism, and electrolyte imbalances [48]. Other mechanisms include pro-apoptotic effects on OBs and osteocytes, accelerated differentiation of bone marrow stromal cells into adipocytes, as well as the impacts of radiotherapy, glucocorticoids, and tyrosine kinase inhibitors [48]. Additionally, premenopausal women diagnosed with breast cancer and undergoing AET may experience amenorrhea, which manifests as ovarian failure and reduced estrogen levels [49]. This condition can exacerbate bone resorption and loss [1, 7], often requiring drug cessation [42, 45, 50–56]. Consequently, the progressive decrease in bone mineral density associated with increased OC activity and OP development *per se* may provide a fertile soil for cancer growth and have been related to the successful settlement of bone metastases [39, 40, 43, 49, 57–60].

1.2 Treatments of bone metastases: Anti-resorptive or bone-protective drugs

Treatment options for bone metastases are available and customized for each patient, often involving multiple therapeutic approaches [61]. Currently, the clinical management of bone metastases in ER+ breast cancer typically includes AET in combination with anti-resorptive or bone-protective agents [62], such as bisphosphonates or denosumab, a monoclonal antibody targeting RANKL [63, 64]. Bisphosphonates, analogs of the inorganic pyrophosphate that is a primary component of bone mineral matrix, exert their action by chelating calcium and selectively targeting the skeleton. They function by inhibiting the activity of osteoclasts, thus reducing bone resorption [65]. In addition, denosumab also negatively regulates bone resorption by blocking the binding of RANKL to $RANK^{+}$ OCs, thereby impeding their differentiation, activation, and function [63].

The use of bone-protecting drugs is clinically important in multiple aspects, including the prevention of both OP induced by cancer treatment and bone metastases, besides improvement of overall survival, particularly as breast cancer evolves to a more chronic disease state [1]. Despite bone protection activity, it was recently shown that the prolonged suppression of bone remodeling can have both beneficial and detrimental effects [66, 67], as patients with minimally invasive bone metastases respond well to high cumulative dosage of anti-resorptive drugs, whereas those with more advanced disease seem to develop resistance to such agents [4, 43, 68]. Furthermore, once bone mass is lost due to metastatic colonization, its restoration with bone-protecting drugs becomes challenging. This difficulty arises because almost all anti-resorptive therapies are accompanied by a concurrent decrease in bone formation, resulting in the suppression of overall bone turnover [69].

For more than two decades, several pre-clinical and clinical studies have shown that the adjuvant use of bisphosphonates, such as clodronate [70], alendronate [71], other bisphosphonates, and zoledronic acid (a third generation of nitrogen-containing bisphosphonate) [72–82], have been shown to lower recurrence rates and mortality in breast cancer patients. These agents also effectively reduce both the incidence and the number of bone metastases arising from breast cancer [72–82]. While adjuvant bisphosphonates have shown efficacy in postmenopausal women with non-metastatic breast cancer [83, 84], their effects in premenopausal women, particularly younger individuals, remain uncertain. Some studies suggest that, although the risk of bone metastases may decrease, there could be an increased dissemination of the disease to other organs, resulting in no significant overall benefit [85, 86]. The lack of efficacy of anti-resorptive drugs in premenopausal or perimenopausal patients has yet to be fully understood, emphasizing the need for preclinical research to explore innovative treatment strategies [61].

In early-stage breast cancer, the application of bisphosphonates as part of adjuvant therapy has yielded inconsistent outcomes [50, 61, 86]. Clinical evidence includes findings where zoledronic acid demonstrated an improvement in disease-free survival for premenopausal patients diagnosed with early ER+ breast cancer [73, 87]. Although many studies reported a decrease in the incidence of bone metastases, the impact of bisphosphonates on overall disease recurrence and breast cancer-related mortality has varied, with observed benefits being limited to specific patient groups or subpopulations identified through subgroup analyses [61, 88, 89]. Finally, some preclinical and clinical studies conducted in breast cancer patients with bone metastases showed that denosumab was superior to zoledronic acid in inhibiting bone resorption and development of SREs, but neither improved patients' clinical outcomes nor altered progression of bone metastases and overall survival [68, 85, 90, 91].

As already mentioned, cancer treatment-induced bone loss may provide a fertile soil for ectopic tumor growth and has been related to the development of osteometastases [39, 40, 49, 57, 58]. However, although some data suggest that pre-cancer OP does not increase the risk of bone metastases, untreated OP has been associated with accelerated progression of bone colonization by tumor cells [39, 57]. In other words, breast cancer patients with pre-cancer treated OP developed bone metastases at a similar pace as those without pre-cancer OP. Nevertheless, women who had never undergone anti-resorptive drug therapy prior to breast cancer diagnosis tended to develop tumor-related bone lesions at a faster rate [57, 71]. Furthermore, the administration of bisphosphonates before the diagnosis of breast cancer, followed by cessation at diagnosis, was linked to a rise in the incidence of bone metastases. In contrast, the administration of bisphosphonates either prior to and following a breast cancer diagnosis, or exclusively post-diagnosis, has been linked to a reduction in the incidence of bone metastases [71, 92]. Hence, it is reasonable to speculate that untreated OP could be linked to the accelerated development of secondary bone lesions, while treated cases might only delay tumor invasion rather than prevent it entirely [43, 68, 71, 86, 93].

2. Pre- and post-osteoporosis in breast cancer disease

Osteoporosis (OP)—a common age-related condition defined by the loss of bone mass and microarchitecture—often results in fractures associated with high socioeconomic burden [94]. OP is particularly worrisome for women with breast cancer, affecting them from diagnosis through treatment to survivorship [94]. The condition has a multifaceted etiology, with primary contributors including endocrine factors such as hyperparathyroidism, vitamin D deficiency, and menopause [94]. The primary driver of OP is the cessation of ovarian function, as declining estrogen levels accelerate bone resorption, resulting in rapid tissue loss [94]. Additionally, both genetic and non-genetic factors exacerbate the detrimental effects of estrogen deficiency on bone health [94]. On a cellular level, the absence of sex steroids promotes bone loss, predominantly by increasing OC formation and extending their lifespan [95].

Both bone and breast tissues are influenced by estrogen, with systemic availability of this hormone identified as a significant risk factor for breast cancer, particularly in women diagnosed with the ER+ histological subtype [96]. Interestingly, surrogate markers for OP often exhibit an inverse correlation with those associated with breast cancer risk [97]. Notably, numerous studies have highlighted a positive association between high bone mineral density and an elevated risk of developing breast cancer [97]. On the other hand, endocrine therapy is associated with OP and muscle weakness and, in some scenarios, likely to accelerate the progression of bone metastases [98]. These observations imply that heightened bone turnover may facilitate the onset of skeletal metastases in the early stages of the disease, potentially occurring even before the dissemination and establishment of tumor cells in the BM [39]. Nevertheless, especially in postmenopausal women with no OP at the moment of breast cancer diagnosis, the AET impact on the risk of fracture and development of bone metastases is still questionable [39]. It is also worth mentioning that the AEP bone impact might be more problematic in younger premenopausal women, but the extent to which this treatment accelerates bone metastases is a matter of study (**Figure 4**) [39].

Therefore, a gap is yet to be crossed over after the analysis of the complex relationship among breast cancer molecular subtypes, estrogen levels, adjuvant therapies, OP status, and the risk of developing bone metastases. Recently, it has been shown that sex steroid deficiency-associated bone loss is microbiota-dependent, alongside the intestinal expansion of bone-damaging $CD4^+$ T cell subtypes, such as Th17 and TNF-α^+ cells, which in turn migrate to BM and disturb the homeostasis of bone remodeling [99]. However, the relationship between pre-cancer OP or cancer treatment-induced OP, which are both influenced by steroidal hormone levels, and the microbiota profile, which might influence the development of bone-damaging $CD4^+$ T cell phenotypes, is currently unknown (**Figure 4**).

3. Microbiota-induced modulation of bone-damaging T cells in osteoporosis

The human body's surface is inhabited by trillions of bacteria, fungi, and viruses, collectively forming a diverse ecosystem referred to as the commensal microbiota [100]. The gastrointestinal tract, being the largest surface area of the human body, houses the most extensive and varied population of these microorganisms that are known to exert numerous beneficial effects on health [100]. For instance, gut microbiota has been shown to mediate the generation of immunomodulatory factors that regulate local and distal physiological processes, ranging from intestinal inflammatory and tolerogenic responses, epithelial cytoprotection, and enteric barrier integrity to bone homeostasis [101, 102]. Apart from the gut, other anatomical sites harbor sets of specialized microbiota communities that seem to locally modulate several cellular activities in skin [103], lung [104], and uterus [105], and even in bone and breast [106]. Indeed, research has shown that germ-free mice exhibit increased bone mass, accompanied by a reduction in $CD4^+$ T cells and osteoclast precursors within the BM, as well as decreased levels of osteoclastogenic cytokines [107]. Furthermore, administering antibiotics to conventional mice has been found to enhance bone density in young subjects [99], whereas specific probiotics mitigate the bone loss typically observed following ovariectomy [99].

It is now clear that gut microbiota, mainly by influencing the balance between pro- and anti-inflammatory immunocytes, impacts both local and extra-enteric immune responses [102]. Indeed, the microbiota-driven intestinal CD4$^+$Foxp3$^+$ regulatory T cells (Treg), which secrete the immunomodulatory cytokines IL-10 and TGF-β, play locally indispensable roles in mediating tolerance toward beneficial commensals and fine-tuning gut microbiota composition, while suppress osteoclastogenesis and bone resorption at a distal site [37, 108]. On the contrary, gut-resident CD4$^+$Rorγt$^+$ Th17 T cells, which are largely induced in a microbiota- and IL-6-driven manner, secrete the pro-inflammatory mediators IL-17A and TNF-α that mediate *in situ* immunity to antigenic challenges. These immune challenges not only influence local responses but also upregulate RANKL expression on OBs and BM stromal cells, thereby facilitating OC-mediated bone resorption. The delicate equilibrium between Tregs and Th17 cells plays a pivotal role in modulating bone loss observed in OP [37, 99, 109–110].

Importantly, estrogen deficiency may lead to the reduction of some species of bacteria that affect the balance between immune pro- and anti-inflammatory cells, such as Th17 and Treg cells, resulting in increased bone loss [37, 99]. Furthermore, estrogen deficiency has the capacity to promote the differentiation and survival of regulatory T cells (Tregs), which effectively suppresses the production of pro-inflammatory cytokines by Th17 cells, thereby mitigating bone resorption [111]. Consequently, bone loss associated with a deficiency in estrogen may stem from disruptions in a complex network of hormones and cytokines that regulate the bone remodeling process. Of note, estrogen deficiency also promotes, by increasing the levels of the lymphopoietic cytokine IL-7, B cell lymphopoiesis, which has been implicated in intense bone loss [112]. Moreover, it has been reported that RANKL is also expressed by B lymphocytes, and RANKL depletion specifically from B cells led to protection of bone loss after ovariectomy [112]. Altogether, these changes in T and B cell compartments, presumably driven by the dysbiosis resulting from drastic estrogen decay, can severely impact the bone homeostasis.

Recent findings indicate that a deficiency in sex steroids enhances intestinal permeability, enabling gut microbiota to activate and promote the expansion of Th17 and CD4$^+$TNF-α$^+$ T cells [99]. These activated effector lymphocytes, which possess bone-destructive potential, exhibit upregulated expression of S1PR1 (sphingosine-1-phosphate receptor 1), facilitating their migration from the intestine to the bone marrow *via* CXCR3- and CCL20-mediated chemoattraction [37, 99]. Additionally, probiotic interventions have demonstrated efficacy in mitigating bone loss associated with steroid deficiency [37, 99]. In this regard, studies reveal that that *Lactobacillus species* mitigate intestinal inflammation and enhance barrier integrity [113]. Additionally, *Lactobacillus rhamnosus* supplementation has been shown to improve bone density in eugonadal mice [37, 110, 114], suppress osteoclastogenesis, and regulate the balance between Th17 and Treg cells under both *in vitro* and *in vivo* conditions [37, 110]. Collectively, these insights underscore the osteoprotective potential of probiotics, paving the way for innovative strategies in addressing postmenopausal OP and pre-metastatic osteolytic disease.

4. Can we establish a correlation between breast and/or gut microbiota and the development of tumor-specific bone-damaging T cells associated with breast tumor bone metastases establishment?

The colonization of mucosal tissues by microbiota is well-documented to occur shortly after birth, undergoing subsequent diversification influenced by dietary habits and environmental exposures over the course of life [100, 102]. The gut microbiota plays a pivotal role in the modulation of the immune system by interacting directly or indirectly with immune cells, thus influencing their responses throughout the body [100, 102]. More recently, gut microbiota has been implicated in the regulation of bone homeostasis, impacting tissular processes such as hematopoiesis, hematopoietic stem cell function, bone mass and growth (*via* insulin-like growth factor 1), alveolar bone dynamics, and skeletal maturation [107, 110, 115–122]. Furthermore, quantitively and/or qualitatively disturbances in gut microbial composition, known as dysbiosis, have been associated with increased risk of developing malignant diseases, including breast cancer [123–128], affecting responses to adjuvant chemotherapy drugs [125, 129–133] and establishing inflammatory chronic conditions related to impaired bone mass and quality [134–138].

The potential mechanisms linking the microbiome and breast cancer encompass estrogen metabolism, susceptibility to obesity, menopause status, and tumor-triggered immune modulation [139, 140]. Regarding the microbiome's impact on sex steroid hormones, it is widely recognized that gut bacteria secrete β-glucuronidase, which deconjugates estrogen, activating it for biological effects [141, 142]. Notably, these bacteria influence the enterohepatic circulation of estrogens and their reabsorption, potentially heightening the risk of estrogen receptor-positive (ER^+) breast cancer development and maintenance [141, 143, 144]. Interestingly, 14 microbial markers linked to various menopausal statuses of breast cancer have been recently identified [145]. *Bacteroides fragilis*, a beneficial commensal largely associated with immunoregulatory effects through the promotion of gut Treg cell function and differentiation in mouse models [146], was specifically detected in young premenopausal women, suggesting a more favorable prognosis for ER^+ breast cancer, whereas *Klebsiella pneumoniae* was identified in older postmenopausal women, indicating a poorer prognosis for ER^+ breast cancer [145]. These differences between premenopausal and postmenopausal breast cancer patients emphasize the significance of menopausal-specific microbial markers for diagnosis and research. This may provide a noninvasive approach to predict breast cancer progression and introduces a fresh tool for its prevention [145].

A recent investigation has identified alterations in the gut microbiome among individuals who develop bone metastases from breast tumors compared to those with non-invasive breast carcinoma or healthy individuals [147]. Particularly, microbiota members promoting steroid hormone biosynthesis were significantly upregulated in the bone metastases group [147]. Indeed, elevated levels of sex steroids have long been associated with increased risk for breast cancer, with subjects in the highest quintile having nearly double the risk compared to those in the lowest quintile [148]. However, as previously stated, the decrease in estrogen levels leads to the establishment of OP in postmenopausal woman and those undergoing cancer treatment, thereby creating a conducive environment for tumor progression in the bone. Therefore, further investigations are required to assess the link between this bacterial-driven metabolic activity and estrogen levels for the establishment of bone metastases. Additionally, the same study demonstrated a significant decrease in the diversity of alpha-protective gut microrganisms across the groups, with the most pronounced disruption—affecting *Megamonas* and *Akkermansia muciniphila*—observed in patients who developed bone metastases [147]. These bacteria produce butyrate and propionate, respectively, which are short-chain fatty acids (SCFAs) that mitigate ovariectomy-induced bone loss by reducing OC numbers and the levels of serum c-terminal crosslinking telopeptide of type I collagen (CTX-I) [115, 118, 119]. Concurrently, *A. muciniphila* has been linked to decreased gut permeability and inflammation during the initial phases of fracture healing in a mouse model, favoring the restoration of bone mass [122], and attenuated bone degradation resulting from inflammation induced by *Porphyromonas gingivalis* [138]. Taken together, these results suggest that potential interventions, by probiotics and/or target-specific antibiotics alongside conventional treatments, may delay or prevent bone loss, thereby mitigating breast cancer progression to the bone. However, several unanswered questions persist regarding the mechanisms by which the gut microbiota might influence breast cancer bone metastases and the predictive value of their signature [147].

Although traditionally viewed as sterile, the breast tissue in the steady-state was recently shown to be colonized by a diverse community of bacteria, which significantly influences local immune responses [128, 149, 150]. As in the gut, dysbiosis of the mammary microbiota has been attributed to play a role in the induction of breast carcinogenesis and tumor dissemination [149, 151]. Variations in its composition and functions are emerging among the distinct histological subtypes of breast cancer [123, 149, 151, 152], while ongoing studies are investigating the potential of mammary microbiota as a biomarker for breast cancer and therapeutic responses [152, 153]. Particularly, the total bacterial DNA load was reported to be lower both in the tumor mass compared to healthy tissue in cases of advanced-stage breast cancer and in early-stage breast cancer compared to healthy tissue [125, 154]. Despite the tumor-confined reduction in microbial biomass, the breast affected by tumors shows even greater microbial diversity and richness than its healthy counterpart [154]. Remarkably, this mammary microbiota was shown to be viable and significantly influence tumor cell behavior, particularly by shaping migratory characteristics towards metastatic sites [154]. Considered collectively, these findings highlight that breast and/or gut local dysbiosis may create an environment favorable to breast tumor carcinogenesis and/or to the tumor-driven selection of microorganisms adapted to such specific microenvironments [124]. Therefore, given that the microbiota and its metabolites are increasingly recognized as potential risk factors for breast cancer development and progression, therapeutic and clinical approaches targeting the microbiota are ongoing.

Multiple studies have demonstrated that the immunophenotypic composition of the primary tumor microenvironment (TME), encompassing both innate and adaptive immune cells, differs across molecular and histological subtypes of breast tumors [155]. These cells are regarded as prognostic factors for survival [156] and predictive indicators of therapy response [156] and in some cases, despite being pro-tumorigenic, can either promote or inhibit the formation of pre-metastatic niches in the lungs [157] and bone [28, 30]. More recently, the interplay between the microbiota and immune cells in breast cancer has emerged as a topic of considerable interest and research [151]. Pre-clinical and clinical evidence suggest that specific microbial taxa can influence the immune landscape within the breast tumor microenvironment, such as tumor infiltration by leukocytes, antitumor immunity, and response to therapy, thereby impacting disease progression and treatment outcomes [158–161]. Of note, the microbiome regulates anticancer immunity through direct contact with immune cells, or *via* metabolites, as reported in mouse experiments [158]. Experiments using the orthotopic 4 T1 BALB/c mouse breast carcinoma demonstrated that tumor colonization by *Fusobacterium nucleatum* fosters tumorigenesis and diminishes $CD4^+$ and $CD8^+$ T cell infiltration, leading to larger lung metastases compared to control mice [162, 163]. Additionally, *F. nucleatum* DNA has been also detected in human breast cancer tissue [164]. Thus, understanding the mechanisms by which different bacterial species boost tumor progression and metastatic spread through immune tumor landscape modulation is likely to be significant not just for the diagnosis, prognosis, and treatment of breast cancer, but also for a range of other cancer types.

Besides their role in bone loss, Th17 cells also exhibit pro-tumoral effects. Tumors secrete several factors associated with the recruitment, induction, and expansion of Th17 cells [165]. The infiltration of Th17 cells into human tumors has been reported in various conditions, including melanoma, lymphomas and breast, ovarian, pancreatic, prostate, and gastric and colon cancers [166–170]. Tumor cells and tumor-associated fibroblasts produce molecules such as monocyte chemoattractant protein-1 (MCP-1) and regulated on activation, normal T-cell expressed and secreted (RANTES) that strongly attract migrating Th17 cells [166]. Additionally, a tumor microenvironment (TME) enriched in IL-1β, IL-6, IL-23, and TGF-β creates a suitable milieu for the differentiation and expansion of Th17 cells [165].

Due to the phenotypic plasticity of Th17 cells and the vast heterogeneity of neoplasms, these cells can exhibit either protective or pathogenic roles [171]. Regarding their pathogenic properties, Th17 cells are involved in inflammatory and immunosuppressive mechanisms within tumors. Th17 cells produce IL-17, which induces the expression of pro-angiogenic factors such as vascular endothelial growth factor (VEGF), nitric oxide (NO), and prostaglandin E2 (PGE2). They also promote the expression of membrane-associated metalloproteinases (MMPs), which are essential for the effective migration of malignant cells [172, 173]. Moreover, cytokines secreted by Th17 cells activate oncogenic signaling pathways in tumor cells, particularly *via* the IL-6/STAT3 axis [174, 175]. Th17 cells also promote the recruitment of pro-tumorigenic suppressive myeloid cells, amplifying cancer-promoting effects [176, 177]. Collectively, these components underscore the contribution of Th17 cells to the progression of primary tumors and metastases.

In breast cancer (BC), the presence of intratumoral IL-17-producing cells, assessed *via* immunohistochemistry, correlates with unfavorable clinical outcomes, with similar findings reported in other solid tumors [165, 166]. A clinical study demonstrated that Th17 cell infiltration decreases gradually as disease progresses, while Treg cells accumulate [167]. Interestingly, in tumor biopsies from patients with invasive ductal carcinoma (IDC), both Th17 and Treg cells were elevated compared to healthy individuals. In these IDC patients, a significant positive correlation has been identified between the expression levels of Foxp3, IL-17A, and RAR-related orphan receptor gamma (RORc) [168]. These findings underscore the critical need to further explore the Th17/Treg axis within this specific context [168].

The peripheral differentiation of both Treg and Th17 cells requires signaling by the cytokine TGF-β [165–169] whose production and function were shown to be under control by the gut microbiota [170–173]. In this scenario, the levels of IL-6, reported to be decisively influenced by the microbiota [174–180], are central to define whether a conventional $CD4^+$ T cell clone will differentiate towards the Treg or Th17 fate [181–184]. In addition, it is now widely known that Treg cells may be converted to the Th17 profile under inflammatory settings [185–188]. However, it is not known whether, besides imposing an immunosuppressive milieu unfavorable to anti-tumoral immunity [189–193], Treg cells within the tumor microenvironment act as precursors of Th17 lymphocytes that, under the influence of tumoral-derived signals, may be functionally deviated towards pro-tumorigenic and/or pro-metatastic players. Particularly, individuals with different malignancies have poor survival outcomes and disease progression that correlate with elevated intratumoral Treg cell numbers [194, 195]. Not surprisingly, immunotherapeutic strategies aiming to inhibit suppressive Treg cell activity through blockade of cytotoxic T-lymphocyte associated protein 4 (CTLA-4-) and/or programmed cell death ligand 1 (PDL-1-related) immune checkpoints have been successful in antagonizing both Treg- and Th17-dependent programs while promoting Th1/IFN-γ-mediated immunoreactivity against tumors [196–203]. Interestingly, it has been extensively reported that effective antitumoral response induced by immune checkpoint blockade is experimentally hampered by microbiota depletion [130, 196, 204–208]. Therefore, uncovering the contribution of local and distal microbiota communities for the emergence of pro- and anti-tumoral T cell phenotypes is currently urgent.

A cross-sectional clinical research showed that patients diagnosed with different breast cancer molecular subtypes had increased plasmatic levels of MIF and Th17-related cytokines when compared to healthy women, as macrophage migration inhibitory factor (MIF) has been described as molecule that favors the polarization of activated T cells towards a Th17 phenotype [169]. In agreement, in orthotopic syngeneic tumor mice models 4 T1 and E0771, increased levels of Th17 cells can be observed within tumors during the progression of the disease [170]. In the 4 T1 model, Th17 cells are associated with tumor growth, angiogenesis, and neutrophil recruitment [171, 172]. Additionally, in polyoma middle T (PyMT)-induced breast tumors, an increased level of Th17 cells in the tumor tissue correlates with increased pro-tumorigenic properties of myeloid-derived suppressor cells and monocytes [173]. In human breast cancer cell lines, IL-17 also induces chemoresistance *via* activation or ERK1/2 pathway [174]. With regard to the microbiome, it has been proposed that intestinal microbiota-propelled Th17 cells play an important role in immune-mediated inflammatory diseases and in tumors [175]. However, the relevance of tumor-resident microbiota for Th17 cell development, maintenance, and/or impact on cancer progression remains unknown. Therefore, further investigations are necessary to elucidate the relationship between local and gut microbiome, Th17-Treg axis, and tumor progression.

Recently, an interesting piece of research has unveiled the presence of microbiota within the primary or secondary human bone tumors, with its metabolic activities closely linked to the release of molecules embedded in bone matrix during resorption [106]. In simple terms, we believe that the process of bone degradation could release factors that facilitate the growth cycle of specific bacteria within the tumor microenvironment. Establishing a causal relationship between the microbiota and bone degradation remains challenging. It is unclear whether the microbiota colonizes the bone and promotes tissue degradation or whether bone degradation *per se* facilitates the establishment of the microbiota. From this perspective, the presence of T and B cells in BM suggests that the migration and colonization of tumor cells might also be influenced not only by bone-damaging pro-osteoclastogenic Th17 cells (and consequently, gut dysbiosis) but also by SCFAs or the microbiota associated with bone metabolism (**Figure 5**).

DOI: http://dx.doi.org/10.5772/intechopen.1010215

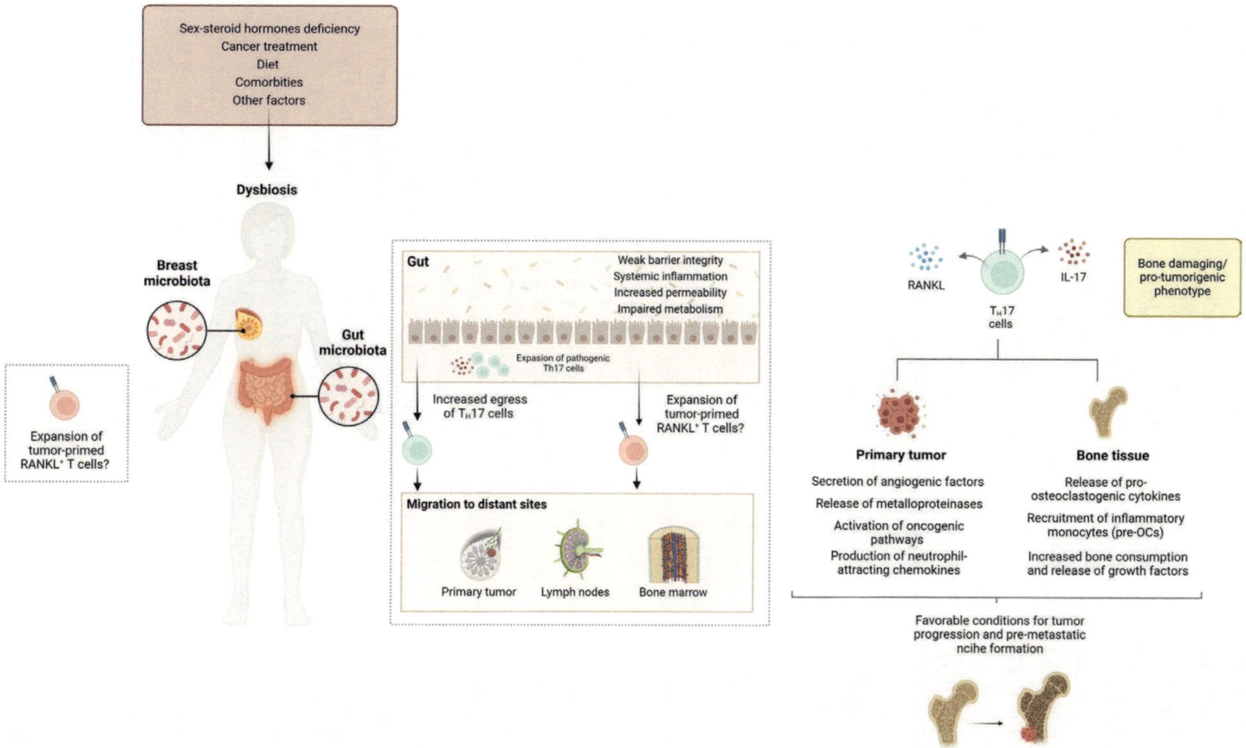

Figure 5.
The possible relationship between microbiota-driven bone-damaging T cells and breast cancer bone metastases. Several factors including sex-steroid hormone deficiency, cancer treatments, and comorbidities may contribute to the generation of dysbiosis in the breast and gut microbiota. The dysbiotic gut microbiota induces the expansion and egress of Th17 cells to distal tissues. Currently, it is already known that intestinal Th17 cells migrate to the bone marrow in experimental primary osteoporosis; whether these cells reach the primary tumor, lymph nodes, and the bone marrow in the context of mammary tumors require further investigation. Besides having catabolic effects on the bone tissue, Th17 cells also exhibit pro-tumorigenic effects such as the production of pro-angiogenic factors, metalloproteinases, molecules associated with activation of oncogenic signaling pathways, and chemokines that can attract immunosuppressive cells, for example, tumor-associated neutrophils. Altogether, the association of bone-damaging and pro-tumoral outcomes, with the activity of pathogenic Th17 cells, could induce bone consumption prior to tumor metastatic colonization, generating a rich microenvironment that license further colonization of the bone cavity by the metastatic tumor clones.

5. Conclusion

A question that remains to be answered is whether bone loss associated with estrogen deficiency, pre-existing or induced by cancer treatment, promotes or influences tumor cells homing and growth in bone, since osteometastases show a close relationship with sex hormones. Moreover, and based on all aspects that have been discussed, we are currently investigating if breast and/or intestinal microbiota control the pro- and anti-breast tumor-specific T cell phenotypes associated with bone metastases (**Figure 5**). Since some pre-clinical and clinical evidences have pointed out that an intense osteoclastic activity may enhance the risk for developing bone metastases perhaps prior to the establishment of disseminated tumor cells in the bone marrow [39, 57], it seems plausible to think that there may be a bridge between microbiota profile and the activation/expansion of bone-specific pro-osteolytic and pre−/anti-metastatic immunophenotypes (**Figure 5**). We are also suggesting that treatment with probiotics, by reducing gut permeability, adsorption of tumor antigens into the circulation, damping mammary gland, and modulating T cell phenotypes, could clear up mammary gland, gut and bone marrow inflammation, and, consequently, bone loss. Blunting the development of inflammation by using probiotics could be a simple complement to pharmacological regimens.

Herein, we provide a mechanistic hypothesis connecting bone-damaging T cells (associated with gut and/or mammary gland microbiota dysbiosis) with increased risk for bone metastases development (**Figure 5**). We postulate that triple-negative breast tumor (TNBC) microenvironment, associated with mammary gland microbiota profile, stimulate the priming of tumor-specific bone-damaging $CD3^+$ T cells expressing RANKL. The priming of these tumor-specific bone-damaging T cells may also be influenced by mammary gland and/or gut microbiota dysbiosis due to the deficiency of steroidal sex hormones associated with conventional OP or that associated with cancer-induced treatment, obesity, diet, or other comorbities. The migration of tumor-specific bone-damaging T cells to the BM, occurring before metastatic tumor colonization, drives intense bone degradation and establishes a favorable microenvironment that facilitates subsequent colonization of the bone cavity by metastatic clones (**Figure 5**). The current challenges and potential biases in microbiota research pose significant barriers to advancing translational and clinical studies aimed at unraveling the intricate interactions among host, microbiota, pharmacological agents, and disease progression in breast cancer. Nonetheless, akin to osteoporosis research, there is a pressing need to further explore the osteoprotective potential of probiotics in the context of bone health and metastatic disease of breast cancer patients at higher risk to develop bone metastases. This knowledge would also support new therapeutic and/or prophylactic strategies to deal with such a relevant threat to women's health.

Author contributions

MEGM contributed to conception and design the figures and final approval of the version of the manuscript; FBC contributed to textual revision of the chapter, interpretation of the data, drafting the manuscript, and final approval of the version to be published; ACM contributed to conception and design of the work, interpretation of the data, drafting the manuscript, and final approval of the version to be published.

Funding

This work was supported with funding granted by FAPERJ (Carlos Chagas Filho Research Support Foundation of Rio de Janeiro State, E-26/311.264/2021, E-26/211.585/2021, E-26/211.223/2019, E-26/210.276/2019), FOPESQ (Programa de Fomento à Pesquisa - UFF/2021 and 2022), Cancer Foundation, and CNPq (National Council for Scientific and Technological Development, 436591/2018–9). Maria Eduarda Globa Masset was granted undegraduation and MSc. scholarships by CNPq.

Declaration of competing interest

The authors state no conflict of interest.

Abbreviations

RANKL	receptor activator of nuclear factor kappa-B ligand
OPG	osteoprotegerin
HER2	human epidermal growth factor receptor 2
ER	estrogen receptor
PR	progesterone receptor
TNBC	triple-negative breast cancer
S1PR1	sphingosine-1-phosphate receptor 1
AIs	aromatase inhibitors
AET	adjuvant endocrine therapy
SCFA	short chain fatty acids
BM	bone marrow
OC	osteoclast
OB	osteoblast
DC	dendritic cells
DC-OC	dendritic cells differentiated into OC
APC	antigen presenting cell
TILs	tumor-infiltrating lymphocytes
TME	tumor microenvironment
SREs	skeletal-related events
CTX-1	c-terminal crosslinking telopeptide of type I collagen
RANK	receptor activator of nuclear factor Kappa-B
CTLA-4	Cytotoxic T-lymphocyte associated protein 4
PDL-1	programmed cell death ligand 1
PyMT	polyoma middle T
MIF	Macrophage Migration Inhibitory Factor
RORc	RAR-related orphan receptor gamma
VEGF	vascular endothelial growth factor

NO	nitric oxide
PGE2	prostaglandin E2
MMPs	membrane-associated metalloproteinases
IDC	invasive ductal carcinoma
Treg	regulatory T cells
BC	breast tumor
OP	osteoporosis

Author details

Maria Eduarda Globa Masset[1], Fábio B. Canto[2] and Ana Carolina Monteiro[1*]

1 Osteo and Tumor Immunology Laboratory (LOIT), Department of Immunobiology, Biology Institute (EGB), Federal Fluminense University (UFF), Brazil

2 Laboratory of Immune Tolerance and Lymphocyte Homeostasis, Department of Immunobiology, Biology Institute (EGB), Federal Fluminense University (UFF), Brazil

*Address all correspondence to: anacarolinadossantosmonteiro@id.uff.br

References

[1] Harbeck N, Penault-Llorca F, Cortes J, Gnant M, Houssami N, Poortmans P, et al. Breast cancer. Nature Reviews Disease Primers. 2019;**5**:66. DOI: 10.1038/s41572-019-0111-2

[2] Amiri Souri E, Chenoweth A, Cheung A, Karagiannis SN, Tsoka S. Cancer grade model: A multi-gene machine learning-based risk classification for improving prognosis in breast cancer. British Journal of Cancer. 2021;**125**(5):748-758. DOI: 10.1038/s41416-021-01455-1

[3] Korde LA, Somerfield MR, Carey LA, Crews JR, Denduluri N, Hwang ES, et al. Neoadjuvant chemotherapy, endocrine therapy, and targeted therapy for breast cancer: ASCO guideline. Journal of Clinical Oncology. 2021;**39**:1485-1505. DOI: 10.1200/JCO.20.03399

[4] Coleman RE, Croucher PI, Padhani AR, Clézardin P, Chow E, Fallon M, et al. Bone metastases. Nature Reviews Disease Primers. 2020;**6**(1):83. DOI: 10.1038/s41572-020-00216-3

[5] David Roodman G, Silbermann R. Mechanisms of osteolytic and osteoblastic skeletal lesions. Bonekey Reports. 2015;**4**:1-7. DOI: 10.1038/bonekey.2015.122

[6] Esposito M, Guise T, Kang Y. The biology of bone metastasis. Cold Spring Harbor Perspectives in Medicine. 2018;**8**(6):a031252. DOI: 10.1101/cshperspect.a031252

[7] Mathis P-LF, Cortes J, Gnant M, Houssami N, Poortmans P, et al. Breast cancer. Nature Reviews Disease Primers. 2019;**5**(1):66. DOI: 10.1038/s41572-019-0111-2

[8] Roodman GD. Mechanisms of bone metastasis. New England Journal of Medicine. 2004;**350**:1655-1664. DOI: 10.1056/NEJMra030831

[9] Liu H, Zhang X, Zhang S, Wang X, Yu S. Factors associated with bone metastasis in breast cancer: A systematic review and meta-analysis. Annals of Palliative Medicine. 2021;**10**:4435-4452. DOI: 10.21037/apm-21-438

[10] Wu K, Feng J, Lyu F, Xing F, Sharma S, Liu Y, et al. Exosomal miR-19a and IBSP cooperate to induce osteolytic bone metastasis of estrogen receptor-positive breast cancer. Nature Communications. 2021;**12**(1):5196. DOI: 10.1038/s41467-021-25473-y

[11] Chen WZ, Shen JF, Zhou Y, Chen XY, Liu JM, Liu ZL. Clinical characteristics and risk factors for developing bone metastases in patients with breast cancer. Scientific Reports. 2017;**7**(1):11325. DOI: 10.1038/s41598-017-11700-4

[12] Chen F, Han Y, Kang Y. Bone marrow niches in the regulation of bone metastasis. British Journal of Cancer. 2021;**124**:1912-1920. DOI: 10.1038/s41416-021-01329-6

[13] Venetis K, Piciotti R, Sajjadi E, Invernizzi M, Morganti S, Criscitiello C, et al. Breast cancer with bone metastasis: Molecular insights and clinical management. Cells. 2021;**10**(6):1377. DOI: 10.3390/cells10061377

[14] Mundy GR. Metastasis to bone: Causes, consequences and therapeutic opportunities. Nature Reviews. Cancer. 2002;**2**:584-593. DOI: 10.1038/nrc867

[15] Okamoto K, Takayanagi H. Osteoimmunology. Cold Spring Harbor Perspectives in Medicine. 2019;**9**(1):a031245. DOI: 10.1101/cshperspect.a031245

[16] Metzger CE, Anand NS. The role of osteocytes in inflammatory bone loss. Frontiers in Endocrinology (Lausanne). 2019;**10**:285. DOI: 10.3389/fendo.2019.00285

[17] Intemann J, de Gorter DJJ, Naylor AJ, Dankbar B, Wehmeyer C. Importance of osteocyte-mediated regulation of bone remodelling in inflammatory bone disease. Swiss Medical Weekly. 2020;**150**:w20187. DOI: 10.4414/smw.2020.20187

[18] Chen H, Senda T, Kin-ya K. The osteocyte plays multiple roles in bone remodeling and mineral homeostasis. Medical Molecular Morphology. 2015;**48**:61-68. DOI: 10.1007/s00795-015-0099-y

[19] Madel MB, Ibáñez L, Wakkach A, De Vries TJ, Teti A, Apparailly F, et al. Immune function and diversity of osteoclasts in normal and pathological conditions. Frontiers in Immunology. 2019;**10**:1-18. DOI: 10.3389/fimmu.2019.01408

[20] Udagawa N, Koide M, Nakamura M, Nakamichi Y, Yamashita T, Uehara S, et al. Osteoclast differentiation by RANKL and OPG signaling pathways. Journal of Bone and Mineral Metabolism. 2021;**39**:19-26. DOI: 10.1007/s00774-020-01162-6

[21] Sims NA, Vrahnas C. Regulation of cortical and trabecular bone mass by communication between osteoblasts, osteocytes and osteoclasts. Archives of Biochemistry and Biophysics. 2014;**561**:22-28. DOI: 10.1016/j.abb.2014.05.015

[22] Rauch F, Adachi R. Sclerostin: More than a bone formation brake. Science Translational Medicine. 2016;**8**:1-4. DOI: 10.1126/scitranslmed.aaf4628

[23] Tsukasaki M, Takayanagi H. Osteoimmunology: Evolving concepts in bone–immune interactions in health and disease. Nature Reviews. Immunology. 2019;**19**:626-642. DOI: 10.1038/s41577-019-0178-8

[24] Jones DH, Nakashima T, Sanchez OH, Kozieradzki I, Komarova SV, Sarosi I, et al. Regulation of cancer cell migration and bone metastasis by RANKL. Nature. 2006;**440**:692-696. DOI: 10.1038/nature04524

[25] Kähkönen TE, Halleen JM, Bernoulli J. Osteoimmuno-oncology: Therapeutic opportunities for targeting immune cells in bone metastasis. Cells. 2021;**10**(6):1529. DOI: 10.3390/cells10061529

[26] Psailaa B, Kaplana RN, Port ER, Lydena D. Priming the “soil” for breast cancer metastasis: The pre-metastatic niche. Breast Disease. 2006;**26**:65-74. DOI: 10.3233/bd-2007-26106

[27] Peinado H, Zhang H, Matei IR, Costa-Silva B, Hoshino A, Rodrigues G, et al. Pre-metastatic niches: Organ-specific homes for metastases. Nature Reviews. Cancer. 2017;**17**:302-317. DOI: 10.1038/nrc.2017.6

[28] Monteiro AC, Leal AC, Gonçalves-Silva T, Mercadante ACT, Kestelman F, Chaves SB, et al. T cells induce pre-metastatic Osteolytic disease and help bone metastases establishment in a mouse model of metastatic breast cancer. PLoS One. 2013;**8**:1-13. DOI: 10.1371/journal.pone.0068171

[29] Monteiro AC, Bonomo A. Dendritic cells development into osteoclast-type APCs by 4T1 breast tumor T cells milieu boost bone consumption. Bone. 2020;**143**:115755. DOI: 10.1016/j.bone.2020.115755

[30] Monteiro AC, de Andrade GD, Du Rocher B, Fontão APGA, Nogueira LP,

Fidalgo G, et al. Cooperation between T and B cells reinforce the establishment of bone metastases in a mouse model of breast cancer. Bone. 2024;**178**:116932. DOI: 10.1016/j.bone.2023.116932

[31] Monteiro AC, Bonomo A. CD8 + T cells from experimental in situ breast carcinoma interfere with bone homeostasis. Bone. 2021;**150**:116014. DOI: 10.1016/j.bone.2021.116014

[32] Bonomo A, Monteiro AC, Gonçalves-Silva T, Cordeiro-Spinetti E, Galvani RG, Balduino A. A T cell view of the bone marrow. Frontiers in Immunology. 2016;**7**:1-14. DOI: 10.3389/fimmu.2016.00184

[33] Monteiro AC, Bonomo A. Dendritic cells as double-agents for breast tumor pre-metastatic bone disease establishment. Journal of Clinical and Cellular Immunology. 2021;**12**:1000616

[34] Sapra L, Bhardwaj A, Mishra PK, Garg B, Verma B, Mishra GC, et al. Regulatory B cells (Bregs) inhibit osteoclastogenesis and play a potential role in ameliorating ovariectomy-induced bone loss. Frontiers in Immunology. 2021;**12**:1-18. DOI: 10.3389/fimmu.2021.691081

[35] Dar HY, Singh A, Shukla P, Anupam R, Mondal RK, Mishra PK, et al. High dietary salt intake correlates with modulated Th17-Treg cell balance resulting in enhanced bone loss and impaired bone-microarchitecture in male mice. Scientific Reports. 2018;**8**(1):2503. DOI: 10.1038/s41598-018-20896-y

[36] Dar HY, Shukla P, Mishra PK, Anupam R, Mondal RK, Tomar GB, et al. Lactobacillus acidophilus inhibits bone loss and increases bone heterogeneity in osteoporotic mice via modulating Treg-Th17 cell balance. Bone Reports. 2018;**8**:46-56. DOI: 10.1016/j.bonr.2018.02.001

[37] Sapra L, Dar HY, Bhardwaj A, Pandey A, Kumari S, Azam Z, et al. *Lactobacillus rhamnosus* attenuates bone loss and maintains bone health by skewing Treg-Th17 cell balance in Ovx mice. Scientific Reports. 2021;**11**(1):1807. DOI: 10.1038/s41598-020-80536-2

[38] Yu M, Pal S, Paterson CW, Li JY, Tyagi AM, Adams J, et al. Ovariectomy induces bone loss via microbial-dependent trafficking of intestinal TNF+ T cells and Th17 cells. Journal of Clinical Investigation. 2021;**131**(4):e143137. DOI: 10.1172/JCI143137

[39] Salamanna F, Borsari V, Contartese D, Nicoli Aldini N, Fini M. Link between estrogen deficiency osteoporosis and susceptibility to bone metastases: A way towards precision medicine in cancer patients. Breast. 2018;**41**:42-50. DOI: 10.1016/j.breast.2018.06.013

[40] Eastell R, Hannon RA, Cuzick J, Dowsett M, Clack G, Adams JE. Effect of an aromatase inhibitor on BMD and bone turnover markers: 2-year results of the anastrozole, tamoxifen, alone or in combination (ATAC) trial (18233230). Journal of Bone and Mineral Research. 2006;**21**:1215-1223. DOI: 10.1359/jbmr.060508

[41] Núñez NP, Jelovac D, Macedo L, Berrigan D, Perkins SN, Hursting SD, et al. Effects of the antiestrogen tamoxifen and the aromatase inhibitor letrozole on serum hormones and bone characteristics in a preclinical tumor model for breast cancer. Clinical Cancer Research. 2004;**10**:5375-5380. DOI: 10.1158/1078-0432.CCR-04-0261

[42] Rachner TD, Göbel A, Jaschke NP, Hofbauer LC. Challenges in preventing

bone loss induced by aromatase inhibitors. Journal of Clinical Endocrinology and Metabolism. 2020;**105**:1-12. DOI: 10.1210/clinem/dgaa463

[43] Pavese F, Parisi A, Rotondaro S, Cocciolone V, Pierorazio G, Sidoni T, et al. Bone recurrence in early breast cancer patients: The paradox of aromatase inhibitors induced bone resorption. Breast Disease. 2021;**40**:257-262. DOI: 10.3233/BD-201036

[44] Mincey BA, Duh MS, Thomas SK, Moyneur E, Marynchencko M, Boyce SP, et al. Risk of cancer treatment-associated bone loss and fractures among women with breast cancer receiving aromatase inhibitors. Clinical Breast Cancer. 2006;**7**:127-132. DOI: 10.3816/CBC.2006.n.021

[45] Wright LE, Harhash AA, Kozlow WM, Waning DL, Regan JN, She Y, et al. Aromatase inhibitor-induced bone loss increases the progression of estrogen receptor-negative breast cancer in bone and exacerbates muscle weakness in vivo. 2017;**8**(5):8406-8419

[46] Ding H, Field TS. Bone health in postmenopausal women with early breast cancer: How protective is tamoxifen? Cancer Treatment Reviews. 2007;**33**:506-513. DOI: 10.1016/j.ctrv.2007.04.005

[47] Marttunen MB, Hietanen P, Tiitinen A, Ylikorkala O. Comparison of effects of tamoxifen and toremifene on bone biochemistry and bone mineral density in postmenopausal breast cancer patients. Journal of Clinical Endocrinology and Metabolism. 1998;**83**:1158-1162. DOI: 10.1210/jcem.83.4.4688

[48] Shapiro CL. Osteoporosis: A long-term and late-effect of breast cancer treatments. Cancers (Basel). 2020;**12**:1-17. DOI: 10.3390/cancers12113094

[49] Mathis KM, Sturgeon KM, Winkels RM, Wiskemann J, de Souza MJ, Schmitz KH. Bone resorption and bone metastasis risk. Medical Hypotheses. 2018;**118**:36-41. DOI: 10.1016/j.mehy.2018.06.013

[50] Clines GA, Choksi P, Van Poznak C. Adjuvant endocrine therapy and bone health in breast cancer. Current Osteoporosis Reports. 2015;**13**:263-273. DOI: 10.1007/s11914-015-0277-9

[51] Rachner TD, Coleman R, Hadji P, Hofbauer LC. Bone health during endocrine therapy for cancer. The Lancet Diabetes and Endocrinology. 2018;**6**:901-910. DOI: 10.1016/S2213-8587(18)30047-0

[52] Hadji P. Cancer treatment-induced bone loss in women with breast cancer. Bonekey Reports. 2015;**4**:1-5. DOI: 10.1038/bonekey.2015.60

[53] D'Oronzo S, Stucci S, Tucci M, Silvestris F. Cancer treatment-induced bone loss (CTIBL): Pathogenesis and clinical implications. Cancer Treatment Reviews. 2015;**41**:798-808. DOI: 10.1016/j.ctrv.2015.09.003

[54] Garg A, Leitzel K, Ali S, Lipton A. Antiresorptive therapy in the management of cancer treatment-induced bone loss. Current Osteoporosis Reports. 2015;**13**:73-77. DOI: 10.1007/s11914-014-0252-x

[55] Michaud LB. Managing cancer treatment-induced bone loss and osteoporosis in patients with breast or prostate cancer. American Journal of Health-System Pharmacy. 2010;**67**(7 Suppl 3):S20-S30; quiz S31-3. DOI: 10.2146/ajhp100078

[56] Kalder M, Hadji P. Breast cancer and osteoporosis - Management of cancer treatment-induced bone loss in

postmenopausal women with breast cancer. Breast Care. 2014;**9**:312-317. DOI: 10.1159/000368843

[57] Chen HM, Chen FP, Yang KC, Yuan SS. Association of bone metastasis with early-stage breast cancer in women with and without precancer osteoporosis according to osteoporosis therapy status. JAMA Network Open. 2019;**2**(3):e190429. DOI: 10.1001/jamanetworkopen.2019.0429

[58] Pagani S, Fini M, Giavaresi G, Salamanna F, Borsari V. The active role of osteoporosis in the interaction between osteoblasts and bone metastases. Bone. 2015;**79**:176-182. DOI: 10.1016/j.bone.2015.06.002

[59] Salamanna F, Borsari V, Brogini S, Torricelli P, Cepollaro S, Cadossi M, et al. A human 3D in vitro model to assess the relationship between osteoporosis and dissemination to bone of breast cancer tumor cells. Journal of Cellular Physiology. 2017;**232**:1826-1834. DOI: 10.1002/jcp.25708

[60] Salamanna F, Pagani S, Maglio M, Borsari V, Giavaresi G, Martelli AM, et al. Estrogen-deficient osteoporosis enhances the recruitment and activity of osteoclasts by breast cancer cells. Histology and Histopathology. 2016;**31**:83-93. DOI: 10.14670/HH-11-651

[61] D'Oronzo S, Coleman R, Brown J, Silvestris F. Metastatic bone disease: Pathogenesis and therapeutic options: Up-date on bone metastasis management. Journal of Bone Oncology. 2019;**15**:100205. DOI: 10.1016/j.jbo.2018.10.004

[62] von Moos R, Body JJ, Rider A, de Courcy J, Bhowmik D, Gatta F, et al. Bone-targeted agent treatment patterns and the impact of bone metastases on patients with advanced breast cancer in real-world practice in six European countries. Journal of Bone Oncology. 2018;**11**:1-9. DOI: 10.1016/j.jbo.2017.11.004

[63] Lacey DL, Boyle WJ, Simonet WS, Kostenuik PJ, Dougall WC, Sullivan JK, et al. Bench to bedside: Elucidation of the OPG-RANK-RANKL pathway and the development of denosumab. Nature Reviews. Drug Discovery. 2012;**11**:401-419. DOI: 10.1038/nrd3705

[64] Cremers S, Drake MT, Ebetino FH, Bilezikian JP, Russell RGG. Pharmacology of bisphosphonates. British Journal of Clinical Pharmacology. 2019;**85**:1052-1062. DOI: 10.1111/bcp.13867

[65] Shapiro CL. Bone-modifying agents (BMAs) in breast cancer. Clinical Breast Cancer. 2021;**21**:e618-e630. DOI: 10.1016/j.clbc.2021.04.009

[66] Miyashita H, Cruz C, Malamud S. Risk factors for skeletal-related events in patients with bone metastasis from breast cancer undergoing treatment with zoledronate. Breast Cancer Research and Treatment. 2020;**182**:381-388. DOI: 10.1007/s10549-020-05712-4

[67] Holen I, Walker M, Nutter F, Fowles A, Evans CA, Eaton CL, et al. Oestrogen receptor positive breast cancer metastasis to bone: Inhibition by targeting the bone microenvironment in vivo. Clinical & Experimental Metastasis. 2016;**33**:211-224. DOI: 10.1007/s10585-015-9770-x

[68] Cortellini A, Cocciolone V, Irelli A, Pavese F, Sidoni T, Parisi A, et al. The possible different roles of denosumab in prevention and cure breast cancer bone metastases: A 'hypothesis-generator' study from clinical practice. Oncology Letters. 2018;**16**:7195-7203. DOI: 10.3892/ol.2018.9561

[69] Henry D, von Moos R, Body JJ, Rider A, De Courcy J, Bhowmik D, et al. Bone-targeted agent treatment patterns and the impact of bone metastases on patients with advanced breast cancer in the United States. Current Medical Research and Opinion. 2019;**35**:375-381. DOI: 10.1080/03007995.2018.1558849

[70] Diel IJ, Solomayer E-F, Costa SD, Gollan C, Goerner R, Wallwiener D, et al. Reduction in new metastases in breast cancer with adjuvant Clodronate treatment. New England Journal of Medicine. 1998;**339**:357-363. DOI: 10.1056/nejm199808063390601

[71] Rouach V, Goldshtein I, Wolf I, Catane R, Chodick G, Iton A, et al. Exposure to alendronate is associated with a lower risk of bone metastases in osteoporotic women with early breast cancer. Journal of Bone Oncology. 2018;**12**:91-95. DOI: 10.1016/j.jbo.2018.07.011

[72] Coleman RE, Marshall H, Cameron D, Dodwell D, Burkinshaw R, Keane M, et al. Breast-cancer adjuvant therapy with Zoledronic acid. New England Journal of Medicine. 2011;**365**:1396-1405. DOI: 10.1056/nejmoa1105195

[73] Gnant M, Mlineritsch B, Schippinger W, Luschin-Ebengreuth G, Pöstlberger S, Menzel C, et al. Endocrine therapy plus zoledronic acid in premenopausal breast cancer. New England Journal of Medicine. 2009;**360**:679-691. DOI: 10.1056/nejmoa0806285

[74] Hadji P, Gnant M, Aapro M, Lipton A, Coleman R. Dosing of zoledronic acid throughout the treatment continuum in breast cancer. Critical Reviews in Oncology/Hematology. 2011;**79**:175-188. DOI: 10.1016/j.critrevonc.2010.07.017

[75] Hiraga T, Williams PJ, Ueda A, Tamura D, Yoneda T. Zoledronic acid inhibits visceral metastases in the 4T1/luc mouse breast cancer model. Clinical Cancer Research. 2004;**10**:4559-4567. DOI: 10.1158/1078-0432.CCR-03-0325

[76] Wilson C, Bell R, Hinsley S, Marshall H, Brown J, Cameron D, et al. Adjuvant zoledronic acid reduces fractures in breast cancer patients; an AZURE (BIG 01/04) study. European Journal of Cancer. 2018;**94**:70-78. DOI: 10.1016/j.ejca.2018.02.004

[77] Baklaushev VP, Grinenko NF, Yusubalieva GM, Gubskii IL, Burenkov MS, Rabinovich EZ, et al. Mono-and combined therapy of metastasizing breast carcinoma 4T1 with zoledronic acid and doxorubicin. Bulletin of Experimental Biology and Medicine. 2016;**161**:580-586. DOI: 10.1007/s10517-016-3464-5

[78] Ottewell PD, Wang N, Brown HK, Reeves KJ, Fowles CA, Croucher PI, et al. Zoledronic acid has differential antitumor activity in the pre- and postmenopausal bone microenvironment in vivo. Clinical Cancer Research. 2014;**20**:2922-2932. DOI: 10.1158/1078-0432.CCR-13-1246

[79] Lipton A, Cook RJ, Major P, Smith MR, Coleman RE. Zoledronic acid and survival in breast cancer patients with bone metastases and elevated markers of osteoclast activity. The Oncologist. 2007;**12**:1035-1043. DOI: 10.1634/theoncologist.12-9-1035

[80] Wilson C, Hinsley S, Marshall H, Cameron D, Bell R, Dodwell D, et al. Reproductive hormone analyses and effects of adjuvant zoledronic acid in early breast cancer – An AZURE (BIG 01/04) sub-study. Journal of Bone Oncology. 2017;**9**:48-54. DOI: 10.1016/j.jbo.2016.10.005

[81] Neville-Webbe HL, Coleman RE, Holen I. Combined effects of the bisphosphonate, zoledronic acid and the aromatase inhibitor letrozole on breast cancer cells in vitro: Evidence of synergistic interaction. British Journal of Cancer. 2010;**102**:1010-1017. DOI: 10.1038/sj.bjc.6605579

[82] Mundy GR, Yoneda T, Hiraga T. Preclinical studies with zoledronic acid and other bisphosphonates: Impact on the bone microenvironment. Seminars in Oncology. 2001;**28**:asonc0280035c. DOI: 10.1053/sonc.2001.24158

[83] Eisen A, Somerfield MR, Accordino MK, Blanchette PS, Clemons MJ, Dhesy-Thind S, et al. Use of adjuvant bisphosphonates and other bone-modifying agents in breast cancer: ASCO-OH (CCO) guideline update. Journal of Clinical Oncology. 2022;**40**:787-800. DOI: 10.1200/JCO.21

[84] Dhesy-Thind S, Fletcher GG, Blanchette PS, Clemons MJ, Dillmon MS, Frank ES, et al. Use of adjuvant bisphosphonates and other bone-modifying agents in breast cancer: A Cancer Care Ontario and American Society of Clinical Oncology clinical practice guideline. Journal of Clinical Oncology. 2017;**35**(18):2062-2081. DOI: 10.1200/JCO

[85] Coleman R, Finkelstein DM, Barrios C, Martin M, Iwata H, Hegg R, et al. Adjuvant denosumab in early breast cancer (D-CARE): An international, multicentre, randomised, controlled, phase 3 trial. The Lancet Oncology. 2020;**21**:60-72. DOI: 10.1016/S1470-2045(19)30687-4

[86] Coleman R, Gray R, Powles T, Paterson A, Gnant M, Bergh J, et al. Adjuvant bisphosphonate treatment in early breast cancer: Meta-analyses of individual patient data from randomised trials. The Lancet. 2015;**386**:1353-1361. DOI: 10.1016/S0140-6736(15)60908-4

[87] Gnant M, Mlineritsch B, Stoeger H, Luschin-Ebengreuth G, Heck D, Menzel C, et al. Adjuvant endocrine therapy plus zoledronic acid in premenopausal women with early-stage breast cancer: 62-month follow-up from the ABCSG-12 randomised trial. The Lancet Oncology. 2011;**12**:631-641. DOI: 10.1016/S1470-2045(11)70122-X

[88] Coleman R. Bisphosphonates and breast cancer – From cautious palliation to saving lives. Bone. 2020;**140**:115570. DOI: 10.1016/j.bone.2020.115570

[89] D'Oronzo S, Gregory W, Nicholson S, Chong YK, Brown J, Coleman R. Natural history of stage II/III breast cancer, bone metastasis and the impact of adjuvant zoledronate on distribution of recurrences. Journal of Bone Oncology. 2021;**28**:100367. DOI: 10.1016/j.jbo.2021.100367

[90] Kostenuik PJ, Nguyen HQ, McCabe J, Warmington KS, Kurahara C, Sun N, et al. Denosumab, a fully human monoclonal antibody to RANKL, inhibits bone resorption and increases BMD in knock-in mice that express chimeric (murine/human) RANKL. Journal of Bone and Mineral Research. 2009;**24**:182-195. DOI: 10.1359/jbmr.081112

[91] Ishikawa T. Differences between zoledronic acid and denosumab for breast cancer treatment. Journal of Bone and Mineral Metabolism. 2023;**41**:301-306. DOI: 10.1007/s00774-023-01408-z

[92] Kremer R, Gagnon B, Meguerditchian AN, Nadeau L, Mayo N. Effect of oral bisphosphonates for osteoporosis on development of skeletal metastases in women with breast cancer: Results from a pharmaco-epidemiological study.

Journal of the National Cancer Institute. 2014;**106**(11):dju264. DOI: 10.1093/jnci/dju264

[93] Irelli A, Cocciolone V, Cannita K, Zugaro L, Di Staso M, Lanfiuti Baldi P, et al. Bone targeted therapy for preventing skeletal-related events in metastatic breast cancer. Bone. 2016;**87**:169-175. DOI: 10.1016/j.bone.2016.04.006

[94] Drake MT, Clarke BL, Lewiecki EM. The pathophysiology and treatment of osteoporosis. Clinical Therapeutics. 2015;**37**:1837-1850. DOI: 10.1016/j.clinthera.2015.06.006

[95] Föger-Samwald U, Dovjak P, Azizi-Semrad U, Kerschan-Schindl K, Pietschmann P. Osteoporosis: Pathophysiology and therapeutic options. EXCLI Journal. 2020;**19**:1017-1037. DOI: 10.17179/excli2020-2591

[96] Grossmann M, Ramchand SK, Milat F, Vincent A, Lim E, Kotowicz MA, et al. Assessment and management of bone health in women with oestrogen receptor-positive breast cancer receiving endocrine therapy: Position statement summary. Medical Journal of Australia. 2019;**211**:224-229. DOI: 10.5694/mja2.50280

[97] Trémollieres FA. Screening for osteoporosis after breast cancer: For whom, why and when. Maturitas. 2014;**79**:343-348. DOI: 10.1016/j.maturitas.2014.08.001

[98] Handforth C, D'Oronzo S, Coleman R, Brown J. Cancer treatment and bone health. Calcified Tissue International. 2018;**102**:251-264. DOI: 10.1007/s00223-017-0369-x

[99] Li JY, Chassaing B, Tyagi AM, Vaccaro C, Luo T, Adams J, et al. Sex steroid deficiency-associated bone loss is microbiota dependent and prevented by probiotics. Journal of Clinical Investigation. 2016;**126**:2049-2063. DOI: 10.1172/JCI86062

[100] Runge S, Rosshart SP. The mammalian metaorganism: A holistic view on how microbes of all kingdoms and niches shape local and systemic immunity. Frontiers in Immunology. 2021;**12**:1-18. DOI: 10.3389/fimmu.2021.702378

[101] Hsu E, Pacifici R. From osteoimmunology to osteomicrobiology: How the microbiota and the immune system regulate bone. Calcified Tissue International. 2017;**102**(5):512-521. DOI: 10.1007/s00223-017-0321-0

[102] Schluter J, Peled JU, Taylor BP, Markey KA, Smith M, Taur Y, et al. The gut microbiota is associated with immune cell dynamics in humans. Nature. 2020;**588**:303-307. DOI: 10.1038/s41586-020-2971-8

[103] Chen PHGQJZYXR. Potential role of the skin microbiota in inflammatory skin diseases. Journal of Cosmetic Dermatology. 2020;**20**(2):400-409

[104] Whiteside SA, McGinniss JE, Collman RG. The lung microbiome: Progress and promise. Journal of Clinical Investigation. 2021;**131**(15):e150473. DOI: 10.1172/JCI150473

[105] Agostinis C, Mangogna A, Bossi F, Ricci G, Kishore U, Bulla R. Uterine immunity and microbiota: A shifting paradigm. Frontiers in Immunology. 2019;**n10**:2387. DOI: 10.3389/fimmu.2019.02387

[106] Nejman D, Livyatan I, Fuks G, Gavert N, Zwang Y, Geller LT, et al. The human tumor microbiome is composed of tumor type–specific intracellular bacteria. Science. 2020;**368**:973-980. DOI: 10.1126/science.aay9189

[107] Sjögren K, Engdahl C, Henning P, Lerner UH, Tremaroli V, Lagerquist MK, et al. The gut microbiota regulates bone mass in mice. Journal of Bone and Mineral Research. 2012;**27**:1357-1367. DOI: 10.1002/jbmr.1588

[108] Pierini A, Nishikii H, Baker J, Kimura T, Kwon HS, Pan Y, et al. Foxp3+ regulatory T cells maintain the bone marrow microenvironment for B cell lymphopoiesis. Nature Communications. 2017;**8**:1-13. DOI: 10.1038/ncomms15068

[109] Srivastava RK, Dar HY, Mishra PK. Immunoporosis: Immunology of osteoporosis-role of T cells. Frontiers in Immunology. 2018;**9**:1-12. DOI: 10.3389/fimmu.2018.00657

[110] Tyagi AM, Yu M, Darby TM, Vaccaro C, Li JY, Owens JA, et al. The microbial metabolite butyrate stimulates bone formation via T regulatory cell-mediated regulation of WNT10B expression. Immunity. 2018;**49**:1116-1131.e7. DOI: 10.1016/j.immuni.2018.10.013

[111] Zhao R. Immune regulation of bone loss by Th17 cells in oestrogen-deficient osteoporosis. European Journal of Clinical Investigation. 2013;**43**:1195-1202. DOI: 10.1111/eci.12158

[112] Onal M, Xiong J, Chen X, Thostenson JD, Almeida M, Manolagas SC, et al. Receptor activator of nuclear factor κB ligand (RANKL) protein expression by B lymphocytes contributes to ovariectomy-induced bone loss. Journal of Biological Chemistry. 2012;**287**:29851-29860. DOI: 10.1074/jbc.M112.377945

[113] Yousefi B, Eslami M, Ghasemian A, Kokhaei P, Salek Farrokhi A, Darabi N. Probiotics importance and their immunomodulatory properties. Journal of Cellular Physiology. 2019;**234**:8008-8018. DOI: 10.1002/jcp.27559

[114] Yu M, Malik Tyagi A, Li JY, Adams J, Denning TL, Weitzmann MN, et al. PTH induces bone loss via microbial-dependent expansion of intestinal TNF+ T cells and Th17 cells. Nature Communications. 2020;**11**:1-17. DOI: 10.1038/s41467-019-14148-4

[115] Tu Y, Yang R, Xu X, Zhou X. The microbiota-gut-bone axis and bone health. Journal of Leukocyte Biology. 2021;**110**:525-537. DOI: 10.1002/JLB.3MR0321-755R

[116] Lu L, Chen X, Liu Y, Yu X. Gut microbiota and bone metabolism. FASEB Journal. 2021;**35**:1-22. DOI: 10.1096/fj.202100451R

[117] Yan J, Herzog JW, Tsang K, Brennan CA, Bower MA, Garrett WS, et al. Gut microbiota induce IGF-1 and promote bone formation and growth. Proceedings of the National Academy of Sciences. 2016;**113**(47):E7554-E7563. DOI: 10.1073/pnas.1607235113

[118] Liu J, Chen C, Liu Z, Luo Z, Rao S, Jin L, et al. Extracellular vesicles from child gut microbiota enter into bone to preserve bone mass and strength. Advanced Science. 2021;**88**(9):2004831. DOI: 10.1002/advs.202004831

[119] Zaiss MM, Jones RM, Schett G, Pacifici R. The gut-bone axis: How bacterial metabolites bridge the distance. Journal of Clinical Investigation. 2019;**129**:3018-3028. DOI: 10.1172/JCI128521

[120] Tyagi AM, Darby TM, Hsu E, Yu M, Pal S, Dar H, et al. The gut microbiota is a transmissible determinant of skeletal maturation. eLife. 2021;**10**:e64237. DOI: 10.7554/eLife.64237

[121] Hathaway-Schrader JD, Carson MD, Gerasco JE, Warner AJ, Swanson BA, Aguirre JI, et al. Commensal gut bacterium critically regulates alveolar bone homeostasis. Laboratory Investigation. 2022;**102**:363-375. DOI: 10.1038/s41374-021-00697-0

[122] Liu J-H, Yue T, Luo Z-W, Cao J, Yan Z-Q, Jin L, et al. *Akkermansia muciniphila* promotes type H vessels formation and bone fracture healing by reducing gut permeability and inflammation. Disease Models & Mechanisms. 2020;**13**(11):dmm043620. DOI: 10.1242/dmm.043620

[123] Laborda-Illanes A, Sanchez-Alcoholado L, Dominguez-Recio ME, Jimenez-Rodriguez B, Lavado R, Comino-Méndez I, et al. Breast and gut microbiota action mechanisms in breast cancer pathogenesis and treatment. Cancers (Basel). 2020;**12**:1-27. DOI: 10.3390/cancers12092465

[124] Alpuim Costa D, Nobre JG, Batista MV, Ribeiro C, Calle C, Cortes A, et al. Human microbiota and breast cancer—Is there any relevant link?—A literature review and new horizons toward personalised medicine. Frontiers in Microbiology. 2021;**12**:584332. DOI: 10.3389/fmicb.2021.584332

[125] Xuan C, Shamonki JM, Chung A, DiNome ML, Chung M, Sieling PA, et al. Microbial dysbiosis is associated with human breast cancer. PLoS One. 2014;**9**:1-7. DOI: 10.1371/journal.pone.0083744

[126] Urbaniak C, Gloor GB, Brackstone M, Scott L, Tangney M, Reida G. The microbiota of breast tissue and its association with breast cancer. Applied and Environmental Microbiology. 2016;**82**:5039-5048. DOI: 10.1128/AEM.01235-16

[127] Plaza-Díaz J, Álvarez-Mercado AI, Ruiz-Marín CM, Reina-Pérez I, Pérez-Alonso AJ, Sánchez-Andujar MB, et al. Association of breast and gut microbiota dysbiosis and the risk of breast cancer: A case-control clinical study. BMC Cancer. 2019;**19**:495. DOI: 10.1186/s12885-019-5660-y

[128] Fu A, Yao B, Dong T, Chen Y, Yao J, Liu Y, et al. Tumor-resident intracellular microbiota promotes metastatic colonization in breast cancer. Cell. 2022;**185**:1356-1372.e26. DOI: 10.1016/j.cell.2022.02.027

[129] Vétizou M, Pitt JM, Daillère R, Lepage P, Waldschmitt N, Flament C, et al. Anticancer immunotherapy by CTLA-4 blockade relies on the gut microbiota. Science. 2015;**350**:1079-1084. DOI: 10.1126/science.aad1329

[130] Sivan A, Corrales L, Hubert N, Williams JB, Aquino-Michaels K, Earley ZM, et al. Commensal *Bifidobacterium* promotes antitumor immunity and facilitates anti–PD-L1 efficacy. Science. 2015;**350**:1084-1089. DOI: 10.1126/science.aac4255

[131] Viaud S, Saccheri F, Mignot G, Yamazaki T, Daillère R, Hannani D, et al. The intestinal microbiota modulates the anticancer immune effects of cyclophosphamide. Science. 2013;**342**:971-976. DOI: 10.1126/science.1240537

[132] Iida N, Dzutsev A, Stewart CA, Smith L, Bouladoux N, Weingarten RA, et al. Commensal bacteria control cancer response to therapy by modulating the tumor microenvironment. Science. 2013;**342**:967-970. DOI: 10.1126/science.1240527

[133] Terrisse S, Derosa L, Iebba V, Ghiringhelli F, Vaz-Luis I, Kroemer G, et al. Intestinal microbiota influences

clinical outcome and side effects of early breast cancer treatment. Cell Death and Differentiation. 2021;**28**:2778-2796. DOI: 10.1038/s41418-021-00784-1

[134] Lorenzo J. From the gut to bone: Connecting the gut microbiota with Th17 T lymphocytes and postmenopausal osteoporosis. Journal of Clinical Investigation. 2021;**131**:1-3. DOI: 10.1172/JCI146619

[135] Jones RM, Mulle JG, Pacifici R. Osteomicrobiology: The influence of gut microbiota on bone in health and disease. Bone. 2018;**115**:59-67. DOI: 10.1016/j.bone.2017.04.009

[136] Chen Y, Wang X, Zhang C, Liu Z, Li C, Ren Z. Gut microbiota and bone diseases: A growing partnership. Frontiers in Microbiology. 2022;**13**:877776. DOI: 10.3389/fmicb.2022.877776

[137] Qiao X, Li X, Wang Z, Feng Y, Wei X, Li L, et al. Gut microbial community and fecal metabolomic signatures in different types of osteoporosis animal models. Aging. 2024;**16**:1192-1217. DOI: 10.18632/aging.205396

[138] Huck O, Mulhall H, Rubin G, Kizelnik Z, Iyer R, Perpich JD, et al. *Akkermansia muciniphila* reduces *Porphyromonas gingivalis* -induced inflammation and periodontal bone destruction. Journal of Clinical Periodontology. 2020;**47**:202-212. DOI: 10.1111/jcpe.13214

[139] Thu MS, Chotirosniramit K, Nopsopon T, Hirankarn N, Pongpirul K. Human gut, breast, and oral microbiome in breast cancer: A systematic review and meta-analysis. Frontiers in Oncology. 2023;**13**:1144021. DOI: 10.3389/fonc.2023.1144021

[140] Jarman R, Ribeiro-Milograna S, Kalle W. Potential of the microbiome as a biomarker for early diagnosis and prognosis of breast cancer. Journal of Breast Cancer. 2020;**23**:579. DOI: 10.4048/jbc.2020.23.e60

[141] Sui Y, Wu J, Chen J. The role of gut microbial β-Glucuronidase in Estrogen reactivation and breast cancer. Frontiers in Cell and Development Biology. 2021;**9**:631552. DOI: 10.3389/fcell.2021.631552

[142] Chen KLA, Liu X, Zhao YC, Hieronymi K, Rossi G, Auvil LS, et al. Long-term Administration of Conjugated Estrogen and Bazedoxifene Decreased Murine Fecal β-Glucuronidase activity without impacting overall microbiome community. Scientific Reports. 2018;**8**:8166. DOI: 10.1038/s41598-018-26506-1

[143] Parida S, Sharma D. The microbiome-Estrogen connection and breast cancer risk. Cells. 2019;**8**(12):1642. DOI: 10.3390/cells8121642

[144] Flores R, Shi J, Fuhrman B, Xu X, Veenstra TD, Gail MH, et al. Fecal microbial determinants of fecal and systemic estrogens and estrogen metabolites: A cross-sectional study. Journal of Translational Medicine. 2012;**10**:253. DOI: 10.1186/1479-5876-10-253

[145] Hou M-F, Ou-Yang F, Li C-L, Chen F-M, Chuang C-H, Kan J-Y, et al. Comprehensive profiles and diagnostic value of menopausal-specific gut microbiota in premenopausal breast cancer. Experimental & Molecular Medicine. 2021;**53**:1636-1646. DOI: 10.1038/s12276-021-00686-9

[146] Mazmanian SK, Round JL, Kasper DL. A microbial symbiosis factor prevents intestinal inflammatory disease. Nature. 2008;**453**:620-625. DOI: 10.1038/nature07008

[147] Wenhui Y, Zhongyu X, Kai C, Zhaopeng C, Jinteng L, Mengjun M, et al. Variations in the gut microbiota in breast cancer occurrence and bone metastasis. Frontiers in Microbiology. 2022;**13**:894283. DOI: 10.3389/fmicb.2022.894283

[148] Picon-Ruiz M, Morata-Tarifa C, Valle-Goffin JJ, Friedman ER, Slingerland JM. Obesity and adverse breast cancer risk and outcome: Mechanistic insights and strategies for intervention. CA: A Cancer Journal for Clinicians. 2017;**67**:378-397. DOI: 10.3322/caac.21405

[149] German R, Marino N, Hemmerich C, Podicheti R, Rusch DB, Stiemsma LT, et al. Exploring breast tissue microbial composition and the association with breast cancer risk factors. Breast Cancer Research. 2023;**25**:82. DOI: 10.1186/s13058-023-01677-6

[150] Hieken TJ, Chen J, Hoskin TL, Walther-Antonio M, Johnson S, Ramaker S, et al. The microbiome of aseptically collected human breast tissue in benign and malignant disease. Scientific Reports. 2016;**6**:30751. DOI: 10.1038/srep30751

[151] Summer M, Sajjad A, Ali S, Hussain T. Exploring the underlying correlation between microbiota, immune system, hormones, and inflammation with breast cancer and the role of probiotics, prebiotics and postbiotics. Archives of Microbiology. 2024;**206**:145. DOI: 10.1007/s00203-024-03868-x

[152] Dieleman S, Aarnoutse R, Ziemons J, Kooreman L, Boleij A, Smidt M. Exploring the potential of breast microbiota as biomarker for breast cancer and therapeutic response. American Journal of Pathology. 2021;**191**:968-982. DOI: 10.1016/j.ajpath.2021.02.020

[153] Banerjee S, Tian T, Wei Z, Shih N, Feldman MD, Peck KN, et al. Distinct microbial signatures associated with different breast cancer types. Frontiers in Microbiology. 2018;**9**:1-20. DOI: 10.3389/fmicb.2018.00951

[154] Al-Ansari MM, Almalki RH, Dahabiyeh LA, Abdel Rahman AM. Metabolomics-microbiome crosstalk in the breast cancer microenvironment. Metabolites. 2021;**11**(11):758. DOI: 10.3390/metabo11110758

[155] El Bairi K, Haynes HR, Blackley E, Fineberg S, Shear J, Turner S, et al. The tale of TILs in breast cancer: A report from the international Immuno-oncology biomarker working group. npj Breast Cancer. 2021;7(1):150. DOI: 10.1038/s41523-021-00346-1

[156] Monteiro AC, Lepique AP, Bonamino M, Fuertes MB. Editorial: Tumor microenvironment immunophenotypes and disease progression. Frontiers in Immunology. 2023;**14**:1141084. DOI: 10.3389/fimmu.2023.1141084

[157] DeNardo DG, Barreto JB, Andreu P, Vasquez L, Tawfik D, Kolhatkar N, et al. CD4+ T cells regulate pulmonary metastasis of mammary carcinomas by enhancing protumor properties of macrophages. Cancer Cell. 2009;**16**:91-102. DOI: 10.1016/j.ccr.2009.06.018

[158] Zheng D, Liwinski T, Elinav E. Interaction between microbiota and immunity in health and disease. Cell Research. 2020;**30**:492-506. DOI: 10.1038/s41422-020-0332-7

[159] Hou K, Wu Z-X, Chen X-Y, Wang J-Q, Zhang D, Xiao C, et al. Microbiota in health and diseases. Signal Transduction

and Targeted Therapy. 2022;**7**:135. DOI: 10.1038/s41392-022-00974-4

[160] El Tekle G, Garrett WS. Bacteria in cancer initiation, promotion and progression. Nature Reviews. Cancer. 2023;**23**:600-618. DOI: 10.1038/s41568-023-00594-2

[161] Villemin C, Six A, Neville BA, Lawley TD, Robinson MJ, Bakdash G. The heightened importance of the microbiome in cancer immunotherapy. Trends in Immunology. 2023;**44**:44-59. DOI: 10.1016/j.it.2022.11.002

[162] Li G, Sun Y, Huang Y, Lian J, Wu S, Luo D, et al. Fusobacterium nucleatum-derived small extracellular vesicles facilitate tumor growth and metastasis via TLR4 in breast cancer. BMC Cancer. 2023;**23**:473. DOI: 10.1186/s12885-023-10844-z

[163] Parhi L, Alon-Maimon T, Sol A, Nejman D, Shhadeh A, Fainsod-Levi T, et al. Breast cancer colonization by *Fusobacterium nucleatum* accelerates tumor growth and metastatic progression. Nature Communications. 2020;**11**:3259. DOI: 10.1038/s41467-020-16967-2

[164] Little A, Tangney M, Tunney MM, Buckley NE. *Fusobacterium nucleatum* : a novel immune modulator in breast cancer? Expert Reviews in Molecular Medicine. 2023;**25**:e15. DOI: 10.1017/erm.2023.9

[165] Chen W, Jin W, Hardegen N, Lei K, Li L, Marinos N, et al. Conversion of peripheral CD4+CD25− naive T cells to CD4+CD25+ regulatory T cells by TGF-β induction of transcription factor *Foxp3*. The Journal of Experimental Medicine. 2003;**198**:1875-1886. DOI: 10.1084/jem.20030152

[166] Veldhoen M, Hocking RJ, Atkins CJ, Locksley RM, Stockinger B. TGFβ in the context of an inflammatory cytokine milieu supports de novo differentiation of IL-17-producing T cells. Immunity. 2006;**24**:179-189. DOI: 10.1016/j.immuni.2006.01.001

[167] Ivanov II, McKenzie BS, Zhou L, Tadokoro CE, Lepelley A, Lafaille JJ, et al. The orphan nuclear receptor RORγt directs the differentiation program of proinflammatory IL-17+ T helper cells. Cell. 2006;**126**:1121-1133. DOI: 10.1016/j.cell.2006.07.035

[168] Zhou L, Lopes JE, Chong MMW, Ivanov II, Min R, Victora GD, et al. TGF-β-induced Foxp3 inhibits TH17 cell differentiation by antagonizing RORγt function. Nature. 2008;**453**:236-240. DOI: 10.1038/nature06878

[169] Wang J, Zhao X, Wan YY. Intricacies of TGF-β signaling in Treg and Th17 cell biology. Cellular & Molecular Immunology. 2023;**20**:1002-1022. DOI: 10.1038/s41423-023-01036-7

[170] Iliev ID, Mileti E, Matteoli G, Chieppa M, Rescigno M. Intestinal epithelial cells promote colitis-protective regulatory T-cell differentiation through dendritic cell conditioning. Mucosal Immunology. 2009;**2**:340-350. DOI: 10.1038/mi.2009.13

[171] Atarashi K, Tanoue T, Shima T, Imaoka A, Kuwahara T, Momose Y, et al. Induction of colonic regulatory T cells by indigenous *Clostridium* species. Science. 2011;**331**:337-341. DOI: 10.1126/science.1198469

[172] Atarashi K, Tanoue T, Oshima K, Suda W, Nagano Y, Nishikawa H, et al. Treg induction by a rationally selected mixture of clostridia strains from the human microbiota. Nature. 2013;**500**:232-236. DOI: 10.1038/nature12331

[173] Martin-Gallausiaux C, Béguet-Crespel F, Marinelli L, Jamet A, Ledue F, Blottière HM, et al. Butyrate produced by gut commensal bacteria activates TGF-beta1 expression through the transcription factor SP1 in human intestinal epithelial cells. Scientific Reports. 2018;**8**:9742. DOI: 10.1038/s41598-018-28048-y

[174] Yan Y, Ramanan D, Rozenberg M, McGovern K, Rastelli D, Vijaykumar B, et al. Interleukin-6 produced by enteric neurons regulates the number and phenotype of microbe-responsive regulatory T cells in the gut. Immunity. 2021;**54**:499-513.e5. DOI: 10.1016/j.immuni.2021.02.002

[175] Xu M, Pokrovskii M, Ding Y, Yi R, Au C, Harrison OJ, et al. c-MAF-dependent regulatory T cells mediate immunological tolerance to a gut pathobiont. Nature. 2018;**554**:373-377. DOI: 10.1038/nature25500

[176] Hunter CA, Jones SA. IL-6 as a keystone cytokine in health and disease. Nature Immunology. 2015;**16**:448-457. DOI: 10.1038/ni.3153

[177] Sefik E, Geva-Zatorsky N, Oh S, Konnikova L, Zemmour D, McGuire AM, et al. Individual intestinal symbionts induce a distinct population of RORγ $^{+}$ regulatory T cells. Science. 2015;**349**:993-997. DOI: 10.1126/science.aaa9420

[178] Rosser EC, Oleinika K, Tonon S, Doyle R, Bosma A, Carter NA, et al. Regulatory B cells are induced by gut microbiota–driven interleukin-1β and interleukin-6 production. Nature Medicine. 2014;**20**:1334-1339. DOI: 10.1038/nm.3680

[179] Ivanov II, Atarashi K, Manel N, Brodie EL, Shima T, Karaoz U, et al. Induction of intestinal Th17 cells by segmented filamentous bacteria. Cell. 2009;**139**:485-498. DOI: 10.1016/j.cell.2009.09.033

[180] Hall JA, Bouladoux N, Sun CM, Wohlfert EA, Blank RB, Zhu Q, et al. Commensal DNA limits regulatory T cell conversion and is a natural adjuvant of intestinal immune responses. Immunity. 2008;**29**:637-649. DOI: 10.1016/j.immuni.2008.08.009

[181] Sun C-M, Hall JA, Blank RB, Bouladoux N, Oukka M, Mora JR, et al. Small intestine lamina propria dendritic cells promote de novo generation of Foxp3 T reg cells via retinoic acid. The Journal of Experimental Medicine. 2007;**204**:1775-1785. DOI: 10.1084/jem.20070602

[182] Coombes JL, Siddiqui KRR, Arancibia-Cárcamo CV, Hall J, Sun C-M, Belkaid Y, et al. A functionally specialized population of mucosal CD103+ DCs induces Foxp3+ regulatory T cells via a TGF-β– and retinoic acid–dependent mechanism. The Journal of Experimental Medicine. 2007;**204**:1757-1764. DOI: 10.1084/jem.20070590

[183] Mucida D, Park Y, Kim G, Turovskaya O, Scott I, Kronenberg M, et al. Reciprocal T_H 17 and regulatory T cell differentiation mediated by retinoic acid. Science. 2007;**317**:256-260. DOI: 10.1126/science.1145697

[184] Bettelli E, Carrier Y, Gao W, Korn T, Strom TB, Oukka M, et al. Reciprocal developmental pathways for the generation of pathogenic effector TH17 and regulatory T cells. Nature. 2006;**441**:235-238. DOI: 10.1038/nature04753

[185] Komatsu N, Okamoto K, Sawa S, Nakashima T, Oh-hora M, Kodama T, et al. Pathogenic conversion of Foxp3+ T cells into TH17 cells in autoimmune arthritis. Nature Medicine. 2014;**20**:62-68. DOI: 10.1038/nm.3432

[186] Lee YK, Turner H, Maynard CL, Oliver JR, Chen D, Elson CO, et al. Late developmental plasticity in the T helper 17 lineage. Immunity. 2009;**30**:92-107. DOI: 10.1016/j.immuni.2008.11.005

[187] Zhou X, Bailey-Bucktrout SL, Jeker LT, Penaranda C, Martínez-Llordella M, Ashby M, et al. Instability of the transcription factor Foxp3 leads to the generation of pathogenic memory T cells in vivo. Nature Immunology. 2009;**10**:1000-1007. DOI: 10.1038/ni.1774

[188] Xu L, Kitani A, Fuss I, Strober W. Cutting edge: Regulatory T cells induce CD4+CD25−Foxp3− T cells or are self-induced to become Th17 cells in the absence of exogenous TGF-β. The Journal of Immunology. 2007;**178**:6725-6729. DOI: 10.4049/jimmunol.178.11.6725

[189] Yan Y, Huang L, Liu Y, Yi M, Chu Q, Jiao D, et al. Metabolic profiles of regulatory T cells and their adaptations to the tumor microenvironment: Implications for antitumor immunity. Journal of Hematology & Oncology. 2022;**15**:104. DOI: 10.1186/s13045-022-01322-3

[190] Scott EN, Gocher AM, Workman CJ, Vignali DAA. Regulatory T cells: Barriers of immune infiltration into the tumor microenvironment. Frontiers in Immunology. 2021;**12**:702726. DOI: 10.3389/fimmu.2021.702726

[191] Wing JB, Tanaka A, Sakaguchi S. Human FOXP3+ regulatory T cell heterogeneity and function in autoimmunity and cancer. Immunity. 2019;**50**:302-316. DOI: 10.1016/j.immuni.2019.01.020

[192] Togashi Y, Shitara K, Nishikawa H. Regulatory T cells in cancer immunosuppression — Implications for anticancer therapy. Nature Reviews. Clinical Oncology. 2019;**16**:356-371. DOI: 10.1038/s41571-019-0175-7

[193] Tanaka A, Sakaguchi S. Regulatory T cells in cancer immunotherapy. Cell Research. 2017;**27**:109-118. DOI: 10.1038/cr.2016.151

[194] Saleh R, Elkord E. FoxP3+ T regulatory cells in cancer: Prognostic biomarkers and therapeutic targets. Cancer Letters. 2020;**490**:174-185. DOI: 10.1016/j.canlet.2020.07.022

[195] Shang B, Liu Y, Jiang S, Liu Y. Prognostic value of tumor-infiltrating FoxP3+ regulatory T cells in cancers: A systematic review and meta-analysis. Scientific Reports. 2015;**5**:15179. DOI: 10.1038/srep15179

[196] Nishimura H, Nose M, Hiai H, Minato N, Honjo T. Development of lupus-like autoimmune diseases by disruption of the PD-1 gene encoding an ITIM motif-carrying Immunoreceptor. Immunity. 1999;**11**:141-151. DOI: 10.1016/S1074-7613(00)80089-8

[197] Kumagai S, Togashi Y, Kamada T, Sugiyama E, Nishinakamura H, Takeuchi Y, et al. The PD-1 expression balance between effector and regulatory T cells predicts the clinical efficacy of PD-1 blockade therapies. Nature Immunology. 2020;**21**:1346-1358. DOI: 10.1038/s41590-020-0769-3

[198] Wei SC, Anang N-AAS, Sharma R, Andrews MC, Reuben A, Levine JH, et al. Combination anti–CTLA-4 plus anti–PD-1 checkpoint blockade utilizes cellular mechanisms partially distinct from monotherapies. Proceedings of the National Academy of Sciences. 2019;**116**:22699-22709. DOI: 10.1073/pnas.1821218116

[199] Wei SC, Levine JH, Cogdill AP, Zhao Y, Anang N-AAS, Andrews MC,

et al. Distinct cellular mechanisms underlie anti-CTLA-4 and anti-PD-1 checkpoint blockade. Cell. 2017;**170**:1120-1133.e17. DOI: 10.1016/j.cell.2017.07.024

[200] Sharma P, Allison JP. The future of immune checkpoint therapy. Science. 2015;**348**:56-61. DOI: 10.1126/science.aaa8172

[201] Curran MA, Montalvo W, Yagita H, Allison JP. PD-1 and CTLA-4 combination blockade expands infiltrating T cells and reduces regulatory T and myeloid cells within B16 melanoma tumors. Proceedings of the National Academy of Sciences. 2010;**107**:4275-4280. DOI: 10.1073/pnas.0915174107

[202] Okazaki T, Honjo T. PD-1 and PD-1 ligands: From discovery to clinical application. International Immunology. 2007;**19**:813-824. DOI: 10.1093/intimm/dxm057

[203] Leach DR, Krummel MF, Allison JP. Enhancement of antitumor immunity by CTLA-4 blockade. Science. 1996;**271**:1734-1736. DOI: 10.1126/science.271.5256.1734

[204] Xia L, Zhu X, Wang Y, Lu S. The gut microbiota improves the efficacy of immune-checkpoint inhibitor immunotherapy against tumors: From association to cause and effect. Cancer Letters. 2024;**598**:217123. DOI: 10.1016/j.canlet.2024.217123

[205] Mager LF, Burkhard R, Pett N, Cooke NCA, Brown K, Ramay H, et al. Microbiome-derived inosine modulates response to checkpoint inhibitor immunotherapy. Science. 2020;**369**:1481-1489. DOI: 10.1126/science.abc3421

[206] Gopalakrishnan V, Spencer CN, Nezi L, Reuben A, Andrews MC, Karpinets TV, et al. Gut microbiome modulates response to anti–PD-1 immunotherapy in melanoma patients. Science. 2018;**359**:97-103. DOI: 10.1126/science.aan4236

[207] Matson V, Fessler J, Bao R, Chongsuwat T, Zha Y, Alegre M-L, et al. The commensal microbiome is associated with anti–PD-1 efficacy in metastatic melanoma patients. Science. 2018;**359**:104-108. DOI: 10.1126/science.aao3290

[208] Routy B, Le Chatelier E, Derosa L, Duong CPM, Alou MT, Daillère R, et al. Gut microbiome influences efficacy of PD-1–based immunotherapy against epithelial tumors. Science. 2018;**359**:91-97. DOI: 10.1126/science.aan3706